Research Methodologies in Human Diabetes
Part 2

Research Methodologies in Human Diabetes
Part 2

Editors: C. E. Mogensen, E. Standl

Walter de Gruyter
Berlin · New York 1995

Deutsche Bibliothek — Cataloging-in-Publication-Data

Research methodologies in human diabetes. — Berlin ; New York : de Gruyter.
Literaturangaben

Pt. 2. Ed.: C. E. Mogensen ; E. Standl. — 1995
ISBN 3-11-014555-3
NE: Mogensen, Carl E. [Hrsg.]

Medical science is constantly developing. Research and clinical experience expand our knowledge, especially with regard to treatment and medication.

For dosages and applications mentioned in this work, the reader may rely on the authors, editors and publisher having taken great pains to ensure that these indications reflect the standard of knowledge at the time this work was completed.

Nevertheless, all users are requested to check the package leaflet of the medication, in order to determine for themselves whether the recommentations given for the dosages or the likely contraindications differ from those given in this book. This is especially true for medication which is seldom used or has recently been put on the market and for medication whose application has been restricted by the German Ministry of Health.

Typesetting and Printing: Arthur Collignon GmbH, Berlin. — Binding: Lüderitz & Bauer GmbH, Berlin. — Printed in Germany.

Editors

Prof. Dr. C. E. Mogensen
Medical Department M
Second University Clinic
of Internal Medicine
(Diabetes and Endocrinology)
Kommunehospitalet
DK-8000 Aarhus C
Denmark

Prof. Dr. E. Standl
Third Medical Department
City Hospital Schwabing
and Diabetes Research Unit
Kölner Platz 1
D-80804 München
Germany

List of first-mentioned contributors

K. G. M. M. Alberti, M. D.
The University of Newcastle
upon Tyne
Department of Medicine
Floor 4 – Clinical Block
The Medical School
Framlington Place
Newcastle upon Tyne NE2 4HH
England

T. P. Almdal, M. D.
Department of Endocrinology 157
Hvidovre University Hospital
DK-2650 Hvidovre
Denmark

J. M. Amatruda, M. D.
Miles Inc.
400 Morgan Lane
Building IC
West Haven, CT 06516-4175
USA

R. N. Bergman, Ph. D.
Department of Physiology
and Biophysics
University of Southern California
Medical School
1333 San Pablo Street
Los Angeles
California 90033
USA

K. Borch-Johnsen, M. D.
Glostrup Population Studies
Glostrup Hospital
University of Copenhagen
DK-2600 Glostrup
Denmark

R. G. Bretzel, M. D.
Universität Gießen
III. Medizinische Klinik
und Poliklinik
Rodthohl 6
D-35392 Gießen
Germany

M. Daffertshofer, M. D.
Abteilung für Neurologie
Universität Heidelberg
Klinikum Mannheim
Theodor-Kutzer-Ufer
D-68167 Mannheim
Germany

F. H. M. Derkx, M. D.
Department of Internal Medicine I
University Hospital Dijkzigt,
Room L242
Dr. Molewaterplein 40
30 15 GD Rotterdam
The Netherlands

U. J. Eriksson, M. D.
Department of Medical
Cell Biology
Uppsala University
Biomedicum, Box 571
Husargatan 3
S-751 23 Uppsala
Sverige

E. Ferrannini, M. D.
Istituto di Fisiologia Clinical
del CNR
Consiglio Nazionale delle
Ricerche – C. N. R.
c/o Università di Pisa
Via Savi, 8
56100 Pisa
Italy

H. Galbo, M. D.
Department of Cardiology
Bispebjerg Hospital
DK-2400 Kobenhavn NV
Denmark

L. Groop, M. D.
University of Lund
Department of Endocrinology
Malmö General Hospital
S-21401 Malmö
Sweden

D. R. Hadden, M. D.
Sir George E. Clark Metabolic Unit
Royal Victoria Hospital
Regional Centre for Endocrinology
and Diabetes
Belfast BT12 6BA
Northern Ireland

K. W. Hansen, M. D.
Medicinsk afdeling M
Aarhus Kommunehospital
DK-8000 Aarhus C
Denmark

J. Ingerslev, M. D.
Koagulationslaboratoriet
Klinisk Immunologisk afdeling
Skejby Sygehus
Brentstrupgaardsvej
DK-8200 Aarhus N
Denmark

J. Mann, M. D.
Department of Human Nutrition
University of Otago
P. O. Box 56
Dunedin
New Zealand

M. Marre, M. D.
Médicine B
Centre Hospitalie Universitaire
F-49033 Angers
France

J. M. Miles, M. D.
Diabetes and Nutritional
Metabolism
Research Laboratory
St. Luke's Hospital
44th & Wornall
Kansas City, MO 64111
USA

N. Møller, M. D.
Medicinsk afdeling M
Aarhus Kommunehospital
DK-8000 Arhus C
Denmark

T. D. O'Brien, M. D.
Endocrine Research Unit
5-164 West Joseph
Mayo Clinic
Rochester
Minnesota
MN 55905
USA

R. Østerby, M. D.
Diabeteslaboratoriet
Medicinsk Forskningslaborator. M
Aarhus Kommunehospital
DK-8000 Aarhus C
Denmark

P. Patrignani, M. D.
Department of Medical
Pathophysiology
Cattedra di Farmacologia I
Università di Chieti
"Gabriele D'Annunzio"
Via del Vestini 31
I-66013 Chieti
Italy

T. S. Purewal, M. D.
Diabetic Department
King's College Hospital
Denmark Hill
London SE5 9RS
England

O. Schmitz, M. D.
Medicinsk afdeling M
Aarhus Kommunehospital
DK-8000 Aarhus C
Denmark

J. M. Stephenson, M. D.
Department of Epidemiology and
Population Health
University College London
66-72 Gower Street
London WC1E 6EA
England

List of first-mentioned contributors

P. K. Thomas, M. D.
Royal Free Hospital School of Medicine
University of London
Department of Neurological Science
Pond Street
London NW3 2QG
England

L. Thuesen, M. D.
Cardiologisk afdeling
Skejby Sygehus
DK-8200 Aarhus N
Denmark

J. E. Tooke, M. D.
University of Exeter
Diabetes Research Laboratories
Postgraduate Medical School
Noy Scott House Haldon View Terrace
Exeter EX2 5EQ
England

A. Wessing, M. D.
Klinikum der Universität GH Essen
Klinik und Poliklinik für Augenheilkunde
Hufelandstr. 55
D-45147 Essen
Germany

Preface

The number of research activities in the field of diabetes mellitus have exploded in recent years. This can come as no surprise in light of the complexity of the disorder – or better, family of disorders – with their multiple, yet distinct aetiopathogenic factors and many clinical manifestations and sequelae. The advent of new research technologies, e. g. derived from molecular biology, gene technology, applied biochemistry, computer methodology or refined ultrasound- and electrophysiology, has fostered a host of new theories and concepts on the development of various types of diabetes mellitus and related complications.

The previous three books of the *Diabetes Forum Series*, starting in 1989, have attempted to compile much of the progress made in modern diabetology. It is fascinating to observe the enormous spectrum of diabetes research and the intensive interaction with a diversity of other research areas such as immunology, epidemiology, endocrinology, cardiology, angiology, nephrology, neurology, opththamology, surgery, gynaecology, etc.; in this sense diabetology is truly an interdisciplinary subject. On the other hand, it has become impossible that a single researcher, or even research group, is able to maintain an overview of or provide all the research methodologies necessary for the investigation of human diabetes.

It is to this end that a book on "Research Methodologies in Human Diabetes" comes into play. It is geared to provide ready access to a wide array of investigative techniques in diabetology. In contrast to laboratory methods, mainly clinically oriented procedures quite often cannot be broken down into step-by-step instructions. Hence, for the various topics on research methodologies contained in this book, rather variable and individual organisations of each chapter have been chosen. We feel, however, that this is a strength of this book and has led to the best possible approach to each topic. In any case, the standard for investigative techniques within a given field of research has become quite apparent and also demarcates the present frontline of further research.

As editors, we feel highly privileged that top researchers in diabetology throughout the world have so willingly shared their particular expertise with the international community of diabetologists. As a result, a unique book has been made possible, representing the true state of the art of human diabetes research. In fact, during the preparation of this book it became obvious that the magnitude of material to be covered is so enormous that only two volumes could accommodate the present state of knowledge. The first volume has been published in 1994.

Above all, it should be remembered, but goes without saying, that research into human diabetes always deals with human beings and that the highest ethical standards have to be applied at all times. Therefore, the Declaration of Helsinki, which gives the ethical framework for any research in humans, concludes this volume of "Research Methodologies in Human Diabetes".

We wish the diabetologists and the many friends throughout the world, a successful and meaningful use of these volumes on diabetes research methodologies.

Carl Erik Mogensen　　　　Eberhard Standl

Contents

Discovery of photocoagulation treatment in diabetic eye disease

A. Wessing

In 1967, Sir Stewart Duke-Elder wrote in his book System of Ophthalmology; "Diabetic retinopathy is one of the major tragedies of ophthamology in our present generation; always common and rapidly becoming still more common, affecting the young as well as the aged, predictable but not preventable and relatively untreatable, chronic and progressive in its course and leading to blindness in a distressing percentage of cases, it is not surprising that it has stimulated speculation and research on a vast scale" [1].

At that time, however, a transition was already underway. Hypophysectomy had sparked interest and found avid proponents [2]. It was clear from the outset, however, that this procedure could only be considered in a few selected cases, if at all. For this reason, more interest was raised by the first sporadic reports of the success of photocoagulation and laser treatment. This seemed to present a treatment possibility, which was relatively easy to use and which could be implemented in the constantly growing number of patients at acceptable costs, both financial and in terms of personnel.

The development of photocoagulation

It is thanks to the work of Meyer-Schwickerath that photocoagulation was developed and made clinically available. With this procedure, he ushered in a new era in the treatment of retinal diseases. The indirect cause was the solar eclipse on July 10, 1945. Burning of the retina by sunlight has been known of since antiquity (Plato: Phaedon). Cases increase as a result of solar eclipses. In the spring of 1946, Meyer-Schwickerath examined a patient, who had viewed the solar eclipse the year before without eye protection and suffered a retinal burn. Meyer-Schwickerath recalled his thoughts, "The question presented itself of whether it might not be possible, using light rays, to create a strong coagulative exudate, which would be suitable to induce an adhesive chorioretinitis and as a result the closure of retinal holes" [3].

There had been previous reports on experimental light damage of the retina, such as those by Czerny (1867), Deutschmann (1882), Widmark (1893) and Maggiore (1927) [4–7]. Practical coagulation trials on rabbit eyes conducted by Móron-Salas in 1945 and 1946 were not published and were first made known on 1950 [8]. Meyer-Schwickerath had spontaneously grasped the entire scope of the idea and, in spite of manifold setbacks, he did not stop until he was able to make it available for practical use in the clinic.

The basic principle was to combine the light source with an ophthalmoscope in such a way that one could exactly place the coagulation on the retina. While this optical combination was relatively easy to achieve, the search for an adequate light source proved to be significantly more difficult. In animal trials on rabbits, it was not difficult to attain an adequate coagulation effect with a simple carbon arc lamp [9]. However, in human eyes, it was not effective due to morphological optical particularities.

In the search for a brighter light, Meyer-Schwickerath again used sunlight, which via a heliostat was reflected into the coagulation apparatus [10]. In the early sixties an improved carbon arc lamp was developed, which simplified use significantly. The breakthrough came in 1955 with the introduction of the Xenon high intensity lamp. Under the expert direction of Dr. Hans Littmann of the Carl Zeiss company in Oberkochen, Germany, a coagulator was developed which became popular around the world within a few years [11]. More than 1200 devices were in use world-wide.

Although simple in construction – or precisely for that reason – the device underwent little change in 20 years of successful use. Fankhauser and Lotmar [12] replaced the original ophthalmoscope with a slit lamp and contact lens to provide a better visualization of the retina. Other coagulators, such as those from Comberg [13] and O'Malley [14] have found only restricted use in the clinic.

A new chapter was begun with the introduction of the laser. After a slow start, it has now fully replaced the standard xenon coagulator. The basic principle of coagulation has, however, remained the same. It always involves focusing light energy on the retina, where it causes a burn and consequently a scar on a pre-planned site. The monochromatic light of the laser also seemed to offer promise of an essentially tissue-specific affect, however, these hopes have not been fulfilled. The success of the laser lies rather in the fact that its use is simpler and the treatment can be more easily integrated into the routine of an ophthalmological practice.

The first milestone in laser coagulation was the introduction of the ruby laser in ophthamology by Campell in 1963 [15]. The decisive step was taken by L'Esperance in 1968 with the argon ion laser, which today is the standard instrument of ophthalmological laser therapy [16]. The red krypton laser, the tunable dye laser and the double frequency YAG laser have only played a subordinate role, in comparison.

Photocoagulation in diabetic retinopathy

In his monograph on photocoagulation published in 1959, Meyer-Schwickerath described five cases of diabetic retinopathy, which had been treated up to then: "Four cases in the late proliferative stage were treated with coagulation without any effect, but in the case presenting microaneuryms and exudates partial disappearance of the latter was achieved by coagulation of the microaneuryms" [11].

Photocoagulation was originally envisioned as a prophylaxis for retinal detachment and in individual cases for its treatment as well [3, 10]. First around 1955 with the introduction of xenon coagulator were blood vessels and vessel proliferations also treated. The goal here was to exclude these as a source of recurring vitreous hemorrhage. In early 1956, Meyer-Schwickerath reported on 6 successfully treated eyes with periphlebitis retinae (morbus Eales) [18]. By the end of the year he was able to present 18 cases with retinitis proliferans. He made the indication more precise in his determination that, (1) "peripheral proliferative and phlebitic regions can be obliterated by photocoagulation"; (2) photocoagulation can "make the vascular trees growing in the vitreous body disappear through the coagulation of the roots" and (3) "old cases with ablatio" cannot be successfully treated [19]. These were the obvious prerequisites for using photocoagulation in diabetic retinopathy as well.

The next contribution to the subject of diabetic retinopathy was presented in Heidelberg in 1964 at a conference of the German Ophthalmological Society. Meyer-Schwickerath still seemed to view the developments with a certain degree of skepticism: "the attempt over many years to influence the progress of diabetic retinopathy by photocoagulation is very problematic" [20]. The same conference saw a presentation by Schott, who would contribute significantly to the further development [21]. Schott was a close colleague of Meyer-Schwickerath's and chief physician at the Eye Clinic in Essen, Germany. In his presentation, he gave an overview of the experiences gathered up to that point in Essen.

In the mean time, there were some basal indications that photocoagulation could have a possible positive effect on diabetic retinopathy. Almaric [22] observed that eyes with extended chorioretinal scars, such as occur with excessive myopia or after a severe chorioretinitis, are less susceptible to diabetic retinopathy. He used this as a reason to treat exudative diabetic retinopathy with episcleral diathermy and achieved respectable improvements [23].

Schott counted 58 diabetics which had been treated with photocoagulation in the Essen Eye Clinic by 1964. He was able to follow-up 33 patients with a

Table 1 Results of photocoagulation [21]

	Treated	Untreated
Vision improved	4	1
Vision unchanged	8	3
Vision worsened	2	6
Total	14	10

total of 50 coagulated eyes. For 21 of these, the observation time lasted between 2 and 5 years. The eyes treated in these patients showed a clear improvement when compared to non-treated partner eyes (Table 1).

In this work, Schott provided the essential criteria for photocoagulation, criteria which were later repeatedly substantiated and which are still used today. In his opinion, the advanced background retinopathy – as it is called today – and the early proliferative phase are appropriate for a coagulation. In advanced vessel proliferation, the coagulation is too late. He is also aware of the fact that the coagulation requires significant intensity and includes 2 or 3 sessions each with up to 200 individual coagulations. The procedure developed by the Essen school was later named pan-retinal coagulation and is still a standard procedure today. Many of the early failures were doubtlessly due to the fact that this rule was not adhered to and coagulations were not performed in sufficient number.

In the early 1960s, photocoagulation had already attained widespread use. From other regions as well came the first reports of experiences with coagulation in diabetic retinopathy. Pischel and Colyear (1960), like Clark (1961), found no practical use [24, 25]; Moura-Brazil and DeRezende (1961) as well as Lopez de Andrade and de Sá (1962) were more successful [26, 27]; François and Weekers (1965) remained undecided [28]. The reports by Wetzig and later those by Okun proved to be important for the further extension of coagulation therapy, especially in the USA. Wetzig, Jepson, and Worlton presented a series with 28 treated diabetics who showed a significant stabilization tendency after coagulation [29]. In 1966 and 1967, they were able to successfully increase this number [30, 31]. In 1966, Okun and Cibis reported their first successes, which were further supplemented by Okun in 1968 [32, 33].

Developments in Essen had proceeded as well. After his initial hesitation, by 1963/64 Meyer-Schwickerath became firmly convinced of the utility of photocoagulation. With hundreds of photographs, he had documented the results and he did not hesitate to share his offering with the ophthalmological world in numerous lectures and publications [34–41] (Figs 1 and 2).

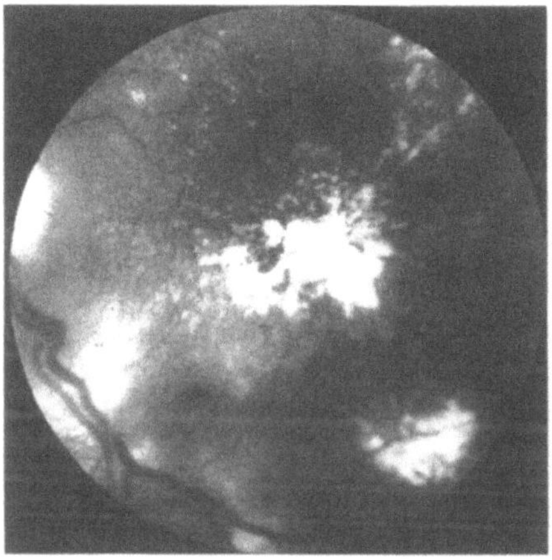

Fig. 1a Exudative diabetic retinopathy, photo from 1960 (reprinted from [21])

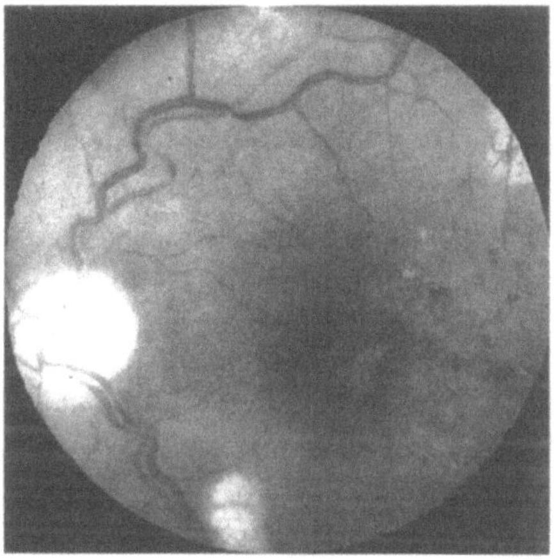

Fig. 1b The same eye, regression of diabetic leasons following photocoagulation, 1962

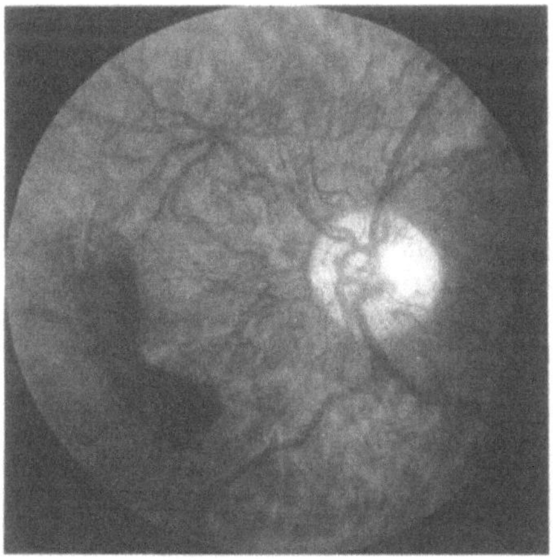

Fig. 2a Proliferative diabetic retinopathy with new vascular formations on the optic disc 1963 (reprinted from the Meyer-Schwickerath collection)

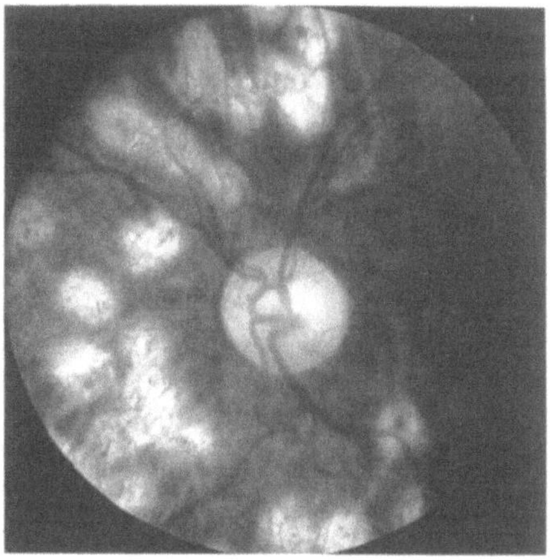

Fig. 2b The same eye, complete regression of the proliferation following intensive coagulation

This development culminated in the Airlie House Symposium, which took place in Warrenton, Virginia in the fall of 1968. The fact that diabetic retinopathy is the leading cause of blindness in adults and the uncertainty in the evaluation of hypophysectomy and photocoagulation were reason enough for the US Public Health Service to assume sponsorship of the event [42]. In the discussion, there was a vigorous clash of opinion between the proponents of photocoagulation and its opponents.

The conference was to serve as the springboard for further development, which was characterized by the increasing use of the argon laser and – more importantly – by a well-founded statistical-scientific discussion.

What Meyer-Schwickerath set into motion with the development of photocoagulation and his first coagulation trials in diabetic retinopathy, found final complete substantiation and a crowning completion in the Diabetic Retinopathy Study (DRS) [43] and in the Early Treatment Diabetic Retinopathy Study (ETDRS) [44]. Even though it was not possible for him to provide this confirmation himself, he did inspire an entire generation of ophthalmologists and fundamental researchers to intensively and fruitfully examine and treat diabetic eye disease.

References

[1] Duke-Elder St. System of Ophthalmology. Vol X, Duke-Elder St, Dobree JH, eds London: Henry Kimpton, 1967: 410.
[2] Luft R, Oliveciona H, Sjögren B. Hypophysectomy in man. Nord Med 1952; 47: 351–354.
[3] Meyer-Schwickerath G. Lichtkoagulation. Eine Methode zur Behandlung und Verhütung der Netzhautablösung. Graefes Arch 1954; 156: 2–34.
[4] Czerny. Über Blendung der Netzhaut durch Sonnenlicht. Ber Wien Acad Wiss 1867; 56/2.
[5] Deutschmann R. Über die Blendung der Netzhaut durch direktes Sonnenlicht. Graefes Arch 1882; 28/3: 241–254.
[6] Widmark. Skand Arch 1893; 4: 281. (Meyer-Schwickerath).
[7] Maggiore L. Soc Ital d'Oftalm (1927). (Meyer-Schwickerath).
[8] Móron Salas J. Arch Soc Oftalm Hisp Amer 1950; 10: 566. (Meyer-Schwickerath).
[9] Meyer-Schwickerath G. Über die Möglichkeiten der Koagulation der Netzhaut mit Lichtstrahlen. 18. Tagung der Vereinigung Nordwestdeutscher Augenärzte. Göttingen 1949 Ref: Klin Mbl Augenheilk 1951; 118: 194.
[10] Meyer-Schwickerath G. Koagulation der Netzhaut mit Sonnenlicht. Ber Deutsche Ophthalmol Ges 1949; 55: 256–259.
[11] Meyer-Schwickerath G. Lichtkoagulation. Bücherei des Augenarztes, Heft 33. Stuttgart: Enke, 1959.
[12] Fankhauser F, Lotmar W. Photocoagulation through the Goldmann contact glas. Arch Ophthalmol 1967; 77: 320–330.
[13] Comberg D. Lichtkoagulation mit einem neuen Gerät. Ber Deutsche Ophthalmol Ges 1964; 66: 355–359.
[14] O'Malley P. Portable xenon are light coagulator. Br J Ophthalmol 1973; 57: 935–944.
[15] Campell CJ, Ritter MC, Koester CJ. Optical maser as retinal coagulator. An evaluation. Tr Am Acad Ophthalmol Otolaryng 1963; 67: 58–67.
[16] L'Esperance FA jr. An ophthalmological argon laser photocoagulation system: design, construction and laboratory investigations. Tr Am Ophthalmol Soc 1968; 66: 827–904.
[17] Meyer-Schwickerath G, Drance SM. Light Coagulation. St. Louis: Mosby Comp, 1960.
[18] Meyer-Schwickerath G. Erfahrungen mit der Lichtkoagulation der Netzhaut und Iris. Doc Ophthalmol 1956; 10: 91–118/131.
[19] Meyer-Schwickerath G. Neue Indikationen der Lichtkoagulation. Ber Deutsche Ophthalmol Ges 1956; 60: 197–201.

[20] Meyer-Schwickerath G. Lichtkoagulation. Ber Deutsche Ophthalmol Ges 1964; 66: 313–324.
[21] Schott K. Weitere Erfahrungen mit der Lichtkoagulation bei Retinopathia diabetica. Ber Deutsche Ophthalmol Ges. 1964; 66: 349–355.
[22] Amalric P. Essai de traitement de la rétinopathie diabétique exsudative. Bull Soc Ophthalmol France 66: 359–363 (1960). Int Ophthalmol Clin 1963; 3: 3.
[23] Amalric P. Nouvelles considérations concernant l'évolution et le traitement de la rétinopathie diabétique. Ophthalmologica 1967; 154: 151–160.
[24] Pischel DK, Colyear BH. Clinical results of lightcoagulation therapy. Am J Ophthalmol 1960; 50: 590–595.
[25] Clark G. Evaluation of photocoagulation. Am J Ophthalmol 1961; 51: 714–715.
[26] Moura-Brazil N, DeRezende J. The role of photocoagulation in ophthalmology. Bull Soc Ophthalm France 1961; 74: 699–710.
[27] Lopez de Andrade A, DeSà S. Clinical results of photocoagulation. Arq Portug Oftal 1962; 14: 63–73.
[28] Francois J, Weekers R. La photocoagulation en ophthalmologie. Bull Soc Belge Ophthalmol 1965; 139: 135–138.
[29] Wetzig PC, Jepson CN, Worlton JT. Treatment of diabetic retinopathy by light coagulation. Br J Ophthal 1963; 47: 539–541.
[30] Wetzig PC, Worlton JT. The treatment of diabetic retinopathy by light Coagulation. Mod Probl Ophthalmol 1966; 4: 19–23.
[31] Wetzig, PC, Worlton JT. The treatment of diabetic retinopathy by light Coagulation. Am J Ophthalmol 1966; 62: 459–465.
[32] Okun E, Cibis PA. The role of photocoagulation in the therapy of proliferative diabetic retinopathy. Arch Ophthalmol 1966; 75: 337–352.
[33] Okun E. The effectiveness of photocoagulation in the therapy of proliferative diabetic retinopathy (PDR). (A controlled study in 50 patients). Tr Am Acad Ophthalmol Otolaryng 1968; 72: 246–252.
[34] Meyer-Schwickerath G. Treatment of vascular diseases of the retina with light Coagulation. Tr Can Ophthal Soc 1963; 26: 137–147.
[35] Meyer-Schwickerath G. Treatment of Eales' disease and diabetic retinopathy with photocoagulation. West J Surgery 1964; 72: 76–81.
[36] Meyer-Schwickerath G. Treatment of Eales' disease and diabetic retinopathy with photocoagulation. Tr Ophthal Soc UK 1965; 84: 67–76.
[37] Meyer-Schwickerath G. Prevention of detachment and proliferation in diabetic retinopathy. New Orleans: 1968.
[38] Meyer-Schwickerath G. Rétinopathie diabétique et photocoagulation. Bull Soc Franc Ophthalmol 1968; 81: 551–564.
[39] Meyer-Schwickerath G, Schott K. Diabetische Retinopathie und Lichtkoagulation. Klin Mbl Augenheilk 1968; 153: 173–179.
[40] Schott K, Meyer-Schickerath G. Diabetic retinopathy and photocoagulation. Am J Ophthal 1968; 66: 597–603.
[41] Wessing A, Meyer-Schwickerath G. Results of photocoagulation in diabetic retinopathy. In: Goldberg MF, Fine SL, eds Treatment of Diabetic Retinopathy. US Public Health Service Publication 1969; No 1890: 569–601.
[42] Goldberg MF, Fine SL. Treatment of Diabetic Retinopathy. US Public Health Service Publication 1969; No 1890.
[43] Diabetic Retinopathy Study Research Group. Preliminary report on effects of photocoagulation therapy. Am J Ophthalmol 1976; 81: 383–396.
[44] Early Treatment Diabetic Retinopathy Study Research Group. ETDRS report No 4: Photocoagulation for diabetic macular edema. Int Ophthalmol Clin 1987; 27: 265–272.

Research methodologies in measuring blood glucose and in defining diabetes

K. G. M. M. Alberti, J. M. Burrin

Introduction

Objective measurements of blood glucose are required for diagnosing diabetes and for direct short-term assessment of glucose control. The methodological approach taken to measure glucose may differ between clinical and research purposes; the former requiring enough information to make diagnostic decisions or treatment judgements whereas the latter may require more accurate information for epidemiological studies of diabetes prevalence or for detecting small alterations in glucose values. Measurement of blood glucose remains an analytical challenge and the choice of method requires careful consideration dependent on the purpose of the measurement.

Blood glucose – the analytical challenge

Glycaemic behaviour in diabetes especially IDDM when treated with conventional therapy is usually erratic so that the range of blood glucose concentrations to be measured may fluctuate widely [1]. In diabetic emergencies it is necessary to measure both high and low levels of blood glucose rapidly. Quantification of hypoglycaemic episodes has also achieved predominance recently with the use of human insulin preparations and some methods of glucose measurement may be inadequate for this purpose [2]. Studies of novel treatments or regimes that have the potential to achieve normoglycaemia or evaluation of the role of glycaemia in degenerative complications of diabetes require accurate and precise measurements of blood glucose.

Most techniques for assessment of glucose control require periodic blood glucose measurement. Twenty years ago, quantitative measurements of glycosuria were frequently used as an additional measure of glucose control to supplement intermittent blood glucose measurement. The utility of these measurements was soon found to be limited by the individual variation of the two processes, glomerular filtration and tubular reabsorption, controlling glycosuria. In addition, information obtained was limited to an indication of hyperglycaemia and gave no warning of impending hypoglycaemia. Continuous monitoring of blood glucose enabled the researcher to record diurnal glycaemic profiles continuously but only in an in-patient setting for short time periods due to the difficulties of maintaining chronic venous access. It remains a useful technique for assessing the effects of new treatments on glycaemic control and the development of biosenors offers the exciting opportunity of completing the feed back loop needed in the development of artificial biofeedback systems for blood glucose control. The use of subcutaneously implanted wicks may circumvent some of the problems [3].

At the other extreme glucose measurements need to be performed by the patient under ordinary life conditions of meals, exercise etc. Perhaps the greatest advance in blood glucose measurement has been the development of test strip methodology. This has made possible home-monitoring of blood glucose enabling the patient to aim for treatment targets near the physiological range. However, confirmation of nocturnal hypoglycaemia or early morning hyperglycaemia requires either constant glucose monitoring or frequent intermittent blood sampling. Since self-monitoring of blood glucose carries risks of falsification [4], long-term research studies to assess the efficiency of novel treatments have achieved a workable compromise of self-collection of blood specimens into capillary tubes or onto filter paper [5]. Samples are subsequently analysed in a local or central laboratory.

The development of blood glucose testing strips has already shifted responsibility for diabetes control from the hospital and the doctor to the patient. This in turn has led to a demand from general practitioners for desk top analysers for glucose monitoring. Tests using desk top laboratory technology bring increased convenience and may be appropriate for monitoring, but a recent study emphasised the financial costs compared to laboratory testing [6]. However, portable blood glucose systems may have uses in the research situation where a method of comparable quality to that in a laboratory is needed for field based epidemiological studies.

Thus, methods for bloods glucose measurement may need to be sensitive, specific, accurate, precise, in wet or dry chemistry format and laboratory or home-based. Fortunately, not all these requirements are needed simultaneously and the rest of this review will examine the analytical methods available for blood glucose measurement and indicate their appropriate applications.

Laboratory methods for glucose determination

Many methods or method modifications for glucose assay have been described and reviewed previously [7–9]. The principle approaches are summarised in Table 1 and fall into two major categories, namely the early chemical methods and the more recent enzymatic methods. In the older chemical reducing methods (Somogyi-Nelson, Folin-Wu, Benedict, Hagedorn-Jensen), the highly reactive 1,2-enediol form of glucose is oxidised by oxidants under alkaline conditions and the reduced products measured colourimetrically. All these methods, which are based on the reducing properties of glucose are non-specific, however, and interference occurs due to the presence in blood of non-glucose reducing substances such as glutathione, creatinine, uric acid ascorbic acid. As a result of these interferences, results obtained with the chemical reducing methods tend to be higher by a variable amount (up to 10%) when compared with the more specific enzymatic methods [10]. Chemical methods based on the reaction of hexoses with concentrated acids in the presence of phenols (resorcinol, anthrone) are currently of historical interest

Table 1 *Laboratory methods for glucose determination*

Method principle	Method designation
1. *Chemical methods*	
a) Oxidatin-reduction	
cupric → cuprous	Somogyi-Nelson
	Folin-Wu
	Benedict
	Neocuproine
ferricyanide → ferrocyanide	Hagedorn-Jenson
b) Aromatic amine condensation	
aldohexose → glycosylamine	0-toluidine
c) Acid-phenol condensation	
hexose → phenol adduct	Resorcinol
	Anthrone
2. *Enzymatic methods*	
a) Glucose oxidase	
Peroxidase/chromogen	e. g. Trinder
Oxygen electrode	e. g. Beckmann analyser
Peroxide electrode	e. g. YSI analyser
b) Hexokinase/G6PDH	
NADPH measurement	Spectrophotometric
	Fluorimetric
c) Glucose dehydrogenase	
NADH measurement	Spectrophotometric
	Fluorimetric

only. Of the chemical methods described, the o-toluidine method is least affected by interfering substances. This method uses the property of glucse and other aldohexoses to condense with aromatic amines in hot acetic acid to give coloured glycosylamines. Specificity for glucose is high since other aldohexoses such as galactose and mannose do not normally occur in significant amounts in man, and glucose results obtained with the o-toluidine method are virtually identical to those found with enzymatic methods [10].

The specificity of methods for the determination of glucose is usually assessed in terms of quantitative agreement with values obtained by enzymatic methods. These procedures are based on either glucose oxidase, hexokinase or more recently glucose dehydrogenase. Although values obtained using these methods are usually referred to as "true" glucose, the presence of interferents can influence their accuracy, and competing side reactions and contaminants in the reagent enzyme preparations may seriously affect specificity.

Glucose oxidase has been routinely used in clinical chemistry ever since it was applied in the Trinder reaction [11]. In this method the hydrogen peroxide produced by glucose oxidase-catalysed oxidation of glucose is detected through the peroxidase-catalysed oxidation of a chromogenic substance, by measuring the change in absorbance of oxidised chromogen.

$$\beta\text{-D-glucose} + 0_2 \xrightarrow[\text{oxidase}]{\text{glucose}} \text{D-gluconic acid} + H_20_2$$

$$\text{Chromogen} + H_20_2 \xrightarrow{\text{peroxidase}} \text{Coloured Chromogen} + H_20$$

Although the conversion of glucose into gluconic acid is a highly specific reaction, various chemical substances can be used as peroxidase substrates. This lack of substrate specificity of peroxidase has led to numerous alternative chromogens being used in this procedure and is also the reason why many substances (eg. bilirubin, ascorbic acid, uric acid, paracetamol, 4-amino-salicylic acid) are reported to interfere. The interference with glucose oxidase/peroxidase coupled reactions can be avoided by measuring oxygen consumption or hydrogen peroxide formation directly with enzyme electrodes. This approach forms the basis of many of the "stat" glucose analysers available. In the oxygen rate method which is utilised in the Beckman glucose analyser, a direct measure of the glucose level in plasma or serum is obtained by using a polarographic oxygen electrode to measure the rate of oxygen consumption in the glucose oxidase reaction. Although not applicable with whole blood or haemolysed specimens the method is simple and suitable for use in smaller laboratories or outpatient clinics [12].

The Yellow Springs Instruments analyser uses a hydrogen peroxide sensitive electrode [13]. As with direct oxygen measurement, whole blood or haemolysed blood interferes with methods measuring H_2O_2 directly. This problem is overcome with the YSI analyser by immobilising the glucose oxidase enzyme inside a polycarbonate membrane with a pore size sufficiently large to allow the passage of glucose, oxygen, and H_2O_2, but small enough to exclude proteins and cells. This allows measurements to be performed in whole blood, serum or plasma. The YSI is amongst the most popular analysers now available for research laboratory outpatient use, and for use in epidemiological studies, where it has been used in remote parts of Africa with the aid of a portable generator [14]. Interferences can occur with this method, most notably from paracetamol [15] and sodium iodoacetate [16].

The hexokinase method for glucose is based on the following reaction sequence, in which the second step is responsible for the high specificity of the assay.

$$\text{D-glucose} + \text{ATP} \xrightarrow{\text{hexokinase}} \text{glucose-6-phosphate} + \text{ADP}$$

$$\begin{matrix}\text{glucose-6-phosphate} \\ + \text{NADP}\end{matrix} \xrightarrow[\text{dehydrogenase}]{\text{glucose-6-phosphate}} \begin{matrix}\text{6-phosphogluconate} \\ + \text{NADPH} + \text{H}^+\end{matrix}$$

The NADPH generated in the second reaction can be measured spectrophotometrically or fluorimetrically [17]. This method is currently regarded worldwide as the reference method for glucose [10]. However, even this method is not totally specific and fructose can interfere. It is converted to fructose-6-phosphate by hexokinase and then to glucose-6-phosphate by phosphofructoiosomerase present in plasma or as a contaminant of the reagent enzymes. This may explain why some authors have found values 1–2.5% higher with this method compared to glucose oxidase [18].

The enzyme glucose dehydrogenase is also used to measure glucose in a single step reaction.

$$\beta\text{-D-glucose} + \text{NAD} \xrightarrow[\text{dehydrogenase}]{\text{glucose}} \text{D-gluconic acid} + \text{NADH} + \text{H}^+$$

Glucose dehydrogenase has a high specificity for ß-D-glucose and the enzyme mutarotase which catalyses the interconversion of the anomeric forms of glucose is included as an auxiliary enzyme in commercial reagent kits to facilitate the overall reaction with glucose. In a similar manner to the hexokinase procedures, the NADH generated can be measured spectrophotometrically or fluorimetrically. Good correlations with both glucose oxidase and hexokinase methods are reported [19, 20) and values are consistently 0.1−0.2 mmol/l lower than with the hexokinase method. Only D-xylose (at a level greater than 2 mmol/l) and mannose are reported as interferents.

Today, most clinical laboratories use enzymatic methods based on hexokinase or glucose oxidase. In the UK, use of hexokinase has overtaken glucose oxidase over the last ten years with approximately 45% of laboratories in the UK National External Quality Assessment Scheme (NEQAS) using hexokinase, 30% using glucose oxidase wet chemistry procedures and the remaining 25%, glucose dehydrogenase or glucose oxidase elextrode methods (DG Bullock, NEQAS, Birmingham, UK – personal communication). The popularity of glucose dehydrogenase methods is increasing slowly, hindered perhaps by the current increased cost of this method compared to the other two enzymatic procedures. All of the enzymatic methods are used on a wide variety of continuous analysers as well as automated discrete analysers and the majority of these laboratory methods are capable of achieving a within-laboratory between-batch imprecision (coefficient of variation) of 2.5%.

Dry reagent methods for glucose determination

Background and principle

Dry chemistry systems for glucose analysis have opened a new area in user convenience. They are designed to be self-contained analytical devices, with analysis being initiated by the user applying the same sample to the system; results are usually available within a few minutes. The dry reagents are stable for long periods of time (months to years) and require no user preparation.

Early systems were designed to detect glucose in urine; the approach has subsequently been extended to the measurement of glucose (and other analytes) in plasma and whole blood. The first dry reagent systems were based on reagent strips; these were later combined with simple reflectance meters and more recently dry reagent chemistry systems have been developed for glucose and other analytes using automated microprocessor-controlled reflectance photometers. It is envisaged that these portable desk-top analysers might be used in the smaller laboratory, the doctor's office or on the ward. Numerous reagent strips (Table 2) and desk-top analysers (Table 3) are available, all are based on a similar functional approach but with different constructional configurations. The basic principles of dry reagent chemistry systems have been discussed in a recent review [21].

Table 2 Details of dry reagent strips/meters

Test strip (manufacturer)	Visual	Meter	Glucose method	Test time	Blood removal
Glucostix (Bayer Diagnostics)	Yes	Glucometer II	GOD and Coloured indicator	50 sec	Yes
BM 1-44 (Boehringer Mannheim UK)	Yes	Reflolux II	GOD and Coloured indicator	50 sec	Yes
Exactech (Medisense)	No	Exactech pen	GOD and Ferrocene electrode	30 sec	No
GA (Hypoguard)	Yes	Hypoguard GA	GOD and Coloured indicator	90 sec	Yes
Supreme (Hypoguard)	Yes	Hypoguard Supreme	GOD and Coloured indicator	60 sec	No
Glucotide (Bayer Diagnostics)	Yes	Glucometer 4	GOD and Coloured indicator	60 sec	No
Glucocard (Kyoto)	No	Glucocard	GOD and Ferricyanide electrode	60 sec	No

Table 3 Details of desktop analysers

Instrument (manufacturer)	Sample	Glucose method	Dry reagent format	Other tests
Ektachem DT (Kodak)	10 µl plasma	GOD	Slides	Yes
Reflotron (Boehringer Mannheim UK)	32 µl whole blood	GOD	Strips	Yes
Analyst (DuPont)	10 µl plasma	HK/G6PDH	Tablets	Yes
Easy ST (Merck Ltd)	79 µl plasma	GDH	Cuvettes	Yes
Vision (Abbott Diagnostics)	150 µl whole blood	HK/G6PDH	Cassettes	Yes
Seralyser (Ames)	10 µl serum	GOD	Strips	Yes
Hemocue B (Hemocue Ltd)	5 µl whole blood	GDH	Cuvettes	No
Satellite G (Medisense)	10–50 µl whole blood	GOD	Strips	No

GOD = glucose oxidase
HK/G6PDH = hexokinase/glucose-6-phosphate dehydrogenase
GDH = glucose dehydrogenase

Reagent strip methods

Each of the reagent strip systems comprises several components and a cross-section of a typical system is shown in Figure 1. A sample of whole blood is applied to the surface of the strip where plasma glucose is separated from red blood cells by a sample handling surface matrix. Plasma diffuses into the reagent layer, reconstituting and activating the enzymes, buffer and indicator dyes. After a short reaction time (30 sec−2 minutes), red blood cells are removed by washing or wiping (in some systems this is not required) and the developed colour is monitored from above with a reflectance meter and translated to glucose concentration or visually compared to a colour chart.

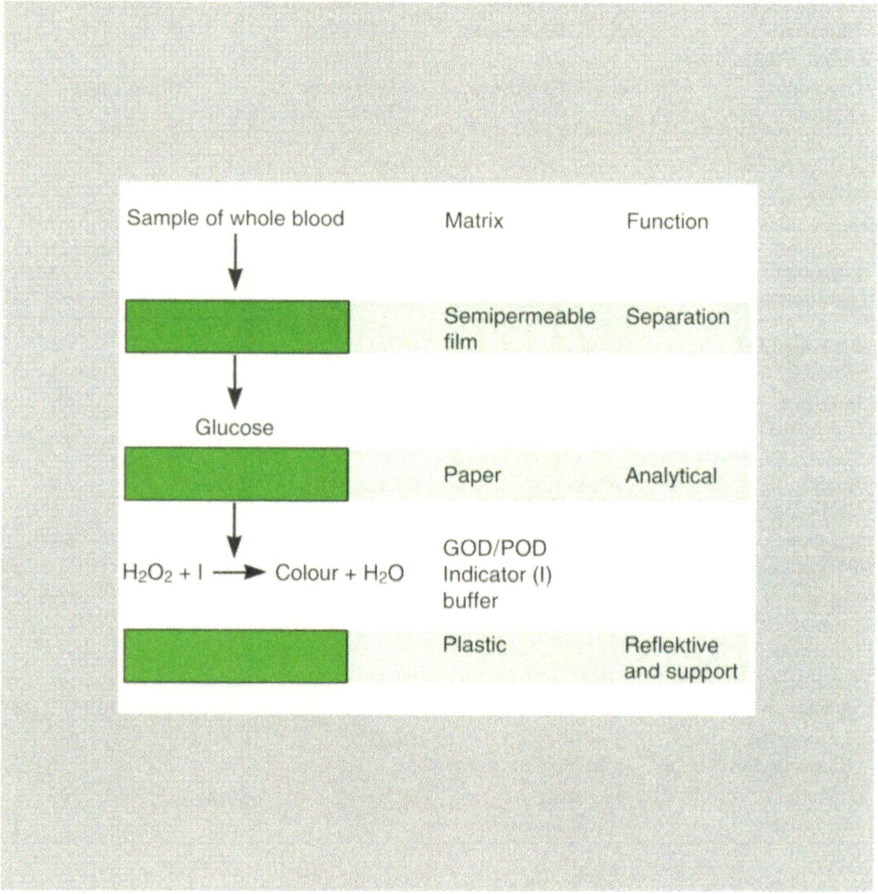

Fig. 1 Cross-section of an example of a dry reagent strip for glucose

Calibration of the meter systems occurs automatically by transmitting reagent lot information contained on each strip (or a separate calibration strip) to the instrument during the test procedure. This overcomes the problem of user calibration and prevents some potential user error.

Most of the reagent strip systems are based on glucose oxidase/peroxidase/chromogen chemistry (Table 2). One exception is the Exactech strip (Medisense, Abingdon, UK). These single-use disposable test strips are actually electrodes containing an enzyme complex with glucose oxidase and ferrocene as the principal components. When a drop of blood is applied to the electrode strip, glucose oxidase calatyses the oxidation of glucose to gluconic acid with the electrons generated being absorbed by the mediator ferrocene in its oxidised state of ferrocinium to form ferrocene. The resulting current of electrons is transferred to the electrode and is proportional to the glucose level of the blood. The system is fast and eminently portable; the meter being only pen-size, and has proved popular with some diabetic patients [22]. Another similar system is the Glucocard^{TM} [22a].

Glucose results obtained with dry reagent strips and meters are reported as accurate and precise when appropriate training and instruction are given [23, 24]. However, numerous reports exist in the literature where poor results have been obtained [25, 26] due to inappropriate [27] and incorrect [28] use of the meter. It is imperative that manufacturers instructions are followed exactly and several countries have produced reports containing recommendations on various aspects of reagent strip glucose monitoring [29–31]. These reports emphasise the need for laboratory-based quality assessment schemes to examine the performance of extra-laboratory instruments. Several schemes have been proposed where parallel samples are collected using a capillary tube or filter paper collection system which is then sent to the laboratory for analysis, together with the result obtained by the reagent strip method [32–34]. These results should be within ± 15% of the laboratory result.

There are several potential sources of error when blood glucose is determined using a test strip [35]. In addition to performing the technique correctly, the same types of chemical interference may be expected in these glucose oxidase systems as described for the wet chemistry version of the enzyme reaction. This interference maybe exacerbated in glucose strip tests where the plasma acts as the solvent for the dry reagents, the relative concentration of interferent consequently being higher than in the conventional wet chemistry system. We have recently completed a study which looked at the effects of ascorbic acid, paracetamol, salicylate uric acid, urea and creatinine on Glucostix, BM 1–44, and Exactech strips [36]. Statistically significant decreases in glucose concentration were observed in the case of ascorbic acid and salicylate on Glucostix and a significant increase in glucose in the case of paracetamol and the Exactech strips. The influence of ascorbic acid on glucose oxidase systems has been documented on several occasions and is thought to be due either to direct competition with the redox indicator system or in the case of O-tolidine (the chromogen used in Glucostix), a lag in colour development [37].

Another major area for concern with the use of reagent strips is the effect of haematocrit on the glucose value obtained. Several reports in the literature have shown some influence of haematocrit on Glucostix, BM 1–44, Hypoguard GA and Exactech strips [38, 39]. In all cases low haematocrits produce higher glucose results on these systems and vice versa. These findings are particularly relevant to diabetic patients with end-stage renal failure who have low haematocrits but depend on blood glucose monitoring since urine testing is unreliable due to altered renal threshold. A recent study in diabetic patients with low haematocrits (24±4%) showed that all reagent strips tested over-read by a variable amount (18–63%), and the percentage over-read was negatively correlated with the haematocrit for each strip [40].

Desktop analysers

Despite the improvements in reagent strips and meter methodology, their performance has not yet matched laboratory-based wet chemistry methods for precision and accuracy. There remains a need for systems which can be used away from the laboratory but which provide the same quality of results as those obtained within the laboratory. These analysers are required for diagnostic and monitoring purposes in the outpatient clinic and the doctor's surgery and also for screening purposes in the community.

Several desktop portable analysers are now available which are designed to measure several analytes (including glucose) or are dedicated to glucose determination only (Table 3). These systems all use dry reagents with the resultant lack of user preparation and long shelf-life, although the format in which the dry reagents are presented may differ (Table 3). Data are available that confirm the accuracy and ease of use of such analysers in the laboratory [41–44], although the is little data on their use outside the laboratory by non-laboratory staff. A study comparing there is little data on their use outside the laboratory by non-labortory staff. A study comparing the use of four desktop analysers in six urban general practices [6] suggested that although the cost per test of using such machines did not compete favourably with laboratory testing, quality control tests were within the specified limits on 98% of occasions. However, laboratory back-up facilities were still required to deal with problems that arose. As noted above for the dry reagent glucose strip tests, interferences can occur with these systems. Thus, positive interference in the HemoCue measurement of blood glucose was noted with both ascorbic acid and triglyceride although there was no effect of changing haematocrit from 35 to 65% [44]. There is no doubt that further improvements of these analysers and expansion of their test repertoires will lead to increased use in both clinical situations and research studies.

The diagnosis of diabetes

As stated above the main use of blood glucose measurement is in the diagnosis of and control of diabetes. Diabetes mellitus has been known since antiquity. Diagnosis was based in ancient times purely on symptoms and signs and referred purely to insulin-dependent diabetes (IDDM) although the Indian name, *Mahudma*, meaning "honey-urine" suggests the beginnings of chemical diagnosis. In the 17th century it was shown that diabetes was associated with sugar in the urine and Matthew Dobson in the 18th century showed excess sugar in the blood. By the 19th century non-fatal diabetes was being recognised in the older age groups i. e. non-insulin dependent diabetes (NIDDM), as well as IDDM in young people. By the 20th century routine clinical diagnosis of diabetes was made using glycosuria initially by cumbersome chemical testing but more recently by tablet or test strip testing. When more accurate testing was required blood glucose levels were measured either in the fasting or random states or following an oral glucose load-the oral glucose tolerance test (OGTT).

It is necessary to establish the reasons for making a diagnosis. In a symptomatic individual it is obvious. However, largely one is trying to identify those at risk of developing the long term complications of diabetes and in the early stages many diabetic subjects will be asymptomatic. This should be borne in mind when attempting to assess or establish diagnostic criteria.

What sample?

Before describing diagnostic levels for the diagnosis a few comments on the sample type and site of sampling are necessary. Considerable confusion has occurred about the differences in apparent glucose level in plasma and whole blood and between different sampling sites e. g. capillary, venous [45]. There is an approximate 12% higher value in plasma than whole blood – inevitable when one considers the water content of whole blood which is lower than plasma because of the red cell mass. Obviously the size of this difference will vary according to the haematocrit. Confusion arises particularly with test strips where it is the glucose content of filtered plasma which is measured, but several meters allow for this and give a whole blood result.

Sample site makes a trivial difference to glucose values in the basal state as there is a low peripheral arterio-venouos difference. In the fed state or following a glucose load, however, there is a sharp increase in muscle glucose uptake and at a circulating glucose level of 10–11 mM there is a 1 mM higher glucose level in capillary compared with venus blood. This difference will, however, be less in insulin resistant subjects, such as those with NIDDM, giving higher venous values. A further point concerns ambient temperature. When comparing OGTTs performed at 32–33 °C with those at 22–23 ° Akanji and Oputa [46] found 1 hour venous plasma glucose levels to be 0.5 mM higher in normal subjects but up to 5 mM higher in those with diabetes. This may be due to arterialisation of venous blood, but whatever the cause has major diagnostic implications for studies in hot climates. Use of arterialised or capillary blood would obviously be safer.

It is obviously important for proper diagnosis of diabetes that both the sample type and the sample site are clearly specified.

Random blood glucose

In many cases where diabetes is suspected measurement of a random blood (or plasma) glucose level will suffice. Thus there is little doubt if a value in excess of 20 mM is found. On the other hand results are often equivocal. The World Health Organisation in its Study Group Report in 1985 [47] stated that venous blood glucose levels of more than 10.0 mM (for venous plasma glucose more than 11.1 mM) were diagnostic but below these levels lies a large grey area which is non-diagnostic. Most asymptomatic individuals fall in this range and other tests are then necessary. Random testing is indeed much too nonspecific and insensitive for screening or for research use.

Fasting blood glucose

Measurement of fasting blood glucose is a highly specific but relatively insensitive method for population screening and diagnosis, although much preferable to random measurements. There are several problems. First there is considerable research interest in impaired glucose tolerance (IGT) – a category promulgated by WHO in 1979 [48] of individuals at increased risk of developing diabetes and macrovascular disease and with a normal fasting glucose by definition. This can only be diagnosed by glucose tolerance test, although the

National Diabetes Data Group [49] refers to plasma glucose between 6.4 and 7.8 mM in the fasting state as non-diagnostic and some refer to this, illogically, as IGT. Second, the initial definition of a diagnostic blood glucose level by WHO and NDDG was done largely by guesswork rather than through its prognostic significance. We have indeed suggested that the levels are too high when looked at in comparison with the 2 hour post oral glucose load levels [50].

Nonetheless a recent interesting study in the Pima Indians [51] has suggested that the fasting glucose is as precise as the 2 h level prognostically and can be used for diagnosis. The suggested cut off level for maximum sensitivity and specificity (81 and 80% respectively) was 7.2 mM for venous plasma glucose compared with the WHO and NDDG criterion of 7.8 mM.

The oral glucose tolerance test

The OGTT was first introduced as a research tool in 1889 [52]. The actual test was not difficult but measuring the glucose content in blood was a long and tedious process at that time. The OGTT continued in research use until after the second World War when more refined and simpler blood glucose measurements became available (see above). Since then the OGTT has became the gold standard for defining diabetes, albeit somewhat tarnished [53].

The benefit of the OGTT is that it is cheap and easy to perform and can be carried out in a wide variety of settings. It is particularly suitable for epidemological studies, aided greatly by the availability of the near patient blood glucose measuring systems now available.

There are, however, problems. In earlier days there was no consistency in either the size of the glucose load or the interpretation of the results. Glucose loads varied from 50 g to 100 g to body weight related doses and West, for example, sites 17 sets of different criteria to interpret the results [54]. The situation was, however, greatly eased in 1979, when international criteria were agreed by both the National Diabetes Data Group (NDDG) in the USA and WHO [48, 49], although there were still some differences between the two organisations. These were in part clarified by WHO in 1985 [47] although the NDDG criteria still contain an unhelpful "non-diagnostic" category.

More important perhaps is that the criteria were now based on risk ie. the chances of developing the specific diabetic complications, particularly retinopathy, as well as the bimodality of glucose distribution in two high prevalence population. The data were derived from long-term studies in Bedford in the UK, the Pima Indians in the USA and Nauruans in the Pacific.

Even this was not without problems as the new oral glucose load was 75 g whereas the previous studies had been performed with 50 g in the UK and 100 g in the USA. The weight of the new test was placed on the 2 hour post-load value, and this alone was deemed suitable for epidemiological studies. For diagnostic purposes, however, it was recommended that there should be at least an additional high value during the test or a high value on a second test. The now accepted criteria are shown in Table 4.

Table 4 Diagnostic values for the oral glucose tolerance test

	Glucose concentration (mM) Whole blood V	C	Plasma V	C
Diabetes				
Fasting	≥ 6.7	≥ 6.7	≥ 7.8	≥ 7.8
2 hours	≥ 10.0	≥ 11.1	≥ 11.1	≥ 12.2
IGT				
Fasting	≥ 6.7	≥ 6.7	≥ 7.8	≥ 7.8
2 hours	6.7–9.9	7.8–11.0	7.8–11.0	8.9–12.1

V = venous; C = capillary; IGT = impaired glucose tolerance.
Adapted from [47].

An additional category of abnormality was introduced by NDDG and WHO, that of IGT. By definition subjects with IGT have a normal fasting glucose and a 2 hour value intermediate between normal and diabetic (Table 4). This group would have been classified as diabetic with many of the pre-1979 criteria, but are not at risk of the specific complications. They are, however, important as they have a greatly increased risk of subsequent development of NIDDM and are thus a target for primary prevention, whilst they also have an increased risk of developing macrovascular disease and are a component part of the Metabolic Syndrome or Syndrome X [55].

Despite these welcome clarifications of a confused situation major difficulties remain. Thus the OGTT has poor reproducibility even within normal subjects with a CV of between 18 and 40% [56, 57]. There is thus considerable movement of individuals between normal, IGT and NIDDM categories emphasizing the need for more than one abnormal test before assigning a firm diagnosis. In some populations unaccustomed to blood tests thee may also be a stress response, so that we found a halving of the apparent diabetes prevalence on repeat testing in rural Tanzania [58] and a significant downward shift of the glucose curve on retesting subjects in Saudi Arabia [59]. The conduct of the test is also critical. The subject must be fasting, which is hard to prove. If the glucose load is consumed in 1 minute compared with 10 minutes there is a 1 mM lower 2 hour glucose value. There is also need for precision in the timing of the 2 hour samples as this can cause a variation of 1 mM [57]. The conduct of the test is indeed laid down precisely by WHO [47], although it is likely that the instructions are not often strictly adhered to. Thus, although the OGTT is the standard method for diagnosing diabetes it is far from perfect as glucose tolerance is also affected by many drugs, and other disorders so interpretation should be cautious. This is becoming increasingly important as attempts are made to diagnose NIDDM earlier in largely asymptomatic individuals. Symptomatic subjects will (fortunately) rarely require the OGTT.

A final points concerns the method of glucose measurement. It is tempting to use test-strips with meters for diagnostic purposes. In our hands these have proved insufficiently precise or accurate under field conditions. The new Hemocue test [44] does, however, appear to be robust and accurate enough for diagnostic use.

Other tests

It is obvious that it would be high advantageous to have available a single blood test suitable for diagnosis. It is beyond the scope of this Chapter to discuss alternatives in detail. It was hoped that the glycated protein tests, HbA_1 and fructosamine, would fill this role. However, most have found that both are too intensitive, although highly specific. Nonetheless McCance et al [51] found HbA_{1C} to be of equal predictive value to the 2 hour post-load glucose, although this was in a high prevalence population. In our own hands fructosamine [60] and another analyte, 1,5-anhydroglucitol [61], were unsatisfactory, so glucose tolerance testing is likely to remain for NIDDM.

For IDDM HLA typing, antibody testing and perhaps measurement of first phase insulin secretion, C-peptide, proinsulin, and proinsulin intermediates are of use, particularly in defining those at risk and for distinguishing these with IDDM from those with NIDDM. Here also, for clinical diagnosis, blood glucose testing is likely to remain.

Conclusions

Despite its apparent simplicity the measurement of glucose in blood samples continues to offer problems of precision and accuracy. These can be overcome but meticulous care and attention to detail is required. The rapid and "simple" extra-laboratory methods require particular care and rarely approach the precision of standard laboratory methods. The application of glucose measurement to the diagnosis of diabetes is also beset by problems concerning the appropriate diagnostic levels, the best method to use and the appropriate sample and site of sampling. The ideal one sample method for simple diagnosis remains elusive.

References

[1] Service FJ, Molnar GD, Rosevear JW et al. Mean amplitude of glycaemic excursions: a measure of diabetic instability. Diabetes 1970; 19: 644–655.

[2] Southgate HJ, Marks V. Measurement of hypoglycaemia by Reflocheck. Practical Diabetes 1986; 3: 206–207.

[3] Ungestedt U, Arner P. Long-term continuous glucose monitoring with microdialysis in amulatory insulin-dependent diabetic patients. Lancet 1993; ii: 1080–1085.

[4] Petranyi G, Burrin JM, Alberti KGMM. What is wrong with home blood glucose monitoring? Use of memory meters in problem patients in a diabetes outpatient clinic. Diab Nutr Metab 1988; 1: 119–123.

[5] Watts GF, Thaker P, West P et al. Filter paper spot blood glucose. Laboratory and patient methodology. Practical Diabetes 1985; 2: 41–44.

[6] Hobbs FDR, Broughton PMG, Kenkre JE et al. Comparison of the use of four desktop analysers in six urban general practices. Br J Gen Practice 1992; 42: 317–321.

[7] Cooper GF. Methods for determining the amount of glucose in blood. CRC Crit Rev Clin Lab Sci 1973; 4: 101–145.

[8] Burrin JM, Price CP. Measurement of blood glucose. Ann Clin Biochem 1985; 22: 327–342.

[9] Farrance I. Plasma glucose methods, a review. Clin Biochem Revs 1987; 8: 55–68.

[10] Passey RB, Gillum RL, Fuller JB et al. Evaluation and comparison of 10 glucose methods and the reference method recommended in the proposed product class standard (1974). Clin Chem 1977; 23: 131–139.

[11] Trinder P. Determination of glucose in blood using glucose oxidase with and alternative oxygen acceptor. Ann Clin Biochem 1969; 6: 24–27.

[12] Morrison B, Scotland CJ, Fleck A. The determination of plasma glucose in a diabetic clinic. Clin Chim Acta 1972; 39: 301–306.

[13] Chua KS, Tan IK. Plasma glucose measurement with the yellow springs glucose analyser. Clin Chem 1978; 24: 150–154.

[14] McLarty DG, Swai ABM, Kitange HM et al. Prevalence of diabetes and impaired glucose tolerance in rural Tanzania. Lancet 1989; i: 871–875.

[15] Sostman HE. Paracetemol interference with blood glucose analysis (letter). Br Med J 1982; 285: 1581.

[16] Hall PM, Cook JGH. Fluoride and iodoacetate interference with glucose determination with the Yellow Springs glucose analyser. Clin Chem 1982; 28: 387–388.

[17] Lloyd B, Burrin JM, Smythe P et al. Enzymic fluorimetric continuous flow assays for blood glucose, lactate, pyruvate, alanine, glycerol and 3-hydroxybutyrate. Clin Chem 1979; 24: 1724–1729.

[18] Wright WR, Rainwater JC, Toile LD. Glucose assay systems: evaluation of a colourimetric hexokinase procedure. Clin Chem 1971; 17: 1010–1015.

[19] Lutz RA, Fluckiger J. Kinetic determination of glucose with the GEMSAEC (ENI) centrifugal analyser by the glucose dehydrogenase reaction and comparison with two commonly used procedures. Clin Chem 1975; 21: 1372–1377.

[20] Burrin JM, Price CP. Performance of three enzymic methods for filter paper glucose determination. Ann Clin Biochem 1984; 21: 411–416.

[21] Walter B, Fundamentals of dry reagent chemistries: the role of enzymes. In Suelter CH (ed): Bio-analytical Application of Enzymes 36. London: John Wiley 1992; 35–62.

[22] Spivey RS, Davies G, Matthews DR. Patient evaluation of a pen-sized glucose meter. Practical Diabetes 1988; 5: 204–206.
[22a] Lewis BD. Laboratory evaluation of the Glucocard^{TM} blood glucose test meter. Clin Chem 1992; 38: 2093–2095.
[23] Walford S, Home PD, Alberti KGMM. A laboratory trial of two new blood glucose meters featuring autonomic external calibration. Ann Clin Biochem 1984; 21: 116–119.
[24] Brooks KE, Runwal N, Henderson AR. Laboratory assessment of three new monitors of blood glucose: AccuChek II, Glucometer II and Glucoscan 2000. Clin Chem 1986; 32: 2195–2200.
[25] Burrin JM, Newton-Adair I, Fyffe JA. Performance of the Reflocheck system used outside the laboratory by trained non-laboratory personnel. Practical Diabetes 1987; 4: 167–169.
[26] Ting C, Nanji AA. Evaluation of the quality of bedside monitoring of the blood glucose level in a teaching hospital. Can Med Assoc J 1988; 138: 23–26.
[27] NHS Procurement Directorate, DHSS. Blood glucose measurements: reliability of results produced in extra-laboratory areas. Health Notice (Hazard) (87) 13. London: DHSS, 1987.
[28] Campbell LV, Ashwell SM, Borkman M et al. White coat hyperglycaemia: disparity between diabetes clinic and home blood glucose concentrations. Br Med J 1992; 305: 1194–1196.
[29] Consensus Development Panel. Consensus statement on self-monitoring of blood glucose. Diabetes Care 1987; 10: 95–99.
[30] Price CP, Burrin JM, Nattrass M. Extra-laboratory blood glucose measurement: a policy statement. Diabetic Med 1988; 5: 705–709.
[31] Committee on Monitoring Devices: Candaian Association of Pathologists. Guidelines on the use of blood glucose meter and non-meter blood glucose reagent strips in hospitals. Can Med Assoc J 1988; 138: 27–29.
[32] Burrin JM, Williams DDR, Price CP. Performance of a quality assessment scheme for blood glucose meters in general practice. Ann Clin Biochem 1985; 22: 148–151.
[33] Thaker, P, Cradock S, Conan ME et al. A quality assurance programme for blood glucose measuring meters used in clinical areas. Practical Diabetes 1986; 3: 307–309.
[34] Forest JC, Rousseau F, Carrier R. et al. Quality control: scheme for blood glucose measured outside the laboratory. Clin Chem 1987; 33: 1233–1235.
[35] Rayman G, Hospital in-patient monitoring of diabetes. Practical Diabetes 1989; 6: 62–64.
[36] Sylvester ECJ, Price CP, Burrin JM. Investigation of the potential for interference with whole blood glucose strips. Ann Clin Biochem 1994; 31: 94–96.
[37] White-Stevens RH. Interference by ascorbic acid in test systems involving peroxidase. Reversible indicators and the effects of copper, iron and mercury. Clin Chem 1982; 28: 578–588.
[38] Barreau PB, Buttery JE. The effect of haematocrit value on the determination of glucose levels by reagent strip methods. Med J Austr 1987; 147: 286–288.
[39] Wiener K. The effect of haematocrit on reagent strip tests for glucose. Diabetic Med 1991; 8: 172–175.
[40] Clark JDA, Goldberg L, Jones K, Hartog M. Are blood glucose reagent strips reliable in renal failure? Diabetic Med 1991; 8: 168–171.
[41] Hicks JM, Iosefsohn M. Haemoglobin, electrolytes and other major clinical laboratory analyses as measure with a physician's office analyser, the Kodak DT60. Clin Chem 1986; 32: 2201–2203.
[42] Price CP, Koller PU. A multicentre study of the new Reflotron system for the measurement of urea, glucose, triglycerides, cholesterol, glutamyltransferase and haemoglobin. J Clin Chem Clin Biochem 1988; 26: 233–250.
[43] Hicks JM, Iosefsohn M. Another physician's office analyser: the Abbott "Vision" evaluated. Clin Chem 1987; 33: 817–819.
[44] Ashworth L, Gibb I, Alberti KGMM. Hemocue: Evaluation of a portable photometric system for determining glucose in whole blood. Clin Chem 1992; 38: 1479–1482.
[45] Burrin JM, Alberti KGMM. What is blood glucose: can it be measured? Diabetic Med 1990; 7: 199–206.

[46] Akanji AO, Oputa RA. The effect of ambient temperature on glucose tolerance and its implications for the tropics. Trop Geogr Med 1991; 43: 283–287.
[47] WHO Study Group on Diabetes Mellitus. World Heath Organisation Technical Report Series 727, WHO, Geneva, 1985.
[48] WHO Expert Committee on Diabetes Mellitus. World Heath Organisation Technical Report Series 646, WHO, Geneva, 1980.
[49] National Diabetes Data Group. Classification and diagnosis of diabetes mellitus and other categories of glucose intolerance. Diabetes 1979; 28: 1039–1057.
[50] Finch CF, Zimmet PZ, Alberti KGMM. Determining diabetes prevalence: a rational basis for the use of fasting plasma glucose concentrations. Diabetic Med 1990; 7: 603–610.
[51] McCance DR, Hanson RL, Charles M-A et al. Comparison of tests for glycated haemoglobin and fasting and two hour plasma glucose concentrations as diagnostic methods for diabetes. Br Med J 1994; 308: 1323–1328.
[52] Hofmeister F. Über Resorption und Assimilation der Nährstoffe. Über den Hungerdiabetes. Arch Exp Path U Pharm 1889–90; 26: 355.
[53] Home PD. The OGTT: gold that does not shine. Diabetic Med 1988; 5: 313–314.
[54] West KM. The epidemiology of Diabetes. New York: Elseveier 1978; 94.
[55] Reaven GM. Role of insulin resistance in human disease. Diabetes 1988; 37: 1595–1607.
[56] McDonald GW, Fisher GF, Burnham C. Reproducibility of the oral glucose toleranc test. Diabetes 1965; 14: 473–480.
[57] Harris PE, Kitange HM, Fulcher G et al. The oral glucose tolerance test: Effects of different glucose loads, reproducibility and the timing of blood glucose measurements. Diab Nutr Metab 1991; 4: 293–296.
[58] Swai ABM, McLarty DG, Kitange HM et al. Study in Tanzania of impaired glucose tolerance – methodological myth? Diabetes 1991; 40: 516–520.
[59] Gazzaz ZJA, Home PD, Alberti KGMM. The reliability of the oral glucose tolerance test in subjects with varying degrees of glucose intolerance in Saudi Arabia. International Diabetes Digest 1992; 3: 71–75.
[60] Swai ABM, Harrison K, Chuwa LM et al. Screening for diabetes: does measurement of fructosamine help? Diabetic Med 1988; 5: 648–652.
[61] Robertson DA, Alberti KGMM, Dowse GK et al. Is serum anhydroglucitol an alternative to the oral glucose tolerance test for diabetes screening? Diabetic Med 1993; 10: 56–60.

Immunhistochemical methods in the study of islet amyloid polypeptide

T. D. O'Brien, M. J. Hukee, P. C. Butler

Background

The two most characteristic morphologic lesions in the pancreas of patients with non-insulin-dependent diabetes mellitus are the progressive loss of up to 50% of β-cells and the concomitant deposition of an approximately equal volume of extracellular amyloid (islet amyloid) [1]. Isolation, purification, and amino acid sequence analysis of amyloid deposits from the pancreatic islets of humans and cats with NIDDM and amyloid from insulinomas revealed the primary constituent to be a previously unknown polypeptide, islet amyloid polypeptide (IAPP) [2, 3]. The mature form of human IAPP (which forms the characteristic amyloid deposits) is comprised of 37 amino acid prepropeptide [4, 5]. The secreted form of human IAPP is cleaved at pairs of basic amino acids from an 89 amino acid prepropeptide [4, 5]. IAPP is a unique polypeptide but it shares approximately 45% amino acid sequence identity with the neuropeptide calcitonin gene-related peptide (CGRP) [2]. Most of the amino acid identity occurs in the amino- and carboxy-terminal regions of the molecules. Subsequent to the initial discovery of IAPP, morphologic studies were essential in demonstrating that IAPP is a normal product of the pancreatic β-cells [2, 6, 7]. Furthermore, immuno-electron microscopic studies showed that IAPP is co-localized with insulin in the β-cell secretory vesicles [6, 7]. These findings suggested, and later physiologic studies confirmed, that IAPP is co-secreted with insulin, in response to a variety of known insulin secretogogues [8, 9, 10]. Future immunohistochemical studies may identify the initial sites of IAPP-derived amyloid formation and elucidate the precise secretory pathway(s) of this peptide in normal β-cells and pinpoint sites of defective handling of IAPP leading to islet amyloid formation in NIDDM.

Light microscopic methods (Fig. 1)

IAPP is fixed tissue sections

As with many other polypeptides and proteins, optimal demonstration of IAPP immunoreactivity in pancreatic tissue sections is dependent upon minimizing autolysis. This consideration is especially important for IAPP and other pancreatic islet hormones since they reside among the exocrine pancreatic acini which are filled with various degradative enzymes. The rate of autolysis depends upon several variables including pre-existing pancreatic disease (e. g., pancreatitis), rate of post mortem cooling of the body, body temperature prior to death, and interval between death and autopsy. In our experience, IAPP immunoreactivity in β-cells diminishes with increasing severity of autolysis, which may lead to complete abolishment of IAPP immunoreactivity. In contrast, islet amyloid deposits are relatively resistant to effects of autolysis and will retain antigenicity even in the face of severe autoly-

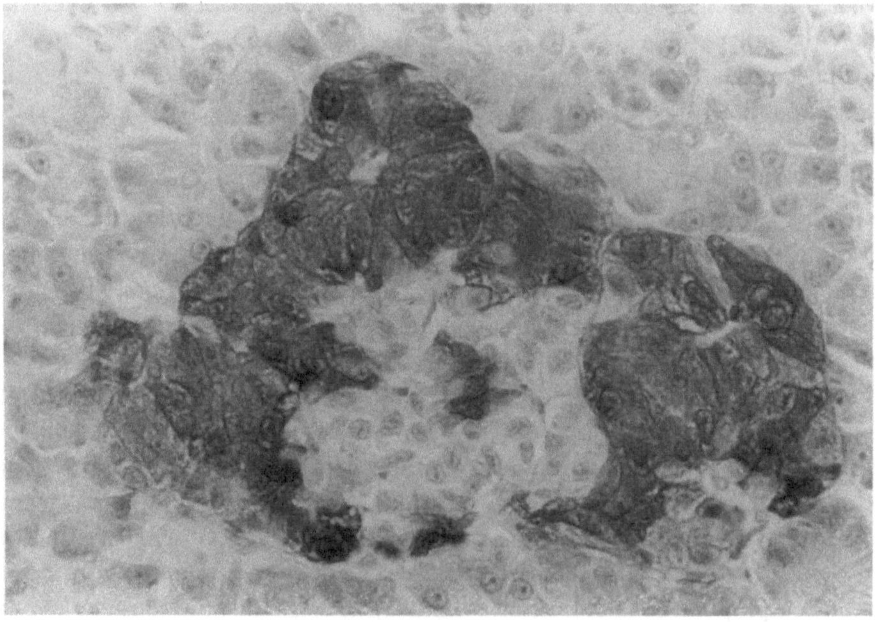

Fig. 1 Photomicrograph of a normal feline pancreatic islet immunohistochemically stained for islet amyloid polypeptide using the peroxidase-antiperoxidase method. The dark staining reaction product (diaminobenzidine) demonstrates β-cells at the periphery of the cat islet; centrally located α-cells are not stained

sis. This is likely due to the high insolubility of islet amyloid fibrils and their high resistance to enzymatic degradation.

Optimal preservation of IAPP immunoreactivity in tissue secretions is also dependent upon proper fixation. Sections of pancreas fixed by immersion should be no more than 3 mm thick to ensure adequate penetration of fixative. In experimental animals, optimal preservation of pancreatic morphology can be assured by collection of pancreas under general anesthesia or immediately after euthanasia with immediate immersion of tissue slices in appropriate fixative. Perfusion fixation of the pancreas may also be considered for optimal tissue preservation for both light and electron microscopy. We have experimented with several fixatives including 10% neutral buffered formalin (NBF), B-5, and Bouin's solution, and also varied the duration of fixation. None of the fixatives were found to have any significant advantages over controlled NBF fixation with respect to antigen preservation. Duration of fixation was also found to be of critical importance in preservation of IAPP immunoreactivity within islet β-cells. IAPP immunocreativity was found to decrease in sections fixed for more than 6 hours in NBF [6]. Optimal fixation, in which antigenicity of IAPP and tissue structure were both adequately preserved, was found to be between 4 and 6 hours. As with autolysis, islet amyloid deposits are more resistant to effects of prolonged fixation and may retain some IAPP immunoreactivity even following weeks of fixation in NBF [6]. After fixation in NBF we hold tissues in 70% ethanol until processed for paraffin embedding. Ethanol may also be used as a primary fixative, however, morphologic detail is more severely altered than with any of the other fixatives mentioned.

The most commonly employed immunostaining methods used on tissue sections are the peroxidase-antiperoxidase (PAP) and avidin-biotin (AB) methods. These methods provide high sensitivity and generate permanent or long-lasting preparations. In either case, the specificity of the staining reaction is dependent upon the primary antibody which is directed against the antigen of interest. The primary antibody may be either polyclonal or monoclonal. Polyclonal antisera may be developed against synthetic peptides corresponding to selected portions of the peptide of interest or may be developed against the entire polypeptide. We have had success with both types of polyclonal antisera for IAPP immunohistochemistry. Advantages of polyclonal antisera over monoclonal antibodies include greater ease of generating antisera (and therefore lower cost), and by virtue of being directed against multiple epitopes, polyclonals generally give more intense labeling at greater antibody dilutions than monoclonals. The disadvantage of polyclonal antisera is the potential for cross-reactivity with other antigens. For example, islet amyloid may cross-react with polyclonal antisera directed against calcitonin gene related peptide (CGRP), probably due to extensive amino acid identity between IAPP and CGRP. The principal advantage of monoclonal antisera is in their high specificity for a particular epitope. Thus, the potential for cross-reactivity with other antigens is greatly reduced. The main disadvantage of monoclonal antibodies is related to the much greater amount of time and effort needed to develop hybrid plasmacyte clones and screen the antibodies generated by clones for specificity. Because monoclonal antibodies are directed against only one epitope, they often show less avidity for the antigen than do polyclonal antisera which necessitates their use at high concentration.

Once a suitable primary antibody is obtained, an optimal working dilution of the antibody should be determined. An optimal dilution of the antibody is the maximal dilution at which an easily detectable color reaction is developed (within a reasonable amount of time, usually less than 15 minutes) and at which there is minimal background or non-specific color development. When using the PAP technique, optimization can be complex due the use of 3 layers of antibody. However, generally the concentrations of the secondary and PAP layers will remain standard once they have been determined to be optimal in a given laboratory, such that only the dilution optimal for the primary antibody need be determined.

In the PAP technique, visualization of the binding sites of the primary antibody is accomplished by application of a secondary antibody directed against the immunoglobulin of the primary antibody. For example, if the primary polyclonal antiserum is generated by inoculating rabbits with IAPP, then the secondary antiserum will be an antibody directed against rabbit IgG. This secondary antibody is developed in a second species such as a goat, sheep, donkey, or pig. Under some conditions, especially if the antigen of interest is abundant (e. g., insulin), the secondary antibody may be directly bound to an enzyme such as horseradish peroxidase (HRP) (or another enzyme such as alkaline phosphatase) which catalyzes a color generating reaction. HRP in the presence of hydrogen peroxide catalyses the oxidation of diaminobenzidine, AEC, or other chromogens which generates the colored precipitate characteristic of each chromogen. However, in the case of antigens such as IAPP which are less abundant, it is often useful to use the PAP technique to amplify the staining reaction [11]. This is accomplished by the addition of a third layer which is comprised of HRP and an antibody directed against HRP (made in the same species as is the primary antibody). The secondary antibody then binds the anti-peroxidase antibody to form the three-layer complex. This complex is generated such that there is a 3 : 2 ratio between the HRP and HRP antibody [11]. Thus, each binding site of the primary antibody is represented by 3 HRP molecules rather than 1, as when the secondary antibody is directly labeled. We have successfully used this technique on pancreas from many species as well as human, dog, and cat pancreatic endocrine tumors.

The AB procedure, in the form most often used, relies upon a secondary antibody which has been conjugated to biotin. The third step in this procedure makes use of the strong binding that occurs spontaneously between biotin and avidin. Avidin used in this procedure is conjugated to HRP which is then used to catalyze the color reaction as in the PAP procedure. Since avidin may be bound to up to 5 molecules of HRP, this method, like the PAP method, amplifies the primary antibody binding signal by up to 5-fold.

IAPP immunofluorescent labeling

Immunofluorescent (IF) staining methods may be classified as direct, in which the primary antibody is labeled with fluorochrome, or indirect, in which a secondary antibody directed against the primary antibody IgG is labeled. IF methods may be used on paraffin-embedded tissue sections as with the PAP technique but are less often used in this manner due to less sensitivity, background fluorescence problems, and because slide preparations with this method are not permanent. However, advantages of IF methods include simplicity of the staining procedures, a high signal to noise ratio in samples lacking background fluorescence (as in isolated cells and islets), lack of non-specific staining due to endogenous peroxidase (problem encountered in methods using HRP), the ability to simultaneously label 2 (or more) antigens in the same sample for co-localization studies, and their use in laser scanning confocal microscopy.

We have employed indirect IF to study IAPP co-localization with insulin in pancreatic islet cells. We have found that adequate fixation and antigen preservation in freshly isolated rat pancreatic islets is accomplished by immersion in 10% NBF for 30 minutes, although other fixatives such as 4% paraformaldehyde or Zamboni's (4% paraformaldehyde/picric acid) may also suffice.

Controls for each of these immunolabeling techniques typically consist of conducting the labeling method but with the omission of the primary antibody and substituting non-immune serum from the same species in which the primary antibody was generated. This assures that the labeling is indeed directed by the primary antibody and is not a consequence of non-specific binding by the primary, secondary, or PAP/avidin-HRP layers. Furthermore, to control for specificity of the primary antibody, it may be incubated (at the working dilution) with excess of the corresponding antigen in solution. Following appropriate incubation time, the solution is centrifuged and the supernatant removed. The "absorbed" antiserum is then used in the labeling procedure as the primary antiserum. Specific staining should be quenched by the absorption procedure.

Transmission electron microscopic methods (Fig. 2)

Considerations regarding minimization of autolysis and proper tissue fixation are similar to those discussed under Light microscopic methods. However, for electron microscopy, these considerations are even more critical due to the rapidity at which ultrastructural autoanalysis occurs. For optimal preservation of ultrastructural detail, it is essential that samples of pancreas be obtained as a biopsy or, in experimental animals, removed immediately following euthanasia. Appropriate tissue samples should then be immediately minced into cubic pieces no greater than 1 mm on edge in cold (4 °C) fixative using a clean, sharp, razor blade. Care should be taken not to macerate tissue in this process. Alternatively, in experimental animals, excellent morphologic preservation may be obtained by perfusion of the pancreas with cold saline followed immediately by cold fixative via the arterial vasculature. Following perfusion fixation, tissue samples are minced into 1 mm cubes in the same fixative as used in perfusion (e. g., 4% paraformaldehyde).

As with light microscopic techniques, control of the fixation time is necessary for preservation of IAPP antigenicity for EM immunolabeling techniques. We have used both Karnovsky's (0.5% glutaraldehyde/2.5% paraformaldehyde) and Trump's (1% glutaraldehyde/4% formaldehyde) fixatives with excellent results. With both Karnovsky's and Trump's solutions, immersion fixation time is optimal between 1.5 and 3 hours at 4 °C. Following aldehyde fixation, some of our specimens have been postfixed in osmium tetroxide and uranyl acetate. While postfixation does not seem to decrease the antigenicity of IAPP, it is necessary to pretreat the sections from osmium-fixed tissue with saturated sodium metaperiodate for successful labeling of IAPP [12].

To dehydrate tissues, we have used a graded series of either ethanol or acetone, and both have shown adequate preservation of ultrastructural detail and IAPP antigenicity. We have successfully used a variety of embedding resins including Epon-Araldite, Spurr, Lowicryl K4M, LR Gold and Quetol 651 to immunolabel IAPP. While a discussion of the advantages of each embedding media is beyond the scope of this paper, little has been published

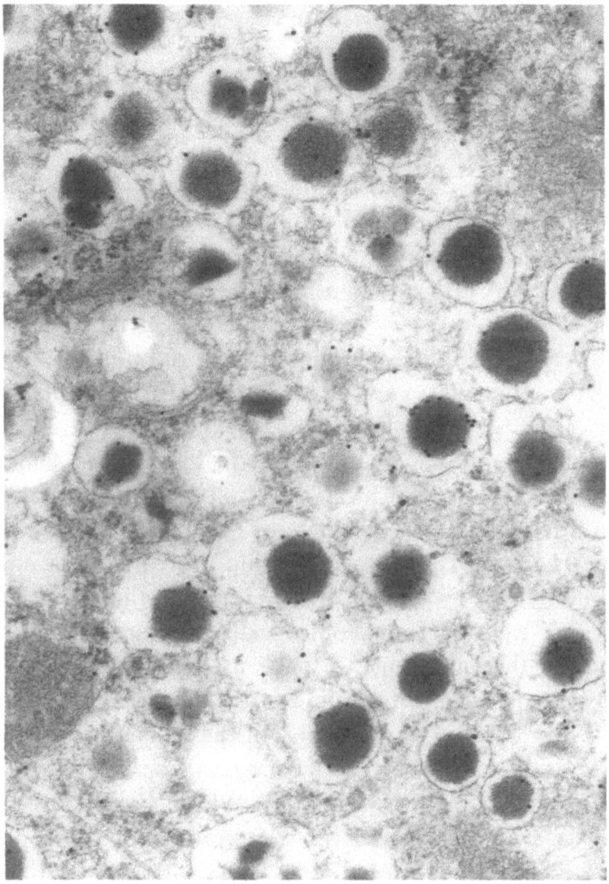

Fig. 2 Transmission electron micrograph of a normal human β-cell showing immunogold labelling (15 nm gold particles) for islet amyloid polypeptide. Note that immunogold labelling is almost completely confined to the β-cell secretory vesicles and principally resides on the dense core of the secretory vesicles. Bar = 200 nm

concerning the attributes of Quetol 651. In our hands, this resin is very tolerant of water (up to 1%), is compatible with acetone dehydration, sections easily, polymerizes at 40 °C and preserves the antigenicity of IAPP.

EM labeling is generally done by mounting thin sections of the tissue on nickel or gold grids and floating grids on bubbles of labeling reagents. This method is technically intensive, and contamination is often visible near the grid bars. We coat a microscope slide with a collodion film and attach sections to the film. When labeling and staining processes are completed, the film and the sections are removed and mounted on a copper grid. This process has proved to be cleaner, faster, and more efficient than the labeling of individual grids.

The blocking of non-specific sites appears to be adequate with bovine serum albumin and Tween 20 incorporated into phosphate buffered saline or tris buffered saline at pH 7.4. When control sections are labeled without primary antibody, the absence of gold label indicates that the blocking buffers prevent the non-specific binding of gold conjugate to the tissue.

EM immunolabeling also requires an empirical determination of optimal antibody dilution. If an LM procedure has been developed, the optimal antibody dilution for LM is a good starting point for the EM labeling. If LM is not possible or available, information about antibody dilution and the effects of various fixatives on antigenicity can sometimes be extrapolated from Western blots.

We have employed two gold conjugates with equal success to demonstrate IAPP labeling at the ultrastructural level. The first, a colloidal gold conjugated to protein A is commercially available or can be easily conjugated in the laboratory [13]. The major advantage of using protein A-gold conjugate is the reactivity of many IgGs with protein A. However, this universal binding to the Fc region of many IgGs becomes a disadvantages when double-labeling is required. In this situation, we have used a gold conjugate of a secondary antibody directed against the IgG of the species in which the primary antiserum was generated. The specificity of the secondary antibody for a particular species of IgG assures that labeling will be specific when the primary antisera are made in different species. When the primary antisera are from similar species where crossreactivity cannot be eliminated, double-labeling of insulin and IAPP has been done by exposing each of side of the section to different antibodies and gold conjugate combinations. This method has been described in detail by Bendayan [14].

Gold conjugates are available in a wide range of particle sizes (1 to 50 nm in diameter). The smaller gold particles give a higher labeling efficiency and more accurate localization of the antigen, but often need to be silver-enhanced to be seen at low magnifications. We find that 15 nm gold adequately demonstrates the localization of IAPP and is easily found at low magnifications. When double-labeling, the sizes of gold particles used to localize each antigen must be different enough to assure differentiation of the labeling sites. A difference of 10 to 15 nm is generally sufficient.

In summary, IAPP is a recently identified polypeptide which is co-secreted with insulin from the pancreatic β-cells. Our knowledge concerning the normal biology and pathology of this polypeptide has been greatly advanced by the application of immunohistochemical methods to human and animal pancreas. The immunohistochemical demonstration of IAPP in tissue sections at either the light or electron microscopic level is critically dependent upon prevention of tissue autolysis, proper tissue fixation, and appropriate staining methodology. Further application of these techniques will undoubtedly help to advance our understanding of the normal processing and secretion of prepro-IAPP as well as to help to identify potential defects in this system which lead to the development of islet amyloidosis in NIDDM.

Acknowledgements

Supported by PHS DK 44341

References

[1] Johnson KH, O'Brien TD, Westermark P. Medical Intelligence. Islet amyloid, islet amyloid polypeptide and diabetes mellitus. N. Engl J Med 1989; 321: 513–518.
[2] Westermark P, Wernstedt C, Heldin C-H et al. Amyloid fibrils in human insulinoma and islets of Langerhans of the diabetic cat are derived from a novel neuropeptide-like protein also present in normal iselt cells. Proc Natl Acad Sci USA 1987; 84: 3881–3885.
[3] Westermark P, Wernstedt C, O'Brien TD et al. Islet amyloid in type 2 human diabetes mellitus and adult diabetic cats is composed of a novel putative polypeptide hormone. Am J. Pathol 1987; 127: 414–417.
[4] Betsholz C, Svensson V, Rorsmann F et al. Islet amyloid polypeptide (IAPP): cDNA cloning and identification of an amyloidogenic region associated with the species-specific occurrence of age-related diabetes mellitus. Exp Cell Res 1989; 183: 484–493.
[5] Sanke T, Bell GI, Sample C et al. An islet amyloid peptide is derived from an 89-amino acid precursor by proteolytic processing. J Biol Chem 1988; 263: 17243–17246.
[6] Johnson KH, O'Brien TD, Hayden DW et al. Immunolocalization of islet amyloid polypeptide (IAPP) in pancreatic beta cells by means of peroxidase-antiperoxidase (PAP) and protein A-gold techniques. Am J Pathol 1988; 130: 1–8.
[7] Lukinius A, Wilander E, Westermark GT et al. Co-localization of islet amyloid polypeptide and insulin in the B cell sectory granules of the human pancreatic islets. Diabetologia 1989; 32: 240–244.
[8] Butler PC, Chou J, Carter WB et al. Effects of meal ingestion on plasma amylin concentration in NIDDM and nondiabetic humans. Diabetes 1990; 39: 752–756.
[9] Inoue K, Hisatomi A, Umeda F et al. Release of amylin from perfused rat pancreas in response to glucose, arginine, ß-hydroxybutyrate, and gliclazide. Diabetes 1991; 40: 1005–1009.
[10] O'Brien TD, Westermark P, Johnson KH. Islet amyloid polypeptide (IAPP) and insulin secretion from isolated perfused pancreas of fed, fasted, glucose-treated and dexamethasone-treated rats. Diabetes 1991; 40: 1701–1706.
[11] Sternberger LA, Hardy PH, Cuculis JJ et al. The unlabeled antibody enzyme method of immunohistochemistry. J Histochem Cytochem 1970; 18: 315–333.
[12] Bendayan M, Zollinger M. Ultrastructural localization of antigenic sites on osmium-fixed tissues applying the protein A technique. J Histochem Cytochem 1981; 31: 101–109.
[13] Ghitescu L, Benadayan M. Immunolabeling efficiency of protein A-gold complexes. J. Histochem Cytochem 1990; 38: 1523–1530.
[14] Bendayan M. Double immunocytochemical labeling applying the protein A-gold technique. J Histochem Cytochem 1982; 30: 81–85.

Determination of insulin sensitivity by the glucose clamp technique

O. Schmitz

Introduction

More than fifty years have elapsed since Himsworth [1] classified diabetes mellitus in insulin-sensitive and insulin-insensitive types based upon an approach consisting of an oral glucose tolerance test and an intravenous insulin injection. Since then, several methods have been employed to measure insulin sensitivity, such as the intravenous glucose tolerance test, the insulin tolerance test, the forearm perfusion technique, the insulin suppression test or the quadruple infusion technique as proposed by Reaven et al. [2], the insulin suppression test in combination with somatostatin, the CIGMA model, the minimal model invented by Bergman et al. [3] and the glucose clamp technique [4–6].

During the last decade, the number of reports dealing with insulin sensitivity has grown exponentially, especially after the proposal of the concept of the metabolic syndrome [7, 8]. The two techniques almost universally employed for assessment of insulin sensitivity are the minimal model and the glucose clamp technique. The minimal model, especially the simplified "12 sample protocol" [9] may seem advantageous for the measurement of insulin sensitivity in large populations, while the clamp is a powerful probe and the "gold standard" in physiologic and pathophysiologic studies of metabolism. Several reviews have meticulously described the different methods available for evaluation of insulin sensitivity in vivo (e.g., [10, 11]). This chapter will only deal with the glucose clamp technique. In addition, it will outline some mainly environmental factors which are able to influence insulin sensitivity, but which are nevertheless often ignored when studying insulin action.

The glucose clamp technique

The glucose clamp technique was originally introduced by Andres et al. in 1966 [4] and developed to its present form by Sherwin et al. [5] and DeFronzo et al. in 1979 [6]. DeFronzo also popularized the method through many investigations in healthy subjects and patients with diabetes mellitus [12]. The classic paper on the glucose clamp technique describes both hyperinsulinemic euglycemic clamping and hyperglycemic clamping [6]. The first allows one to reliably assess whole-body insulin sensitivity under "steady-state" conditions at a predetermined glucose and insulin concentration without potential hazards of hypoglycemic reactions and a confounding release of counter-regulatory hormones, while the hyperglycemic clamp primarily allows one to determine the β-cell response to glucose. Together with infusion of somatostatin the latter methodology is able to assess non-insulin-mediated glucose uptake (NIMGU). One major advantage of the clamp technique is the possibility of combining it with several other methodologies such as the tracer dilution technique (e. g., labelled glucose to quantitate hepatic glucose production, labelled fatty acids to evaluate lipid homeostasis or labelled amino acids), indirect calorimetry, the forearm (or leg) technique, needle biopsies of skeletal muscle or fat tissue, nuclear magnetic resonance spectroscopy and positron emitting tomography scanning.

The hyperinsulinemic clamp technique (Fig. 1 and 2)

Circulating insulin concentration is acutely raised to a pre-determined level by a constant intravenous infusion of insulin, while *plasma glucose* is clamped at a pre-planned level (most often euglycemia) by an intravenous *infusion of glucose*. The amount of glucose necessary to infuse during "steady-state" is the result of insulin-stimulated glucose uptake in peripheral tissues (mainly skeletal muscle, [13]) and insulin-mediated suppression of endogenous (hepatic) glucose production. Glucose uptake in splanchnic tissue is only slightly modified by insulin [14].

Insulin infusion: After basal blood sampling, insulin is administered intravenously. The infusion rate of insulin depends on the desired insulin concentration, e. g. in the low, medium, high, supraphysiological or pharmacological range which normally is achieved by infusion rates of approximately 0.3, 0.6, 1.0 ($\approx$ 40 mU/m^2), 2.0 or 5.0 to 10 mU/kg/min. One should keep in mind that there are large interindividual variations in insulin clearance. In our laboratory, insulin infusates are prepared in 50 ml of isotonic saline to which 2 ml of the subjects blood is added. The infusion rate is kept constant at between 5 to 7 ml/h. A 10- to 15-minute priming dose given in an exponentially declining manner is used by many groups [6], but stable insulin levels

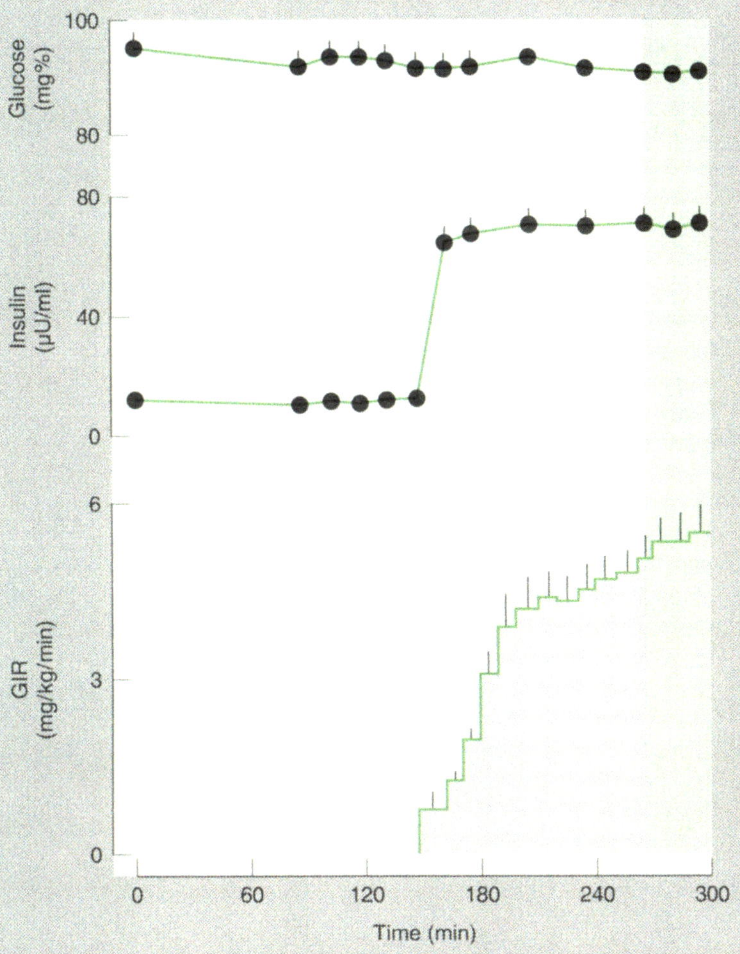

Fig. 1 Plasma glucose, serum insulin and glucose infusion rates (GIR) (mean ± SE) in a 150 min hyperinsulinemic (insulin infusion rate: 0.8 mU/kg/min) euglycemic clamp in 8 healthy subjects (The clamp was preceded by a 150 min period for tracer equilibration)

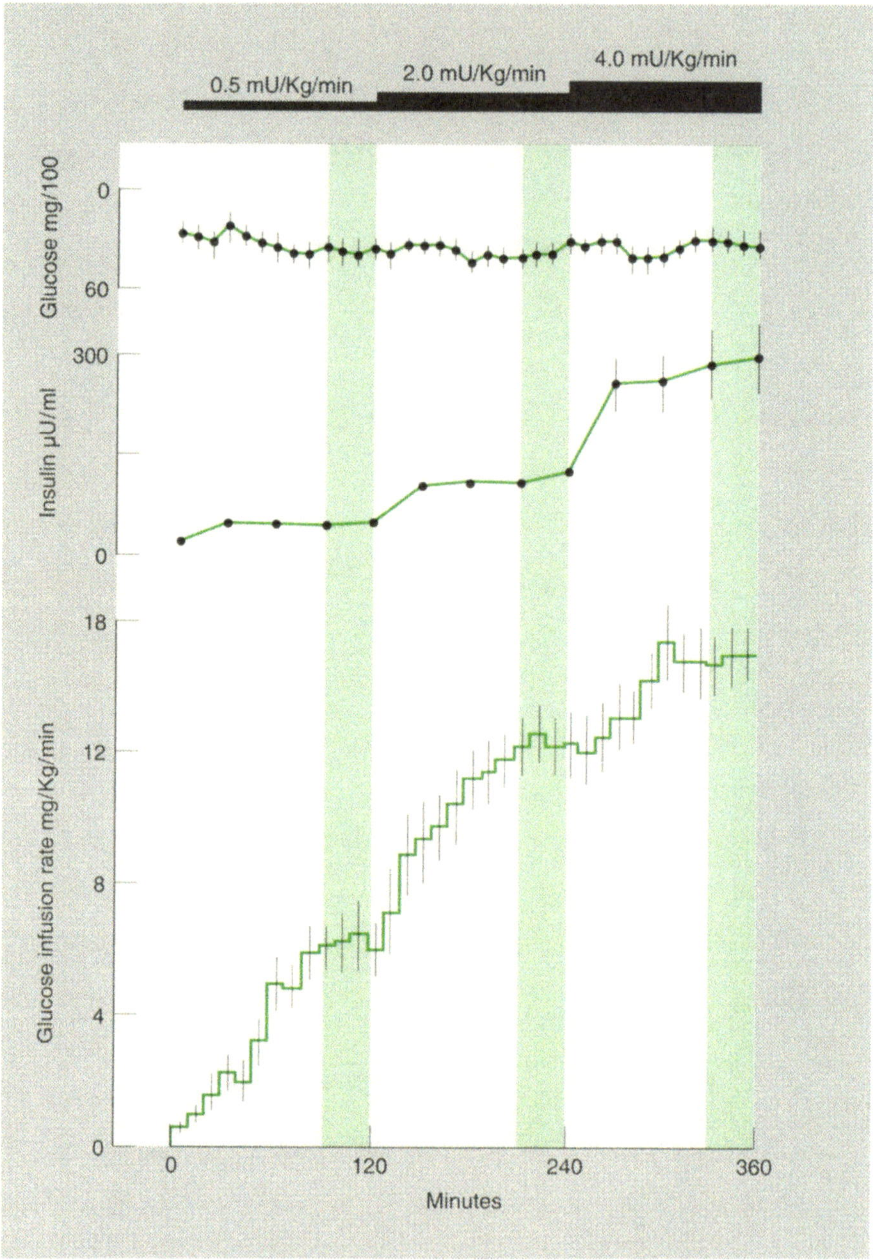

Fig. 2 Blood glucose, serum insulin and glucose infusion rates (mean ± SE) during a sequential 3-step euglycemic clamp in 10 healthy subjects. Insulin infusion rates were 0.5, 2.0 and 4.0 mU/kg/min. The last 30 min of each step (hatched columns) were considered as steady-state

are hardly obtained earlier with this approach, as compared to a constant insulin infusion throughout the study [15].

To enhance insight into insulin action, several investigators examine glucose metabolism at more than one level of insulin and some define relevant Michaelis-Menten parameters in vivo (V_{max} and K_m; designated insulin responsiveness and insulin sensitivity) and attempt to relate changes in vivo and in vitro. Determination of glucose metabolism at multiple insulin concentrations may be done either through clamps performed on separate days [16] or through a single sequential euglycemic clamp over several hours [17].

In healthy individuals, the maximal effect of insulin on whole-body glucose metabolism occurs at insulin concentrations of between 200 and 700 mU/l while the half-maximal effect of insulin is found to occur already at insulin concentrations of around 55 mU/l. Similarly, the insulin concentration necessary for half-maximal suppression of endogenous glucose production is around 30 mU/l and complete suppression is obtained at approximately 50 mU/l [17]. However, data on endogenous glucose production should be interpreted cautiously, because portal insulin concentrations are unknown and due to limitations in tracer methodology. The liver is probably not as sensitive to insulin as previously assumed.

Plasma glucose: In many conditions it is desirable to compare insulin action in individuals with variable glycemia, e. g. healthy versus diabetic subjects. Such comparisons demand that one take into consideration the effect of plasma glucose itself on glucose uptake, a phenomenon described by Soskin and Levine more than 50 years ago [18]. It was previously widely attempted to circumvent this hindrance by expressing insulin sensitivity as the metabolic clearance rate of glucose (MCRG), i. e. the rate of glucose uptake divided by the glucose concentration. The validity of MCRG as an index of insulin sensitivity was, however, based on the assumption that glucose uptake is proportional to plasma glucose concentration. There is now evidence that this is not correct; MCRG depends significantly on the glucose concentration as reviewed by Gottesman et al. [19]. MCRG declines approximately by 10 to 40% when glucose is raised from euglycemia to physiological hyperglycemia. From a mathematical viewpoint plasma glucose plotted against glucose disposal rate at various insulin concentrations takes the form of a hyperbolic curve. Consequently, although the inhibitory effect of hyperglycemia on MCRG is clearly minimized in the well-insulinized state [20, 21], as it is generally not possible to show differences in glucose clearance at small changes in plasma glucose, MCRG as a measure for tissue sensitivity to insulin should be applied only with prudence. Bergman et al., however, suggested that an insulin sensitivity index determined as MCR/I (I: steady-state serum insulin) may be employed at different levels of glycemia [22]. This index appears independent of both insulin and glucose at insulin concentrations of up to 100 mU/l and plasma glucose in the range between 5.5 and 16 mmol/l.

In nondiabetic subjects it is advisable to perform the clamp at basal glycemia or 0.1 mmol/l below fasting glucose to avoid endogenous insulin release. In diabetic subjects with fasting hyperglycemia, we prefer to bring all subjects to comparable (eu)glycemia, either overnight by means of a Biostator or "manually". It may be even better to simply allow plasma glucose to decline to euglycemia during the hyperinsulinemic clamping. The latter protocol is burdened by the fact that even moderate hyperglycemia in insulin-resistant subjects requires a considerable extension of the clamp procedure. Obviously, the time of insulin exposure must be identical in all subjects examined to ensure matched periods of insulin infusion (vide infra).

It has been proposed that blood glucose lowering might provoke the release of counteracting hormones even when blood glucose is in the euglycemic or hyperglycemic level. Fear of such a spurious and confounding anti-insulin effect was grounded on clinical experience of hypoglycemia-like symptoms occurring in the response to a fall in plasma glucose in absence of biochemical hypoglycemia. Two reports have failed to confirm this hypothesis despite a vigorous decline in plasma glucose [23, 24]. Amiel et al. [24] showed that in both healthy and insulin-dependent diabetic subjects the plasma glucose threshold at which hormonal response began was below 4.2 mmol/l. However, the diabetic subjects studied all had blood glucose around 7 to 8 mmol/l. Whether this finding can be extrapolated to a condition of long-standing and pronounced hyperglycemia remains to be clarified. Therefore, rates of glucose decline in the "pre-clamp period" should be kept at a moderate level, and measurements of counter-regulatory hormones should be carried out.

Finally the hyperinsulinemic clamp may also be performed under stepwise lowering of plasma glucose to hypoglycemia to investigate the counter-regulatory response, recovery from hypoglycemia, metabolism under hypoglycemia etc.

Precise and rapid measurements of blood or plasma glucose during the clamp are crucial. Most groups use glucose analyzers from Beckman or Yellow Springs. The artificial endocrine pancreas (Biostator, Life Science Instruments, Miles Laboratories, Elkhart, IN) has also been applied in a large number of clamp experiments especially in the early 1980s. One claimed drawback of the Biostator is a short-coming in blood glucose determinations owing to variations in the dilution of blood drawn to the glucose analyzer [25]. Similarly, the precision of stix as a tool for analyses of blood glucose during clamping is not adequate.

Blood for determination of glucose should be arterialized (oxygen saturation > 90%) achieved from a hand or a wrist vein heated in a box to approximately 55 °C. A heated hand vein has been shown to be an acceptable surrogate for direct arterial sampling [26]. Arterial sampling is important because blood glucose may differ 1 to 2 mmol/l between arterial and deep venous blood under marked glucose uptake.

Glucose infusion: The amount of glucose necessary to infuse into a deep vein to maintain the desired plasma glucose level is dependent on the prevailing insulinemia and glycemia, duration of the clamp and the subjects tissue sensitivity to insulin. For glucose infusions, our laboratory employs concentrations not higher than 20% to reduce risk of phlebitis. Likewise, we add KCl (20 mmol/l glucose) to avoid hypokalemia during the insulin stimulation. It can be difficult to keep plasma glucose constant during pronounced hyperinsulinemia in insulin-sensitive subjects. DeFronzo et al. [6, 11] designed a rather simple and empirically based algorithm for calculating the rate of glucose infusion which has been employed successfully in numerous studies. Previously, the Biostator was used to a large extent both with and without the special developed glucose clamping algorithm [27].

Many laboratories with experience in clamping and a skilled "clamper", however, prefer to use a manual control to further minimize the coefficient of variation of plasma or blood glucose measurements.

Reproducibility: Shortly after the introduction of the clamp technique, it was suggested by Greenfield et al. [28] that it may be possible to trick glucose disposal rates by a manual overriding of the glucose infusion rates. This objection has, however, not been confirmed. On the contrary, a systematic increase or decrease in the glucose infusion rate, amounting to only 10% from the predicted infusion, results in considerable hyper- or hypoglycemia [6]. The reproducibility of the hyperinsulinemic clamp technique is high. DeFronzo et al. [6] found almost identical amounts of insulin-stimulated glucose uptake during similar insulinemia (8.5 ± 0.8 and 8.4 ± 0.8 mg/kg/min) in a group of healthy subjects undergoing a repeat clamp within a period of 3–4 weeks. Similarly, in 6 healthy subjects receiving a repeat euglycemic clamp (blood glucose: 5 mmol/l, insulin infusion rate: 1.0 mg/kg/min) at an interval of two to four weeks, we found M-values (glucose infusion rates) between 90 and 120 min at 9.4 ± 0.4 and 8.8 ± 0.2 mg/kg/min (mean ± SE) and serum insulin concentrations of 86 ± 12 and 84 ± 14 mU/l. The average difference in M-values was 0.9 mg/kg/min. Generally, the expression of insulin sensitivity as an M-value divided by steady-state serum insulin (I) fails to narrow the measure. It may, however, be used cautiously in the limited range of the insulin dose-response curve, where glucose disposal is linearly related to insulin, to compare M-values achieved at slightly different serum insulin concentrations.

Duration: While circulating insulin achieves steady-state within approximately 30 minutes after commencement of insulin infusion, a stable rate of glucose infusion is probably not attainable due to dynamics in distribution volume, up and down regulation of receptors, glucose transporters, intracellular enzymes, etc. Though the amount of glucose necessary to infuse to maintain euglycemia increases gradually over the initial 5 to 6 hours of insulin (and glucose) infusion [29], the increment of increase is only modest after 120 min of insulin exposure. In the pioneering days of the clamping "steady-state glucose infusion rate" was commonly defined as time, 40 to 120 min, 80 to 120 min or 90 to 120 min. Now, the clamp is often prolonged and "steady-state" values based upon the periods 120 to 150 min or even to 180 min. The problem may not be that important when comparing subjects with normal body composition, but Prager et al. [30] have demonstrated that activation by insulin is significantly slower in obese subjects than in lean subjects. Therefore, it is crucial that the clamp periods are identical in all subjects and long enough to ensure a condition characterized by a rather stable glucose infusion rate. In obese objects, this may be 180 min and in hyperglycemic diabetics who are to be examined at normoglycemia, even 240 min.

The hyperglycemic clamp

In this variation of the glucose clamp technique, plasma glucose is acutely raised to a given plateau and maintained at this level for a period of 120 to 180 minutes by intravenous infusion of glucose. To fill the glucose space rapidly and without overshooting plasma glucose, it is necessary to give a priming dose of glucose over 15 minutes in a logarithmically decreasing manner depending on the prevailing plasma glucose, assayed every 2 minutes. Guidance for glucose priming has been delineated elsewhere [6]. When the desired level of glycemia is achieved, infusion of glucose and measurements of plasma glucose proceed as in the hyperinsulinemic euglycemic clamp. Conducted properly, the hyperglycemic clamp provokes a biphasic insulin release in healthy subjects, namely an early burst characterized by a peak serum insulin within 4 to 8 minutes after start of glucose administration (*first* or *early-phase response*) followed by a decline to a nadir after 10 to 15 minutes. The initial peak is then replaced by a gradual rise in serum insulin (*second* or *late-phase response*) which at best approaches a plateau after 90 to 120 minutes [31]. From a cell kinetic point of view, early-phase insulin release was formerly thought to represent the liberation of an intracellular pool from β-cells, while the late-phase secretion was assumed to be mainly dependent on new synthesis of insulin. But the actual mechanisms underlying the glucose-induced insulin release are still unclear. High reproducibility of both the first- and second-phase response has been found when blood was drawn from an arterialized vein [6, 32]. Similar to the euglycemic clamp, it is not possible to bias insulin responses or rates of glucose infusion. It should be borne in mind that pheripheral serum insulin concentrations reflect the balance between insulin secretion and hepatic and extrahepatic insulin clearance rather than β-cell secretion itself. Approximately 50% of the insulin delivered to the portal vein is extracted during the first pass, but this fraction as well as insulin clearance in peripheral tissues and the kidneys may decline at substantial hyperinsulinemia. Whether hyperglycemia is capable of influencing insulin kinetics is controversial. Nevertheless, provided that insulin clearance is within normal range, frequent measurements of serum insulin are for descriptive purposes adequate to appraise the β-cell function. Plasma C-peptide may be measured to substantiate or extend insulin-derived data.

Tissue sensitivity to endogenously released insulin during late-phase response may be expressed as a glucose disposal (M)/I ratio. Because both glucose infusion rate and serum insulin are often characterized by non-steady-state conditions as the M-value is influenced by mass action of glucose, M/I calculated on basis of hyperglycemic clamp derived data is a less reliable indicator of tissue sensitivity to insulin than the M-value obtained from the euglycemic clamp. Thus it is important to note that the hyperglycemic clamp is feasible primarily in the assessment of insulin secretion, while the primary method for determination of insulin sensitivity is the euglycemic clamp technique.

Hyperglycemic clamp with concomitant somatostatin infusion: In addition to circulating insulin concentrations, glucose uptake in tissues is considerably influenced by changes in glucose concentrations. In the basal state this mass action is predominant, accounting for approximately 75% of the post-absorptive glucose uptake in healthy male subjects [33, 34]. The best way to measure mass action of glucose in vivo has, however, not been agreed upon. One approach has been introduced by Olefsky's group, namely the method of 'zero-insulin' [34], where somatostatin is given during a hyperglycemic clamp in a dose sufficient to suppress endogenous insulin secretion completely. This protocol is, however, impeded by two major limitations. First, glucose uptake systems, even those responsible for 'non-insulin' mediated glucose uptake (NIMGU) may be dependent on the presence of minimal amounts of insulin. Consequently, complete insulin deprivation may induce unpredictable down regulation of intracellular enzymatic processes critically dependent on insulin and possible disruption of the integrity of the glucose transport system may occur. Second, insulin depletion implies a change in the fluxes of substrates (FFA, ketone bodies, amino acids) and ions which may affect glucose uptake, thus rendering assessment of true NIMGU difficult. The Mayo group [35] introduced a similar protocol, but used a small replacement dose of insulin to avoid the potential drawbacks described above. Because insulin modulates the mass action of glucose considerably, glucose uptake measured through this experimental design is not solely ascribable to NIMGU, but does in part also involve insulin-stimulated glucose uptake. Therefore, applying this design, glucose uptake may more cautiously be termed glucose-induced glucose uptake (GIGU).

In the two designs, somatostatin infusion is mandatory to restrain endogenous insulin secretion. Apart from suppression of growth hormone, glucagon, several gastrointestinal hormones and peptides, somatostatin may further induce drawbacks by diminishing splanchnic blood flow and even by having a direct positive intrinsic effect on glucose clearance. Employing these designs, subjects with NIDDM have been characterized by normal NIMGU [34], but decreased GIGU (DelPrato et al., unpublished data), while GIGU has been found reduced in subjects with IDDM [36], the latter group thus being characterized by both insulin and glucose resistance.

Variations in insulin action in healthy individuals

When comparing insulin sensitivity in two groups or in subjects exposed to different conditions it is important to be cognizant of the many and mainly environmental factors capable of influencing insulin sensitivity in man. They may be responsible for a great deal of the variation in insulin action observed in healthy male subjects (Fig. 3). Body composition, physical activity, stimulants, acute infections, mental and physical stress, and sodium intake all affect insulin sensitivity.

Body composition: Obese subjects are characterized by a pronounced insulin resistance [37]. However, when data are given per kg lean body mass

Fig. 3 Steady-state glucose infusion rates in 18 lean (BMI < 25 kg/m²), healthy subjects, between 20 and 38 years of age. None had a family history of diabetes

instead of per m^2 body surface, the impairment of insulin sensitivity in obese subjects is less prominent. When expressing glucose disposal per kg lean body mass in considerably obese objects, fat distribution (Waist/Hip ratio) seems more important than BMI as a predictor of insulin sensitivity [38]. Yki-Järvinen and Koivisto [39] have nicely demonstrated a positive relationship between per cent muscle mass and insulin-stimulated glucose uptake and an inverse one as regards fat content in non-obese healthy subjects. The progressive increase in insulin resistance associated with aging is probably also closely related to an altered body composition [40]. Consequently, it is crucial to be aware of fat-free mass (e. g., determined by bioimpedance) and other anthropometric measures of subjects in studies dealing with insulin action.

Physical activity: Another fundamental factor affecting insulin sensitivity in humans is physical fitness. The low insulin levels in the fasting state and reduced insulin levels following an oral glucose tolerance test in the face of a normal glucose tolerance in trained athletes have for decades been explained by an enhanced insulin sensitivity [41]. Employing the hyperinsulinemic clamp technique several groups have found a strong correlation between whole-body glucose uptake and maximal aerobic capacity in healthy subjects, with a R-value above 0.6 [42–44]. (Fig. 4). In addition to chronic training, acute exercise affects insulin sensitivity for days. Conversely, detraining or bed rest deteriorate insulin sensitivity significantly [45]. Unless one

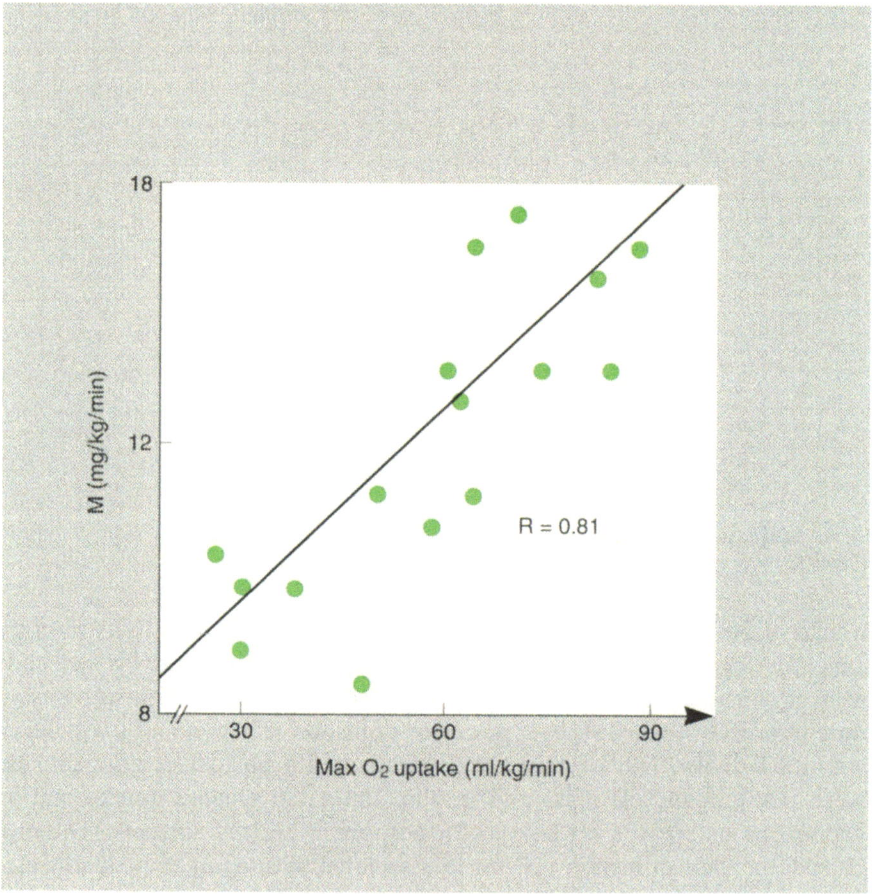

Fig. 4 Correlation between maximal aerobic uptake and insulin-stimulated glucose uptake (M-value) as assessed during a hyperinsulinemic euglycemic clamp in 16 healthy subjects. (Based upon data from Andersen PH et al., Ref. [44])

is examining effects of physical activity on insulin action, it is essential to ensure that the pattern of physical activity has not changed prior to assessment of insulin sensitivity and subjects have avoided heavy exercise for 3 days prior to the tests. Determination of maximal O_2 uptake is normally mandatory, and clearly, it is not advisable to measure maximal O_2 the last few days prior to the clamp procedure.

The significance of physical activity on insulin resistance may be highlighted by the fact that, to the knowledge of this author, only one of the many reports showing insulin resistance in relatives of NIDDM subjects have so far determined maximal aerobic capacity of these relatives and compared it to the capacity of the control group.

Stimulants: It is well known that acute alcohol exposure deteriorates insulin action [46], and it has recently been demonstrated that chronic cigarette smoking is also associated by hyperinsulinemia, dyslipidemia and deranged insulin action [47]: changes which may be ascribable to a perturbed blood flow in skeletal muscle.

Sodium intake: Recently, Donovan et al. [48] demonstrated that short-term variations in sodium intake influence insulin sensitivity inversely. The change in insulin action seemed independent of changes in the counter-regulatory hormones and potassium, but was probably mediated by altered levels of FFA.

Stress: It has been established that mental stress is followed by an increase in the production of epinephrine and norepinephrine, which may deteriorate glucose metabolism [49].

During the last decade, needle biopsies from the vastus lateralis have been performed in a huge number of studies in a search for the cellular mechanism in skeletal muscle responsible for insulin resistance. Biopsies have been taken before, during, and at the end of the clamping. Taylor et al. [50] found that performance of a muscle biopsy was accompanied by a transient rise in FFA, epinephrine and norepinephrine. Whether the procedure is able to influence insulin action has only been sparsely tested. The question is relevant as intracellular findings from a basal biopsy are often related to the insulin sensitivity determined in the subsequent insulin clamp. Recent data from our laboratory suggest that the procedure of drawing a muscle biopsy (250 mg) – employing a Bergström needle – reduces insulin-stimulated non-oxidative glucose disposal at physiological insulinemia [51]. Whether the acute insulin resistance was due to the muscle biopsy per se, or was actually provoked by the local anesthesia needle is not clear.

Other factors: Many other events are able to influence insulin action, including acute infections [52] and puberty [53]. It is uncertain whether insulin sensitivity is affected by the phase of the menstrual cycle in healthy women. However, hormone replacement therapy (progesterone) seems to decrease insulin sensitivity [54]. Finally, various medication may interfere with insulin action; e. g. ACE-inhibitors and prazosin are suggested to improve insulin action while ß-adrenergic blockers probably blunt insulin action slightly.

Epilogue

The hyperinsulinemic euglycemic clamp is a reliable and potent approach to the investigation of glucose, lipid, amino acid and electrolyte metabolism in man. As regards insulin sensitivity, a high reproducibility of the method can be further increased by taking into account the many – and mainly environmental – factors which affect insulin action. Whether an investigator prefers a study design involving the insulin clamp or the minimal model for assessment of insulin sensitivity depends on the specific questions to be addressed and the population size. When compared, the measures of insulin sensitivity achieved by the two methods often show a high coefficient of correlation. However, it should always be kept in mind, that though these methods are currently the best available to assess insulin sensitivity, both are invalidated in many aspects by not representing a physiologic condition.

References

[1] Himsworth HP, Kerr RB. Insulin-sensitive and insulin-insensitive types of diabetes mellitus. Clin Sci 1939–1942; 4: 119–152.

[2] Shen S-W, Reaven GM, Farquhar JW et al. Comparison of impedance to insulin-mediated glucose uptake in normal subjects and in subjects with latent diabetes. J Clin Invest 1970; 49: 2151–2159.

[3] Bergman RN, Phillips LS, Cobelli C. Physiologic evaluation of factors controlling glucose tolerance in man. Measurement of insulin sensitivity and ß-cell glucose sensitivity from the response to intravenous glucose. J Clin Invest 1981; 68: 1456–1467.

[4] Andres R, Swerdloff R, Pozefsky T et al.Manual feedback technique for the control of blood glucose concentration. In: Skeggs Jr LT, ed. Automation in Analytical Chemistry. New York: Mediad Inc, 1966; 486–491.

[5] Sherwin RS, Kramer KJ, Tobin JD et al. A model of the kinetics of insulin in man. J Clin Invest 1974; 53: 1481–1492.

[6] DeFronzo RA, Tobin JD, Andreas R. Glucose clamp technique: a method for quantifying insulin secretion and resistance. Am J Physiol 1979; 237: E214–223.

[7] Reaven GM. Role of insulin resistance in human disease. Diabetes 1988; 37: 1595–1607.

[8] DeFronzo RA, Ferrannini E. Insulin resistance. A multifaceted syndrome responsible for NIDDM, obesity, hypertension, dyslipidemia, and atherosclerotic cardiovascular disease. Diabetes Care 1991; 14: 173–194.
[9] Steil GM, Volund AA, Kahn SE et al. Reduced sample number for calculation of insulin sensitivity and glucose effectiveness from the minimal model. Suitability for use in population studies. Diabetes 1993; 42: 250–256.
[10] Bergman RN, Finegood DT, Ader M. Assessment of insulin sensitivity in vivo. Endocrine Rev 1985; 6: 45–86.
[11] Del Prato S, Ferrannini E, DeFronzo RA. Evaluation of insulin sensitivity in man. In: Clarke WL, Larner J, Pohl SL, eds. Methods in Diabetes Research. Volume II: Clinical Methods. John Wiley & Sons, 1986; 35–76.
[12] DeFronzo RA. The triumvirate: ß-cell, muscle, liver. A collusion responsible for NIDDM. Diabetes 1988; 37: 667–687.
[13] DeFronzo RA, Jacot E, Jequier E et al. The effect of insulin on the disposal of intravenous glucose. Results from indirect calorimetry and hepatic and femoral venous catheterization. Diabetes 1981; 30: 1000–1007.
[14] DeFronzo RA, Ferrannini E, Hendler R et al. Influence of hyperinsulinemia, hyperglycemia, and the route of glucose administration on splanchnic glucose exchange. Proc Natl Acad Sci USA 1978; 75– 5173–5177.
[15] Poncher M, Heine RJ, Pernet A et al. A comparison of the artificial pancreas (glucose controlled insulin infusion system) and a manual technique for assessing insulin sensitivity during euglycaemic clamping. Diabetologia 1984; 26: 420–425.
[16] Kolterman OG, Insel J, Saekow M et al. Mechanisms of insulin resistance in human obesity. Evidence for receptor and postreceptor defects. J Clin Invest 1980; 65: 1272–1284.
[17] Rizza RA, Mandarino LJ, Gerich JE. Dose-response characteristics for effects of insulin on production and utlization of glucose in man. Am J Physiol 1981; 240: E630–E639.
[18] Soskin S, Levine R. A relationship between the blood sugar level and the rate of sugar utilization, affecting the theories of diabetes. Am J Physiol 1937; 120: 761–770.
[19] Gottesman I, Mandarino L. Gerich J. Use of glucose uptake and glucose clearance for the evaluation of insulin action in vivo. Diabetes 1984; 33: 184–191.
[20] DeFronzo RA, Ferrannini E. Influence of plasma glucose and insulin concentration on plasma glucose clearance in man. Diabetes 1982; 31: 683–688.
[21] Best JD, Taborsky J, Halter JB et al. Glucose disposal is not proportional to plasma glucose level in man. Diabetes 1981; 30: 847–850.
[22] Bergman RN, Hope ID, Yang YJ et al. Assessment of insulin sensitivity in vivo: A critical review. Diabetes/Metabolim Rev 1989; 5: 411–429.
[23] DeFronzo RA, Andres R, Bledsoe TA et al. A test of the hypothesis that the rate of fall in glucose concentration triggers counterregulatory hormonal responses in man. Diabetes 1977; 26: 445–452.
[24] Amiel SA, Simonson DC, Tamborlane WV et al. Rate of glucose fall does not affect counterregulatory hormone responses to hypoglycemia in normal and diabetic humans. Diabetes 1987; 36: 518–522.
[25] Christiansen JS, Svendsn PAa, Søegaard U et al. An artificial betacell: assessment of the glucose analyser, infusion system and optimization of constants for the algorithms. Scand J Clin Lab Invest 1981; 41: 647–654.
[26] Copeland KC, Kenney FA, Nair KS. Heated dorsal hand vein sampling for metabolic studies: a reappraisal. Am J Physiol 1992; 263: E1010–E1014.
[27] Clemens AH, Hough DN, D'Orazio PA. Development of the Biostator glucose clamping algorithm. Clin Chem 1982; 28: 1899–1903.
[28] Greenfield MS, Doberne L, Kraemer F et al. Assessment of insulin resistance with the insulin suppression test and the euglycemic clamp. Diabetes 1981; 30: 387–392.
[29] Doberne L, Greenfield MS, Schulz B et al. Enhanced glucose utilization during prolonged glucose clamp studies. Diabetes 1981; 30: 829–835.

[30] Prager R, Wallace P, Olefsky JM. In vivo kinetics of insulin action on peripheral glucose disposal and hepatic glucose output in normal and obese subjects. J Clin Invest 1986; 78: 472–481.
[31] Rudenski AS, Hosker JP, Burnett MA et al. The beta cell glucose stimulus-response curve in normal humans assessed by insulin and C-peptide secretion rates. Metabolism 1988; 37: 526–534.
[32] Rayman G, Clark P, Schneider AE et al. The first phase insulin response to intravenous glucose is highly reproducible. Diabetologia 1990; 33: 631–634.
[33] Felber JP, Thiebaud D, Maeder E et al. Effect of somatostatin-induced insulinopenia on glucose oxidation in man. Diabetologia 1983; 25: 325–330.
[34] Baron AD, Kolterman OG, Bell et al. Rates of non-insulin-mediated glucose uptake are elevated in type 2 diabetic subjects. J Clin Invest 1985; 76: 1782–1788.
[35] Hansen IL, Cryer PE, Rizza RA. Comparison of insulin-mediated and glucose-mediated glucose disposal in patients with insulin-independent diabetes mellitus and in nondiabetic subjects. Diabetes 1985; 34: 751–755.
[36] Arnfred J, Schmitz O, Hother-Nielsen O et al. Marked impairment of the effect of hyperglycemia on glucose uptake and glucose production in insulin-dependent diabetes. Diabetic Med 1988; 5: 755–760.
[37] Bonadonna RC, Groop L, Kraemer N et al. Obesity and insulin resistance in humans: A dose-response study. Metabolism 1990; 39: 452–459.
[38] Pedersen SB, Børglum JD, Schmitz O et al. Abdominal obesity is associated with insulin resistance and reduced glycogen synthase activity in skeletal muscle. Metabolism 1993; 42: 998–1005.
[39] Yki-Järvinen H, Koivisto VA. Effects of body composition on insulin sensitivity. Diabetes 1983; 32: 965–969.
[40] Coon PJ, Rogus EM, Drinkwater D et al. Role of body fat distribution in the decline in insulin sensitivity and glucose tolerance with age. J Clin Endocrinal Metab 1992; 75: 1125–1132.
[41] Björntorp P, Fahlén M, Grimby G et al. Carbohydrate und lipid metabolism in middle-aged, physically well-trained men. Metabolism 1972; 21: 1037–1044.
[42] Devlin JT, Horton ES. Effects of prior high-intensity exercise on glucose metabolism in normal and insulin-resistant men. Diabetes 1985; 34: 973–979.
[43] Rosenthal M, Haskell WL, Solomon R et al. Demonstration of a relationship between level of physical training and insulin-stimulated glucose utilization in normal humans. Diabetes 1983; 32: 408–411.
[44] Andersen PH, Lund S, Schmitz O et al. Increased insulin-stimulated glucose uptake in athletes: the importance of GLUT4 mRNA, GLUT4 protein and fibre type composition of skeletal muscle. Acta Physiol Scand 1993; 149: 393–404.
[45] Mikines KJ, Sonne B, Farrell PA et al. Effect of physical exercise on sensitivity and responsiveness to insulin in humans. Am J Physiol 1988; 254: E248–E259.
[46] Yki-Järvinen H, Nikkilä EA. Ethanol decreases glucose utlization in healthy man. J Clin Endocrinol Metab 1985; 61: 941–945.
[47] Facchini FS, Hollenbeck CB, Jeppesen J et al. Insulin resistance and cigarette smoking. Lancet 1992; 339: 1128–1130.
[48] Donovan DS, Solomon CG, Seely EW et al. Effect of sodium intake on insulin sensitivity. Am J Physiol 1993; 264: E730–E734.
[49] Lönnqvist F, Wennlund A, Wahrenberg H et al. Effects of mental stress on lipolysis in humans. Metabolism 1992; 41: 622–630.
[50] Taylor R, Price TB, Rothman DL et al. Validation of 13C NMR measurement of human skeletal muscle glycogen by direct biochemical assay of needle biopsy samples. Magn Reson Med 1992; 27: 13–20.
[51] Holck P, Pørksen N, Nielsen MF et al. Effect of needle biopsy from the vastus lateralis muscle on insulin-stimulated glucose metabolism in humans. Am J Physiol 1994; 267: E544–548.

[52] Yki-Järvinen H, Sammalkorpi K, Koivisto VA et al. Severity, duration, and mechanisms of insulin resistance during acute infections. J Clin Endocrinol Metab 1989; 69: 317–323.
[53] Amiel SA, Sherwin RS, Simonson DC et al. Impaired insulin action in puberti. A contributing factor to poor glycemic control in adolescents with diabetes. N Engl J Med 1986; 315: 215–219.
[54] Elkind-Hirsch KE, Sherman LD, Malinak R. Hormone replacement therapy alters insulin sensitivity in young women with premature ovarian failure. J Clin Endocrinol Metab 1993; 76: 472–475.

Insulin sensitivity from the minimal model

R. N. Bergman

Introduction

The existence of insulin resistance in subjects at risk for non-insulin-dependent diabetes mellitus (NIDDM) was inferred from the apparent basal hyperinsulinemia in obese subjects first observed by Yalow and Berson [53]. Due to controversy regarding the significance of insulin-like activity from the insulin radioimmunoassay, the significance of the hyperinsulinemia remained controversial until the introduction of methods for direct assessment of insulin action in vivo. Qualitative early methods [26] eventually gave way to the glucose clamp, introduced by Andres [5] and widely exploited by DeFronzo [16, 18, 19] and others. To this day, the glucose clamp is a highly regarded approach to direct assessment of in vivo insulin action, and it has been referred to as a "gold standard" for this measurement. However, others have pointed out limitations in the interpretation of glucose clamp-based indicators of insulin action [9, 20].

Given the existence of the glucose clamp, it is of interest to consider why additional methodology for insulin sensitivity assessment might be useful. This need arises from recent observations of associations between insulin resistance and a variety of high risk chronic conditions such as hypertension [39] and atherosclerosis [46]. A major limitation of the glucose clamp methodology is its cost and the substantial labor that must be invested to use it. With few exceptions, only small populations have been studied using this methodology, generally less than 25 subjects per group (e. g., refs. [15, 31, 38]. Additionally, in metabolic studies information concerning insulin secretory function and insulin-independent glucose utilization rates are useful, and these are not easily obtainable from simple clamp protocols, although they may be procured with more complex approaches [35, 40].

Insulin sensitivity in large cohorts

The apparent association of chronic illnesses with insulin resistance has led to the hypothesis that insulin resistance per se may be a causative factor. For example, it has been proposed that insulin resistance leads to a cluster of risk factors, including an unfavorable lipid profile, elevated blood pressure, and diabetes, which ally to yield cardiovascular disease. To assess the importance of insulin resistance in the pathogenesis of these factors, in populations which vary with respect to genetic and environmental risk factors, it is necessary to assess insulin action in large population groups. These cohorts, not infrequently, exceed 1000 in number.

There are few options for assessment of insulin sensitivity in large populations. One possible candidate is fasting insulin level, which has been shown to be associated with insulin resistance in nondiabetic subjects [11]. This is an attractive approach, in that it requires only accurate (and preferably repeated) assessment of fasting plasma insulin levels. Clearly, insulin secretory response will increase in insulin resistant states to maintain normal glucose tolerance [7]. However, the relationship between insulin resistance and b-cell function will be altered in states of subtle or overt b-cell dysfunction, including not only NIDDM andd gestational diabetes, but also in GDM subjects after delivery, when diabetes recedes [14], as well as in pre-Type 1 diabetic individuals [27]. Thus, it will not be appropriate to interpret fasting or stimulated insulin (or C-peptide) levels as insulin resistance in any population in which a subtle or overt b-cell defect may be present. As it is generally not possible to state a priori whether such a defect may be present, the use of fasting insulin may be misleading.

Other approaches have been put forward for assessment of insulin sensitivity in larger groups, including the insulin suppression test [44] and the insulin injection test [36]. While a detailed exposition of these methods is inappropriate here (c. f., refs. [2, 9]), suffice it to say that serious risk concerns may attach to the use in large groups of procedures which allow for a substantial "free fall" of plasma glucose into the hypoglycemic range or which allow termination of a glucose infusion with a substantial quantity of insulin in the interstitial compartment [4].

Conceptual background

When added directly to cells in vitro, insulin acts rapidly to stimulate glucose uptake, achieving steady-state effects within a few minutes. However, when infused into animals or human volunteers, insulin acts surprisingly slowly, failing to achieve steady-state activation of glucose uptake for several hours [45]. The reason for the delay in insulin action in vivo in normal individuals is apparently due to the time necessary for insulin to cross the endothelial barrier separating blood and interstitial fluid. When insulin sensitivity is considered, this dynamic delay in its action cannot be ignored. Because the dynamic delay may differ between normal subjects and individuals with diabetes [42], we attempted to devise a method for assessment of insulin sensitivity which encapsulated the dynamic as well as the steady-state effect of insulin on carbohydrate utilization. Because it was necessary to interpret complex dynamic relationships between insulin and glucose in blood, mathematical modeling was used and implemented on the digital computer.

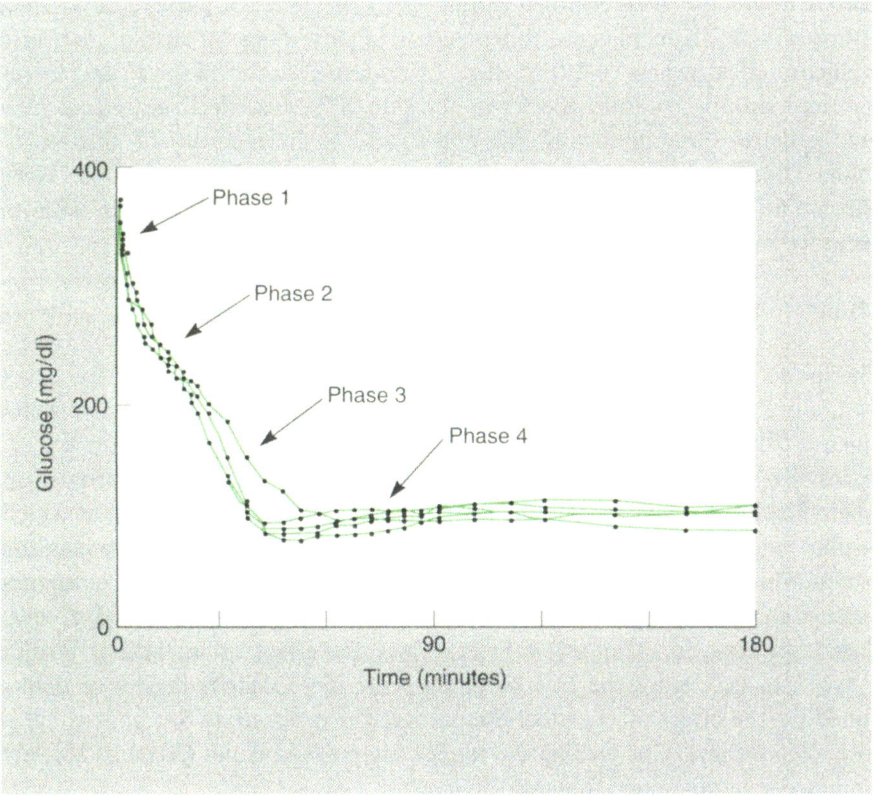

Fig. 1 Phases of glucose decline following glucose injection in dogs. The insulin response (not shown) was delayed several minutes by a somatostatin injection preceding the glucose injection (0.3 g/kg) at time 0. Phase 1 is dominated by the mixing of glucose in the extracellular space. Phase 2 is dominated by glucose effectiveness, i. e., the effect of glucose per se on its own renormalization. Phase 3 is associated with an acceleration of glucose decline caused by dynamic insulin response. Phase 4 is associated with the slow dynamics of insulin action. Maximum insulin effect is associated with minimum glucose concentration at 45 minutes; reestablishment of basal glucose at 180 is caused by the slow decay in insulin action between 45 and 180 minutes. Slow dynamics of insulin action are due to time necessary for insulin to enter the interstitial space from plasma

Theory

Rapid blood sampling after glucose injection in animals revealed that the decline in glucose in lean dogs was not exponential, but followed a complex pattern. This pattern can best be elucidated by experiments in which the insulin secretory response is delayed a few minutes with somatostatin (Fig. 1). The re-establishment of basal glucose following injection includes 4 phases: 1. immediately after injection there is a rapid decline in glucose explained by extracellular mixing, 2. a short period intervenes (8–15 minutes) when the decline in glucose is determined primarily by the effect of glucose on its own disappearance from plasma, independent of any dynamic insulin response ("glucose effectiveness"), 3. the effect of an increment in plasma (and therefore interstitial) insulin to accelerate the rate of glucose decline; glucose may plunge below baseline during this phase, and 4. the recovery of glucose, to achieve basal values by 180 minutes. The question we addressed was "How may we utilize modelling to account for injection glucose dynamics, with an accurate assessment of insulin sensitivity as a byproduct?".

Minimal model

The model itself is 2 differential equations (Fig. 2) which describe the effect of a suprabasal plasma insulin response to accelerate the decline in plasma glucose following injection. One equation (Equation 2) incorporates the kinetics of insulin transfer between the plasma and the interstitial compartment where insulin acts [10, 11, 54]. One coefficient (p_2) describes the rate at which insulin enters the interstitial compartment; the second (p_3) determines the rate at which insulin is removed from the interstitial (i. e., remote) compartment; i. e., the rate of irreversible internalization by insulin-sensitive cells. The other equation (Equation 1) expresses the effect of interstitial insulin ("X(t)") to accelerate the rate of glucose decline. Glucose decline is determined by the effect of elevated glucose itself (expressed as S_G; coined "glucose effectiveness"), as well as the rate of interstitial insulin (X(t)) to accelerate glucose uptake and suppress the liver.

When the model is fitted to intravenous glucose injection data (see below), several metabolic parameters are calculated by the computer (Table 1). Of particular interest are S_I, the insulin sensitivity index, and S_G, glucose effectiveness. Parameter S_I is calculated as $\frac{p_2}{p_3}$. Intuitively, it is possible to understand why this ratio affects in vivo insulin sensitivity. An increase in p_2 will increase insulin sensitivity – this would represent an increased efficiency of

$$\frac{dG}{dt} = -\left\{S_G + X(t)\right\} \cdot G$$

$$\frac{dX}{dt} = p_2 \cdot I(t) - p_3 \cdot X(t)$$

$$S_I = p_2/p_3$$

$$\text{Glucose restoration rate} = -\left\{\text{Glucose effectiveness} + \text{Remote insulin}\right\} \cdot G$$

$$\text{Increase in remote insulin} = p_2 \cdot \text{Plasma insulin} - p_3 \cdot \text{Remote insulin}$$

Fig. 2 The minimal model equations. The first equation describes the effect of glucose per se (S_G) to enhance glucose disappearance; $X(t)$ is the effect of insulin in a remote (i. e., interstitial) compartment to enhance glucose disappearance. The second equation describes the slow dynamics by which insulin ($I(t)$) enters the remote compartment ($X(t)$). Parameter p_2 describes the ability of insulin to cross the endothelial barrier and enter interstitium; p_3 is the fractional disappearance rate of insulin from the interstitial compartment. It is assumed that p_3 is determined by cellular internalization and degradation of the hormone

plasma insulin to cross the endothelial barrier and stimulate glucose uptake. It is also possible to see why increasing p_3, in the denominator of the S_I calculation, would reduce insulin sensitivity – increased p_3 is associated with a faster rate of insulin elimination from the interstitial active compartment. Such elimination (presumably due to cellular insulin internalization and lysosomal degradation) would lower steady-state interstitial insulin, and decrease the overall efficiency of plasma insulin to enhance glucose utilization.

Table 1 Parameters from the minimal model

Metabolic parameter	Definition from model	Meaning	Mean value
S_I	$\frac{p_2}{p_3}$	Insulin sensitivity. Fractional increase in net glucose utilization per unit increase in insulin	5.1×10^4 min^{-1} per μU/ml
S_G	p_1	Glucose effectiveness. Effect of glucose per se to enhance net glucose disappearance at basal insulin	0.021 min^{-1}
GEZI	$S_G - S_I \times I_b$ (I_b = basal insulin)	Glucose effectiveness at zero insulin. Effect of glucose on its own net disappearance, corrected for the effect of basal insulin on glucose disappearance	0.017 min^{-1}
G_0	G_0	Initial glucose. Value of plasma glucose immediately following injection, assuming instantaneous distribution in ECF	279 mg/dl
V_D	$\frac{\text{Glucose dose}}{G_0}$	Glucose distribution volume. One-compartment apparent glucose distribution space	150 dl
$AIR_{glucose}$	$\int_0^{10} \Delta\text{Insulin}\, dt$	Acute insulin response, 0 to 10 minutes	915 μU/ml × min

Parameter S_G, glucose effectiveness, represents the effect of hyperglycemia itself to increase the net rate of glucose utilization. Thus, if glucose is elevated, but concomitant insulin elevation is prevented (c. f., refs. [3, 49]), glucose will renormalize, although at a slow rate. S_G determines the rate of normalization, independent of the dynamic insulin response. While S_G does include a component which is determined by basal insulin, this component is relatively minor (20%) when compared with the overall glucose effectiveness. Glucose effectiveness independent of the basal insulin effect has been termed "GEZI" (glucose effectiveness at zero insulin) by Kahn et al. [28].

Experimental protocol

When originally introduced, it was hoped that the injection of glucose alone would be a sufficient stimulus for accurate calculation of insulin sensitivity from the minimal model in all individuals. However, it soon became clear that alternative protocols were needed. This need resulted from relative imprecision of the original protocol in very insulin resistant or insulinopenic subjects [21]. Various protocols that have been utilized are in Table 2.

Table 2 Protocols used for minimal model testing

Protocol	Description
PI. Original	Glucose injected (0.3 g/kg); 28 samples over 180 minutes
PII. Increased glucose injection	Same as I, but 0.5 g/kg glucose injection
PIII. Tolbutamide-modified protocol	Glucose (0.3 g/kg); tolbutamide (300–500 mg) injected at 20 min; 28 samples over 180 min
PIV. Reduced sample protocol	Same as III, but only 12 samples taken over 180 min. Tailored for epidemiological studies
PV. Insulin-modified protocol	Same as III, but tolbutamide replaced with regular human insulin injection (0.02–0.05 U/kg). Applicable in diabetics
PVI. Insulin Infusion protocol	Same as V, but insulin infused over 5 minutes
PVII. Somatostatin protocol	Somatostatin (16 μg/kg) injected 1 min before 0.3 g/kg glucose injection. Used in dogs

The most commonly utilized protocol (Fig. 3) is the tolbutamide assisted version (Protocol III in Table 2). Subjects are tested in the morning after an overnight fast, and carbohydrate intake of at least 150 g/day is recommended for 3 days prior to the test. Indwelling cannulae are inserted in antecubital or hand veins in both arms (heating of the hand veins is not necessary [8]. Following at least 15 minutes of rest, 1 or 2 basal samples are collected. It is important to have an anti-oxidant such as NaF in the tubes to prevent glycolysis, as the results of the calculation are very dependent upon the glucose concentration. Assay error in our hands for the automated glucose assay is ± 2.0% or less (C. V.). At $t = 0$ glucose (0.3 g/kg) is injected over 60 seconds ($t = 0$ to $t = 1$). Blood samples are then collected at the following times: 2, 3, 4, 5, 6, 8, 10, 12, 14, 16, 19, 22, 24, 25, 27, 30, 40, 50, 60, 70, 90, 100, 120, 140, 160 and 180 min. During sample collection, at $t = 20$ min, tolbutamide (Orinase, Upjohn, Kalamazoo Michigan, USA) is injected (300 mg for BMI < 30 kg/m^2, 500 mg for BMI > 30 kg/m^2). Kahn and his colleagues have recommended doses normalized to surface area [21]: 11.4 g/m^2 glucose and 125 mg/m^2 tolbutamide. Blood samples are collected and immediately cooled to 4 °C until separation of plasma by centrifugation. Keeping blood samples on ice is necessary to retard possible insulin degradation which can result if erythrocytes are even moderately hemolyzed [37]. Plasma samples are assayed for glucose and insulin by autoanalyzer and radioimmunoassay, respectively. As the insulin levels are utilized in the calculation of S_I (unlike with other methods such as the glucose clamp or insulin injection test), it is strongly recommended that insulin assays be compared to an international standard.

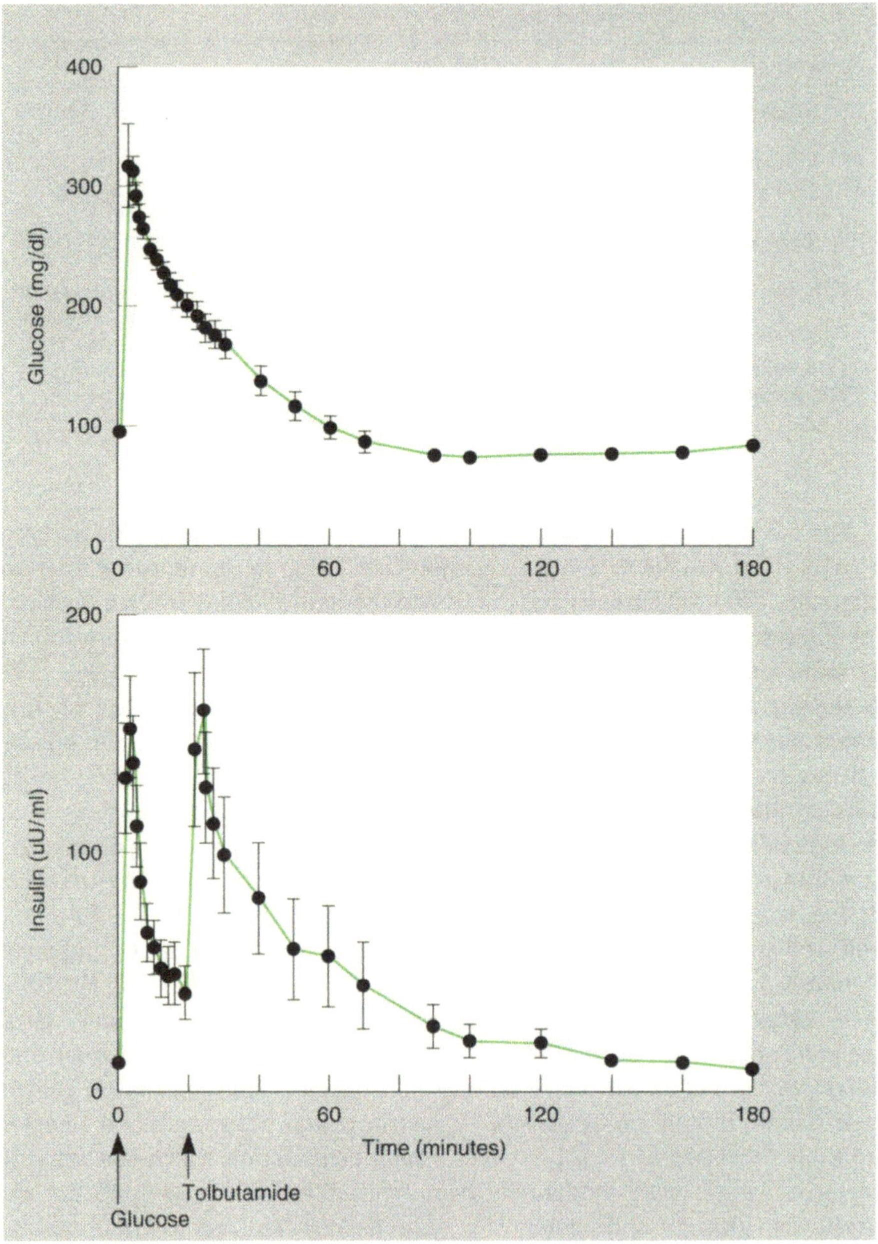

Fig. 3 Tolbutamide-modified protocol (PIII in Table 2). Glucose 0.3 g/kg) is injected at t = 0; tolbutamide (300–500 mg) is injected at 20 minutes. The tolbutamide injection induces a secondary insulin peak, which enables the computer to make a more accurate assessment of S_I. This protocol has 27 samples; S_I can also be calculated from 12 samples (PIV in Table 2)

Parameter calculation

Metabolic parameters (Table 1) may be calculated using the program MINMOD (copyright R. N. Bergman). This software uses standard parameter identification techniques to fit the minimal model to measured results. All parameters are calculated from the entered data per se; no assumptions regarding the physiologic status of the tested individual are necessary. In essence, the program makes initial guesses as to the model parameters (S_G, p_2, p_3, G_0). Plasma insulin is regarded as an "input" to the model, and the computer simulates the model to predict the glucose concentration. The program then compares the plasma glucose time course predicted by the model to the real (measured) glucose data, and generates a new, and presumably better (i. e., more accurate) set of parameter values. This process is repeated, using traditional algorithms, until a "best" fit of the model to the data is achieved. The parameters S_I, S_G and V_D are then calculated as indicated in Table 1.

Validation

The value of insulin sensitivity from the minimal model, S_I, has been validated many times (Table 3, refs. [6, 12, 24]). The approach to validation has been to compare S_I with a similar value emanating from the glucose clamp procedure. This was originally done by Finegood et al., using dogs, for the original (PI, Table 2) protocol. Beard et al., however, showed that the glucose-only protocol yields imprecise results in man [6]; therefore the tolbutamide (PIII) protocol was introduced. The purpose of a tolbutamide injection 20 minutes after glucose is to elicit a secondary insulin response. The added

Table 3 Comparison of S_I from the minimal model with glucose utilization from glucose clamp experiments

Investigators (reference)	Subjects	Protocol	r-value
Beard et al. [6]	Lean	PIII (from Table 2)	0.84
Bergman et al. [12]	Lean, obese	PIII	0.89
Dunaif et al. [48]	Normals, PCO	PIII	0.79
Korytkowski et al. [32]	Normals, PCO	PIII	0.93
Saad et al. [43]	Normals, nicotinic acid treated	PIII	0.78
Kruszynska et al. [33]	Normals, cirrhotics	PIII	0.90
Finegood et al. [23]	Normal dogs	PVI	0.82
Godsland et al. [47]	Normals, heart failure patients	PII	0.91
Mean			0.86

insulin at a later time increases the ability of the computer to achieve accurate estimates of the parameters of the minimal model.

Using the tolbutamide-modified protocol (Protocol III), various groups have compared S_I from the model with glucose utilization using the clamp. In these 8 independent studies, the correlation coefficient ranged from 0.78 to 0.93, with a mean of 0.86. Thus, if the glucose clamp is taken as a "gold standard" for insulin sensitivity, there can be little doubt that the minimal model yields an accurate measure of insulin sensitivity in normal and insulin resistant subjects. However, the measurement of S_I in individuals with overt diabetes is more problematic (see below).

Reproducibility of S_I

Power calculations are indispensable for calculation for population sizes needed to test specific quantitative hypotheses in population studies. To make such calculations in studies exploiting the minimal model, the reproducibility of minimal model parameters must be available. This reproducibility was first reported by Ferrari et al. [22], and has since been also described in a paper by Abbate et al. [1]. Reproducibility of S_I was similar in these two publications which utilized the tolbutamide Protocol III: 14.4% and 16.9%. Additionally, Abbate et al. reported coefficients of variation for S_G (18.3%), GEZI (20.6%) and first phase insulin release ($AIR_{glucose}$, 20.6%). Based upon these numbers, it can be calculated that to detect a 10% change in S_I 50 subjects per group would be needed, but only 20 per group is necessary for a 20% change, and 8 per group is necessary to demonstrate a 50% change in insulin sensitivity with a significance level of $P < 0.05$.*

* As recently reported by Steil et al. (Diabetes 43: 1365–1371, 1994), reproducibility of minimal model parameters S_I and S_G obtained with the standard IVGTT protocol (three tests/subject) averaged 20.2% and 25.1%, respectively. When the reduced sample schedule was employed, repeatability of S_I and S_G increased to 27.2% and 28.4%, respectively.

Application of the minimal model to large population studies

The large number of blood samples required for the standard or modified protocols (25–30 samples) severely limits the use of the method in large studies due to cost and requisite assay labor. Therefore, we considered that it would be helpful to examine the possibility of reducing the sample number in an individual test, so that multiple tests could be performed without undue labor or assay costs. However, it is not obvious exactly which samples could be eliminated from the protocols while optimizing the ability to obtain accurate and precise estimates of S_I and other parameters. Standard approaches to this problem utilize optimal sampling theory which could, in theory, be applied directly to the minimal model to determine which are the most important samples to collect. However, the special problem in this case is that reducing samples not only reduces the number of glucose measurements which are necessary for "fitting" the model to data, but also limits information about the plasma insulin time course, which is the all-important "input" to the minimal model, and which must be accurately known to calculate parameters. Despite this theoretical problem, we have been able to define a specific "reduced sampling protocol" which yields accurate S_I and S_G parameters from tolbutamide Protocol III, with 12 blood samples only (PIV, Table 2). Sample times are pre-injection, 2, 4, 8, 19, 22, 30, 40, 50, 70, 90, and 180 min. (Recent considerations have led us to recommend an additional sample at 24 min.) Of course, there is a reduction in accuracy with reduction in sample number. Reduction in sample number to 12 is associated with a mean 20% error in the calculated value of S_I compared to a full 28-sample test. However, overall there is an excellent correlation ($r = 0.95$) and no apparent bias between S_I values measured with full versus reduced sample schedules (PIII versus PIV). Similar results were found for S_G ($r = 0.85$). The reduced sample protocol is now being applied in a population study (The Insulin Resistance and Atherosclerosis Study; "IRAS") with 1600 participants. The IRAS is the first in which insulin sensitivity is directly measured in a large cohort.

Assessment of insulin sensitivity in diabetic subjects

There is little debate today that most subjects with NIDDM are insulin resistant. However, the importance of resistance to the disease is controversial. While some investigators have envisioned insulin resistance as being the primary factor [17, 34], which leads to "exhaustion" of the b-cells, others have championed the view that a b-cell defect is either involved or primary [41]. The b-cell theory has been helped along by demonstrations of numerous mutations in the glucokinase gene in maturity-onset diabetes of the young (MODY). However, such mutations have not yet been uncovered in "garden variety" NIDDM.

The assessment of insulin sensitivity in diabetics is complex. If the glucose clamp is employed, problems arise due to the difficulty of comparing diabetics with individuals with normal fasting blood glucose levels. Should subjects be tested at their ambient glucose, and the glucose utilization rate normalized using a clearance calculation [13], or should blood glucose should be prenormalized with an overnight insulin infusion [30]? Is it possible that hyperinsulinemia itself, or pre-normalization of the blood glucose will reduce the insulin resistance of diabetic subjects? Clearly, hyperglycemia alone, even in normal individuals will lead to relative insulin resistance [29], and insulin treatment improves the metabolic status of diabetic individuals [25].

Similar questions arise when the minimal model is applied to diabetics. A requirement of the model approach is a robust insulin response, so that the effect of the dynamic insulin on the blood glucose decline may be used to calculate S_I. However, first-phase insulin response is totally absent in NIDDM subjects [50]. Therefore, the rate of decline of blood glucose after glucose injection is determined by glucose effectiveness alone (as well as the urinary loss of glucose, which is only a minor contributor). How then to determine insulin sensitivity in diabetic subjects?

With Welch and Gebhart and their colleagues, we introduced the insulin injection protocol (Protocol V, Table 2) for assessment of insulin sensitivity in diabetics. When we compared in normal subjects S_I calculated with insulin injection to the same parameter calculated with tolbutamide, a close relationship was found ($r = 0.87$), although S_I with insulin averaged about 15% lower than that from the tolbutamide protocol. One potential reason for the lower S_I with insulin injection is that tobutamide induces greater hyperinsulinemia in portal compared to peripheral blood, whereas insulin injection yields similar hyperinsulinemia in the portal and peripheral blood. To the extent that S_I is determined by insulin suppression of hepatic glucose production, rather than stimulation of peripheral glucose utilization, the value from tolbutamide injection may exceed the value from peripheral injection. Regardless of these relatively minor differences, in normals there appears to be a close association between S_I from protocols exploiting insulin versus tolbutamide injection 20 min after glucose.

Based upon the limited data of Welch et al., the insulin injection protocol has been applied to diabetic subjects in a few studies. Welch reported a mean S_I value of 0.65×10^4 min^{-1} per μU/ml, approximately 90% reduced from S_I in normal, young subjects. Wing et al. [52] used the insulin protocol to examine the effects of weight loss on insulin sensitivity in obese NIDDM subjects. She has reported that S_I increased from 0.58 (similar to Welch et al.'s value) to 1.6×10^4 min^{-1} per μU/ml with an 11 kg weight loss.

Limitations

The application of the minimal model to assesses insulin action in diabetics is in its infancy. Certain real problems must be addressed. First, because of possible inaccuracies in measuring insulin action in diabetes using the euglycemic clamp, no gold standard may exist for the diabetic state. Thus, it is not clear to what standard the model based S_I assessment in diabetics must adhere. Second, in some very resistant diabetics, hyperinsulinemia induced by exogenous insulin injection, even up to supra-physiologic levels (500 μU/ml), has no apparent effect on the blood glucose pattern. Insulin sensitivity from the minimal model is indeterminate in such a case, and we have chosen to term this "insulin sensitivity not different from 0." However, it is certainly possibly that increased insulin dose, or a more prolonged infusion (such as in the euglycemic, hyperinsulinemic clamp) would elicit an increase in glucose utilization. What is the significance of such a very reduced sensitivity? Clearly, as the injection even exceeding the physiologie range does not affect the plasma glucose curve, and since the NIDDM has a very suppressed insulin response, it is quite clear that insulin per se has little role in enhancing glucose uptake in such an individual. Given this it may be moot what the exact degree of insulin resistance is in an NIDDM subject! Nevertheless, future investigation is sorely needed to re-examine insulin resistance in individuals with NIDDM to determine if values provided by different methods reflect insulin's potential role in a normal physiological setting.

Final comments

It seems clear that the minimal model is an accurate approach to assessment of insulin action in normal as well as insulin resistant subjects. It has the advantage that it is based upon known physiology of glucose control, and is therefore a mechanistic as opposed to a strictly empirical approach. Parameters gleaned from the model, S_I, S_G, V_D, and AIR can be readily interpreted in terms of physiological mechanisms. Thus, the insulin sensitivity index is the degree to which a given increment in the plasma insulin concentration will increase the net fractional disappearance of glucose from the extracellular fluid. S_G is the effect of an increment in glucose on its own net disappearance from plasma independent of an increase in plasma insulin. Thus, insulin-dependent and insulin-independent mechanisms can be separately assessed using this methodology. An additional advantage is that the first phase insulin response ($AIR_{glucose}$) can be calculated directly from the response to the intravenous injection. Additionally, exploitation of plasma insulin and C-peptide measurements can allow for calculation of the mass of first phase insulin release (c.f. ref. [51]). Thus, the minimal model provides accurate estimates of the 3 factors which coalesce to determine the intravenous glucose tolerance, insulin sensitivity (S_I), glucose effectiveness, (S_G) and b-cell sensitivity ($AIR_{glucose}$). Thus, it is possible to obtain a comprehensive metabolic profile from a single individual using the minimal model test.

There are clear challenges remaining with regard to application of the minimal model approach. The method yields no explicit information regarding the separate insulin (or glucose) sensitivities of liver versus periphery. Also, the use of the insulin-injection protocol has not been validated to the extent of the tolbutamide-modified protocol, and further validation is justified. Finally, the meaning of the very reduced S_I values in NIDDM patients remains unclear, given the ability of insulin to increase glucose utilization by most diabetics during prolonged insulin infusion during euglycemic clamps. Despite these inadequacies, however, it appears that the minimal model is now an accepted and widespread method for assessment of insulin sensitivity in vivo. Given that reduced S_I and S_G is associated with a great increase in risk for NIDDM among non-diabetic individuals [34], it seems likely that this methodology will be widely applied for purposes of establishing risk from genetic and environmental causes in the immediate future.

References

[1] Abbate SL, Fujimoto WY, Brunzell JD et al. Effect of heparin on insulin-glucose interactions measured by the minimal model technique: implications for reproducibility using this method. Metabolism 1993; 42: 353–357.

[2] Ader M, Bergman RN. Insulin sensitivity in the intact organism. In: Bailliere's Clinics in Endocrinology and Metabolism. Alberti KGMM, Home PD, Taylor R, eds. London: Bailliere Tindall, 1987: 879–910.

[3] Ader M, Pacini G, Yang YJ et al. Importance of glucose per se to intravenous glucose tolerance: comparison of the minimal model prediction with direct measurements. Diabetes 1985; 34: 1092–1103.

[4] Ader M, Poulin RA, Yang YJ et al. Dose response relationship between lymph insulin and glucose uptake reveals enhanced insulin sensitivity of peripheral tissues. Diabetes 1992; 41: 241–253.

[5] Andres R, Swerdloff R, Pozefsky T et al. Manual feedback technique for the control of blood glucose concentration. In: Automation in Analytical Chemistry. Skeggs J, ed. New York: Mediad Inc, 1966: 486–491.

[6] Beard JC, Bergman RN, Ward WK et al. The insulin sensitivity index in nondiabetic man: correlation between clamp-derived and IVGTT-derived values. Diabetes: 1986; 35: 362–369.

[7] Bergman RN. Toward physiological understanding of glucose tolerance: minimal-model approach (Lilly Lecture). Diabetes 1989; 38: 1512–1527.

[8] Bergman RN, Beard JC, Chen M. The minimal modelling method: assessment of insulin sensitivity and B-cell function in vivo. In: Methods in Diabetes Research: Clinical Methods. Clarke WL, Larner J, Pohl SL, eds. John Wiley and Sons Inc, 1986: 15–34.

[9] Bergman RN, Finegood DT, Ader M. Assessment of insulin sensitivity in vivo. Endocr Rev 1985; 6: 45–86.

[10] Bergman RN, Ider YZ, Bowden CR et al. Quantitative estimation of insulin sensitivity. Am J Physiol 1979; 236: E667–E677.

[11] Bergman RN, Phillips LS, Cobelli C. Physiologic evaluation of factors controlling glucose tolerance in man: measurement of insulin sensitivity and B-cell glucose sensitivity from the response to intravenous glucose. J Clin Invest 1981; 68: 1456–1467.

[12] Bergman RN, Prager R, Volund A et al. Equivalence of the insulin sensitivity index in man derived by the minimal model method and the euglycemic glucose clamp. J Clin Invest 1987; 79: 790–800.
[13] Best JD, Taborsky GJ, Halter JB et al. Glucose disposal is not proportional to plasma glucose level in man. Diabetes 1981; 30: 847–850.
[14] Buchanan TA. Glucose metabolism during pregnancy: normal physiology and implications for diabetes mellitus. Isr J Med Sci 1991; 27: 432–441.
[15] Chen YDI, Jeng CY, Hollenbeck CB et al. Relationship between plasma glucose and insulin concentration, glucose production, and glucose disposal in normal subjects and patients with non-insulin dependent diabetes. J Clin Invest 1988; 82: 21–25.
[16] DeFronzo RA, Alvestrand A, Smith D et al. Insulin resistance in uremia. J Clin Invest 1981; 67: 563–568.
[17] DeFronzo RA, Bonadonna RC, Ferrannini E. Pathogenesis of NIDDM: a balanced overview. Diab Care 1992; 15: 318–368.
[18] DeFronzo RA, Hendler R, Simonson D. Insulin resistance is a prominent feature of insulin-dependent diabetes. Diabetes 1982; 31: 795–801.
[19] DeFronzo RA, Tobin JD, Andres R. Glucose clamp technique: a method for quantifying insulin secretion and resistance. Am J Physiol 1979; 237: E214–E223.
[20] Doberne L, Greenfield MS, Schulz B et al. Enhanced glucose utilization during prolonged glucose clamp studies. Diabetes 1981; 30: 829–835.
[21] Donner CC, Fraze E, Chen YDI et al. Presentation of a new method for specific measurement of in vivo insulin-stimulated glucose disposal in humans: comparison of this approach with the insulin clamp and minimal model techniques. J Clin Endocrinol Metab 1985; 60: 723–726.
[22] Ferrari P, Alleman Y, Shaw S et al. Reproducibility of insulin sensitivity measured by the minimal model. Diabetologia 1991; 34: 527–530.
[23] Finegood DT, Hramiak IM, Dupre J. A modified protocol for estimation of insulin sensitivity with the minimal model of glucose kinetics in patients with insulin-dependent diabetes. J Clin Endocrinol Metab 1990; 70: 1538–1549.
[24] Finegood DT, Pacini G, Bergman RN. The insulin sensitivity index. Correlation in dogs between values determined from the intravenous glucose tolerance test and the euglycemic glucose clamp. Diabetes 1984; 33: 362–368.
[25] Ginsberg HN. Investigation of insulin resistance during diabetic ketoacidosis: role of counter-regulatory substances and effect of insulin therapy. Metabolism 1977; 26: 1135–1146.
[26] Himsworth HP. The syndrome of diabetes mellitus and its causes. Lancet 1949; 2: 465–473.
[27] Hollander PH, Asplin SM, Kniaz D et al. Beta-cell dysfunction in nondiabetic HLA identical siblings of insulin-dependent diabetics. Diabetes 1982; 31: 149–153.
[28] Kahn SE, Beard JC, Schwartz MW et al. Increased B-cell secretory capacity as mechanism for islet adaptation to nicotinic-acid-induced insulin resistance. Diabetes 1989; 38: 562–568.
[29] Klip A, Paquet MR. Glucose transport and glucose transporters in muscle and their metabolic regulation. Diab Care 1990; 13: 228–243.
[30] Kolterman OG, Gray RS, Burstein P et al. Receptor and postreceptor defects contribute to the insulin resistance in noninsulin-dependent diabetes mellitus. J Clin Invest 1981; 68: 957–969.
[31] Kolterman OG, Insel J, Saekow M et al. Mechanisms of insulin resistance in human obesity: evidence for receptor and postreceptor defects. J Clin Invest 1980; 65: 1272–1284.
[32] Korytkowski M, Berga S, Horwitz M. Comparison of the minimal model and hyperglycemic clamp techniques for measuring insulin sensitivity. Diabetes 1993; 42: 169A. (Abstract).
[33] Kruszynska YT, Harry DS, Bergman RN et al. Insulin sensitivity, insulin secretion and glucose effectiveness in diabetic and non-diabetic cirrhotic patients. Diabetologia 1993; 36: 121–128.

[34] Martin BC, Warram JH, Krolewski AS et al. Role of glucose and insulin resistance in development of type 2 diabetes mellitus: results of a 25-year follow up study. Lancet 1992; 340: 925–929.
[35] Mitrakou A, Kelley D, Mokan M et al. Role of reduced suppression of glucose production and diminished early insulin release in impaired glucose tolerance. N Engl J Med 1992; 326: 22–29.
[36] Mitsukawa T, Takemura J, Asai M et al. Insulin amyloid polypeptide response to glucose, insulin, and somatostatin analogue administration. Diabetes 1990; 39: 639–642.
[37] O'Rahilly S, Burnett MA, Smith RF et al. Haemolysis affects insulin but not C-peptide immunoassay. Diabetologia 1987; 30: 394–396.
[38] Olefsky JM, Kolterman OG. Mechanisms of insulin resistance in obesity and noninsulin-dependent (Type II) diabetes. Am J Med 1981; 70: 151–168.
[39] Pollare T, Lithell H, Berne C. Insulin resistance is a characteristic feature of primary hypertension independent of obesity. Metabolism 1990; 39: 167–174.
[40] Polonsky KS, Given BD, Hirsch LJ et al. Abnormal patterns of insulin secretion in non-insulin-dependent diabetes mellitus. N Engl J Med 1988; 318: 1231–1239.
[41] Porte D, Jr. Beta cells in type II diabetes mellitus (Banting lecture). Diabetes 1993; 40: 166–180.
[42] Prager R, Wallace P, Olefsky JM. In vivo kinetics of insulin action on peripheral glucose disposal and hepatic glucose output in normal and obese subjects. J Clin Invest 1986; 78: 472–481.
[43] Saad MF, Bergman RN, Degregorio M et al. Inability of normal beta-cells to compensate completely for experimentally-induced insulin resistance. Proc 14th IDF Congress 1991; 374. (Abstract).
[44] Shen SW, Reaven GM, Farquhar JW. Comparison of impedance to insulin-mediated glucose uptake in normal subjects and in subjects with latent diabetes. J Clin Invest 1970; 49: 2151–2160.
[45] Sherwin RS, Kramer KJ, Tobin JD et al. A model of the kinetics of insulin in man. J Clin Invest 1974; 53: 1481–1492.
[46] Sowers JR. Insulin resistance, hyperinsulinemia, dyslipidemia, hypertension, and accelerated atherosclerosis. J Clin Pharm 1992; 32: 529–535.
[47] Swann JW, Godsland I. Assessment of insulin sensitivity in man: a comparison of the minimal model with the glucose clamp in normal subjects and those with heart disease. Clin Sci 1993; (in press).
[48] Tarlin N, Finegood D, Green G et al. Use of the minimal model to determine insulin action in an insulin resistant population. Proc Endo Soc 1991; 786. (Abstract).
[49] Vranic M, Fono P, Kovacevic N et al. Glucose kinetics and fatty acids in dogs on matched insulin infusion after glucose load. Metabolism 1971; 20: 954–967.
[50] Ward WK, Bolgiano DC, McKnight B et al. Diminished B cell secretory capacity in patients with noninsulin-dependent diabetes mellitus. J Clin Invest 1984; 74: 1318–1328.
[51] Watanabe RM, Volund A, Roy S et al. Prehepatic B-cell secretion during the intravenous glucose tolerance test in humans: application of a combined model of insulin and C-peptide kinetics. J Clin Endocrinol Metab 1989; 69: 790–797.
[52] Wing RR, Blair EH, Bononi P et al. Caloric restriction per se is a significant factor in improvements in glycemic control and insulin sensitivity during weight loss in obese NIDDM patients. Diab Care 1994; 17: 30–36.
[53] Yalow RS, Glick SM, Roth J et al. Plasma insulin and growth hormone levels in obesity and diabetes. Ann NY Acad Sci 1965; 131: 357–373.
[54] Yang YJ, Youn JH, Bergman RN. Modified protocols improve insulin sensitivity estimation using the minimal model. Am J Physiol 1987; 253: E595–E602.

Methodological issues in dietary studies of diabetes

J. Mann, M. Ball

Introduction

This chapter addresses aspects of experimental design, assessment of nutrient intake and outcome measurements which are particularly relevant to studies of diet in the aetiology and treatment of diabetes.

Study hypothesis and experimental design

Nutritional studies in diabetes have included cross sectional surveys, case control studies, prospective (cohort) observational studies, and both large and small scale intervention trials. Any meaningful study must have a clear statement of the hypothesis being tested. This hypothesis usually either relates dietary "exposure" to the probability of developing diabetes, or concerns the extent to which dietary factors can modify the severity of the disease. Understanding the methodological issues requires careful considerations of the hypothesis being tested. If causation is being examined, the hypothesis should include: exposure to a food nutrient, or a deficiency for X years between ages A and B leads, after a latent period of C years, to an increased risk of P in the probability of developing diabetes. For intervention studies, the effect of dietary change should be able to be reasonably related to differences in morbidity.

Cross sectional and case-control studies

Many surveys have been carried out in diabetes research either to compare the diets of people with diagnosed diabetes in different countries, for example the EURODIAB study [1] or to characterize the diet of populations with different rates of diabetes. West's classical studies observing association between sucrose intake and diabetes [2] are examples of the latter. The most important methodological issues are identifying the hypothesis, correct selection of the population to be surveyed, and ensuring that the sampling is both representative of the total population and of sufficient size to draw meaningful conclusions. The epidemological considerations are identical with those of all surveys in diabetes and are discussed in more detail by other authors in this book. The range of dietary instruments which may be used in such studies is discussed later.

If the purpose of the survey is to relate dietary characteristics or nutritional intake to the risk of having diabetes it is extremely important to ensure that dietary data are obtained before the subject knows whether (s)he has diabetes, impaired glucose tolerance (IGT) or a normal glucose tolerance. Knowledge of the presence or absence of diabetes or IGT could influence reported intakes to the extent that this bias could produce meaningless results. This may also be the case in studies comparing diabetics with and without complications. In case control studies attempts are made to compare dietary practices before the onset of symptoms in diabetics and controls. Such studies are often uninterpretable because biases are inevitable, including recall bias in those aware they have developed the disease, and because the "exposure" is unknown and could be so many possible factors. Data from studies correlating disease with diet, as in the early studies of Himsworth [3] stimulated much research. This should facilitate formulation of new hypotheses that can be tested by studies using more rigorous methodologies.

Prospective studies

Prospective investigations may be either observational, where no attempt is made to alter dietary practices, or interventional (clinical trials) where there is an attempt to alter eating practices. Prospective (cohort) observational involve collection of dietary information and baseline measurements on large population samples of disease free individuals who are then followed for a sufficient period of time so that the initial characteristics may be related to subsequent risk of developing diabetes. Baseline characteristics of those who develop diabetes may also be contrasted with those who do not in a nested case control study within a prospective observational study. Relatively few prospective studies involving dietary intake have been published – one example is the Israel prospective study [4] which studied almost 10,000 male government employees over age 40, three times in 5 years, and showed no individual dietary characteristics to be related to subsequent risk of developing non insulin dependent diabetes (NIDDM). However in this and many other studies, increasing obesity, particularly with a high waist/hip ratio, is strikingly associated with an increasing risk of diabetes. Major limitations of the prospective approach are that baseline data collection may not coincide with the relevant exposure or reflect the average severity of that exposure over the exposure period. Dietary practices reported at a single point in time do not necessarily reflect those in the past and may also change between the baseline and the time of outcome measurements, although repeated measurement in intervening years may reduce this problem. Failure to show an association with dietary factors does not necessarily mean that one does not exist, it may just reflect the fact that the study design did not allow its identification. An exposure may potentially be well before the time of investigation, such as in utero or in early childhood [5]. Recent suggestions from case control studies [6] that early introduction of cow's milk in the diet of infants may be associated with the later development of insulin dependent diabetes (IDDM), raise methodological concerns as to further investigation. This could be obtaining detailed information on infant feeding practices, with appropriate diet methodology, from a large cohort of children who can then be followed prospectively until sufficient numbers have developed IDDM. Alternatively, in a country such as New Zealand where there are detailed records of infant feeding practices, a nested case control study may be appropriate, although the potentially confounding effects of diet, weight, etc. in the intervening period cannot then be evaluated carefully.

Documentation of prevailing diet in people with diagnosed diabetes is influenced by their knowledge of their disease and the advice they have received, and this may be affected by whether they have complications. Collecting such data as a baseline is, however, part of the EURODIAB study, and data on outcomes will then be added in a prospective manner.

Intervention studies

The literature includes many intervention studies in which different diets have been compared in the management of diabetes in order to modify the severity of the disease. Most of these studies have been short term (a few days to a few months) and the outcomes have, for expediency, been those which can be measured in the clinic and the laboratory such as the effect on weight, glycaemic control and plasma lipids, rather than true morbidity measures. Such studies may involve simple randomisation into groups studies in parallel or utilise a cross over design. A common difficulty in both approaches is maintaining compliance with the dietary advice, and indeed this is probably a major reason why most studies have been carried out over a short time frame. It is beyond the scope of this chapter to consider in detail the various techniques which have been used to encourage compliance in such experiments but constant reinforcement by an appropriate person appears the single most important factor.

In short term studies a cross over design is frequently employed. This has the advantage that each subjects acts as their own control, the comparisons are more sensitive and the same degree of statistical power may be achieved with a smaller number of subjects. The disadvantages are that participants may become confused by the change from one experimental diet to another. Carry over effects may also complicate the interpretation of results, although a washout period between different diets (which lengthens the study) may reduce this effect, and an order effect can be evaluated mathematically. Randomisation into parallel groups is also used, and is obviously the only possible design for studies involving the clinical endpoints of morbidity and mortality or when one wishes to continue the experiment for a prolonged period of time. It is perhaps not surprising that no examples of the morbidity or mortality outcome studies have been published and few long-term, surrogate-outcome studies. When contemplating such studies it is important to ensure that the groups are large enough to answer the study hypothesis, and are of similar age, gender, type and duration of diabetes, and the degree of glycaemic control is considered.

We recently attempted an 18 month study of three different diets, a fat modified diet, a high fibre-low fat diet and a simple weight reducing diet, in order to determine the optimal dietary prescription for people with NIDDM. This highlighted two methodological considerations. The most striking finding was the improvement in glycaemic control between the time of recruitment and of randomisation. This "entry to trial" phenomenon was almost certainly explained by participants adhering to diet and other lifestyle measures which they had been taught earlier. Secondly differences in the diet groups were smaller than predicted by the experimental design because preexisting knowledge, ongoing media publicity and discussion amongst participants in different diet groups resulted in individuals in one group making additional changes which had been suggested to another group. Another issue is study length, as the question regarding the most appropriate dietary prescription for people with diabetes can only be answered by long term studies. Short term changes (e.g. the transient increase in triglyceride and fall in high density lipoprotein on a high refined carbohydrate diet) means that the findings of short term studies may differ from those of longer ones and results cannot be directly extrapolated to the clinical situation. These observations indicate just how difficult it will be to obtain a clinically relevant answer.

Methods for assessing nutrient intake

There are three main methods used in research for assessing nutrient intake and each is appropriate for different purposes. Use of an inappropriate method may invalidate a study. Total energy intake is more difficult to assess accurately than the proportion of total energy derived from the various macronutrients so calculation of the latter is useful. Accuracy of reporting must always be considered when any form of nutrient assessment is made. Studies comparing reported energy intake with energy output (measured by double labelled water) indicate that obese people tend to underreport their energy intake.

Twenty four hour recall

The 24 hour recall involves asking participants to recall everything eaten or drunk during the 24 hour period immediately preceding the interview. The interview is structured to reduce memory lapses and bias by using questions such as "what did you eat when you woke up, between waking and breakfast, at midday etc."? The recall is followed by standard questions which provide a food frequency checklist to jolt participants memory, and questions on areas such as the types of milk used (e. g. skimmed, partially skimmed, full cream), type of fats used for cooking, baking and spreading, quantities of sugar added to beverages, and usual size of food portions. Ideally the interview should be carried out as above by a dietitian or nutritionist; occasionally respondents have been asked to complete a self-administered questionnaire requesting similar information. This approach is a reasonable second best among well educated individuals.

The main advantage of the 24 hour recall is that it is simplest and quickest of the three approaches and makes the least demands on participants. It can be repeated on several occasions to improve the reliability of the results, but this makes it more demanding. In large epidemiological studies it may be used to provide a reasonable estimate of mean nutrient intakes of groups of people or populations. It should not be used to assess the intake of individuals, as dietary intake is rarely consistent on a day to day basis (as exemplified in Fig. 1), and it depends on short term memory which may be particularly poor in elderly diabetics. Misleading conclusions may thus be drawn when this dietary instrument is used for any purpose other than in large scale surveys. Even in large surveys the data should not be used in correlation analysis or to estimate the proportions of subjects above or below specified intakes, as the method overestimates the number of people at the extremes of the nutrient intake distribution [7].

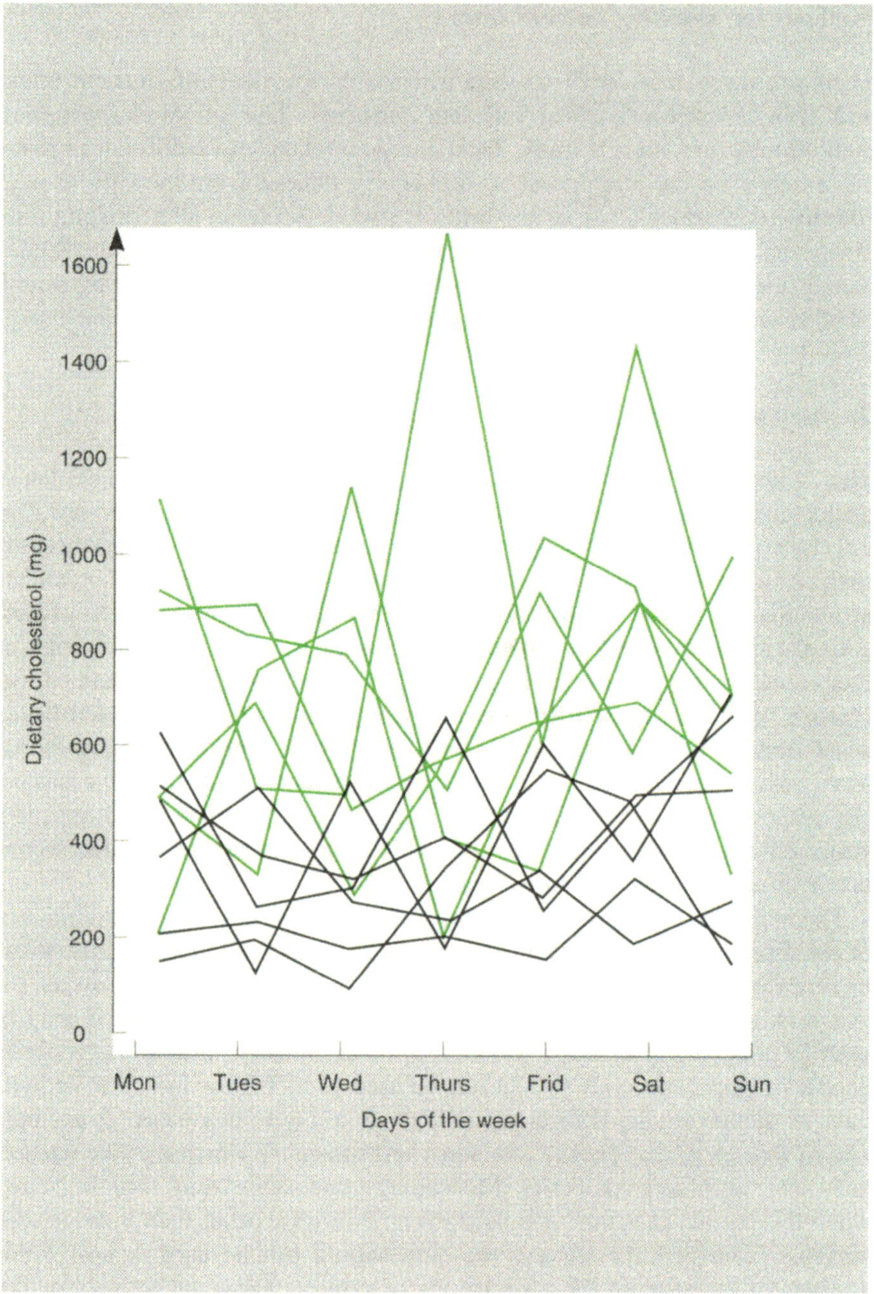

Fig. 1 The variable intake of dietary cholesterol (mg/day) for men with a high intake (green line) compared to men with a lower weekly intake (solid line)

Dietary diaries or records

In this approach study participants are required to record, usually in clearly structured booklets, everything eaten or drunk for periods ranging from 3 to 12 days, and sometimes longer. The period concerned will depend upon the nutrient of particular interest. The intake of some nutrients is fairly consistent and records maintained over a relatively short period of time provide reasonably reliable estimates. For example, a three day record will provide a reasonable estimate of intake of sucrose. However, to be reasonably confident about intake of iron the record needs to be kept for at least 12 days [8]. Table 1 provides an indication of the number of days required for reliable estimate of most nutrients [9]. In general 7 day records are regarded as fairly reliable for assessing the majority of important nutrients and 4 day records (including weekend days) have been shown to provide a reasonable estimate of macronutrient intake [10]. The decision regarding the time of recording is usually a compromise between what might be regarded as ideal and what might reasonably be expected of research participants. The individuals need to fill in the record as soon as possible after they have eaten to reduce reliance on memory. Clear instructions are needed on how to record types and brands

Table 1 Number of days required to classify 80% of the population into their appropriate tertiles with 95% confidence[a]

Nutrient	Men	Women
Energy	5	4
Fat	9	6
Protein	5	5
Carbohydrate	3	2
Sucrose	2	3
Fibre	10	5
Vitamin A	46	64
Vitamin C	6	6
Thiamin	6	9
Sodium	11	7
Calcium	4	4
Iron	12	19
Nutrient intake per MJ energy intake		
Fat	18	7
Protein	10	11
Carbohydrate	7	5
Fibre	11	4
Vitamin C	14	3

[a] Data based on Bingham et al. 1981

of food and the quantity eaten. Even diabetics who have had considerable dietary advice may find it difficult to assess portion size [11]. The size of portions may be described in terms of household measures (cups and spoons, which need to be described), by comparison with photographs or they may be weighed. The weighed record is of course the most accurate and a seven day weighed dietary record is usually regarded as the "gold standard" against which other methods are compared. However, it is also the most inconvenient for participants and may reduce the number of days for which one can reasonably expect people to record intakes. Furthermore the need to weigh individual food items may discourage people from eating foods they might otherwise have eaten, particularly between meal snacks, or reduce the size of portion selected. This may be particularly true if studies are conducted in a diet-conscious society or group, particularly one with a high prevalence of obesity.

The diet record may be used in surveys where there is a need to describe the intake of groups with a higher degree of accuracy than is possible with 24 hour recalls. For example, a 4 day records has been used for the EURODIAB study. It is also the assessment of choice in all studies where there is a need to characterize the intake of individuals rather than of groups. For example, when intake needs to be compared to recommended allowances or when individual nutrient intakes need to be correlated with metabolic variables or when compliance to an experimental diet is being assessed. It can also provide a timed record of food intake for assessment relative to insulin therapy in IDDM if this is relevant. The disadvantages of the method lie in the level of literacy and compliance needed by the respondents.

Food frequency questionnaires

Food frequency questionnaires (FFQs) consist of lists of food and the respondent is asked to indicate the frequency with which individual foods are eaten, usually by circling one of a number of options, over a specified period eg. 1–3 months. The number of food and drink items is variable. Initially these questionnaires were used to provide a broad indication of dietary patterns in epidemiological studies in order to relate dietary practices to the risk of disease. For example, in studies of Seventh Day Adventist vegetarians the frequency of meat consumption was related to subsequent risk of developing diabetes. However, recently more sophisticated approaches have been developed which enable food frequency questionnaires to be used to generate quantitative dietary data which, although less accurate than that from food records, may certainly be used to compare intakes by decile or quartile [12]. It is essential that these questionnaires be developed in the society in which they are to be used since the foods which provide the important nutrients differ from one country to another. Data used for their analysis, such as portion size, is usually based on recalls or records gathered from large random population samples. FFQs should generally be validated against extended periods of diet recording, preferably in the subgroup of the population they are to be used to study. Thus an FFQ to be used to assess intake in elderly people should be validated against records from such individuals before being used in research studies [13]. FFQs have the advantage of being less time consuming for the respondent to complete which improves study participation. They are also convenient for the investigator since they are readily computerised and analysed once the initial programme has been written. In theory, they provide a better indication of usual dietary intake than diet records which are restricted to a certain number of days. Some people find recall of usual frequency of intake difficult but in general validation studies of the newer questionnaires has been encouraging. FFQs are generally used only in epidemiological studies and are most reliable in conjunction with other dietary techniques. Simplified questionnaires have been developed to assess intake of one particular nutrient, e. g. calcium, using any questions about foods high in this nutrient, but they provide limited information and must be validated before use.

Analysis of recalls, records and food frequency questionnaires

The essential requirement for the analysis of all dietary data is an accurate food table based principally on the analysis of locally available foods. The composition of food varies and may differ appreciably from that in the widely used "international" food tables. For example, cereals and bread are fortified in some countries and this will influence iron intake, and trace elements in foods may vary widely depending on the soil they are grown in. The development of country specific tables is being facilitated by the international organisation INTERFOODS. Given that most nutritional studies involve fairly large groups of participants it is also necessary to have a available computer software to translate recalls, records and food frequency questionnaires into nutrient intakes. Many software packages are now available, but important considerations are appropriateness and completeness of the food composition database. A high percentage of missing data on the nutrients of concern will lead to serious underestimation of intake. Missing data should be stated, not entered as zero.

Specific methodological considerations

It must be remembered that the results obtained by any of these diet methods only represent the quantity of food injested over the time period reviewed.

Table 2 Monthly coefficients of variation % in dietary fibre intake in regions of the European Economic Community[a]

Area	Vegetables (and potatoes)	Cereal	Total
Friesland	8.1	13.1	7.3
Ghent	8.2	14.3	7.4
Leige	7.2	6.4	4.7
Luxembourg	17.1	6.9	13.7
Normandy	10.9	8.9	7.4
Bretagne	17.2	13.1	11.8
Campania	23.0	13.4	12.3
(Between 11 regions)	30.0	26.1	9.1

[a] Data from Bingham and Cummings, 1981 [13]

Food intake can vary considerably during different seasons (as shown in Table 2), and the timing of assessment(s) must be considered. The results may also differ considerably from what is actually absorbed into the body. Reduced absorption may occur in diabetics with disordered gastrointestinal function. Bioavailability is a particularly important consideration for some nutrients, e. g. iron, yet this cannot be adequately addressed. The issue of dietary fibre is also important. The effect of fibre, particularly foods high in soluble fibre, on glycaemic control and plasma lipids has been the subject of much research [14]. Yet there is no real agreement on methods of measuring dietary fibre, food tables vary in their designation and the issue of digestability is not addressed. Diabetics are also frequently taking medication of various types, and the possibility of drugs/nutrient interactions must be considered.

Surrogate biological methods for assessing nutrient intake

All methods of assessing nutrient intake have potential difficulties. It is therefore very useful to have measurements with which to correlate dietary intake data or to relate to outcome measurements. One example is measurement of 24 hour urinary sodium which if repeated on a number of occasions provides a reasonably accurate reflection of intake of a nutrient which is almost impossible to assess by dietary methodology except by chemical analysis of a duplicate diet. Reported intake almost invariably underestimates true intake because of the difficulties in measuring the amount of salt added in cooking or at the table and because the salt content of manufactured food can seldom be assessed. An approach used to obtain an indication of the profile of fatty acids in the diet, or confirm a change in dietary fat composition is the measurement of the fatty acid composition of lipids in the plasma, red cell membranes, platelets or adipose tissue. Although this does not provide information on total fat intake it reflects changes in the relative intake of saturated and polyunsaturated fats. The tissue examined must reflect the time period under investigation, e. g. adipose tissue fatty acid composition provides an indication of long term dietary intake whereas the fatty acid composition of plasma triglyceride reflects very recent fat intake. The dietary fatty acids of interest or under study must also determine the tissue analysed. For example the long chain unsaturated fatty acids, eicosapentaenoic acid, C20 : 5, and docosahexaenoic acid C22 : 6 are only found in readily measurable amounts in the phospholipid fraction of red cell membrane or platelets, but not in cholesterol esters.

It can be seen from Table 1 that assessment of intake of vitamin A using diet records is impractical. An "evaluation" may thus be made by measuring the plasma concentration. Assessment of vitamin C by dietary methods may also be unreliable, because of variability in the content of vitamin C in foods and variable losses during cooking. As antioxidant intake may be of interest in diabetics, a 'biological marker' would seem valuable. The choice may however require careful consideration as different measures may best reflect short or long term intake or overall status.

Outcome measurements in dietary studies

In most dietary studies in diabetes the usual outcome measurements are indicators of glycaemic control (glucose, fructosamine, and glycated haemoglobin and perhaps dynamic tests such as GTTs) or measurements of cardiovascular risk factors (lipids, lipoproteins, haemostatic factors, membrane fatty acid composition, blood pressure) although a wide range of other outcomes including renal function may also be of interest.

Studies using intermediate outcome measures must be viewed with caution since the changes may not necessarily produce meaningful changes in clinical outcome. It is possible for hard clinical endpoints (e. g. death, diabetes complications) to be used in dietary studies. However this has only been the case in a small number of studies such as the United Kingdom Prospective Study of NIDDMs where dietary treatment alone has been compared with diet and the additional use of oral hypoglycaemic therapy or insulin. The principles of assessing all outcomes are the same as in other prospective studies or clinical trials, with perhaps the most important being that the assessor of the outcome should not be aware of the dietary treatment received.

Statistical issues and interpretation of nutritional issues

The starting point of testing a study hypothesis is the calculation of the sample size needed to achieve a definitive result. The calculation is based on the variance of the measured variables, which is the unknown quantity to be measured in the study, the minimum difference one wishes to detect, and the likelihood of false-positive (p value, confidence intervals) and false-negative (study power) results one is prepared to accept. Measurements are subject to a variable degree of assay error (which should be minimised) and often to diurnal and seasonal variation. It is important to minimise measurement variance at baseline and for each study period. This usually entails standardising measurement conditions and making several measurements of each parameter, for example fasting lipid and blood pressure measurements on two or three days a few days apart under similar conditions. Small changes may be clinically important, as meta-analyses suggest a 5% fall in cholesterol might result in a 10% fall in CHD risk, although this has not been demonstrated in diabetics. The minimum difference to be detected is an a priori judgement that should be made before any sample size calculations are made. The power of a study to detect a particular change is often not stated, but is vital to allow interpretation, particularly of 'negative' results.

Other issues are particularly relevant to the statistical analysis and interpretation of nutritional studies. Nutrients are closely interrelated and attempts to disentangle the effects of individual nutrients can lead to confusing and sometimes misleading conclusions. Even sophisticated statistical analyses cannot resolve this problem. For example a diet which contains large amounts of fresh fruit, vegetables and lightly processed cereals will be low in fat and extrinsic sugars and high in non starch polysaccharides, starches, intrinsic sugars and antioxidant nutrients and it may be impossible to be certain whether any protective or untoward effect is explained by one or more of these characteristics. Similarly in intervention studies if one intentionally alters one nutrient there are inevitably changes in others so nutritional interventions are almost invariably multifactorial. Alterations in diet may also have an effect on weight and this may have an effect on outcome measures. Interactions between the effects of diet and other lifestyle factors, such as exercise, must also be considered.

Dietary factors may be involved in the aetiology of diabetes, which could provide potential for prevention, and diet is currently a major part of diabetes management. It is thus vital that studies in this area are methodologically sound with clear hypotheses being investigated, that results are given with their limitations, and that any changes resulting from dietary intervention can reasonably be linked with an expected change in wellbeing or clinical outcome.

References

[1] Microvascular and acute complications in IDDM: the EURODIAB IDDM complications study. Diabetologia 1994: 37 (3): 278–285.
[2) West KM. Epidemology of diabetes and its vascular lesions. New York: Elsevier North Holland, 1978; 321–341.
[3] Himsworth H, Marshall E. The diet of diabets prior to the onset of the disease. Clin Sci 1935; 2: 67–115.
[4] Medalie J, Papier C, Goldbourt et al. Major factors in the development of diabetes. Arch Intern Med 1975; 135: 811–817.
[5] Hales C, Barker D, Clark P et al. Fetal and infant growth and impaired glucose tolerance at age 64 years. Brit Med J 1991; 303: 1019–1022.
[6] Virtanen S, Rosanor L, Aro A et al. Infant feeding in Finnish children < 7 years of age with newly diagnosed IDDM. Diabetes Care 1991; 14: 415–417.
[7] Gam S, Larkin F, Cole P. The problem with one-day dietary intakes. Ecol Food Nutr 1976; 5: 245–247.
[8] Marr J, Heady J. Within and between person variation in dietary surveys: number of days needed to classify individuals. Human Nutrition: Applied Nutrition 1986; 40A: 347–364.
[9] James WP, Bingham S, Cole T. Epidemiological Assessment of Dietary intake. Nutrition and Cancer 1984; 2: 203–212.
[10] Edington J, Thorogood M, Geckie K et al. Assessment of nutritional intake using dietary records with estimated weights. J Human Nutrition and Dietetics 1989; 2: 407–414.
[11] Rapp S, Dubbert P, Burkett P et al. Food portion size estimation by men with Type 2 diabetes. J Am Diet Assoc 1986; 86: 249–251.
[12] Harworth CC. Validity of a short food frequency questionnaire for estimating nutrient intake in elderly people. Brit J Nutrition 1993; 70: 3–14.
[13] Bingham S, Cummings J. Sources and intakes of "Dietary Fibre in man". In: Spiller G, Kay R, eds. Medical Aspects of Dietary Fibre. New York: Plenom Publishing Corporation, 1981.
[14] Vinik A, Jenkins D. Dietary fibre in management of Diabetes. Diabetes Care 1988; 2: 160–173.

Assessment of body composition

J. M. Amatruda

Body composition measurements are primarily used as a research tool for reference in metabolic studies. Accurate measurements are critical since body composition varies substantially among individuals of the same age, sex, height and weight in addition to the expected variation with these parameters. Most of the inexpensive, easily obtainable measures of body composition that are used for population studies do not actually measure body composition and those noted for more detailed clinical investigations are expensive or inconvenient and require considerable expertise and equipment. Because of the latter considerations, investigators have searched for accurate and precise measurements that are both convenient and inexpensive. In addition to measures of overall body composition, the ability to measure the composition of body segments or organs is sometimes important. New, more sophisticated techniques for this purpose are now being validated. For all techniques a serious flaw is a lack of a standard in man to validate methods. However, many studies comparing different methods have found good correlations between body density, ^{40}K, and total body water and nitrogen [1–8]. Many other studies have shown good correlations between other methods [2, 4–6, 9–12]. Measures of body composition have assumed increased importance recently because of the demonstration of multiple metabolic disorders related to abdominal obesity and the increasing importance of body composition as it relates to the metabolic effects of aging. The association of insulin resistance with primarily upon body obesity [13] and the relationship between insulin resistance, hyperinsulinemia, hypertriglyceridemia and hypertension [14] have drawn increasing attention to measures of body composition.

In all studies, an understanding of the normal relationship between lean body mass (LBM) and body fat is important. Forbes [15] recently reviewed the data from several studies involving women and found that LBM is related to the logarithm of body weight over a wide range of body weights. With a change in weight, the change in LBM is inversely related to the initial body weight. Conversely, changes in weight in thin individuals are accompanied by greater changes in LBM than in obese individuals.

Table 1 Body composition measurement techniques: advantages and disadvantages

	Advantages	Disadvantages
Density	Apparatus inexpensive Estimates LBM and fat simultaneously Nonhazardous Can be repeated frequently	Subject cooperation necessary for underwater weighing Unsuitable for young children and the elderly Error from intestinal gas Must measure residual lung volume Assumes bone mineral/fat free mass and hydration constant
^{40}K counting	No hazard Minimal subject cooperation Can be repeated frequently	Instrument expensive Proper calibration necessary Problem in interpretation in subjects with K deficiency Assumes constant K content of body
Total body water	Estimate body fluid volumes ^{3}H, ^{2}H or ^{18}O	Radiation exposure (^{3}H); overestimation by $^{2}H_2O$, $^{3}H_2O$; value for ECF depends on method used; ^{18}O and ^{2}H assays require elaborate equipment; ^{18}O difficult to obtain
Creatinine excretion	No hazard Estimate of muscle mass	Meticulous subject cooperation Influenced by diet; collection time critical Day-to-day variation (5 to 10%)
3-Methylhistidine excretion	Estimate of muscle mass	Meat-free diet 2 days before collection Subject cooperation Variable contribution from gastrointestinal tissue
Electrical impedance	Noninvasive Easy to perform Minimal patient cooperation Quick	Inaccurate when weight or body H_2O is changing

Table 1 Continued

	Advantages	Disadvantages
Anthropometry (skin fold)	Inexpensive	Poor precision in obese subjects and those with firm subcutaneous tissue Regional differences in subcutaneous fat depots Different ratios of subcutaneous/total fat
Functions of height and weight (BMI)	Easy Quick	Magnitude of day-to-day variations Not an accurate measure of body composition
height-weight tables	Easy Quick	Do not measure body composition
MRI and CT	Validated Ability to measure different adipose tissue pools	Expensive X-ray exposure (CT)
Waist/hip ratio	Easy Quick Inexpensive Can assign risk based on waist/hip ratio Useful as adjunctive information for metabolic studies	Doesn't measure body composition
Dual-Photon absorptiometry	Easy Quick Can be repeated often Less affected by body dimensions, body water and bone density Few assumptions necessary Low coefficient of variation Good correlation with established techniques Measures bone density	Expensive equipment Not widely used Need to estimate soft tissue composition overlaying bone

The "gold standard" for body composition has been and continues to be underwater weighing. At body temperature, fat has a specific gravity of 0.90 and the fat free tissues have an average specific gravity of 1.10. The subject is weighed in air and when completely submerged under water. Body density calculated as the weight in air divided by the weight in air minus the weight in water after a adjusting for the residual lung volume and the air in the intestine which is assumed to be 100 ml [16]. The actual air in the intestine can vary from 50 to 300 ml, however these differences as well as those in determining residual lung volume give potential differences in fat-free mass which are within the error of the procedure [17]. This procedure can also be performed be measuring water displacement or with a plethysmograph [1] and does not require immersion of the head. As stated in Table 1, the procedure requires considerable patient cooperation, an accurate measure of residual lung volume and a large immersion tank. It also assumes that the proportion of bone mineral to fat-free mass and the degree of hydration is constant. The two assumptions can lead to an error of 3–5% in the estimation of fat-free mass [18]. The error in measurement of % body fat varies considerably depending on the % fat of the individual with a greater error in less obese individuals. Nevertheless, despite the cumbersome nature of the technique underwater weighing is still the most accepted method of measuring body composition. The coefficient of variation is 0.0023 to 0.0063 g/cm^3 [19]. Percent body fat is calculated from body density (D) by one of two equations: $f = (4570/D) - 4.142$ [20] or $f = (4950/D) - 4.50$ [18].

While requiring equipment that is available in few institutions i.e. a lead lined steel room and detector, measurement of the naturally occurring isotope, ^{40}K, is widely used where available but dependent on the assumption that the K content of tissue remains constant with age and changes in nutritional status. Calibration for body size and adiposity and background radiation [19, 21] is necessary. While the potassium content of lean tissue varies little, the data in humans is based on only a few subjects. Nevertheless, our own data indicate a close correlation between ^{40}K and total body water measurements and support the usefulness of ^{40}K as an index of LBM [22, 23]. The ease of measurement, the noninvasiveness and the ability to repeat measurements at frequent intervals conveniently and with little cost (once one has already invested in the counting room) make the procedure very useful. The average K content of fat free tissue in men is 66 mmol (2.57 g)/kg fat free mass and in women 60 mmol (2.34 g)/kg fat free mass [1]. Others have estimated the potassium content per kg of fat free mass to vary between 2.46–2.66 g for men and 2.28–2.50 g for women [21]. In women, we have assumed that the K content of the fat-free body was 64.2 mmol/kg [22, 23, 24]. The coefficient of variation for ^{40}K counting is 2–4.8% [19].

Total body water measurements also rely on the assumption that the water composition of lean body mass is constant between individuals and within an individual over time and with changes in weight. Again, few human carcasses have been evaluated, but there is extensive data in animals. The percentage of LBM that is water in humans and animals ranges from approximately 70 to 78%. While the usual % used in calculating LBM is 73%, an error of 3% would lead to an approximately 4% error in calculating LBM. The error in calculating % body fat decreases as the % body fat increases. There is little difference between males and females and the % of LBM that is water is nearly constant over wide variations in body fat. Total body water can be determined with ^3H, ^2H, or ^{18}O through the simple relationship stating that $C_1V_1 = C_2V_2$ where C_1V_1 is the amount of tracer given, C_2 is the final concentration of tracer in biological fluid and V_2 is the volume of TBW. Because of exchange of H with nonaqueous Hydrogen, approximately 95% of the administered dose is exchangeable and LBM is calculated as TBM $\times$ 0.95/0.73. $H_2{}^{18}O$ has the advantage of the lack of exchange with nonaqueous body constituents leading to an approximately 3% lower TBW and the ability to measure ^{18}O as breath CO_2. The most commonly used technique measures serum isotope, however saliva and urine can also be used [25]. The equilibrium is achieved within 3 hours [21] making the procedure convenient as a research tool [22, 23].

A simpler and less expensive method of estimating LBM is to measure the 24 h excretion of creatinine. Forbes and Bruining [26] found that on an ad lib diet, LBM in Kg = 0.0291 Cr (mg/day) + 7.38, with an r value of 0.97. This technique gives different results depending on the meat content of the diet and varies with the day to day variation in creatine excretion (5 to 10%). The technique also requires meticulous subject cooperation with accurate timing of the urine collection, assurance of a complete collection and assurance that the bladder is completely empty which may be a problem especially in patients with diabetes and neuropathy. For accurate estimates of LBM, subjects should eat a meat free diet for two days prior to the urine collection. The coefficient of variation of urinary creatinine is 2–19%. Urinary 3-methyl histidine can also be used but is more difficult to measure [7], varies with the rate of muscle protein turnover [27], and is contained in tissues other than muscle [28].

Biolectrical impedance [21] has recently become popular because it is inexpensive, can be measured quickly, is portable and shows a high correlation (0.9 to 0.97) with fat-free mass by density measurements [29]. The technique is useful for static measurements, however biolectrical impedance is not a good predictor of change in body composition [3, 29–33] and is not useful under circumstances where weight is changing. In a recent study evaluating our own data in sixteen subjects as well as data from six other studies evaluating ninety two subjects we found that the correlation between the measured change in resistance and the change in lean body mass measured by total body water, body density or ^{40}K counting was -0.559 while the r value for the change in LBM against the change in weight was 0.690. In fact, there is question as to the validity of the basic equation used to calculate LBM when weight is changing [31].

Total body electrical conductivity (TOBEC) requires more elaborate apparatus than bioimpedance. It is based on the principle that an object placed in an electromagnetic field will perturb the field based on the quantity of conducting material present [34]. This method correlates very well with other established methods including hydrostatic weighing, total body water, ^{40}K, and electrical impedance ($r = 0.80-0.92$, [35–37]). This method is subject to the same problems as bioimpedance with regard to changes in hydration.

Skinfold thickness is a widely used method to estimate body fat. Several studies have compared skinfold thickness measurements to densitometry [38] and neutron activation [39, 40] in people and have generally found good correlations between skinfold thickness and LBM. These correlations are not as good in the elderly, ill patients or in subjects with easily compressible subcutaneous tissue. In one study, LBM could be estimated from height and weight as well as it could from skinfold measurements [41]. Other problems with the method are that it is indirect, that the amount of subcutaneous fat as a function of total body fat varies from individual to individual and from region to region and the method assumes that the thickness of all subcutaneous sites is the same. For these reasons I do not believe that skinfold thickness measurements are a valid or precise measure of fat mass in individuals and at best represent a qualitative and not a quantitative measure by which to compare individuals. Skinfold measurements should not be converted into measures of body fat but should rather be expressed in their original units i. e. mm. The coefficient of variation of this technique is 6–24% [21].

Body mass index [$BMI = weight(kg)/height^2(m)$] is the most common measure of obesity but is also not a true measure of fatness. As such it is also useful in evaluating populations because of the ease of measurement of height and weight but is not useful to study or compare individuals.

Height-weight tables are based on the levels of overweight associated with excess mortality. The most commonly used tables are the Metropolitan Life Insurance Tables based on the 1979 Build Study published by the Society of Actuaries and the Association of Life Insurance Medical Directors [42]. These tables report relative body weights which do not necessarily reflect adiposity. As discussed, [1] the studies on which these tables are based were flawed in many ways including the skewed population studied, the unit of analysis i.e. the policy, the length of time of followup, the failure to consider important variables such as smoking, the failure to actually measure frame size, and the fact that approximately 10% of the data were self reported. None of the studies considered the distribution of body fat. Height weight tables are useful clinically to estimate ideal body weight for patients and for consideration for entry into research studies prior to more precise measures of body composition. Height-weight tables should not be used alone to determine the degree of obesity either for clinical or research purposes but are usually qualitatively correct in assigning a patient as obese.

Newer methods of measuring body fat and the distribution of body fat are MRI and CT scanning [43–48]. These methods have been validated by comparison to ^{40}K, and water space. In animals, both techniques have been validated by dissection and analysis of carcass fat [48, 49]. The disadvantage of these techniques for measuring body composition is the expensive computer hardware and software required as well as the expense of the techniques themselves which is considerably more for MRI than for CT. CT scanning, however, is complicated by the attendant x-ray exposure which is difficult to justify for studies of body composition. The two techniques give different absolute values for visceral fat, however the ranking of individuals is similar using the two techniques [47]. A major advantage of these techniques is the ability to evaluate different adipose tissue pools in the body, specifically subcutaneous and intra-abdominal fat. Using CT scanning, Fujioka et al. [50] and Peiris et al. [51] have demonstrated that intra-abdominal visceral fat is more closely related to fasting plasma glucose, glucose and insulin area under the plasma glucose and insulin curves after a glucose tolerance test, triglyceride levels and blood pressure than is subcutaneous adipose tissue or total body fat mass as measured by underwater weighing.

While not as sophisticated as CT or MRI scanning and while not providing specific information concerning body composition or fat distribution, the measurement of waist/hip ratios has proven useful in assigning risk related to body type and obesity. Vague [52] first drew our attention to the relationship between "android" obesity and diabetes and atherosclerosis. Since then several studies have confirmed and extended these observations and demonstrated relationships between the waist/hip ratio and diabetes, hyperinsulinemia, insulin resistance, hypertension, hyperlipidemia, gallbladder disease, ischemic heart disease, myocardial infarction, stroke and death [51, 53–60]. These relationships with waist/hip ratio are often present even in those with the same total body fat [53]. Waist and hip measurements are easily made by measuring the smallest circumference at the waist and dividing it by the largest circumference at the buttocks. In metabolic and epidemiologic studies as well as in clinical practice I recommend making this measurement to allow for classification of patients into risk groups.

Dual-photon absorptiometry is now a widely used technique to measure bone density and is very helpful in the evaluation of osteoporosis. Recently, dual photon absorptiometry has also been studied as a method to assess lean and fat mass. This method is less affected by differences in body dimensions, body water and bone density than many other methods making it especially acceptable when comparing subjects of different ages, ethnic backgrounds or with illnesses affecting body composition. No assumptions need be made about the density of tissue, its hydration or its potassium content [61] and the technique is useful even in malnourished patients with AIDS [62]. Using ^{153}Gd, the ratio of attenuation at 44 keV to that at 100 keV directly indicates the fat content of tissue [63, 64]. Mazess et al. [63] and Pierson et al. [61] reported that the correlation between dual photon absorptiometry and underwater weighing was 0.87 and 0.82 respectively. Furthermore, the coefficient of variation for DPA was the lowest of seven traditional methods used [61]. The deviation of %fat measured by density from that measured by absorptiometry was due to variation in skeletal mass which can also be measured by absorptiometry [63]. With correction of the underwater weighing or DPA measurements for bone mineral content, the correlation of %fat by density and underwater weighing was 0.90 [63] and 0.92 [65]. The advantage of DPA is the ability to make both bone and soft tissue measurements. This overcomes the major error in underwater weighing i. e. the variation in bone density between individuals. An error in the DPA technique includes the need to estimate the soft tissue composition overlying bone since it cannot be measured directly. A recent study compared two four-compartment models, one using DPA, ^3H_2O dilution and hydrodensitometry and the other using neutron activation and ^3H_2O dilution [66]. The correlation between the estimates of fat, protein and mineral between the two models were $r = 0.98, 0.72$ and 0.94, respectively.

Several methods such as neutron-activation, ultrasound, and uptake of fat soluble gases are techniques which either require very expensive and not readily available apparatus as for neutron activation [67]; are no better than skinfold thickness in predicting body fat as for ultrasound [68] or require significant instrumentation, complicated mathematical treatment and long measurement times as for fat soluble gases [19].

Conclusions

There are many acceptable methods of assessing body composition and the method of choice depends on the information needed and the population to be studied. In large population studies where expense and ease of measurement is important and where body composition is static, anthropometric methods such as BMI, height weight tables, and electrical conductivity supplemented with waist hip ratios are reasonable approaches. In more sophisticated research studies where metabolic data needs to be normalized to body composition, the most accepted methods are underwater weighing, total body potassium and total body water. MRI, while expensive, will likely replace these methods in the future at institutions where the technique is readily available since it provides information about body fat that cannot be obtained by other methods except CT scanning but has the advantage of not exposing the patient to any radiation. DPA will also likely become more accepted in the future with further studies confirming the validation relative to more accepted methods. Bioelectrical impedance and TOBEC are useful only under static conditions. Skinfold measurements, creatine excretion and 3-methylhistidine excretion are supplemental methods which should not be used alone because of their lack of precision and accuracy.

References

[1] Garrow JS, Stalley S, Diethelm R et al. A new method for measuring the body density of obese adults. Br J Nutr 1979; 42: 173–183.

[2] Krzywicki HJ, Ward GM, Rahman DP et al. A comparison of the methods of measuring human body composition. Am J Clin Nutr 1974; 27: 1380–1385.

[3] Cohn SH. How valid are biolectrical impedance measurements in body composition studies. Am J Clin Nutr 1985; 42: 889–890.

[4] Wormersley J, Boddy K, King PC et al. A comparison of the fat-free mass of young adults estimated by anthropometry, body density and total body potassium. Clinical Sciences 1972; 43: 469–475.

[5] Wormersley J, Durnin JVGA, Boddy K et al. Influence of muscular development, obesity, and age on the fat-free mass of adults. J of Applied Physiology 1976; 41: 223–229.

[6] Morgan DB, Burkinshaw L. Estimation of non-fat body tissues from measurements of skinfold thickness, total body potassium and total body nitrogen. Clinical Science 1983; 65: 407–414.

[7] Lukaski H, Mendez J. Relation between fat-free weight and urinary 3-methylhistidine excretion in man. Metabolism 1980; 29: 758–761.

[8] Clark DA, Kay TD, Tatsch RF et al. Estimations of body composition by various methods. Aviation, Space and Environmental Medicine 1978; 48: 701–704.

[9] Lukaski HC, Mendez J, Buskirk ER et al. Relationship between endogenous 3-methylhistidine excretion and body composition. Am J Physiol 1981; 240: E302–E307.

[10] Lukaski HC, Mendez J, Buskirk ER et al. A comparison of methods of assessment of body composition including neutron activation analysis of total body nitrogen. Metabolism 1981; 30: 777–782.

[11] Cohn SH, Vartsky D, Yasumura S et al. Compartmental body composition based on total-body nitrogen, potassium and calcium. Am J Physiol 1980; 239: E524–E530.

[12] Cohn SH, ed. Non-invasive measurements of bone mass and their clinical application. Boca Raton, FL: CRC Press 1981.

[13] Peiris A, Struve MF, Mueller RA et al. Glucose metabolism in obesity: Influence of body fat distribution. J Clin Endocrinol Metab 1988; 67: 760–767.
[14] Amatruda J, Welle M, Obesity S. In: Felig P, Baxter JD, Frohman LA, eds. Endocrinology and metabolism, 3rd edn., 1993; (in press).
[15] Forbes GB. Lean body mass-body fat interrelationships in humans. Nutr Rev 1987; 45: 225–231.
[16] Akers R, Buskirk ER. An underwater weighing system utilizing "force cube" transducers. J Appl Physiol 1969; 26: 649–652.
[17] Durnin JVGA, Satwanti BH. Variations in the assessment of the fat content of the human body due to experimental technique in measuring body density. Ann Hum Biol 1982; 9: 221–225.
[18] Siri WB. The gross composition of the body. In: Tobias CA, Lawrence JH, eds. Advances in biological and medical physics. New York: Academic Press, 1956; 239–280.
[19] Forbes GB. Techniques for estimating body composition. In: Human Body Composition. New York: Springer Verlag, 1987; 5–100.
[20] Brozek J, Grande F, Anderson JT et al. Densinometric analysis of body composition: revision of some quantitative assumptions. Ann NY Acad Sci 1963; 110: 113–140.
[21] Lukaski HC. Methods for the assessment of human body composition: traditional and new. Am J Physiol 1987; 46: 537–556.
[22] Amatruda JM, Statt MC, Welle SL. Total and resting energy expenditure in obese women reduced to ideal body weight. J Clin Invest 1993; 92: 1236–1242.
[23] Welle S, Statt M, Barnard R et al. The Differential Effects of Insulin on Whole-Body Proteolysis and Glucose Metabolism in Normal-Weight, Obese and Reduced-Obese Women. Metabolism Metabolism 1994; 43: 441–445.
[24] Forbes GB, Schultz F, CaFarelli G et al. Effects of body size in potassium-40 measurement on the whole body counter (title chair technique) Health Physics 1968; 15: 435–442.
[25] Schoeller DA, van Santen E, Peterson DW et al. Total body water measurement in humans with 180 and 2H labeled water. Am J Clin Nutr 1980; 33: 2686–2693.
[26] Forbes GB, Bruining GJ. Urinary creatinine excretion and lean body mass. Am J Clin Nutr 1976; 29: 1359–1366.
[27] McKeran RO, Halliday D, Purkiss P. Comparison of human myofibrillar protein catabolic rate derived from 3-methylhistidine excretion with synthetic rate from muscle biopsies during L-(a-15N)lysine infusion. Clin Sci 1978; 54: 471–475.
[28] Elia M, Carter A, Smith R. The 3-methylhistidine content of human tissues. Br J Nutr 1979; 42: 567–570.
[29] Gray DS. Changes in bioelectrical impedance during fasting. Am J Clin Nutr 1988; 48: 1184.
[30] Kushner RF, Kunigk A, Alspaugh M et al. Validation of bioelectrical-impedance analysis as a measure of change in body composition in obesity. Am J Clin Nutr 1990; 52: 219.
[31] Forbes GB, Simon W, Amatruda JM. Is bioelectrical impedance a good predictor of body-composition change. Am J Clin Nutr 1992; 56: 4–6.
[32] Pennock BE. Sensitivity of bioelectrical impedance to detect changes in human body composition. J Appl Physiol 1990; 68: 2246–2247.
[33] Vasquez JA, Janosky JE. Validity of bioelectrical-impedance analysis in measuring changes in lean body mass duting weight reduction. Am J Clin Nutr 1991; 54: 970–975.
[34] Brodie DA. Techniques of measurement of body composition: Part II. Sports Medicine 1988; 5: 74–98.
[35] Presta E, Wang J, Harrison GG et al. Measurement of total body electrical conductivity: a new method for estimation of body composition. Am J Clin Nutr 1983; 37: 735–739.
[36] Presta E, Segal KR, Gutin B et al. Comparison in man of total body electrical conductivity and lean body mass derived from body density: validation of a new body composition method. Metabolism 1983; 32: 524–527.
[37] Segal KR, Gutin B, Presta E et al. Estimation of human body composition by electrical impedance methods: a comparative study. J Appl Physiol 1985; 58: 1565–1571.

[38] Pollock ML, Whitmore JH, Fox SMIII. Exercise in Health and Disease. Philadelphia: W. B. Saunders, 1984.

[39] Hill GL, M ID, Collins JP et al. A new method for the rapid measurement of body composition in critically ill patients. Br J Surgery 1978; 65: 732–735.

[40] Almond DJ, King RFGJ, Burkinshaw L et al. Measurement of short-term changes in the fat content of the body: a comparison of three methods in patients receiving intravenous nutrition. Br J Nutr 1984; 52: 215–222.

[41] Hume R. Prediction of lean body mass from height and weight. J Clin Pathol 1966; 19: 389–391.

[42] Build Study, 1979. Chicago: Society of Actuaries and Association of Life Insurance Medical Directors, 1980.

[43] Grauer WO, Moss AA, Cann CE et al. Quantification of body fat distribution in the abdomen using computed tomography. Am J Clin Nutr 1984; 39: 631–637.

[44] Borkan GA, Gerzof SG, Robbins AH et al. Assessment of abdominal fat content by computed tomography. Am J Clin Nutr 1982; 36: 172–177.

[45] Tonkunaga K, Matsuzawa Y, Ishikawa K et al. A novel technique for the determination of body fat by computed tomography. Int J Obesity 1983; 7: 437–445.

[46] Sjostrom L, Kvist H, Cederblad et al. Determination of total adipose tissue and body fat in women by computed tomography, 40K and tritium. Am J Physiol 1986; 250: E737–E745.

[47] Seidell JC, Bakker CJG, van der Kooy K. Imaging techniques for measuring adipose-tissue distribution – a comparison between computed tomography and 1.5-T magnetic resonance. Am J Clin Nutr 1990; 51: 953–957.

[48] Fowler PA, Fuller MF, Glasbey CA et al. Validation of the in vivo measurement of adipose tissue by magnetic resonance imaging of lean and obese pigs. Am J Clin Nutr 1992; 56: 7–13.

[49] Young MJ, Garden KL, Knopp TC. Computer aided tomography – comprehensive compositional data from live animals. Proc N Z Soc Anim Prod 1987; 47: 69–71.

[50] Fujikoka S, Matsuzawa Y, Tokunaja K et al. Contribution of intra-abdominal fat accumulation to the impairment of glucose and lipid metabolism in human obesity. Metabolism 1987; 36: 54–59.

[51] Peiris AN, Sothmann MS, Hoffman RG et al. Adiposity, fat distribution and cardiovascular risk. Ann Int Med 1989; 110: 867–872.

[52] Vague J. The degree of masculine differentiation of obesities: A factor determining predisposition to diabetes, atherosclerosis, gout and uric calculous disease. Am J Clin Nutr 1956; 4: 20–34.

[53] Hartz AJ, Rupley DC, Rimm AA. The association of girth measurements with disease in 32,856 women. Am J Epidemiology 1984; 119.

[54] Kissebah AH, Nardarajen V, Murray R et al. Relation of body fat distribution to metabolic complications of obesity. J Clin Endocrinol Metab 1982; 54: 254–260.

[55] Krotkiewski M, Bjorntorp P, Sjostrom L et al. Impact of obesity on metabolism in men and women: Importance of regional adipose tissue distribution. J Clin Invest 1983; 72: 1150–1162.

[56] Evans DJ, Hoffman RG, Kalkhoff RK et al. Relationship of androgenic activity to body fat topography, fat cell morphology, and metabolic aberrations in premenopausal women. J Clin Endocrinol Metab 1983; 57: 304–310.

[57] Haffner SM, Fong D, Hazuda HP et al. Hyperinsulinemia, upper body adiposity and cardiovascular risk factors in non-diabetics. Metabolism 1988; 37: 338–345.

[58] Anderson AJ, Sobocinski KA, Freedman DS et al. Body fat distribution, plasma lipids, and lipoproteins. Arteriosclerosis 1988; 8: 88–94.

[59] Larsson B, Svardsudd K, Welin L et al. Abdominal adipose tissue distribution, obesity, and risk of cardiovascular disease and death: 13 year follow up of participants in the study of men born in 1913. Br Med J 1984; 288: 1401–1404.

[60] Lapidus L, Bengtsson C, Larsson B et al. Distribution of adipose tissue and risk of cardiovascular disease and death: a 12 year follow up of participants in the population study of women in Gotherburg, Sweden. Br Med J 1984; 289: 1257–1261.

[61] Pierson RNJ, Wang J, Heymsfield SB et al. Measuring body fat: calibrating the rulers. Intermethod comparisons in 389 normal caucasian subjects. Am J Physiol 1991; 261: E103–E108.
[62] Wang J, Kotler DP, Russell M et al. Body-fat measurement in patients with acquired immunodeficiency syndrome: which method should be used? Am J Clin Nutr 1992; 56: 963–967.
[63] Mazess RB, Peppler WW, Gibbons M. Total body composition by dual-photon (153Gd) absorptiometry. Am J Clin Nutr 1984; 40: 834–839.
[64] Wang J, Heymsfield SB, Aulet M et al. Body fat from body density: underwater weighing vs. dual-photon absorptiometry. Am J Physiol 1989; 256: E829–E834.
[65] Heymsfield SB, Wang J, Heshka S et al. Dual-photon absorptiometry: comparison of bone mineral and soft tissue mass measurements in vivo with established methods. 1989; 49: 1283–1289.
[66] Heymsfield SB, Lichtman S, Baumgartner RN et al. Body composition of humans: comparison of two improved four-compartment models that differ in expense, technical complexity, and radiation exposure. Am J Clin Nutr 1990; 52: 52–58.
[67] Heymsfield SB, Waki M, Kehayias J et al. Chemical and elemental analysis of humans in vivo using improved body composition models. Am J Physiol 1991; 261: E190–E198.
[68] Fanelli MT, Kuczmarski RJ. Ultrasound as an approach to assessing body composition. Am J Clin Nutr 1984; 39: 703–709.

Calorimetry

E. Ferrannini

Energy metabolism

Unlike plants, which convert the energy of solar photons into chemical energy, animals depend entirely on chemical bonds as an energy source. In this regard, the only significant bond is the one between carbon and hydrogen (C−H), found in carbohydrates, edible fats, and certain amino acids. The reaction of molecular oxygen with C−H bonds generates carbon dioxide (CO_2) and water (H_2O), and releases energy. When this combustion occurs in biological systems, it is customarily referred to as biological oxidation. The energy thus released is used for mechanical, osmotic, and biosynthetic work; the balance between the energy produced and that utilized is called energy metabolism. According to the first law of thermodynamics, energy metabolism is strictly conservative, in that any closed system neither gains nor loses, but only transforms energy. Energy metabolism also obeys the second principle of thermodynamics, which states that the change in total heat content (enthalpy, ΔH) of a substance or physical system equals the change in free (expendable) energy (ΔG) plus the change in entropy (ΔS) (randomness or non-expendable energy). It follows that the efficiency ($\Delta G/\Delta H$) of energy transformation is inevitably less than 100%, and that after all inter-conversions the common fate of the different types of energy (chemical, kinetic, electrical, thermal) is heat. Accordingly, energy metabolism is measured in calories (= 4.18 joules), i. e., a thermal quantity.

The adult human body contains different amounts of the main components of energy metabolism. Thus, water (42 L) and total energy (150 Mcal) are abundant and slowly renewed (5% and 2% per day, respectively), whereas the body pools of oxygen (1.5 L) and heat (1 Mcal) are small and rapidly turned over (240 and 3 times a day, respectively). Intuitively, maintenance of easily exhaustible pools must involve finer regulation than conservation of large depots. Thus, we can lose half of the total energy pool (or ~ 10 kg of adipose tissue) without compromising bodily functions (indeed, often with some advantage), while failure to replace ~ 10% of body heat would lead to fatal hypothermia.

Energy exchange is made possible through the reversible trapping of energy packets in a variety of so-called high-energy compounds, the most important of which is ATP. As would be expected of a carrier molecule, ATP has a very high turnover rate (66 kg per day) but only a minuscule pool (43 mg), totally renewed in < 1 min. The standard free-energy change of ATP in vivo (in erythrocytes) is -12.5 kcal/mol: hydrolysis of its triphosphate bond to form ADP and inorganic phosphorus yields enough energy to activate glucose to glucose-6-phosphate, the first committed step in glucose metabolism.

If complete oxidation of nutrients is the quantitatively dominant source of animal energy, other degenerative chemical reactions not involving oxygen can also produce energy. For example, anaerobic breakdown of glucose to pyruvate is associated with the net production of 2 ATP moles per mole of glucose; this pathway of energy production is known as substrate-level phosphorylation. Thus, both oxidation (through oxidative phosphorylation in the mitochondrial respiratory chain) and non-oxidative energy production make use of ATP as the carrier. For this reason, the basic energy data of a biological fuel include its cost in terms of oxygen and its yield in terms of ATP (Table 1). Thus, the caloric equivalent of 1 mole of glucose is 673 kcal, and its complete oxidation yields 36 moles of ATP; since the caloric equivalent of each ATP is 12.5 kcal, the efficiency of this energy transfer is 68% (i. e., $12.5 \times 36/673$). Physiologically more important is the comparison of the energetics of the different biological fuels (Table 1). Fat, for example, is more energy efficient than glucose, as 1 mole of a typical fatty acid (palmitate) contains 3.6 times more calories than 1 mole of glucose. To release this energy by oxidation, however, requires 3.8 times more oxygen for palmitate than glucose; consequently, the cost of producing a mole of ATP in oxygen currency is 6% higher for the former than the latter. Stated otherwise, each

Table 1 Energy balance sheet for the three main biological fuels

	Glucose	Palmitate	AA*
$\Delta G°$ (kcal/mol)	−673	−2,398	−475
O_2 used (L)	134	515	114
CO_2 produced (L)	134	358	92
RQ	1	0.695	0.807
Net ATP yield (mol)	36	131	23
Oxygen cost of ATP (L/mol)	3.72	3.93	4.96
Caloric cost of ATP (kcal/mol)	18.7	18.3	20.7
Caloric yield of oxygen (kcal/L)	5.02	4.66	4.17

* an ideal amino acid, with a molecular weight (116) close to the weighted mean value of biological amino acids

liter of oxygen used has a higher caloric equivalent (5.02 vs. 4.66) when the substrate oxidized is glucose rather than fat. Conversely, oxidation of glucose produces 0.2 L of CO_2 per kcal energy evolved vs. 0.15 L/kcal of palmitate oxidation because of the low respiratory quotient ($RQ = VCO_2/VO_2$) of fat [1–4].

These calorimetric characteristics have physiological and pathophysiological bearing. Thus, external work performed under less than fully aerobic conditions relies on the preferential oxidative use of carbohydrate (substrate-level phosphorylation), the resulting 'oxygen debt' being remitted during the recovery phase. In addition, burning protein is the least parsimonious way of utilizing oxygen, in line with the need to preserve vital cell constituents and enzymes. Myocardial muscle, which normally runs on lipid, responds to hypoxia by switching from fat to carbohydrate oxidation. In this case, radioactive fluorodeoxyglucose will create a hot area on a positron-emission (PET) scan, thereby localizing an ischaemic region even some time after the actual ischaemic episode [5]. Total parenteral nutrition of critically ill patients generates an overload of CO_2 when the nutrient is dextrose rather than a mixed formula, thereby jeopardizing respiration in those who have pulmonary diffusion problems [6].

Calorimetry

The measurement of heat production in living organisms is known as animal calorimetry. Under conditions of thermodynamic equilibrium (constant body temperature and repletion of energy stores), the amount of energy released from chemical bonds equals the amount of energy expended and, ultimately, the amount of heat produced. *Direct calorimetry* measures the total heat lost from an organism to the environment, whereas *indirect calorimetry* measures respiratory gas exchange, from which an inference is made on the rate and type of oxidative reactions that release the free energy of metabolic fuels. Thus, the two calorimetric methods provide estimates for the two sides of the energy balance equation that must coincide when measurements are obtained at equilibrium and are free of systematic errors. Indeed, when the two techniques are combined, the respective estimates of energy turnover become super-imposable within a half hour [1].

Direct calorimetry

The equation upon which direct calorimetry is based is:

$$M = (R + C + K + E) + S$$

where R, C, K, and E are the radiant, convective, conductive, and evaporative heat transfer rates, and S is the rate of body heat storage. For a subject at rest, whose body heat content is constant (S = O), the sum total of all 4 routes of heat dissipation will measure heat production (M).

In practice, an isothermal calorimeter is a thermally insulated chamber surrounded by a shell space in which air is maintained at the same temperature as that of the chamber itself. In this gradient-free system, air temperature and humidity are measured at the chamber inlet and outlet. The body dry and evaporative heat output are then calculated from the temperature and humidity gradient between inlet and outlet and the air flow (corrected for the heat added or substracted by the heat exchanger).

In gradient-layer calorimetry, the body is tightly wrapped in a substance (an epoxy resin) of known thermal conductivity and thickness, and the temperature gradient between the inner and outer layers provide a measure of (R + C + K), while E is measured by condensing out the exact amount of water lost by the subject. Gradient-layer suits have a low thermal inertia and, therefore, a short response time, and are used to measure energy expenditure during various physical activities. Isothermal calorimeters have longer response times, but can be used to obtain measurements over longer periods of time.

Indirect calorimetry

Theory: Heat production (= energy expenditure) can be estimated indirectly from measurements of O_2 consumption and CO_2 production by making use of a set of assumptions, as follows:

a) a separate estimate of protein oxidation can be obtained;
b) all O_2 consumed is utilized for oxidation;
c) all CO_2 produced by oxidation of substrates is recovered promptly and measured;
d) the bicarbonate pool is stable during calorimetric measurements;
e) the only metabolic processes involving respiratory gas exchange are the complete oxidation of carbohydrate, fat and protein.

If a given metabolic state complies with the above constraints, then one can easily derive the standard calorimetric equations from the known stoichiometry of complete oxidation of carbohydrates, lipids, and proteins as they occur in a bomb calorimeter. By drawing up the O_2 and CO_2 balances, it is possible to partition the observed VO_2 and VCO_2 (or RQ = VCO_2/VO_2) between the three substrates (Table 2). Finally, starting from the caloric equivalents of carbohydrate, fat, and protein and their respective oxidation rates, energy expenditure is calculated from the measured variables (i. e., VO_2 and VCO_2). Thus, no actual caloric (heat or temperature) measurement is made in indirect calorimetry; heat production is inferred from the oxidative reactions through the observed pattern of respiratory gas exchange.

*Table 2 Equations of indirect calorimetry**

Standard		
Protein oxidation (g/min)	$= 6.25\ N$	(1)
Glucose oxidation (g/min)	$= 4.55\ VCO_2 - 3.21\ VO_2 - 2.87\ N$	(2)
Lipid oxidation (g/min)	$= 1.67\ (VO_2 - VCO_2) - 1.92\ N$	(3)
NPRQ	$= (VCO_2 - 4.89\ N) / (VO_2 - 6.04\ N)$	(4)
Energy expenditure (kcal/min)	$= 3.91\ VO_2 + 1.10\ VCO_2 - 3.34\ N$	(5)
Modified		
Protein oxidation (g/min)	$= 3.074\ (VO_2 - VCO_2) + 2.714\ N$	(1b)
Protein oxidation (g/min)	$= 6.25\ N - G_a$	(1c)
Glycogen oxidation (g/min)	$= 4.09\ VCO_2 - 2.88\ VO_2 - 2.59\ N$	(2b)
Glucose oxidation (g/min)	$= 1.34\ (VCO_2 - 4.88\ N)$	(2c)
Glucose oxidation (g/min)	$= 4.55\ VCO_2 - 3.21\ VO_2 - 2.87\ N - G_a$	(2d)
Lipid oxidation (g/min)	$= 1.67\ (VCO_2 - VO_2) + 1.92\ N$	(3b)
Lipid oxidation (g/min)	$= 1.67\ (VO_2 - VCO_2) - 1.92\ N - 0.1\ G_a$	(3c)
Energy expenditure (kcal/min)	$= 3.86\ VO_2 + 1.15\ VCO_2 - 3.34\ N - 0.35\ G_a$	(5b)

* N = non-protein urinary nitrogen excretion rate (in g/min); NPRQ = non-protein respiratory quotient; G_a = gluconeogenesis from alanine; VO_2 and VCO_2 are expressed in L/min

The coefficients of the relationships in Table 2 can vary depending on the assumed stoichiometry of the oxidative reactions. The nitrogen content of protein is taken to be 16% by weight, hence the factor 6.25 (1/0.16) used to convert grams of urinary nitrogen into protein. Since the urinary nitrogenous compounds derived from amino acid oxidation (urea, uric acid, creatine, creatinine, ammonia) have an average heat of combustion of 1.26 kcal per g of protein, the metabolizible energy of protein (combustion heat = 5.65 kcal/g) is 4.39 kcal/g. In addition, 1 g of protein yields 1.15 g of constituent amino acids upon hydrolysis. Therefore, the oxidation of free amino acids releases a metabolizable energy of 3.89 kcal/g. The caloric equivalent used in Table 2

(4.1 kcal/g) assumes equal contributions of protein and free amino acids to total protein oxidation.

With regard to carbohydrates, the hydrolysis of 1 g of glycogen yields 1.11 g of glucose because water molecules are removed during the formation of α-1,4 and α-1,6 linkages. Thus, the equation for carbohydrate oxidation must be modified when there is reason to think that glycogen rather than free glucose is the predominant form of carbohydrate being oxidized. While this may typically be the case in the overnight fasting state, there is some controversy as to the exact contribution of glycogenolysis to circulating glucose concentration in normal humans [7]. In any event, assuming exclusive glucose oxidation (with a caloric equivalent of 3.74 kcal/g) is unlikely to introduce a major error. The gas balance for fats in Table 2 is based on the stoichiometry of palmitate (MW = 256). A typical triacylglycerol (palmitoyl-stearoyl-oleyl glyceride or PSOG, MW = 887) has a slightly higher RQ than palmitate (0.731 vs. 0.696) due to the presence of glycerol, and a caloric equivalent that is higher than that of palmitate on a molar basis (8,139 vs. 2,398 kcal/mol) but lower on a per-gram basis (9.2 vs. 9.4 kcal/g). Since triglycerides must be hydrolyzed before oxidation of their FFA moieties, it is convenient to express fat oxidation in palmitate equivalents, as per the equation in Table 2. To express substrate oxidation in molar rates (mmol/min), one simply divides the relationships in Table 2 by 0.18 for glucose, 0.256 for lipid, and 0.116 (the molecular weight of an average constituent amino acid) for protein oxidation.

The assumption that all the O_2 exchanged between ambient air and the alveolar surface is used to oxidize substrates, is verified by the fact that O_2 body stores are small and O_2 diffusion is fast. In addition, O_2 has no sink or slowly exchanging pool. In contrast, cellular CO_2 evolving from oxidative reactions enters the body bicarbonate pool, which is large (0.8 moles, or a blood-equivalent distribution space equal to 40% of body weight) and multicompartmented. The principal loss path of CO_2 from the body is via respiration. However, CO_2 is also lost through the skin and intestine, and is fixed in the bone carbonate pool. Therefore, recovery of CO_2 in the breath is invariably incomplete, if only by a small amount, which predictably leads to an overestimation of fat and protein oxidation at the expense of carbohydrate oxidation. Another problem is the time resolution of the bicarbonate system. If cellular CO_2 must traverse a vast body space before reaching the window (alveolar air) where it is detected, 'actual' and 'apparent' production of the gas will be separated by a significant time lapse. From in vivo experiments, the bicarbonate mean transit time has been estimated to be ~ 90 min. However, it has also been demonstrated [8] that the large majority of the bicarbonate molecules is channeled through relatively fast pathways, so that the effective time resolution of indirect calorimetry for VCO_2 is approximately 30 min.

The requirement that the bicarbonate pool and blood pH are in steady-state during the acquisition of indirect calorimetric measurements stems from the fact that changes in pH, whether induced by hyper/hypoventilation, metabolism, or exogenous administration, will cause a shift in CO_2 between the blood and expired air. Thus, hyperventilation and metabolic acidosis are associated with over-excretion of CO_2 in the breath, whereas hypoventilation and metabolic alkalosis lead to CO_2 retention. Fig. 1 illustrates the quantitative impact of bicarbonate shifts on calorimetric estimates. Sodium lactate (lactic acid neutralized with equimolar sodium hydroxide) is infused into fasting volunteers for 3 hours (at a rate of 25 µmol $min^{-1}kg^{-1}$) during continuous indirect calorimetry. Since lactic acid is a weak acid while sodium hydroxide is a strong base, the rapid removal of the lactate ion by metabolism induces alkalosis. In fact, arterial blood pH and bicarbonate increase in parallel throughout the period of infusion. By indirect calorimetry, the calculated total RQ falls significantly from 0.84 to 0.76, which would indicate a decrease in carbohydrate, and an increase in lipid, oxidation. However, if a correction for retained CO_2 is applied (by multiplying the changes in blood bicarbonate concentration by the bicarbonate distribution volume for each hourly interval, and by adding the result to the observed VCO_2), then the 'true' total RQ actually rises during lactate infusion. In fact, in these subjects total (glucose + lactate) carbohydrate oxidation increases from 10 to 15 µmol $min^{-1}kg^{-1}$, reflecting the prompt oxidation of the exogenous substrate [9].

The assumption that no other metabolic processes contribute to respiratory gas exchange is only an approximation, the direction and size of which it is important to clarify for a critical understanding of indirect calorimetry.

(a) Lipogenesis from glucose is a biosynthetic pathway involving gas exchange. Intuitively, the conversion of an oxygen-rich substrate like glucose (one oxygen per carbon) into an oxygen-poor compound like palmitate (one oxygen per 8 carbons) frees up oxygen. Since an endergonic process does not occur in isolation, concomitant glucose oxidation (RQ = 1) can provide the necessary energy. Thus, the total reaction will have an RQ greater than 1, and, by reverse reasoning, one can surmise the occurrence of lipogenesis whenever the observed RQ exceeds 1. If the stoichiometry of lipogenesis from glucose (0.52 g of fat originating from 1 g of glucose) is included in the gas balance sheet, one finds that glucose conversion into fat can be expressed by eq. 3b in Table 2 (i.e., simply by multiplying both sides of eq. 3 by -1). In other words, when eq. 3 yields a positive number, that indicates lipid oxida-

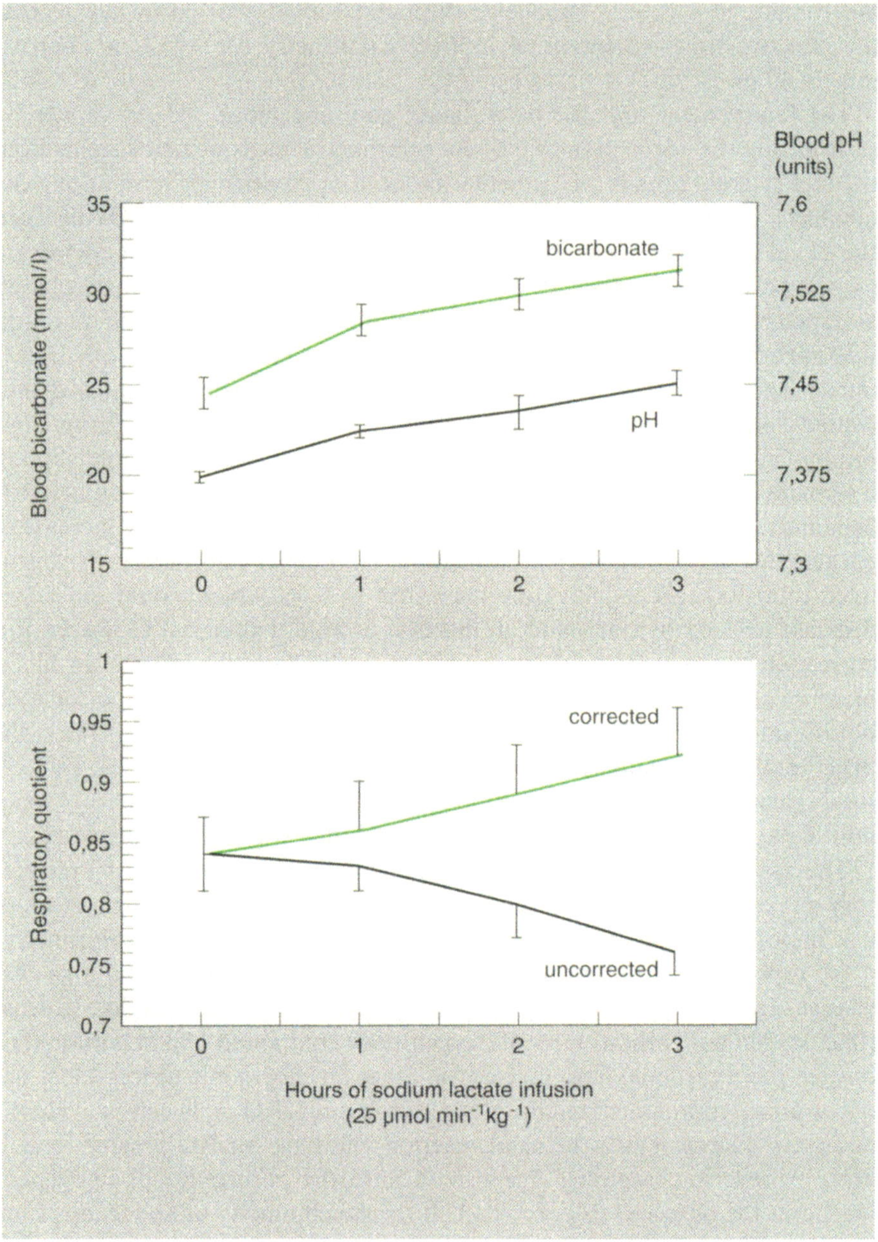

Fig. 1 Changes in blood bicarbonate and pH levels during a 3-hour infusion of sodium lactate (top panel). The bottom panel shows the RQ values calculated from the uncorrected gas balance rates (dotted line) and those recalculated after correcting for the accumulation of bicarbonate in its body pool (full line) drawn from data reference [9].

tion whereas a negative value indicates lipid synthesis. Two key points must be made. First, the biochemical sequence of reactions leading from glucose-derived acetyl-CoA to palmitate may be active also when the RQ calculated from whole-body gas exchange is less than 1: it only becomes quantitatively prevalent over lipid oxidation for RQ's > 1. This is equivalent to saying that indirect calorimetry only estimates the net sum of lipid oxidation and de novo synthesis from glucose, i. e., the net disappearance of lipid from the body by oxidation. Second, in the presence of net lipid synthesis the equation for glucose oxidation becomes eq. 2c in Table 2. The algebraic difference between eq. 2 and eq. 2c is the amount of glucose converted into fat, which, when multiplied by 0.52, is exactly net lipid synthesis as calculated from eq. 3. In other words, in the presence of net lipogenesis, the use of the standard equation for glucose oxidation will overestimate true glucose oxidation by an amount equal to the glucose that is used to synthesize fat. Interestingly, energy expenditure will be correctly estimated by eq. 5 regardless of whether net lipid turnover is positive or negative.

When the acetyl-CoA used to synthesize fat is derived from amino acids rather than glucose, there is the additional complication that the nitrogen cleaved off the amino acid will be excreted into the urine just as the nitrogen derived from protein oxidation. The latter process will therefore be overestimated when judged from the total rate of urine nitrogen excretion. The expression for 'true' protein oxidation then becomes eq. 1b in Table 2. Although this correction looks very simple, the difficulty is that in de novo lipogenesis, the proportions which stem from glucose or amino acids are totally unknown (unless measured by an independent experimental approach). The case of lipogenesis from protein therefore remains undetermined.

(b) Among the gluconeogenic precursors, the conversion of lactate, pyruvate, and glycerol into glucose does not involve gas exchange, and therefore does not affect calorimetric measurements. In contrast, gluconeogenesis from alanine (as well as other amino acids that donate their amino group to alanine) involves CO_2 fixation at the carbamoyl-phosphate step of the urea cycle. Thus, this metabolic pathway has a very low RQ, which leads to an underestimation of both glucose and lipid oxidation, and a gross overestimation of protein oxidation. By considering the stoichiometry of alanine conversion into glucose (1 g of the former giving rise to 1.01 g of the latter with the release of 0.157 g of nitrogen), and by assuming that lipid oxidation provides the energy to finance the process, one can derive the equations (1c, 2d, and 3c, Table 2) that estimate substrate oxidation in the presence of gluconeogenesis from alanine. Unlike the case of lipogenesis from glucose, where adequately modified equations are available, some independent (experimental) measure of the rate of alanine gluconeogenesis is necessary in order to correct the standard calorimetric equations. Otherwise, lipid oxidation will be overestimated only by ~ 10% of the gluconeogenic rate (eq. 3c), and energy expenditure will be overestimated minimally (< 1%, eq. 5b, Table 2), but protein and glucose oxidation will be off by an amount equal to the entire gluconeogenic rate.

Ketogenesis consumes oxygen and releases hydrogen ions, which displace CO_2 from the bicarbonate pool. When formation of ketone bodies exceeds their oxidation, the overall RQ of the pathway is low, resulting is misjudgments of carbohydrate and lipid oxidation qualitatively similar to those caused by gluconeogenesis.

An important corollary to these considerations is that the standard calorimetric relationships estimate the net rate of glucose and lipid excretion from the body, i. e., the algebraic sum of absolute oxidation and de novo synthesis for both carbohydrate and fat. In other words, the measurement of gas exchange can describe the pattern of substrate oxidation reliably only when the actual circumstances deviate from the assumed model minimally. Under the model, indirect calorimetry can partition the observed rate of oxygen consumption and carbon dioxide production to the net disappearance (by oxidation) of carbohydrates and lipids regardless of the metabolic route (direct oxidation or prior conversion into other substrates). If other metabolic processes involving gas exchange take place to a quantitatively significant extent, they will affect the calorimetric estimates in a calculable degree (Table 3). If protein oxidation, or lipogenesis from glucose, or gluconeogenesis from protein or ketogenesis are separately measured (with the use of tracer techniques) and entered into the gas balance with the appropriate stoichiometry, absolute rates of substrate oxidation can be obtained. Importantly, the indirect calorimetric estimates of energy expenditure are invariably more robust, as they depend predominantly on VO_2.

*Table 3 Impact of different metabolic processes on calorimetric estimation**

	Glucose Ox.	Lipid Ox.	Protein Ox.	EE
Lipogenesis	↑	↓	–	–
Gluconeogenesis	↓	↑	↑	↑
Ketogenesis	↓	↑	–	↑

* ↑ = overestimate; ↓ = underestimate; – no effect. Ox = oxidation; EE = energy expenditure

Practical aspects: Direct and indirect calorimetry estimate energy expenditure with equivalent accuracy; both are non-invasive techniques. Direct calorimetry, however, is more cumbersome and usually requires that the subject is isolated and physically confined for long periods of time. In addition, direct calorimetry does not provide any information on the nature of the substrates that are being oxidized. For these reasons, indirect calorimetry has become the method of choice for physiologists and nutritionists.

A closed or open circuit may be used for gas exchange; while the former is still employed for measurements in small animals, human studies are carried out with open-circuit systems. Open-circuit indirect calorimetry can be performed with a mouthpiece, with a canopy, or a respiration chamber. The mouthpiece (a non-rebreathing mask) perturbs ventilation and is poorly tolerated for periods longer than 15–30 min; it is best suited for breath-to-breath measurements during exercise protocols. The canopy consists of a plexiglas chamber which is made airtight around the subject's neck with a drawstring attached to a nylon sheet (Fig. 2). Air is drawn through the hood by an adjustable-speed fan which maintains a slightly negative internal pressure to prevent leakage of expired air. The air flow is maintained at a rate sufficient to 'clamp' CO_2 concentrations at levels (0.6–0.8%) high enough

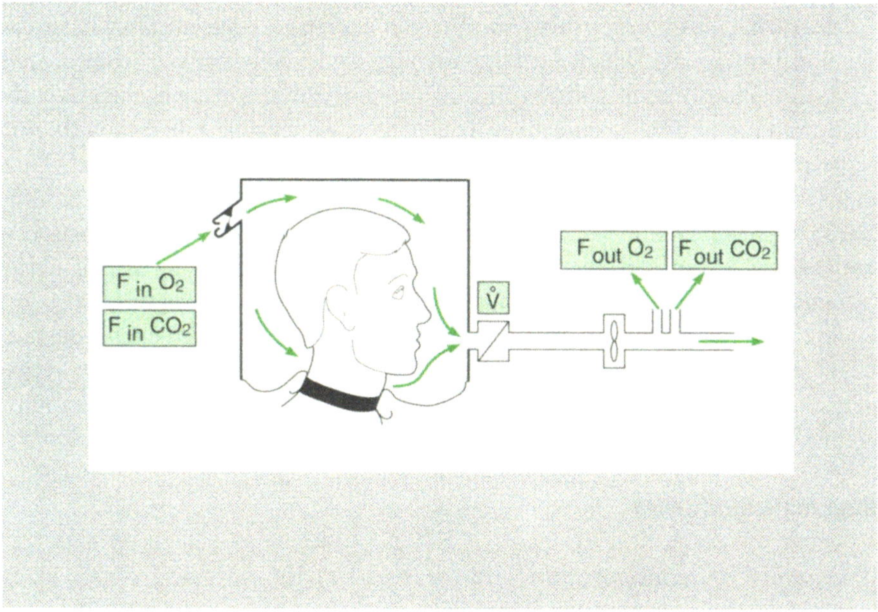

Fig. 2 Indirect calorimetry with the canopy system (from reference [4]).

to allow accurate measurement but lower than those that would stimulate ventilation. A continuous low-flow pump removes expired air samples for analysis by O_2 and CO_2 analyzers.

The operating requirements of a canopy system, open-circuit calorimeter are: 1. sensitive, stable gas analyzers; 2. a calibration routine using standard gas mixtures; 3. some system (a desiccant or an ice bath) to trap or condense out the moisture of the expired air line feeding into the sensors; 4. a software that converts measured volumes to STPD (standard temperature pressure dry) with the Haldane correction for gas mixtures [4]; and 5. software for data storage and manipulation.

For good-quality metabolic studies, subjects should be adapted to the experimental settings for some time before the data acquisition period; each set of measures should be taken under steady-state conditions, and accumulated for at least 30 min. Restlessness, hyper-/hypoventilation, and changes in ambient temperature all violate the assumption that the measured gas exchange only reflects metabolic events.

In the respiration chamber, calorimetric measurements can be extended to an entire day, with the subject performing everyday-life activities inside the chamber. This apparatus, expensive and demanding as it is, makes it possible to measure total energy expenditure and its components (resting expenditure, meal-induced thermogenesis, and external work).

Measuring urinary non-protein nitrogen excretion is essential to calculate the non-protein RQ. Ideally, all the nitrogen exclusively derived from protein oxidation should be quantified. In healthy individuals, urine excretion is the predominant ($> 90\%$) route of nitrogen removal, but in patients with end-stage renal disease gastrointestinal and skin losses become important. Urea alone makes up a large proportion of total urine nitrogen (the remainder being creatine, creatinine, uric acid, and ammonia), but this proportion is unpredictably variable between individuals, and therefore causes error. Chemical determination of total nitrogen in timed urine samples (by the Kjeldhal method) is the method of choice to estimate nitrogen excretion rate. Urine output is another source of error, and is best estimated over longer periods of time. However, protracted urine collections may reflect a changing metabolic state (e. g., prolonged fasting with enhanced protein breakdown).

Regional calorimetry

If O_2 and CO_2 concentrations are measured at the inlet and outlet of an organ, and the flow-through is known, one can apply input-output analysis to measure VO_2 and VCO_2 as the product of the respective concentration gradient and blood flow rate. Since the measured quantities are respiratory gas exchange rates, the equations of regional open-circuit calorimetry are the same as those of whole-body indirect calorimetry (Table 2). The only difference is that regional protein oxidation (P) cannot be estimated from urine nitrogen excretion. In the forearm of healthy volunteers, muscle myofibrillar protein oxidation can be taken to be 85 nmol/min per 100 ml of forearm volume by assuming that endogenous proteolysis is 1.2 μmol/min per 100 ml [10], and that 7% of the resulting amino acids are completely oxidized [11]. The standard calorimetric relationships then take the following form:

$$\text{carbohydrate oxidation} = 0.548\ VCO_2 - 0.381\ VO_2 - 0.302\ P$$
$$\text{lipid oxidation} = 0.143\ (VO_2 - VCO_2 - P)$$
$$\text{energy expenditure} = 0.0869\ VO_2 + 0.0261\ VCO_2 - 0.071\ P$$

where gas flow and substrate oxidation rates are all expressed in μmol/min per 100 ml of forearm volume, and energy expenditure is in cal/min per 100 ml [12].

Much like whole-body calorimetry, the requirements of regional calorimetry are that: a) cells remove O_2 from the inflow and add CO_2 to the outflow at a constant rate (i. e. cellular metabolism is stable); b) O_2 and CO_2 levels in the inflow are constant, and c) the flow rate through the organ is constant. The metabolic model to interpret gas exchange varies from organ to organ. In peripheral tissues (e. g., forearm muscle), gluconeogenesis and ketogenesis are negligible, whereas these processes are quantitatively relevant in the liver.

The full equivalence between whole-body indirect calorimetry and regional calorimetry is best illustrated by Fig. 3. The whole organism can be assimilated into one big compartment containing all living cells, bathed by a homogeneous extra-cellular fluid and renewed by a constant blood flow. The anatomical equivalent of the open system is as follows: cardiac activity provides the flow (i. e., cardiac output), the inlet to the cell compartment is arterial blood whereas its outlet is the right heart (mixed venous blood refluent from organs and tissues). The pulmonary circulation interposed between the two sections of the heart provides a constant supply of O_2 and a large diffusion surface for excess CO_2. Thus, the body can be treated as one big region. By the Fick principle, measurements of cardiac output and O_2 and CO_2 levels in the aorta (or any other accessible artery) and in the right cardiac chambers allows one to calculate VO_2 and VCO_2: these are the same as those derived by multiplying the ventilatory rate by the O_2 and CO_2 gradients between inspired and expired air. Indeed, in 1870 Fick originally proposed (but never actually attempted) to measure VO_2 from gas exchange, and to measure the trans-pulmonary O_2 gradient and cardiac output by heart catheterization [13].

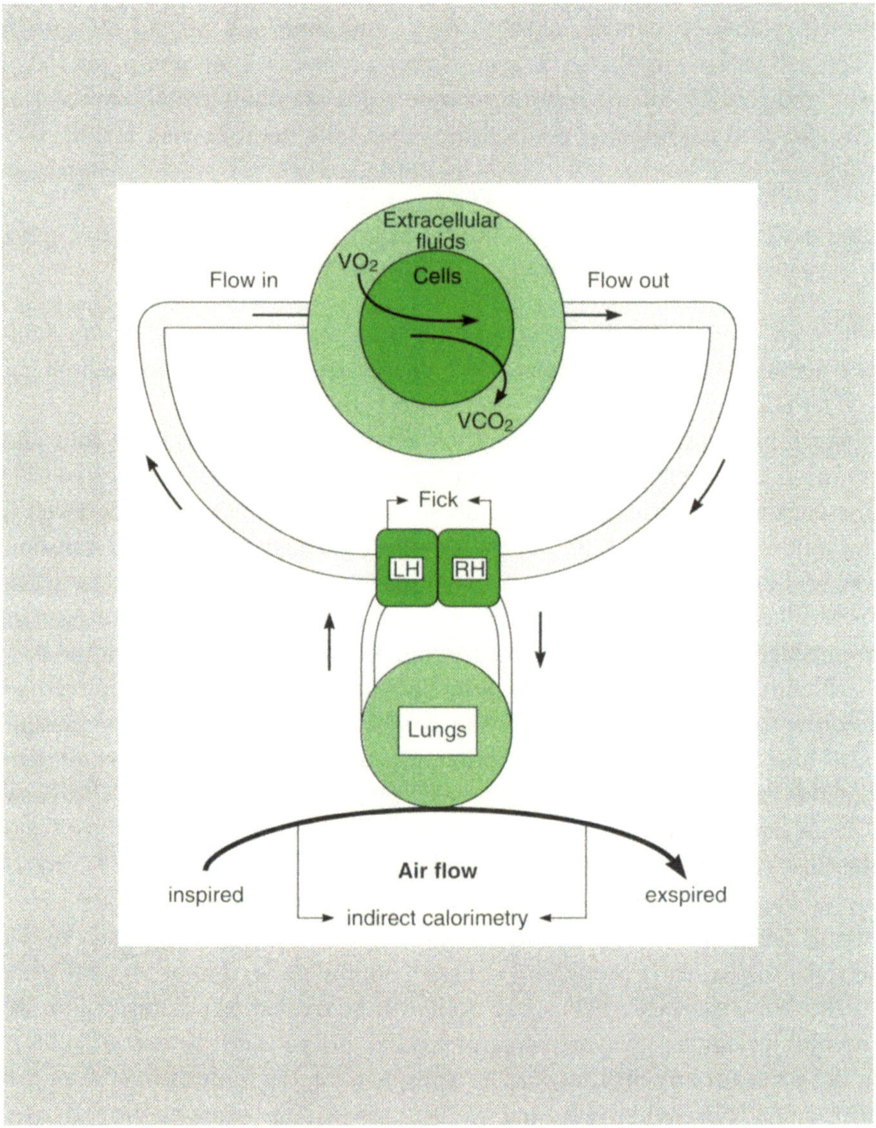

Fig. 3 Diagram showing the equivalence between the Fick principle and indirect calorimetry. LH = left ventricle; RH = right ventricle. See text for further explanation.

When both heart catherization (with measurement of cardiac output by thermodilution) and indirect calorimetry are performed in the same subject, the latter shows better precision than the former, particularly for VCO_2 and RQ [14]. In regional calorimetry, the variability of calorimetric estimates is even higher. In the human forearm, for example, blood flow measurements (by the plethysmographic technique) have a ~ 6% intra-individual variability. This is compounded by the variability of gas concentration measurements in whole blood (the largest, 8.5% being that of deep venous O_2). The variance of the estimates is further increased by the calculation of arterio-venous concentration differences, and by the coefficients of the calorimetric equations (particularly in the case of differential terms). For practical purposes, changes in VO_2, VCO_2, and RQ of $< 15\%$ can be considered conservatively as time-related random fluctuations, changes in energy expenditure should be in excess of 20%, and estimates of substrate oxidation rates are really only semi-quantitative.

Conclusions

Indirect calorimetry is a very useful technique in evaluating metabolism and nutrition. It is completely safe, relatively inexpensive, it combines well with other investigative techniques. When carefully executed and critically interpreted, indirect calorimetry furnishes reliable, reproducible results conveying information that no other in vivo method can provide for the same cost.

References

[1] Jéquier E. Direct and indirect calorimetry in man. In: Garrow JS, Halliday D, eds. Substrate and energy metabolism. London: John Libbey, 1985; 82–92.

[2] Frayn KN. Calculation of substrate oxidation rates in vivo from gaseous exchange. J Appl Physiol 1983; 55: 628–634.

[3] Ben-Porat M, Sideman S, Burzstein S. Energy metabolism rate equation for fasting and postabsorptive subjects. Am J Physiol 1983; 244: R764–R769.

[4] Ferrannini E. The theoretical bases of indirect calorimetry: a review. Metabolism 1988; 37: 287–301.

[5] Camici P, Ferrannini E, Opie LH. Myocardial metabolism in ischemic heart disease: basic principles and application to imaging by positron emission tomography. Progr Cardiovac Dis 1989; 32: 217–227.

[6] Brandi LS, Oleggini M, Frediani M et al. Energy metabolism of surgical patients in the early postoperative period: a reappraisal. Crit Care Med 1988; 16: 18–24.

[7] Barrett EJ, Liu Z. Hepatic glucose metabolism and insulin resistance in NIDDM and obesity. In: Ferrannini E, ed. Insulin resistance and disease. London: Baillière's Clinical Endocrinology and Metabolism, Vol 7 (no 4), 1993; 875–902.

[8] Ferrannini E. Equations and assumptions of indirect calorimetry: some special problems. In: Kinney JM, Tucker HN, eds. Energy Metabolism. Tissue determinants and cellular corollaries. New York: Raven Press, 1992; 1–18.

[9] Ferrannini E, Natali A, Brandi LS et al. Metabolic and thermogenic effects of lactate infusion in humans. Am J Physiol 1993; 265: E504–E512.

[10] Gelfand RA, Barrett EJ. Effect of physiological hyperinsulinemia on skeletal muscle protein synthesis and breakdown in man. J Clin Invest 1987; 80: 1–6.

[11] Tessari P, Trevisan R, Inchiostro S et al. Dose-response curves of effects of insulin on leucine kinetics in humans. Am J Physiol 1986; 251: E334–342.

[12] Natali A, Buzzigoli G, Taddei S et al. Effects of insulin on hemodynamics and metabolism in human forearm. Diabetes 1990; 39: 490–500.

[13] Fick A. Über die Messung des Blutquantums in den Herzventrikeln. Sitz der Physik Med Ges Würtzburg 1870; 16.

[14] Brandi LS, Grana M, Mazzanti T et al. Energy expenditure and gas exchange measurements in postoperative patients: thermodilution versus indirect calorimetry. Crit Care Med 1992; 20: 1273–1277.

Research methodologies for recording blood pressure in diabetic patients

K. W. Hansen, J. S. Christiansen

Introduction

Measurement of arterial blood pressure is used in the majority of epidemiological studies and clinical trials in diabetes, since hypertension is generally accepted as a risk factor for cardiovascular morbidity and as a variable used to determine the progression of diabetic nephropathy. In large scale epidemiological studies, the techniques employed should be simple and the use of time minimized. Therefore, sphygmomanometry is the method of choice, despite a low degree of reproducibility [1]. Methods with a high reproducibility are appropriate in acute, short- or long-term studies with a restricted number or patients.

Direct or indirect measurement

Blood pressure in diabetes research is rarely measured invasively and arterial blood pressure is often regarded as synonymous with the systolic and diastolic values obtained from indirect measurement of the blood pressure in the brachial artery. However, it may be worthwhile to note that important differences exist between systolic blood pressure in the peripheral arteries, the site where it is usually measured, and in the central arteries. The systolic pressure is higher (and diastolic, slightly lower) in peripheral arteries than in the central aorta [2]. This difference between central and peripheral blood pressure is reduced by arterial stiffening, which causes increased pulse wave reflection [2], as seen in aging, in hypertension and in diabetes [3–6]. Mean arterial blood pressure is nearly constant throughout the arterial system.

Clinical blood pressure measurement by sphygmomanometry and automatic monitors

The measurement of blood pressure by sphygmomanometry and a mercury column is the time-honoured method and the basis for our present knowledge of limits for normal blood pressure. It is the method of choice in large scale studies and studies where the actual level of the blood pressure is important, rather than an individual change during time or after intervention. Care should be taken to adopt a uniform procedure for measuring systolic (Korotkoff I) and diastolic blood pressure (Korotkoff V/IV (children and pregnant women)) to be followed by different investigators. However, different interpretations of the Korotkoff sounds do exist and it is wise, whenever possibly, to have the same investigator measure all patients, particularly in intervention trials. Instructive video tapes may be a practical way to standardize the technique for correct auscultatory blood pressure measurements between investigators in large scale studies [7, 10]. Experience has shown that this instruction is a process that needs to be repeated to make investigators adhere to the technique [8].

The important practical questions about choosing the right cuff size, the position of the patient and the arm, the deflation rate of the cuff pressure and maintenance of the manometer are outlined very clearly in the recommendations from the *British Hypertension Society* [9]. It should be specified that anaeroid manometers should be avoided and that an occlusive cuff of the dimensions 12.5 × 35 cm is now highly recommended for all non-obese adults [10]. Also, the *American Heart Association* has published a more extensive (and less clear) review of guidelines for blood pressure measurement [11]. The *American Society of Hypertension* has recently provided guidelines including a useful checklist for publications utilizing blood pressure measurements [12]. The patient should be seated in a comfortable chair with his/her arm supported and talking during the measurement should be discouraged [13]. Care should be taken to read measurements to the nearest two mmHg to minimize digit preference. A quiet room is essential.

In addition to the practical pitfalls associated with auscultatory measurements and individual variation in interpretation of sounds, this method is also handicapped by digit preference and observer bias [14]. In non-blinded intervention trials, or studies where the observer is well aware of the status of the patient as relevant to the investigation, it is advisable to blind the observer by use of a random zero manometer [15]. Recently, the Hawskley random zero manometer has been found to consistently underestimate the systolic and diastolic blood pressure compared with the results from ordinary mercury sphygmomanometers [16]. Although this finding was disputed [17], the Hawskley apparatus should probably not be used in epidemiological research. However, as a method for recording unbiased intrapatient changes in blood pressure during intervention trials, it is still a valuable method.

Alternatively, automatic, non-portable blood pressure monitors may be used as a substitute for auscultatory measurements of clinic blood pressure, thus making the measurement totally unbiased [18, 19]. However, other errors may be introduced, such as the poor quality of some monitors, zeropoint deviation between monitors, or a shift of zero point during the study. Due to different techniques (microphone/oscillometric), the absolute level of blood pressure from automatic monitors may be impossible to compare with auscultatory results from other studies. It is advisable to check the calibration of automatic monitors on a regular basis [12].

Ambulatory blood pressure monitoring

In a previous chapter in this series, we discussed the theoretical and practical arguments favouring the use of ambulatory measurement [20]. Ambulatory monitoring is the only way of obtaining information concerning the prevailing blood pressure during normal daily activities and during the night. Increasing evidence suggests that such blood pressure values more closely reflect the true blood pressure burden on end organs than do clinical blood pressure measurements [21]. In type 1 diabetes, we found a correlation between ambulatory blood pressure and urinary albumin excretion, which had been undetected by clinical measurements [68]. It may be anticipated that the possible effects of anti-hypertensive treatment (e. g. cardiovascular events, urinary albumin excretion, left ventricular mass), attributable to change in blood pressure level *per se*, can be more precisely evaluated by tracking ambulatory blood pressure. This approach avoids the "regression dilution bias" associated to the restricted number of measurements (usually 1–3) obtainable from clinical blood pressure readings [22]. Also, the high number of measurements in a 24-hour ambulatory recording (usually 50–100) are responsible for the greater reproducibility of this method [22]. An important practical implication is that the number of patients in clinical trials can be reduced four-fold without reducing the power of the study [22]. Usually the problem is the opposite; a limited number of patients and controls can be recruited and the investigator has to decide whether his hypothesis can be investigated or whether the magnitude of the type 2 error precludes the study for ethical reasons. Application of ambulatory blood pressure monitoring allows the observation of minor differences in blood pressure (if any) without an unacceptable type 2 error.

Types of ambulatory blood pressure monitors

The modern ambulatory blood pressure monitor is ideally a noiseless, light (< 500 g including batteries), accurate, and durable instrument capable of being programmed to take automatic measurements with varying frequency at different times during a 24-hours measurement period.

Two different types of monitors exist for intermittent blood pressure measurement [23]. One type of monitor measures the Korotkoff sounds over the brachial artery by means of a microphone in the cuff. In order to discriminate between Korotkoff souds and ambient noise, it is necessary to have another microphone in the cuff placed a way from the artery. Alternatively, a continuous electrocardiogram can be recorded to identify relevant sounds ("R

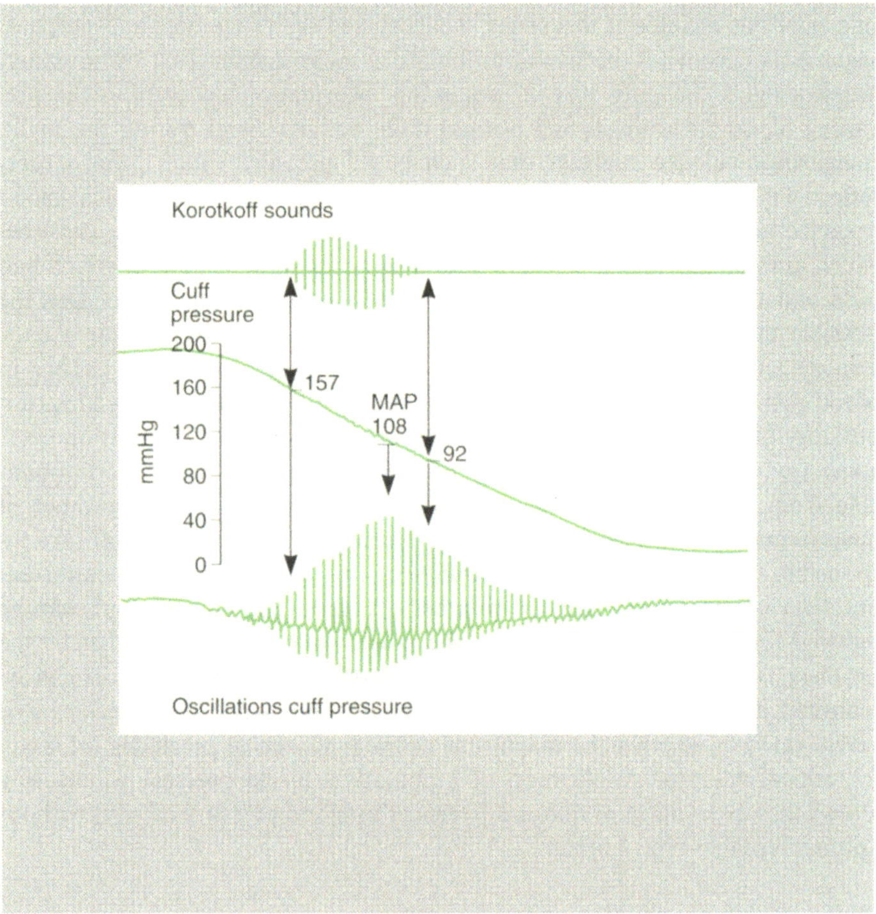

Fig. 1 Proposed relationship between systolic and diastolic blood pressure measured by auscultatory and oscillometric technique. Mean arterial blood pressure (MAP) is defined as the blood pressure corresponding to the maximal amplitude of pressure oscillations in the cuff (from [28] with permission).

wave gating") [24]. The oscillometric technique does not require a microphone. This method is based on the long-held principle that mean arterial blood pressure can be identified as the lowest blood pressure corresponding to the point of maximal oscillations of the cuff [25–28]. Oscillometric monitors do not measure systolic or diastolic blood pressure: these values are calculated from the curve form of the oscillations (Fig. 1). Unfortunately, these algorithms are regarded as industrial secrets, though a continuing demand from the users will hopefully result in the release of more useful information [29]. The oscillations in the cuff begin at a pressure higher than the systolic blood pressure. Using a hypothetical example of an algorithm, the systolic values could be calculated as the blood pressure when the amplitude of oscillations are 45–55% of the maximal (while increasing) and diastolic blood pressure when the amplitude is 74–82% of the maximal (while decreasing) [28] (Fig. 1).

Pros and cons can be stated for both methods. The microphone technique seems more closely related to the auscultatory method, but there have been problems with inaccurate readings in some monitors. This method critically depends on the correct placement of the microphone. If the cuff (and microphone) are displaced during the measurement, the recordings are ruined. For this reason, the microphone is often taped over the brachial artery. This is inconvenient for the patient, because it is not possible to remove the cuff (to have a shower). The oscillometric technique is essentially unsatisfactory, because of the unclear method for calculating systolic and diastolic blood pressure. However, in clinical tests of oscillometric monitors the results have been acceptable. Some manufacturers combine both methods in the same monitor. The oscillometric technique is then used if the microphone fails to detect a clear signal. Obviously, the ideal monitor does not exist. From the user's point of view, it is frustrating that new models are introduced in rapid succession without a proper validation study and without clear documentation that the problems of their predecessors have been solved. Monitors of the same model number have even been updated with new software without notifying the customer [29].

Finally, the possibility of short-term (two-hour), non-invasive, continuous measurement of blood pressure should be mentioned. This can be obtained by means of the Penaz finger cuff method, which is commercially available as the Finapress recorder [23, 24, 30]. While there may exist systematic differences when compared with intra-arterial blood pressure, the method may be well-suited to follow short-term changes in blood pressure (e. g. orthostatic test). In studies of cardiac autonomic neuropathy, this may be combined with simultaneous registration of the sympathovagal balance by means of power spectral analysis. The combination of two alternating occlusive finger cuffs has been introduced as the Portapress system, which allows a full 24-hour recording [24].

Recommendations for the use of ambulatory monitors

No globally-accepted recommendations have been adopted with respect to the practical methodology for ambulatory monitoring and presentation of results. Recently, data from different fields of ambulatory blood pressure monitoring have been summarized [31] and an attempt to provide guidelines has been presented in the form a consensus document [32, 33].

Two protocols exist for validating automatic monitors, the protocol of the *British Hypertension Society* (BHS) [34] and the protocol of the *American Association for the Advancement of Medical Instruments* (AAMI) [35]. The BHS protocol incorporates special features of interest for the user of ambulatory monitors, like assessment of inter-device variability and a grading of the differences between the monitor and auscultatory measurements. A number of the currently available monitors have been validated by the two protocols [36–44]. We strongly advise against purchasing a monitor without having access to the results of a validation study performed by independent observers.

Attention should be directed to the fact that the validations of ambulatory blood pressure measurements have not necessarily included special groups (e. g. old persons or pregnant) [45]. We have not observed any difference in the performance of the oscillometric technique on healthy adults and type 1 diabetic patients [67].

Practical advice

The quality of the blood pressure recordings depends largely on careful instruction regarding equipment use [46]. The patients must be told that an unclear transducing of signals (in some models) triggers a second attempt within few minutes after the failure of the first one. Minor practical advice on how to remove the cuff or monitor when undressing and how to temporarily stop measurement while driving greatly improves the likelihood of a successful 24-hour measurement. It is of utmost importance to instruct the patient to keep the arm motionless when the cuff is deflated. To avoid anxiety, the results of each measurement should be stored in the memory of the monitor without being shown on the display.

Before leaving the laboratory, at least three measurements of the monitor must be compared with auscultatory measurements. If possible, this comparison should be done by simultaneous measurements (by means of a Y valve). Often, however, the investigator can not cope with the rapid or step-wise desufflation, and sequential measurements on the same arm may be used [34 This comparison gives information not only on the discrepancy between the methods in the individual patient, but also allows for comparison between clinic blood pressure and ambulatory values obtained by the same method.

After completion of the measurement, the patient should be asked about the exact night period [47], and whether he was measured on a day off or a work day. It is our experience that people with "flabby" or obese arms very often produce a lot of unsuccessful measurements. At present, ambulatory monitoring is impossible in patients with cardiac arrhythmia such as atrial fibrillation.

Controversies in ambulatory monitoring

A central issue is how to calculate the day and night blood pressure and how to describe the circadian variation. Twenty-four hour average and day and night values are usually calculated by the software supplied by manufacturer. One needs to remain critical when using these values. How is the 24-hour average calculated; as an average of all measurements or as an average of hourly averages? This is of obvious importance if an even frequency of measurements is not maintained. Day and night values are calculated from fixed time points. These values are of no value to describe the diurnal variation, since people do not go to bed and get up at the same time every day [47]. Consequently, true "day" values are erroneously calculated as "night" values and vice versa. The result in a group of patients is a serious underestimation of the nocturnal decline of blood pressure [67]. Differences in nocturnal reduction of blood pressure observed between different groups of patients may be caused simply by different sleeping habits. The individual information of the night period is essential for a correct estimation of the diurnal variation. We have found the night/day ratio of diastolic blood pressure to be 80% in normoalbuminuric type 1 diabetic patients if individual night periods were used, while the ratio was 90% when a fixed period from 22.30 to 6.30 h was applied [67].

Numerous mathematical possibilities exist to describe the diurnal variation in blood pressure or smoothing the curves [48–52]. In general, it is advisable to use simple parameters with a clear clinical meaning [48]. If differences exist between arithmetic mean and the median, a non-parametric approach is recommended. The concept of blood pressure load as the proportion of daytime measurements above 140/190 and nighttime values above 120/80, has been suggested to improve correlation between ambulatory blood pressure and target organ damage [53].

There are no established guidelines for the frequency of measurement. Probably short-term measurement periods (4 hours) cannot precisely substitute for a full day-time measurement period including at least 20 measurements [54]. Most clinics measure 3 to 4 times per hour during the day and from (1) 2 to 3 times per hour at night. The frequency of night measurements seems to be a compromise between the number of measurements achieved and the impact of the quality of the sleep. Contrary to our own experience from the patient's reports, studies have not found that the night blood pressure is altered on a group basis with even 4 measurements per hour [55, 56]. The commonly used criteria for classification of patients as dippers and non-dippers [32, 57] needs a critical reconsideration [47, 67].

Another controversy is how to handle outliers [58]. Most software automatically rejects data which exceed certain limits, however, the criteria vary between monitors. These criteria should either be accepted or no editing should be performed at all. Post-hoc outlier editing by the investigator himself is bound to be biased.

Normal blood pressure data

Whereas large epidemiological studies have provided data on the distribution of auscultatory clinic blood pressure in children [59, 60] and adults [61], no good data exists for ambulatory blood pressure values [62, 63]. Attempts have limited value because of the differences between different monitors. No data of sufficient size exists for diabetic patients.

Update of review of literature

The literature on ambulatory blood pressure in diabetic patients is growing quickly. In addition to the references mentioned in a previous chapter of this series [20], many papers have since appeared which discuss the diurnal variation in NIDDM patients [64–66], IDDM patients [67–72] or mixed populations [73] in relation to autonomic neuropathy or stages of renal disease.

References

[1] Armitage P, Rose GA. The variability of measurements of casual blood pressure. I. A laboratory study Clin Sci 1966; 30: 325–335.
[2] O'Rourke MF. What is blood pressure. Am J Hypertens 1990; 3: 803–810.
[3] Woolam GL, Schnur PL, Vallbona C et al. The pulse wave velocity as an early indicator of atherosclerosis in diabetic subjects. Circulation 1962; 25: 533–539.
[4] Scarpello JHB, Martin TRP, Ward JD. Ultrasound measurements of pulse-wave velocity in the peripheral arteries of diabetic subjects. Clin Sci 1980; 58: 53–57.
[5] Oxlund H, Rasmussen LM, Andreassen TT et al. Increased aortic stiffness in patients with Type 1 (insulin-dependent) diabetes mellitus. Diabetologia 1989; 32: 748–752.
[6] Thordarson H, Thorgeirsson G, Helgason T. Aortic stiffness in insulin-dependent diabetics: An echocardiographic study. Diabetic Med 1986; 3: 449–454.
[7] O'Brien E, Mee F, Tan KS et al. Training and assessment of observers for blood pressure measurement in hypertension research. J Human Hypertens 1991; 5: 7–10.
[8] Bruce NG, Shaper AG, Walker M et al. Observer bias in blood pressure studies. J Hypertens 1988; 6: 375–380.
[9] Petrie JC, O'Brien ET, Littler WA et al. Recommendations on blood pressure measurement. Br Med J 1986; 293: 611–615.
[10] Beevers DG. Sphygmomanometer cuff sizes – new recommendations. J Human Hypertens 1990; 4: 587–588.
[11] Frohlich ED, Grim C, Labarthe DR et al. Recommendations for human blood pressure determination by sphygmomanometers. Report of a special task force appointed by the Steering Committee, American Heart Association. Hypertension 1988; 11: 210A–222A.
[12] American Society of Hypertension. Recommendations for routine blood pressure measurement by indirect cuff sphygmomanometry. Am J Hypertens 1992; 5: 207–209.
[13] Webb GD. Pitfalls in the measurement of blood pressure. Am J Hypertens 1992; 5: 859–861.
[14] Rose GA, Holland WW, Crowley EA. A sphygmomanometer for epidemiologists. Lancet 1964; I: 296–300.
[15] Wright BM, Dore CF. A random-zero sphygmomanometer. Lancet 1970; I: 337–338.
[16] O'Brien E, Mee F, Atkins N et al. Inaccuracy of the Hawksley random zero sphygmomanometer. Lancet 1990; 330: 1465–1468.
[17] Hense HW. Inaccuracy of the Hawksley random zero sphygmomanometer. Lancet 1991; 337: 556–557.
[18] Fowler G, Jamieson MJ, Lyons D et al. Sphygmomanometers in clinical practice and research. In: O'Brien E, O'Malley K, eds. Handbook of Hypertension. Vol 14. Blood pressure measurement. Amsterdam, London, New York, Tokyo: Elsevier Science Publishers 1991; 72–94.
[19] Jamieson MJ, Webster J, Witte K et al. An evaluation of the A & D UA-751 semi-automated cuff-oscillometric sphygmomanometer. J Hypertens 1990; 8: 377–381.
[20] Hansen KW. How to monitor blood pressure changes in the diabetes clinic: office, home or 24 h-ambulatory recordings? In: Mogensen CE, Standl E, eds. Diabetes Forum Series Vol 4. Concepts for the Ideal Diabetes Clinic. Berlin, New York: Walter de Gruyter 1993; 235–248.
[21] Devereux RB, Pickering TG. Relationship between the level, pattern and variability of ambulatory blood pressure and target organ damage in hypertension. J Hypertension 1991; 9 (suppl. 8): S34–S38.
[22] Coats AJS, Radaelli A, Clark SJ et al. The influence of ambulatory blood pressure monitoring on the design and interpretation of trials in hypertension. J Hypertens 1992; 10: 385–391.
[23] Pickering TG, Blank SG. Blood pressure measurement and ambulatory blood pressure monitoring. Evaluation of available equipment. In: Laragh JH, Brenner BM. Hypertension: Pathophysiology, Diagnosis, and Management. New York: Raven Press, Ltd., 1990; 1429–1441.

[24] Meyer-Sabellek WA. Non-invasive ambulatory blood pressure measurement. In: O'Brien E, O'Malley K, eds. Handbook of Hypertension Vol 14. Blood pressure measurement. Amsterdam, London, New York, Tokyo: Elsevier Science Publishers 1991; 184–217.
[25] Posey JA, Geddes LA, Williams H et al. The meaning of the point of maximim oscillations in cuff pressure in the indirect measurement of blood pressure. Part I. Cardiovasc Res Center Bull 1969; 8: 15–25.
[26] Ramsey II M. Non-invasive automatic determination of mean arterial pressure. Med & Biol Eng & Comput 1979; 17: 11–18.
[27] Geddes LA, Voelz M, Combs C et al. Characterization of the oscillometric method for measuring indirect blood pressure. Ann Biomedical Engineering 1982; 10: 271–280.
[28] Geddes LA. The indirect measurement of blood pressure. In: Cardiovascular Instrumentation. Applicability of New Technology to Biobehavioral Research. US Department of Health and Human Services. Public Health Service, National Institute of Health 1984; 5–19.
[29] Hansen KW, Ørskov H. A plea for consistent reliability in ambulatory blood pressure monitors: a reminder. J Hypertens 1992; 10: 1313–1315.
[30] O'Rourke MF, Gallagher DE. Continuous noninvasive recording of arterial pressure. Am J Hypertens 1992; 5: 857–858.
[31] National High Blood Pressure Education Program Coordinating Committee. National High Blood Pressure Education Program Working Group Report on Ambulatory Blood Pressure Monitoring. Arch Intern Med 1990; 150: 2270–2280.
[32] The Scientific Committee. Consensus document on non-invasive ambulatory blood pressure monitoring. J Hypertens 1990; 8 (suppl. 6): S135–S140.
[33] Pickering TG, O'Brien E. Second international consensus meeting on twenty-four-hour ambulatory blood pressure measurement: consensus and conclusions. J Hypertension 1991; 9 (suppl. 8): S2–S6.
[34] O'Brien E, Petrie J, Littler W et al. The British Hypertension Society protocol for the evaluation of automated and semi-automated blood pressure measuring devices with special reference to ambulatory systems. J Hypertens 1990; 8: 607–619.
[35] Association for the advancement of medical instrumentation: American National Standard for Electronic or automated Sphygmomanometers. Washington DC: AAMI; 1987.
[36] O'Brien E, O'Malley K. Twenty-four-hour ambulatory blood pressure monitoring: a review of validation data. J Hypertens 1990; 8 (suppl. 6): S11–S16.
[37] O'Brien E, Mee F, Atkins N et al. Accuracy of the Del Mar Avionics Pressurometer IV determined by the British Hypertension Society protocol. J Hypertens 1991; 9 (suppl. 5): S1–S7.
[38] O'Brien E, Mee F, Atkins N et al. Accuracy of the Novacor DIASYS 200 determined by the British Hypertension Society protocol. J Hypertens 1991; 9 (suppl. 5): S9–S15.
[39] White WB, Pickering TG, Morganroth J et al. A multicenter evaluation of the A & D TM-2420 ambulatory blood pressure recorder. Am J Hypertens 1991; 4: 890–896.
[40] O'Brien E, Mee F, Atkins N et al. Accuracy of the Takeda TM-2420/TM-2020 determined by the British Hypertension Society protocol. J Hypertens 1991; 9 (suppl. 5): S17–S23.
[41] O'Brien E, Mee F, Atkins N et al. Evaluation of the SpaceLabs 90202 non-invasive ambulatory recorder according to the AAMI Standard and BHS criteria. Human Hypertens 1991; 5: 223–226.
[42] O'Brien E, Mee F, Atkins N et al. Accuracy of the SpaceLabs 90207 determined by the British Hypertension Society Protocol. J Hypertens 1991; 9 (suppl. 5): S25–S31.
[43] O'Brien E, Mee F, Atkins N et al. Accuracy of the CH-Druck/Pressure Scan ERKA ambulatory blood pressure measuring system determined by the British Hypertension Society Protocol. J Hypertens 1991; 10: 1283–1284.
[44] O'Brien E, Mee F, Atkins N et al. Short report: Accuracy of the Profilomat ambulatory blood pressure measuring system determined by the British Hypertension Society Protocol. J Hypertens 1991; 10: 1285–1286.
[45] Coats, AJS, Clark SJ. Validation of ambulatory monitors in special populations. Am J Hypertens 1992; 5: 664–669.

[46] Meyer-Sabellek W, Schulte K-L, Distler A et al. Methodological developments and problems of recorders for automatic, indirect, ambulatory 24-hour monitoring of blood pressure. In: Meyer-Sabellek W, Anlauf M, Gotzen R et al.: Blood Pressure Measurements. New Techniques in Automatic and 24-hour Indirect Monitoring. Darmstadt, New York: Steinkopff Verlag; Springer Verlag 1989; 127–140.
[47] Chung MYW, Smits P, Lenders JWM et al. Reproducilibity of the blood pressure fall at night in healthy normotensive volunteers. J Hypertens 1991; 9 (suppl. 6): S324–S325.
[48] Streitberg B, Meyer-Sabellek W, Baumgart P. Statistical analysis of circadian blood pressure recordings in controlled clinical trials. J Hypertens 1989; 7 (suppl. 3): S11–S17.
[49] Streitberg B, Meyer-Sabellek W, Baumgart P. Smoothing twenty-four-hour ambulatory blood pressure profiles: a comparison of alternative methods. J Hypertens 1990; 8 (suppl. 6): S21–S27.
[50] Staessen J, Celis H, De Cort P et al. Methods for describing the diurnal blood pressure curve. J Hypertens 1991; 9 (suppl. 8): S16–S18.
[51] Coats AJS, Clark SJ, Conway J. Analysis of ambulatory blood pressure data. J Hypertens 1991; 9 (suppl. 8): S19–S21.
[52] Dickson D, Hasford J. 24-hour blood pressure measurement in antihypertensive drug trials: data requirements and methods of analysis. Stat Med 1992; 11: 2147–2158.
[53] White WB. Analysis of ambulatory blood pressure data in antihypertensive drug trials. J Hypertens 1991; 9 (suppl. 1): S27–S32.
[54] Conway J, Coats AJS. Ambulatory blood pressure monitoring in the design of antihypertensive drug trials. J Hypertens 1991; 9 (suppl. 8): S57–S58.
[55] Schwan Å, Eriksson G. Effect on sleep – but not on blood pressure – of nocturnal non-invasive blood pressure monitoring. J Hypertens 1992; 10: 189–194.
[56] Degaute J-P, van de Borne P, Kerhofs M et al. Does non-invasive ambulatory blood pressure monitoring disturb sleep? J Hypertens 1992; 10: 879–885.
[57] Verdecchia P, Schillaci G, Porcellati C. Dippers versus non-dippers. J Hypertens 1991; 9 (suppl. 8): S42–S44.
[58] Berardi L, Chau NP, Chanudet et al. Ambulatory blood pressure monitoring: a critical review of the current methods to handle outliers. J Hypertens 1992; 10: 1243–1248.
[59] Voors AW, Foster TA, Frerichs RR et al. Studies of blood pressure in children, ages 5–14 years, in a total biracial community. The Bogalusa Heart Study. Circulation 1976; 54: 319–327.
[60] Dillon MJ. Blood pressure measurement in childhood. In: O'Brien E, O'Malley K, eds. Handbook of Hypertension. Vol 14. Amsterdam, London, New York, Tokyo: Elsevier Science Publishers 1991; 126–138.
[61] Acheson RM. Blood pressure in a national sample of U. S. adults: Percentile distribution by age, sex and race. Int J Epidemiol 1973; 2: 293–301.
[62] Staessen J, Fagard R, Lijnen P et al. Reference values for ambulatory blood pressure: a meta-analysis. J Hypertens 1990; 8 (suppl. 6): S57–S64.
[63] Palatini P, Pessina AC. A new approach to define the upper normal limits of ambulatory blood pressure. J Hypertens 1990; 8 (suppl. 6): S65–S70.
[64] Nielsen FS, Rossing P, Gall M-A et al. Impaired nocturnal decline in arterial blood pressure in type 2 (non-insulin-dependent) diabetic patients with nephropathy (abstract). Diabetologia 1992; 35 (suppl. 1): A48.
[65] Lindsay RS, Stewart MJ, Nairn IM et al. Diurnal variation of blood pressure is reduced in type 2 diabetic patients with microalbuminuria (abstract). Diabetic Med 1992; 9 (suppl. 2): S39–S40.
[66] Fogari R, Zoppi A, Malamani GD et al. Ambulatory blood pressure monitoring in normotensive and hypertensive type 2 diabetics. Prevalence of impaired diurnal blood pressure patterns. Am J Hypertens 1993; 6: 1–7.
[67] Hansen KW, Mau Pedersen M, Christiansen JS et al. Diurnal blood pressure variations in normo-albuminuric type 1 diabetic patients. J Int Med 1993; 234: 175–180.

[68] Hansen KW, Christensen CK, Andersen PH et al. Ambulatory blood pressure microalbuminuric type 1 diabetic patients. Kidney Int 1992; 41: 847–854.
[69] Moore WV, Donaldson DL, Chonko AM et al. Ambulatory blood pressure in type 1 diabetes mellitus. Comparison to presence of incipient nephropathy in adolescents and young adults. Diabetes 1992; 41: 1035–1041.
[70] Benhamou PY, Halimi S, De Gaudemaris R et al. Early disturbances of ambulatory blood pressure load in normotensive type 1 diabetic patients with microalbuminuria. Diabetes Care 1992; 15: 1614–1619.
[71] Hansen KW, Mau Pedersen M, Marshall SM et al. Circadian variation of blood pressure in patients with diabetic nephropathy. Diabetologia 1992; 35: 1074–1079.
[72] Torffvit O, Agardh C-D. Day and night variation in ambulatory blood pressure in type 1 diabetes mellitus with nephropathy and autonomic neuropathy. J Int Med 1993; 233: 131–137.
[73] Gambardella S, Frontini S, Spallone V et al. Increased left ventricular mass in normotensive diabetic patients with autonomic neuropathy. Am J Hyp 1993; 6: 97–102.

Research methodologies in measurement of platelet function, endothelial proteins, coagulation factors and fibrinolysis

J. Ingerslev

Introduction

Increased morbidity and mortality from atherosclerotic vascular disease are common hallmarks of diabetes mellitus [1–5]. Although not entirely uniform in appearance, micro- and macrovascular complications significantly shorten the life-span of diabetic type I and II patients. Understanding these relationships and preventing the progression of vascular lesions is important. A correlation between increased risk of premature death and presence of nephropathy in diabetes has been demonstrated [6–9], but the true nature of this linkage needs clarification. An increasing number of cross-sectional and longitudinal studies have shown that diabetes is accompanied by atherosclerosis, which – when compared with non-diabetics – progresses more rapidly to disabling and fatal endpoints. Cross-sectional studies have repeatedly indicated that the mechanisms of hemostasis and fibrinolysis in diabetics seem altered in favor of arterial thrombus formation. In the following sections these abnormalities will be summarized and discussed as far as present knowledge allows for, accompanied by descriptions of the relevant components of the hemostatic system likely to be involved in the pathophysiology of diabetic vascular disease. Particular emphasis will be placed on study methodologies. Since early clinical studies in this field were based on patient cohorts less stringently defined then they would be with the demographic classification commonly used today, and since relevant controls were lacking in a number of those studies, the present author also wishes to underscore the importance of these particular sides of clinical hemostasiologic research in diabetes.

Natural and pathological variance of hemostatic factors

The hemostatic variables most extensively studied in relationship to vascular complications in diabetes in the past appear in Table 1. In healthy individuals,

Table 1 Haemostatic parameters reported abnormal in diabetes

Main group	characteristic/function	production site
Platelets	size spontaneous aggregation induced aggregation – ADP – collagen – epinephrine – arachidonic acid markers of platelet release – β-thromboglobulin (β-TG) – platelet factor 4 (PF-4)	megakaryocytes
Plasma proteins of primary haemostasis	von Willebrand factor antigen (vWF: Ag) von Willebrand factor (vWF: RcoF)	Endothelial cells & megakaryocytes
Plasma proteins of the coagulation cascade	fibrinogen factor VII (VII: C) factor VIII (VIII: C)	Liver cells
Fibrinolysis	tissue plasminogen activator (tPA) plasminogen activator inhibitor-1 (PAI-1)	Endothelial cells EC + liver
Markers of activated coagulation	Thrombin-Antithrombin(-III) complex Prothrombin fragment F1+2 Fibrinopeptide A	Plasma

Abbreviations in brackets confer with those used in text and the international literature

the majority of these components vary with sex and age. In the case of the von Willebrand factor/factor VIII complex, variation may even be due to ABO blood group characteristics [13]. Some quantities, or their functional behavior, belong to the class of so-called acute-phase reactants (i. e. vWF, fibrinoylitc components and fibrinogen), implying that significantly raised levels may result from ongoing infectious disease, malignancy, recent physical exercise and other conditions of stress not necessarily related to diabetes per se. Significant natural diurnal variations must also be accounted for. Furthermore, atherosclerosis from causes other than diabetes also shifts the plasmatic levels of proteins like vWF, fibrinogen and fibrinolytic reactants. However, as will be discussed in each case, it has been established that certain proteins change in a characteristic way in parallel to the progression of diabetic vascular complications, suggesting a possible pathophysiological linkage between the development of diabetic atherosclerosis and recurrent arterial microthrombosis.

Brief introduction to platelet functions, coagulation and fibrinolysis

The hemostatic system consists of three major classes of functions: primary hemostatis, coagulation and fibrinolysis. Primary hemostasis, and by inference thrombosis, is initiated by attachment of platelets to injured endothelial cells or subendothelial structures exposed to rapidly flowing blood in vessels where high velocity laminar blood flow conditions exist. In the case of an atherosclerotic vessel wall, platelets bind to the endothelial cell basement membrane or subendothelial tissues where endothelial cells are injured or absent on the fissured atherosclerotic plaque. The von Willebrand factor (vWF), a large multi-adhesive endothelial cell glycoprotein, plays a pivotal role in this context since it is the primary platelet adhesive glue acting through distinct binding epitopes simultaneously binding to exposed vessel

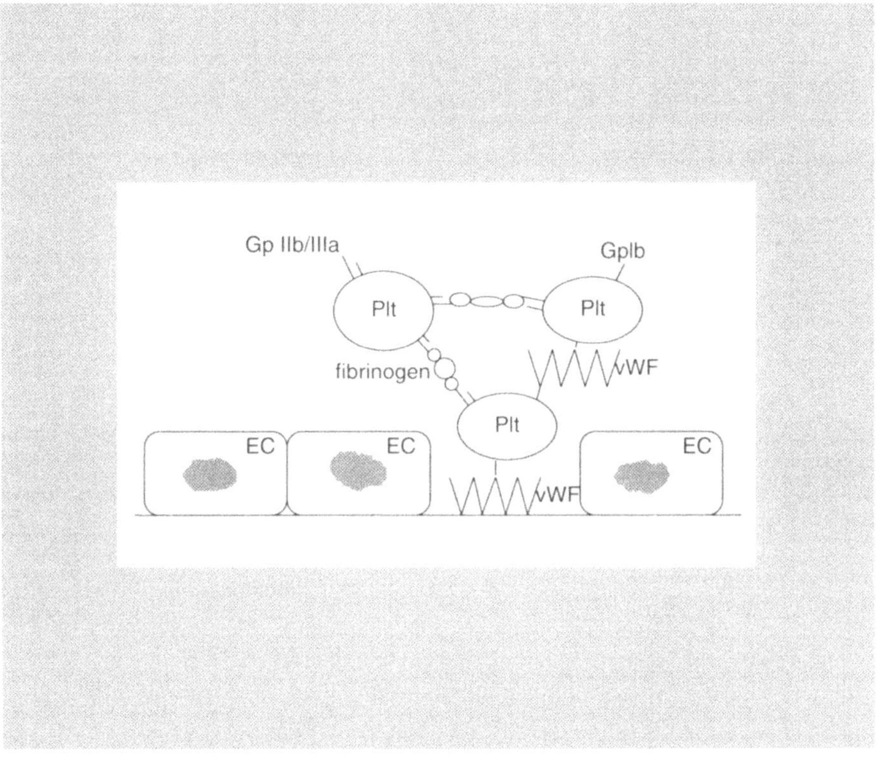

Fig. 1 The mechanisms involved in platelet adhesion and aggregation to a diseased vessel wall. EC: endothelial cell, Plt: platelet, vWF: von Willebrand Factor, GP-Ib: platelet glycoprotein Ib, GP-IIb/IIIa: platelet glycoprotein IIb/IIIa complex, fibrinogen: molecule of fibrinogen spanning between GpIIb/IIIa molecules on adjacent platelets

wall collagens, or other extra-endothelial matter, and glycoprotein Ib of the platelet surface, whereby platelets are anchored to sites devoid of endothelial cell coverage. This process, called platelet adhesion, is followed by the activation of adhered platelets that attract neighbor platelets to accumulate locally through a process called aggregation. As a result, platelets are tied together by bridges of fibrinogen and vWF molecules spanning between platelet surface glycoprotein IIb/IIIa (GpIIb/IIIa) complexes or glycoprotein Ib (GpIb) epitopes on adjacent platelets (Fig. 1). Platelet and endothelial cell surfaces contain phospholipids that support the assembly of coagulation factors, and as a consequence of the coagulation cascade enzyme reactions (Fig. 2), thrombin induces the polymerization of fibrinogen molecules to build up

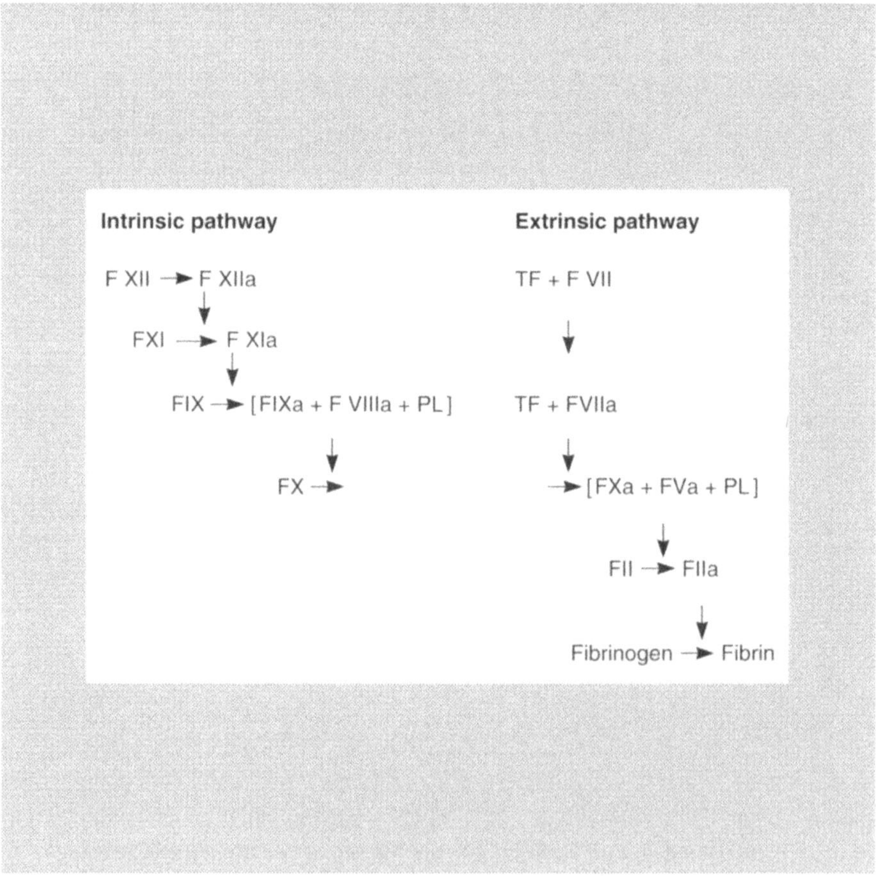

Fig. 2

fibrin in and around platelet aggregates that may eventually constitute the basis for a local mural or occluding thrombus. If attachment is unstable, emboli may occlude the artery downstream of the atherosclerotic lesion. The intrinsic and extrinsic pathways of coagulation are controlled by natural anticoagulants, amongst which the most important known today are the protein S/protein C system, antithrombin-III, heparin co-factor II, and the tissue factor pathway inhibitor (TFPI), each of which distinctly inhibits the coagulation cascade. The majority of coagulation factors and their natural inhibitors are synthesized in the liver, whereas vWF is produced in endothelial cells. The breakdown of preformed fibrin is effected by the fibrinolytic system in which the proenzyme plasminogen is converted into active plasmin after limited proteolysis induced by plasminogen activators. Three major types of plasminogen activators are at work: tissue plasminogen activator (endothelial cell synthesis) t-PA, urokinase plasminogen activator (extravascular cell synthesis) u-PA, and an activating system dependent of the initial contact factors of the intrinsic coagulation system through an – as of yet – incompletely understood mechanism (Fig. 3). An important natural inhibitor of fibrinolysis in blood, denoted the plasminogen activator inhibitor-1 (PAI-1), is synthesized in hepatocytes and endothelial cells. Plasmin is responsible for proteo-

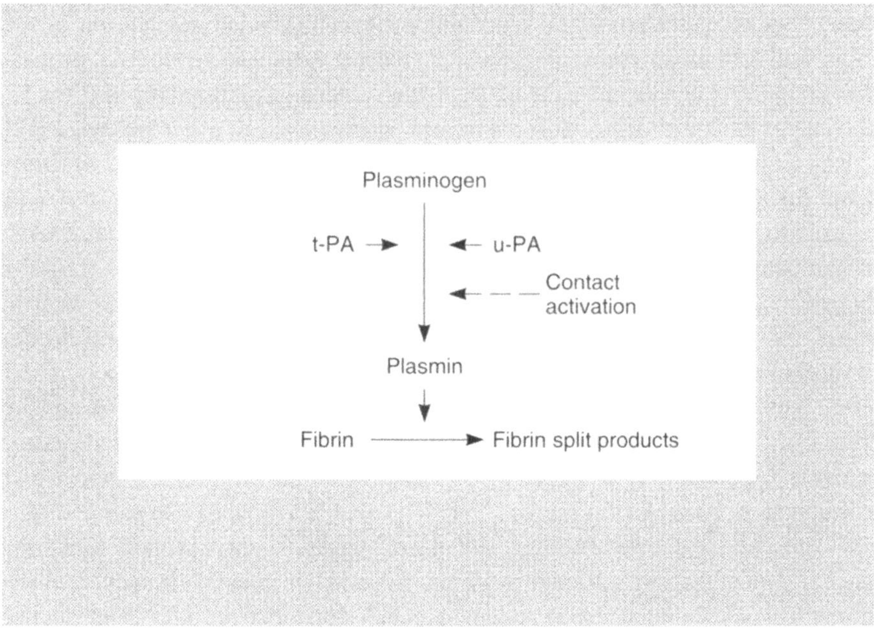

Fig. 3 Activation mechanisms of fibrinolytic pathways

lytical cleavage of fibrin resulting in the formation of various degradation products of fibrin.

The convergence of results of previously published work, based on in vitro analysis, gives the general impression that diabetes is accompanied by multi-faceted abnormalities of the hemostatic system including increased plasmatic levels of von Willebrand factor facilitating platelet adhesion, increased tendency for platelets to form aggregate, diminished endothelial production of anti-aggregatory prostatacyclin (PGI_2), increased coagulation as demonstrated by the presence of markers of coagulation activation like thrombin-antithrombin complexes (TAT), fibrinopeptide A (FPA), and elevated activities of coagulation factors VII and VIII, increased levels of fibrinogen, and reduced fibrinolytic capacity. All of these point to an increased risk of thrombus formation. In some cases, pathological values are more often seen in patients with poor glycemic control or signs of preexisting vascular complications. A number of reviews are available for study.

The involvement of platelets and coagulation in atherosclerosis

The thrombogenic theory of atherosclerosis, as firstly forwarded by Rokitansky in 1852 [14] and rediscovered by Duguid [15], still lends much support. Due to space restrictions in the present context a detailed description of this topic will not be presented. However, recent work points to the primary thrombus as a consistent part of the atherosclerotic plaque [16] and the involvement of fibrin disposition on vessel endothelium in atherosclerosis [17].

Readers of publications in the area reviewed here often meet the term "endothelial dysfunction". This descriptive expression offers no proof with regards to the etiology of mechanisms responsible for altered plasmatic levels of hemostatic endothelial proteins (vWF in particular) in advanced stages of diabetic vascular complications. An accelerated synthesis rate may well be suspected, but prolonged in vivo survival of a particular plasma protein due to diminished natural cleavage in circulation or reduction in number of specific receptors causing internalization and breakdown must also be considered. Furthermore, it is noteworthy that not endothelially-synthesized plasma proteins alone, but also proteins of hepatocellular origin may increase in diabetes (e. g. coagulation factors VII, VIII and fibrinogen). Ongoing studies will attempt to define whether increased synthesis may explain increased plasma concentrations of such proteins. Expression velocity, however, as demonstrable by the amount of specific mRNA, has only recently been studied in relationship with PAI-1, and the target cell compartments that internalize these hemostatic proteins following interaction with their natural receptors are still largely unknown. Until at least some of this has been accomplished, the term "endothelial dysfunction" may raise confusion.

Abnormalities of the hemostatic system in diabetes and methods for analysis

In the following, a number of protein functions and quantities are reported with particular reference to assay methodologies. Readers are advised that early methods were often less accurate than those used today, and that patients were selected according to different standards. Thus, references selected here may not always point out the first investigation that made a significant finding, but rather publications that demonstrated a pathological relationship by stringent clinical, biochemical and analytical criteria. Furthermore, it should be pointed out that results from various laboratories may not prove strictly comparable due to differences in assay methodologies and standardization, and due to heterogeneity of diabetic patient cohorts.

Collection of blood for study

For hemostasiological work, blood is obtained from venipuncture after minimal or no stasis and the first 5 ml of blood is discarded. For investigating platelets, hemostatic components, coagulation and fibrinolysis, trisodium citrate is the primary anticoagulant of choice. For nephelometric methods of protein quantitation however, EDTA plasma is most often recommended. If markers of platelet activation like β-thromboglobulin and platelet factor 4, or plasminogen activator inhibitor-1 (PAI-1) are to be measured, great caution must be taken to avoid activation of platelets in the course of preparation. Hence, inhibitors of platelet activation should be present in the vacuum tube. Specially prepared tubes are available from the manufacturers of the assay kits. Furthermore, blood samples must be kept at around 0 °C until cooling centrifugation is performed, and plasma for study must be pipetted off from the plasma mid-layer in order to prevent an unwanted aspiration of platelets which could contaminate the plasma sample. If a functional assay of plasminogen activator is planned, t-PA must be protected from its rapid degradation in the plasma milieu by using specially prepared tubes containing acidic citrate. Vacuum tubes with acidic citrate are available from the manufacturers of the assay kits. For the collection of blood prior to the assay of fibrinopeptide A, a strong thrombin inhibitor must be present in the aspiration tube. For all other assays reviewed in this article, platelet-poor citrated plasma is used for study, as collected from citrated whole blood obtained after centrifugation at 2000 G for 20 min at ambient temperature or in a cooling centrifuge. For all functional protein assays, plasma should be kept at -80° C if analysis is not performed within a few hours of sampling.

Introductory remarks on laboratory procedures for protein quantitation

When selecting a procedure for determination of given plasma protein, the concentration level of the protein in question is important. In the range of ng/ml to µg/ml, radio-immuno assay, an immuno-radiometric assay, or an enzyme-linked immuno-sorbent assay (ELISA) is generally preferable. If the concentration is in the range of µg/ml to mg/ml, immune electrophoresis or nephelometry may be best suited. The precision of such assays varies greatly, variance being mostly dependent on the quality of the antibodies used, and the principle of analysis. Usually, the coefficient of variation (CV%) for between day analysis in immunoradiometric assays, ELISA's and nephelometry is around 5%, whereas the imprecision of rocket immune electrophoresis is most often near 10%.

The procoagulant function of a protein acting in the coagulation cascade can be recorded by registering its ability to promote coagulation in a plasma base that is complete in every way except for the coagulation factor to be determined (test base: single coagulation factor deficiency plasma). Standardization is based on multiple dilution points of a normal plasma, the activity of which should preferably be calibrated against an international standard for the specific coagulation factor, whenever such a calibrator exists. A double logarithmic plot of the coagulation time recorded for various standard concentrations of the specific coagulation factor serves as the calibration curve into which the coagulation times of each of 4 or more different dilutions of the test sample are plotted either by visual reading or by calculation using a suitable polynomium (most often the least square principle). Alternatively, the function of a procoagulation protein can be estimated by an assay that relies on its protyeolytic properties towards a synthetic peptide containing a peptide bond that is cleavable by the coagulant enzyme in question, or through a coupled enzyme reaction with another coagulation factor and a different zymogen. Close to the cleavage site, the synthetic substrate carries a p-nitroanilin (p-NA) group that is colorless as long as the peptide is uncleaved. When cleavage takes place, the pNA-group turns yellow and a rise in absorbancy at 405 nm will be recorded. This measurement principle, called the amidolytic assay, has been widely used for functional measurement of several human coagulation factors (FVII, FVIII, FIX, FX), factors of the fibrinolytic system (plasminogen, t-PA, PAI-1), and natural anticoagulants (AT-III, protein C). It should be emphasized, that since measurement of coagulant activities is a specialized task that is not routinely performed in most laboratories, it is advisable that such tests are carried out in a laboratory that performs procoagulant assays on a routine basis.

Platelets

Platelets may be studied in numerous ways. The platelet count of whole blood can be estimated using phase-contrast microscopy and a suitable platelet counting chamber. Today, however, platelets are frequently counted electronically using automated equipment for hematological analysis. Here it should be pointed out that the platelet count is based on the electronic recording of single platelets, whereas preformed aggregates of platelets in the sample are not registered. Recently, another type of automated instrument, the FACS (flow assisted cell sorter) analyzer, also called the flow-cytometer has gained increasing interest, since this type of equipment may provide an estimate of the platelet size distribution and, utilizing specific monoclonal antibodies, quantification of various platelet surface markers, the presence of which signify previous platelet activation (e. g. platelet surface glycoprotein 140). This particular option, however, has as yet not been much used in relationship with scientific work related to diabetes. The aggregatory function of platelets may be studied in vitro by their spontaneous tendency to form lumps (spontaneous aggregation) or their aggregatory response to certain chemical stimuli, called aggregation agonists. Indirectly, plasma markers of in vivo platelet α-granule release, like β-thromboglobulin (β-TG) and platelet factor 4 (PF-4), agents that promote aggregation (platelet synthesized thromboxane B_2) or compounds protective against aggregation (endothelially synthesized prostacyclin PGI_2) may also be measured (review, see [11]).

Platelets in diabetes

Numerous publications have pointed out that platelets are hyperfunctional in diabetics, as firstly reported in 1972 by Kwaan et al. [18]. Theoretically, platelet adhesion studies should be of great interest. A number of early reports dealt with platelet adhesion to a glass surface, a methodology bearing the name platelet retention. Today this method is regarded as less useful, since the glass surface is unphysiologic. Platelet adhesion to a biologically relevant surface like denuded arterial wall subendothelium is quite difficult to perform and no large-scale studies have been reported in connection with diabetes. Studies of platelet function and biochemical markers in the platelet functional state have frequently been reviewed in the past [11, 19–23]. However, platelet function studies have suffered problems since standardization is poor, precision low, and significant intraindividual day-to-day variance must be accounted for. In consequence, conflicting results have quite often been produced. Furthermore, platelet behavior is highly influenced by widely-used prescriptions like acetylsalicylic acid and drugs belonging to the group of NSAID's. Applying a meta-analytical approach, however, it can be assumed that platelets in diabetics are hypersensitive to platelet aggregation inducers like ADP, collagen, thrombin and arachidonic acid, even if data is insufficient to draw clear conclusions about the linkage between in vitro platelet aggregatory reactivity and vascular complications. A recent study found that platelet activity towards collagen increased in microalbuminuric patients [24], whereas platelets from patients with manifest albuminuria were no different from normal platelets. It has been speculated that increased platelet aggregation activity in diabetes may be due to increased binding of fibrinogen to diabetic platelets [25] compared to normal platelets. Further, is has been questioned whether the stimuli of platelet aggregation by the arachidonic acid pathway or by thrombin are the more relevant [26] in diabetes. Platelet survival is abnormally short in diabetics.

Methodologies of platelet aggregation

Platelet aggregation studies are performed using the aggregometer, as first reported by Born [27]. In principle, platelet rich plasma or – using a specialized equipment – whole blood, is investigated within two hours of venipuncture. After exposure to several, often 3–5 different, concentrations of a platelet-aggregation-inducing agent like adenosine di-phosphate, platelet activating factor, collagen, thrombin, or arachidonic acid, aggregation in each experiment is recorded as a function of light transmission that increases concomitantly with the diminishment of the plasma turbidity that results when lumps of platelets build up. Manufacturers of equipment for platelet aggregation studies often devise a particular set-up that is most favorably used with their brand of instrument. Since no "gold standard" exists for platelet aggregation procedures and since several types of instruments exist, readers are recommended to seek advice with manufacturers of such instruments and with the local coagulationist. Platelet aggregation is laborious, operator-dependent and -demanding, and only a few patients can be studied during the working day by one full-time technician. As mentioned above, a large intra-subject variability in the response may be found, making interpretation of abnormal results somewhat dubious.

A particular assay for measurement of the function of von Willebrand factor (vWF), called the ristocetin co-factor assay (vWF : R-CoF), utilizes an unexplained ability of the antibiotic, ristocetin, to promote binding of von Willebrand factor to platelet surface glycoprotein Ib. A qualitative assay for this function of von Willebrand factor is performed in the aggregometer utilizing formalin-fixed or freeze-dried platelets that are unable to activate and aggregate. The passive agglutination of platelets is dependent on the amount and quality of von Willebrand factor present in the plasma sample. However, today this assay is rarely used in hemostasiological research of diabetes.

Circulating markers of platelet activation

When platelets are activated in vivo, α-granules of the platelet empty and (amongst others) two proteins specifically indicating platelet activation, β-TG and PF-4, are released. Both of these can be quantitated using a specific radio-immune assay or ELISA, and various series of investigations in diabetes have demonstrated elevated levels of β-TG and PF-4 in diabetes (review, [11, 28].

von Willebrand factor

Numerous studies have detected increased levels of vWF in diabetics [11, 29–33]. Recent cross-sectional investigations have revealed that vWF is increased in type I [34] and type II [35] diabetics, and levels are highest when overt albuminuria is present. In a longitudinal study, 94 patients were followed for 9–59 months. Follow-up analysis revealed that vWF increased in patients who developed a pathological urinary albumin excretion [36]. Increased risk of cardiovascular events were seen in patients with high levels of vWF in whom a pathological urinary albumin excretion was also found.

Readers are advised that in publications prior to 1986, von Willebrand factor was most often designated Factor VIII related antigen, abbreviated FVIII : RAg. Today vWF protein mass is called vWF : Ag, whereas the platelet agglutinating activity is denoted vWF : RcoF [37]. vWF is a large glycoprotein, up to 12×10^6 Da in size, that is synthesized in endothelial cells [38] and megakaryocytes [39]. vWF in plasma and platelets appears as a set of differently sized multimers constructed with a variable number of repeats (n = 4–50) of the 225,000 Da subunits that are tied together by disulphide bonds. Along with the polypeptide, several specific epitopes exist amongst which some are found that bind to collagen, platelet glycoprotein Ib and platelet glycoprotein IIb/IIIa. The importance of these for the biological functions served by vWF has been demonstrated, in particular in relation to platelet function in primary hemostasis (adhesion and aggregation), results here are equally relevant for pathology of thrombus formation. The normal plasma concentration of vWF is around 10 mg/l, but most often results are expressed as relative arbitrary units. Unitage (normal 1.00) is defined as the content of vWF in one ml of plasmapool from a large number healthy persons. Preferably calibration should be performed against a primary international standard (2nd International Standard for plasma factor VIII and von Willebrand factor, National Institute for Biological Standards and Control, Potters Bar, Hertfordshire, UK). In early work, vWF was measured by the rocket immune electrophoresis technique, as devised by Laurell [40], in which standard and test material are applied to separate wells punched out of an agarose electrophoresis gel containing a heterologous (rabbit) antibody to human vWF. During electrophoresis, vWF in standard and test sample proteins moves by electrical forces towards the anode in the gel, where a rocket-like precipitation arch is formed by the collision of vWF with the gel anti-vWF antibody. The height of the rocket is proportional to the amount of vWF present in the sample. This measuring principle has been widely used for the determination of vWF : Ag in plasma. An important limitation is the imprecision of this quantitation principle. As a consequence, more precise quantitation methods have been developed based on the enzyme-linked immuno-sorbent essay (ELISA) principle [41–42], which determines the mass of plasma vWF with an imprecision of around 5–6% (CV%).

Coagulation cascade factors

Coagulation factor VII

Although increased activity of coagulation factor VII was detected as early as 1979 [43], and later confirmed by others [44–46], an important epidemiological relationship between an elevated activity of coagulation factor VII (VII : C) and the development of coronary heart disease was reported by the Northwick Park study [47]. Procoagulant Factor VII (VII : C) can be measured via the tissue factor dependent pathway utilizing a one-stage coagulation assay, or by chromogenic analysis using the amidolytic principle. It should be pointed out that various types of tissue factor may produce different coagulometric results [48]. In order to study whether activation of factor VII is present (VIIa), the ratio is calculated for factor VII procoagulant activity (VII : C) against factor VII antigen (VII : Ag) as measured by ELISA [48].

Coagulation factor VIII

Factor VIII procoagulant activity, today denoted VIII : C, stems from the hepatocyte [49]. In circulation, factor VIII is bound to vWF, which serves as a carrier, protecting it against random proteolysis. Hence, vWF is responsible for the length of the circulating half-life of factor VIII [50], and it is reasonable to assume that fluctuations in factor VIII in the non-hemophilic person predominantly reflect changes in vWF. Numerous investigators have demonstrated that factor VIII is increased in diabetics, as selected by various criteria [11], but that results are somewhat less uniform than for vWF.

Methodologies: Factor VIII can be estimated using a one-stage procoagulant assay (VIII : C) following the general guidelines described above, or by amidolytic assay in which the endpoint is conversion of factor X to its activated form, factor Xa. In order to establish a primary in-house plasma pool standard, an international standard is recommendable (2nd International standard for plasma factor VIII, NISBC, Potters Bar UK). One must bear in mind that a rather high imprecision (CV% ≅ 15–20%) will be encountered. Factor VIII may also be quantitated by the antigen reactive material (VIII : Ag) in an ELISA system, utilizing antibodies from plasma of patients with severe hemophilia A in which a high titer antibody against factor VIII has resulted from treatment with factor VIII concentrate [51]. Suitable antibodies are, however, not commercially available, and only few laboratories perform this assay routinely. Its imprecision is aroung 6% (CV%).

Fibrinogen

It has been unequivocally established that plasma fibrinogen is elevated in diabetes, where its magnitude presumably reflects increased cardiovascular risk as assessed in the Framingham [1] and Northwick Park [47] studies, and in more recent investigations [45, 52, 53].

Fibrinogen, a 340 kDa plasma glycoprotein containing ≅ 3% carbohydrate in normal individuals, is the principle substrate from thrombin. Its construction is complex consisting of a dimer linked by disulphide bonds. Each of the two monomers is formed by three heterologous peptide chains held together by disulphide bonds. When exposed to thrombin, an important off-cleavage of small N-terminal fragments called fibrinopeptides A and B precedes other cleavage exposing polymerization sites in the central regions of fibrinogen. These subsequently react with carboxy-terminal regions of adjacent fibrinogen molecules, leading to one-dimensional polymerization of thrombin-modified fibrinogen molecules. Eventually, tri-dimensional cross-linking of monomeric fibrin is facilitated by the action of coagulation factor XIII.

Fibrinogen is synthesized in the liver. The concentration of fibrinogen in plasma from healthy persons is 2–4 g/l. Traditionally, fibrinogen is measured utilizing either its functional coagulant properties in the presence of thrombin, in the methodology proposed by Clauss [54], or by its antigenic reactivity against monospecific antibodies utilizing the rocket immunelectrophoresis technique of Laurell [40], or nephelometry. In the Clauss principle, a fixed amount of thrombin is added to various dilutions of plasma and standard fibrinogen solution. The coagulation time of each sample is then recorded. Calculation is based on double logarithmic plots of time versus concentration, as mentioned above. A different quantitation principle was recently developed in which fibrinogen is derived as a function of the signal amplitude in a pro-thrombin time reaction in the coagulometer, giving a quite precise estimate of fibrinogen. Standardization is important in fibrinogen measurements. A number of calibrators and control plasmas are available from commercial sources. It is important to observe whether the standard label value refers to one or both of the recording principles (functional or antigenic fibrinogen).

Fibrinolysis

Fibrinolysis (recent review [55]) is precipitated by the action of plasmin on the fibrin network. From its proenzymatic form, called plasminogen, plasmin is derived by the proteolytic attack of plasminogen activators of which two major classes are well known, tissue plasminogen activator and urokinase-type plasminogen activator. In addition, an activating system relating to the contact-phase constituents of intrinsic coagulation has been detected as mentioned above. The steps involved are issues of debate [55]. Plasmin also exhibits proteolytic activity towards other plasma proteins like factor VIII and von Willebrand factor.

Activators and inhibitors of fibrinolysis

Tissue plasminogen activator (t-PA) is synthesized in endothelium from which it is either exported to circulating blood or stored in the subendothelium. t-PA is thought be the most important plasminogen activator in the local vascular environment, and its release from the endothelial cells seems to be increased where a local thrombus is formed. t-PA is a 70,000 Da large polypeptide occurring as a single-chain serine protease. Several isotypes of this protein have been found. The other major plasminogen activator, denoted urokinase (u-PA), presumably stems from several different extravascular tissues from where it is brought to the blood stream and cleared by renal excretion. It was first detected in urine and its name was derived from this finding, regardless of its role in the plasma fibrinolytic activity. Recent studies have revealed that u-PA exists in numerous different types of cells and its physiologic role outside of the vascular compartment seems closely linked to cell migration in health and disease. In the plasma milieu, however, the importance of u-PA is still less-well understood. From investigations attempting to describe the relative contribution of t-PA and u-PA in plasma, it seems that u-PA may be responsible for around 50% of the total fibrinolytic activator capacity in plasma. The relative importance of u-PA, t-PA or other plasminogen activating substances (like the factor XII dependent activator) in diabetic fibrinolysis is unknown.

An inhibitor of plasminogen activation called plasminogen activator inhibitor 1 (PAI-1) has been discovered during the last decade. Synthesis takes place in endothelial and liver cells. PAI-1 blocks the function of t-PA by complex formation, and this protein has gained high interest since increased levels have often been detected in relationship to spontaneous familial thrombosis. Elevated PAI-1 has been found in diabetics [58–60], where it presumably accounts for the reduced functional activity of global fibrinolysis. Another inhibitor of plasminogen activation, denoted PAI-2, is particularly increased during pregnancy, but it is unlikely that PAI-2 has any importance in diabetes.

A number of studies have shown that fibrinolysis, as determined by functional t-PA or fibrin-plate methods, is weakened in diabetes, particularly in the obese type II diabetic. These results have been summarized in reviews [11, 56, 57]. From the numerous clinical studies reviewed, normal fibrinolysis is not infrequent in diabetes, in particular in type I DM males. Normal or supra-normal quantities of t-PA antigen in plasma have often been reported in diabetes, making the suppression of the fibrinolytic activity difficult to understand at first glance. Large variations have been seen in investigations of different groups and cohorts of diabetics. However, investigations in recent years have pointed to the crucial role of increased levels of the natural inhibitor of t-PA function, PAI-1, in diabetes. It is thought that PAI-1 is an important link in the suppression of fibrinolysis in diabetes [55, 58, 60]. Up-regulation of hepatic PAI-1 synthesis may be caused by insulin [61], and – at the endothelial level – possibly by hyperglycemia [62].

Methodologies: The overall functional fibrinolytic activity in plasma can be studied in various ways. Euglobulin lysis time, a method often used in the past but much less popular today, relies on the ability of plasminogen activators present in the plasma sample to resolve a fibrin clot formed in the same plasma sample. Hence, the endpoint of analysis is the time span for an established clot to undergo lysis aided by its own fibrinolytic pathways. This test, however, demands continuous supervision by the technician, and the risk of bias hampers its potential use. In the fibrin plate method, a (fibrino-)lysis zone in preformed bovine fibrin is measured after its exposure to a fixed volume of patients plasma incubated inside the bovine fibrin for a given period of time (20–24 h) at 37 °C. This method records the overall fibrinolytic activity of the test sample but suffers from the lack of an exact control, and a high intra-individual variation has also been found (unpublished observation).

Today, most work in fibrinolysis is performed utilizing either ELISA for quantitation of the antigenic amount of a fibrinolytic component, or chromogenic (amidolytic) assays that determine its functional activity. Early chromogenic methods for determination of t-PA and PAI-1 suffered from imprecision due to several obstacles of analysis. In this context, attention has been paid to the fact that plasma contains a variable mixture of complexes of the two components and that t-PA is notoriously unstable. Guidelines for laboratory practice in this field have been presented [63]. A solution to these difficulties was found by Petersen and coworkers [64] utilizing ELISA technology in which t-PA is extracted by a monoclonal antibody followed by recording of the amidolytic activity of immuno-retained t-PA. Recently, another assay has been reported that measures functional PAI-1 by using a two-site ELISA in which the primary monoclonal antibody is specific for PAI-1, and, after saturating retained PAI-1 with urokinase, an urokinase specific monoclonal antibody is used to detect the amount of urokinase complexed with PAI-1 [65]. In this publication, readers will find a complete list of references for all recently published methods for measuring t-PA and PAI-1. As mentioned above, the antigenic amount of t-PA present in plasma can also be quantitated by a two-site ELISA with a high specificity for t-PA [66]. However, antigen levels do not seem to reflect the biological function of t-PA, as mentioned above. It is likely that u-PA will gather some interest in studies of the diabetic patient, since specific assays for this fibrinolytic activator have recently been developed. However, to the knowledge of this author, no clinical studies on u-PA in relationship with diabetic fibrinolysis have yet been reported. A number of commercial single component assays of fibrinolysis are available from several companies.

The reader is advised that reference intervals in the study of fibrinolytic parameters are generally much broader than those usually seen in clinical biochemistry. This may be due to an imprecision of the assays used or to a large normal variation in healthy people. Since the variation from day to day is also rather large, unknown factors in the regulation of the plasma levels of fibrinolytic factors must also be given attention. In the clinical laboratory setting, overall variation complicates the diagnostic use of fibrinolysis in patients with abnormal tendency to thrombosis [67].

Markers of in vivo enhanced coagulation

Prothrombin fragment 1 + 2, thrombin-antithrombin complex and fibrinopeptide A

When coagulation takes place, the consequence of the activation of prothrombin to thrombin can be registered by the simultaneous increase in the cleavage products of prothrombin, called prothrombin fragments F1 + 2 (F1 + 2). At present, the literature lacks significant information on F1 + 2 in diabetes. The natural inhibitor of thrombin, antithrombin-III, will interact with newly formed thrombin by the formation of an inactive complex, called the thrombin-antithrombin complex (TAT). In the few studies carried out, elevated TAT levels have been observed in diabetic patients [53, 58, 60], in particular in type II diabetics and patients with poor glycemic control. During the process of fibrin formation, activation peptides A and B are cleaved off the fibrinogen molecule. Fibrinogen peptide A (FpA) has proven a useful marker of in vivo fibrin generation in diseases with enhanced in vivo coagulation [69].

Methodologies: Prothrombin fragment F1 + 2 can be measured by ELISA [70], and TAT-complex recording utilizes the same measurement principle [71]. Both assays are available from Behringwerke (Behring AG, Marburg, Germany). FpA may be recorded by non-isotopic methods. An ELISA for FpA is available from Stago (Asnieres-sur-Seine, France, or local branches).

Thrombomodulin

Although thrombomodulin (TM) is an endothelially synthesized protein, and in this context relates more to t-PA and vWF, its natural function belongs to the actions of thrombin, and, for this reason, a summary of very recent experiences regarding its position in diabetic research will be given within the frame of markers of hypercoagulation. TM acts as a natural inhibitor of thrombin on the surface of endothelial cells, where thrombin is bound and inactivated by TM [72]. Simultaneously, the TM-thrombin complex introduces the activation of protein C that, in conjunction with protein S, forms an enzymatic complex (the protein C-S complex) that irreversibly cleaves coagulation factors V abd VIII (the pathology of protein C and S in relationship with diabetes is relatively unclear at present). TM is abnormal in a variety of disease states, including diabetes, where hyperactive coagulation has been identified by other means [73]. In 56 undefined diabetics of Japanese origin, plasma TM was significantly raised in 30%, and a significant correlation to levels of vWF was found. These early observations predict that future research of TM involvement in diabetes will be a worthwhile study object.

Recommendations for future clinical studies

The diagnostic entity of diabetes mellitus includes a variety of heterogeneous disease states as seen from biochemical and clinical perspectives. Although hyperglycemia is a common hallmark, the entity is comprised of both patients with complete lack of functional insulin (type I) and patients with hyperinsulin/insulin resistance (type II). Obesity is more frequent in the latter. In the course of the lifetime of the diabetic patient, numerous stages of complications may set in, affecting smaller or larger arteries in various compartments of circulation. The glycemic control of patients may vary considerably. In the literature, relatively ill-defined groups of diabetic patients have often been compared with healthy volunteers who were much younger (and hence, less atherosclerotic) than the diabetic patients. Since it is well known that the factors of the hemostatic and fibrinolytic system are subject to large variation with age and sex, the present author wishes to stress the importance of a few demographic characteristics that deserve consideration for the younger investigator planning a study of hemostasiologic variables in diabetes:

1. sex- and age matching of study and control persons
2. patient's renal albumin excretion levels
3. glycemic control characteristics
4. coexistence of other disease states like hypertension, veno-occlusive diseases, infections, malignant conditions, etc.
5. sampling time (of day) and previous exercise
6. medications
7. body mass index

Concluding remarks

Numerous publications during the last 10–15 years have amply demonstrated a wide array of disturbances in the hemostasiologic components, signifying an increased risk of thrombosis in diabetes mellitus and its complications. Since increased risk of premature cardiovascular death threatens the life expectancy of the patient with diabetes (type II in particular), a linkage of hemostatic system abnormalities and the clinical endpoint of this disease seems obvious. For further clarification, homologous patient groups of smaller sample size may be preferable to larger-scale investigations of irregularly-defined patient cohorts. The large amount of information available regarding the relationship to diabetes prompts the medical profession to introduce measures that prevent the development of vascular disease in the diabetic. Prospective long-term studies are highly important for the assessment of such markers which may prove helpful in defining risk of the individual patient in future work. Likewise, prospective trials of intervention attempting to reduce the risks associated with development of vascular complications are necessary. It seems overwhelmingly evident that longitudinal monitoring of hemostasiologic parameters will be useful in such studies. In preparing this paper, it was anticipated that the reader would ask: Which, then? The answer is clearly: some, but not all! The author suggests the use of a set of analyses that are relatively easy to perform, precise and illustrative of the hyperfunctional condition of primary hemostasis and coagulation. In this context, vWF : Ag, fibrinogen and a marker of activated coagulation like prothrombin fragment F1 + 2 seems relevant, but only if the study design employs stringency with regard to the pertinent classification of patients.

References

[1] Kannel WB, McGee DL. Diabetes and cardiovascular disease. The Framingham Study. JAMA 1979; 241: 2035–2038.

[2] Morrish NJ, Staqvens LK, Head J et al. A prospective study of mortality among middle-aged diabetic patients (the London Cohort of the WHO Multinational Study of Vascular Disease in Diabetics) I: causes and death rates. Diabetologia 1990; 33: 538–541.

[3] Krolewski AS, Kosinski EJ, Warram JH et al. Magnitude and determinants of coronary artery disease in juvenile-onset insulin dependent diabetes mellitus. Am J Cardiol 1987; 59: 750–755.

[4] Donahue RP, Abbott RD, Reed DM et al. Postchallenge glucose concentration and coronary heart disease in men of Japanese ancestry: Honolulu Heart Program. Diabetes 1987; 36: 689–692.

[5] Melton IJ, Makin KM, Palumbo PJ et al. Incidence of clinical peripheral vascular disease in a population based cohort of diabetic patients. Diabetes Care 1980; 3: 650–654.

[6] Jarrett RJ, Viberti GC, Argyropolous A et al. Microalbuminuris predicts mortality in non-insulin dependent diabetes. Diab Med 1984; 1: 17–19.

[7] Mogensen CE. Microalbuminuria predicts clinical proteinuria and early mortality in maturity onset diabetes. N Engl J Med 1984; 310: 356–360.
[8] Borch-Johansen K, Anderssen PK, Deckert T. The effect of proteinuria on relative mortality in type 1 (insulin-dependent) diabetes mellitus. Diabetologia 1985; 28: 596.
[9] Borch-Johansen K, Kreiner S. Proteinuria: value as predictor of cardiovascular mortality in insulin-dependent diabetes mellitus. Br Med J 1987; 294: 1651–1654.
[10] Greaves M, Preston FE. Haemostatic abnormalities in diabetes. In: Jarrett RJ, ed. Diabetes and heart disease. Amsterdam: Elsevier Science Publishers B. V., 1990; 47–80.
[11] Ostermann H, van de Loo J. Factors of the hemostatic system in diabetic patients. A survey of controlled studies. Haemostasis 1986; 16: 386–416.
[12] Colwell JA. Platelets endothelium and diabetic vascular disease. Paris: Diabete et Metabolisme, 1988; 14: 512–518.
[13] Gill JC, Endes-Brooks J, Bauer PJ et al. The effect of ABO blood group on the diagnosis of von Willebrand disease. Blood 1987; 1691–1695.
[14] Rokitanski K. A manual of Pathological Anatomy (translated by G. E. Day). London: Sydenham Society, 1852; 271–273.
[15] Duguid JB. Thrombosis as a factor in the pathogenesis of coronary atherosclerosis. J Pathol 1946; 58: 207–212.
[16] Schwartz CJ, Valente AJ, Kelley JL et al. Thrombosis and development of atherosclerosis. Rokitanski revisited. Semin Thromb Hemost 1988; 14: 189–195.
[17] Thomsen WD, Smith EB. Atherosclerosis and the coagulation system. J Pathol 1989; 159: 97–106.
[18] Kwaan HC, Colwell JA, Cruz A et al. Increased platelet aggregation in diabetes mellitus. J Lab Clin Mede 1972; 80: 236–246.
[19] Sagel J, Colwell JA, Crook et al. Increased platelet aggregation in early diabetes mellitus. Ann Int Med 1975; 82: 733–738.
[20] Mustard JF, Packham MA. Platelets and Diabetes mellitus. (Editorial) N Engl J Med 1984; 311: 665–667.
[21] Colwell JA, Winocour PD, Halushka PV. Do platelets have anything to do with diabetic microvascular disease? Diabetes 1983; 32 (Suppl. 2): 14–19.
[22] Banga JD, Sixma JJ. Diabetes Mellitus, vascular disease and thrombosis. Clinics in Haematology 1986; 15: 456–492.
[23] Kwaan HC. Changes in blood coagulation, platelet function and plasminogen-plasmin system in diabetes. Diabetes 1992; 41 (Suppl. 2): 32–35.
[24] O'Donnell MJ, Le Guen CA, Lawson N et al. Platelet behaviour and haemostatic variables in type 1 (insulin-dependent) diabetic patients with and without albuminuria. Diab Med 1991; 8: 624–628.
[25] DiMinno G, Silver MJ, Cerbone AM et al. Platelet fibrinogen binding in diabetes mellitus. Diabetes 1986; 35: 182–185.
[26] Winocour P. Platelet abnormalities in diabetes mellitus. Diabetes 1992; 41 (Suppl. 2): 26–31.
[27] Born GVR. Aggregation of blood platelets by adenosine diphosphate and its reversal. Nature 1962; 194: 927–929.
[28] O'Donnell MJ, Le Guen CA, Lawson N et al. Platelet behaviour and haemostatic variables in type 1 (insulin-dependent) diabetic patients with and without albuminuria. Diab Med 1991; 8: 624–628.
[29] Porta M. von Willebrand factor as an indicator of endothelial dysfunction in diabetic microangiopathy: studies in vivo. Diabete et Metabolisme 1988; 14: 523–526.
[30] Fischer BM, Quin JD, Rumley A et al. Effects of scute insulin-induced hypoglycaemia on haemostasis, fibrinolysis and haemorheology in insulin-dependent diabetic subjects and control subjects. Clin Sci 1991; 80: 525–531.
[31] Silveira AMV, Sjöberg S, Blombäck M et al. von Willebrand factor antigen in plasma and urine in patients with type II (insulin-dependent) diabetes mellitus with and without nephropathy. J Diab Compl 1992; 6: 89–95.

[32] Gamba G, Solerte SB, Grignani G et al. Haemostatic variables, serum lipid abnormalities and vascular complications in diabetes mellitus: a 5 year follow-up study. Blut 1988; 56: 257–260.
[33] Nowak-Göttl U, Kreuz WD, Besier E et al. Thrombozytenfunktion bei Kindern mit diabetes mellitus typ I. Querschnittstudie. Monatsschr Kinderheilkd 1991; 139: 821–825.
[34] Jensen T. Increased plasma concentration of von Willebrand factor in insulin dependent diabetics with incipient nephropathy. Brit Med J 1989; 298: 27–28.
[35] Schmitz A, Ingerslev J. Haemostatic measures in type 2 diabetic patients with microalbuminuria. Diabetic Med 1990; 7: 521–525.
[36] Stehouwer CDA, Nauta JJP, Zeldenrust GC et al. Urinary albumin excretion, cardiovascular disease and endothelial dysfunction in non-insulin dependent diabetes mellitus. Lancet 1992; 340: 319–323.
[37] Marder VJ, Mannucci PM, Firkin BG et al. Standard nomenclature for factor VIII and von Willebrand factor. A recommendation by the International Committee on Thrombosis and Haemostasis. Thromb Haemostas 1985; 54: 871–872.
[38] Jaffe EA, Hoyer LW, Nachman R. Synthesis of antihemophilic factor antigen by human endothelial cells. J Clin Invest 1973; 52: 2757–2764.
[39] Nachman RL, Jaffe EA. Subcellular platelet factor VIII antigen and von Willebrand factor. J Exp Med 1975; 141: 1101–1113.
[40] Laurell CB. Quantitative estimation of proteins by electrophoresis in agarose gel containing antibodies. Anal Biochem 1966; 15: 454–462.
[41] Short PE, Williams CE, Enayat S et al. Factor VIII-related antigen: an improved enzyme linked immuno assay. Med Lab Sci 1982; 39: 351–355.
[42] Ingerslev J. A sensitive ELISA for von Willebrand factor antigen (vWF: Ag). Scand J Clin Lab Invest 1987; 47: 143–149.
[43] Fuller JH, Keen H, Jarrett RJ. Haemostatic variables associated with diabetes mellitus and its complications. Br Med J 1979; II: 964–966.
[44] Christie M, Fritschi J, Lammle B et al. Fifteen coagulation and fibrinolysis parameters in diabetes mellitus and in patients with vasculopathy. Thromb Haemostas 1984; 523: 138–143.
[45] Ford I, Singh TP, Kitchen S et al. Activation of coagulation in diabetes mellitus in relation to presence of vascular complications. Diab Med 1991; 8: 322–329.
[46] Carmassi F, Morale M, Puccetti R et al. Coagulation and fibrinolytic system in insulin dependent diabet mellitus. Thromb Res 1992; 67: 643–654.
[47] Meade TW, Brozovic M, Chakrabarti RR et al. Haemostatic function and ischaemic heart disease: Principal results of the Northwick Park Study. Lancet 1986; 2: 533–537.
[48] Kitchen S, Malia RG, Preston FE. A comparison of methods for the measurement of activated factor VII. Thromb Haemostas 1992; 68: 301–305.
[49] Ingerslev J, Sloth Christiansen B, Heickendorff et al. Synthesis of factor VIII by human hepatocytes in culture. Thromb Haemostas 1988; 60: 387–391.
[50] Tuddenham EDG, Lane RS, Rotblat F et al. Response to infusions of polyelectrolyte fractionated human factor VIII concentrate in human haemophilia A and von Willebrand's disease. Brit J Haematol 1982; 52: 259–267.
[51] Ingerslev J, Stenbjerg S. Enzyme linked immuno sorbent assay (ELISA) for the measurement of factor VIII coagulant antigen (CAg) using haemophilic antibodies. Brit J Haematol 1986; 62: 325–332.
[52] Shiabi ZK, Konen JC, McCormick CP. Plasma fibrinogen levels in type II diabetics. Clin Physiol Biochem 1990; 8: 297–300.
[53] Carmassi F, Morale M, Pucetti R et al. Coagulation and fibrinolytic system impairment in insulin dependent diabetes mellitus. Thromb Res 1992; 67: 643–654.
[54] Claus A von. Gerinnungsphysiologische Schnellmethode zur Bestimmung des Fibrinogens. Acta Haematol (Basel) 1957; 17: 237–241.
[55] Bachmann F. Fibrinolysis. In: Verstaete M, Vermylen J, Lijnen R et al., eds. Thrombosis and Haemostasis 1987. Leuven, Belgium: Leuven University Press 1987; 227–265.

[56] Gough SCL, Grant PJ. The fibrinolytic system in diabetes. Diab Med 1991; 8: 898–905.
[57] Vague P, Raccah D, Juhan-Vague I. Hemobiology, vascular disease, and diabetes with special reference to impaired fibrinolysis. Metabolism 1992; 41 (Suppl. 1): 2–6.
[58] Davi G, Violo F, Catalano C et al. Increased plasminogen activator inhibitor antigen levels in diabetic patients with strable angina. Blood Coagul Fibrinolysis 1991; 2: 41–45.
[59] Spannagl M, Drummer C, Fröschl C et al. Plasmatic factors of haemostasis remain essentially unchanged except for PAI activity during n-3 fatty acid intake in type I diabetes mellitus. Blood Coagul Fibrinolysis 1991; 2: 256–259.
[60] Donders SHJ, Lustermans FAT, van Wersch JWJ. Low order correlations of lipoprotein (a) with other blood lipids and with coagulation and fibrinolytic parameters in diabetic patients. Blood Coagul Fibrinolysis 1992; 3: 249–256.
[61] Alessi MC, Juhan-Vague I, Kooistra T et al. Insulin stimulates the synthesis of plasminogen activator inhibitor 1 by the human hepatocellular cell line HepG2. Thromb Haemostas 1988; 60: 491–494.
[62] Maiello M, Boeri D, Podestra F et al. Increased expression of tissue plasminogen activator and its inhibitor and reduced fibrinolysis potential of human endothelial cells cultured in elevated glucose. Diabetes 1992; 41: 1009–1015.
[63] Kluft C, Verheijen JH. Leiden Fibrinolysis Working Party: Blooed collecting and handling procedures for assessment of tissue-type plasminogen activator (t-PA) and plasminogen activator inhibitor-1 (PAI-1). Fibrinolysis 1990; 4 (Suppl. 2): 155–161.
[64] Petersen LC, Handest P, Brender J et al. A sensitive solid-phase immuno sorbent assay for tissue-type plasminogen activator in plasma using tribenzoylated poly-L-lysine as stimulator for plasminogen activation. Thromb Haemostas 1987; 57: 205–211.
[65] Philips M, Juul A-G, Selmer J et al. A specific immunologic assay for functional plasminogen activator inhibitor in plasma – standardized measurements of the inhibitor and related parameters in patients with thromboembolic disease. Thromb Haemostas 1992; 68: 286–494.
[66] Rånby M, Bergsdorf N, Nilsson T. Age dependence of tissueplasminogen activator concentrations in plasma as studied by an improved enzyme-linked immunosorbent assay. Clin Chem 1986; 32: 2160–2165.
[67] Malm J, Laurell M, Nilsson IM et al. Thromboembolic disease – critical evaluation of laboratory investigation. Thromb Haemostas 1992; 68: 7–13.
[68] Fareed J, Bick RL, Squillac G et al. Molecular markers of hemostatic disorders: implications in the diagnosis and therapeutic management of thrombotic and bleeding disorders. Clin Chem 1983; 29: 1641–1658.
[69] Pelzer H, Schwarz A, Stüber W. Determination of human prothrombin fragment 1 + 2 in plasma with an antibody against a synthesic peptide. Thromb Haemostas 1991; 65: 153–159.
[70] Pelzer H, Schwartz A, Heimburger N. Determination of thrombin-antithrombin III complex in plasma with an enzyme-linked immuno sorbent assay. Thromb Haemostas 1988; 59: 101–106.
[71] Amiral J, Walenga JM, Fareed J. Development and performance characteristics of a competitive enzyme immunoassay for fibrinopeptide A. Semin Thromb Haemost 1984; 228–242.
[72] Esmon NL. Thrombomodulin. Progr. Haemostas Thromb 1989; 9: 29.
[73] Takahashi H, Ito S, Masahara H et al. Circulating thrombomodulin as a novel endothelial cell marker. Amer J Haematol 1992; 41: 32–39.

Clinical research methodologies in diabetic pregnancy

D. R. Hadden

Research challenges and methodological problems

It may be helpful to an embryo researcher in the field of diabetic pregnancy to consider what particular questions require to be addressed, and having asked the question, what methodological problems may be expected. Many of these questions and problems are considered in detail in other chapters in this book, but the specific challenge of the fetal/maternal interactions in pregnancy has always attracted intelligent seekers after truth.

The simple clinical challenge is to meet the St. Vincent Declaration statement that the outcome of pregnancy in a diabetic mother should be similar to that of a non diabetic mother. The problem here is to achieve a local, national or international audit of obstetrical outcome; although maternity records are in general good, retrieval of data is often difficult and relatively few attempts have been made to audit consistently in this field apart from recognized centres of excellence.

The challenge of congenital malformations in diabetic pregnancy is generally considered still to be a major problem, although some centres feel they have reduced it to minor proportions. The question remains why there is such a large difference in the incidence of different malformations in different countries in successive years, and how much these background changes are related to a specific diabetic aetiology. Large scale epidemiological studies in this field do not generally identify diabetes as a risk factor. Further studies at local or national level will have to include assessments of food intake, including vitamins and other free radical scavengers as well as measures of blood glucose control.

Big babies have been traditionally associated with diabetic pregnancy. The definition of macrosomia will in the future depend on more than crude birth weight, and more and more sensitive methods of dating the gestation will be used. The distribution of body fat and muscle will also be measured so that a distinction between true "diabetic fetopathy" and a normal healthy big baby can be achieved. Whether the short term obstetric risk of delivering a big baby alone justifies insulin treatment of the mother before delivery will require careful assessment. The possible long term benefits or hazards of having been a big baby can also be assessed in true population studies: as obstetric records of birth weight have been kept for many years in most western countries, more studies of 30, 40 or 50 year outcomes may be expected. Similar challenges for the long-term outcome of the small, or small-for-dates baby have also been identified and are in process of study. Epidemiological investigation in this field is relatively new and many opportunities exist. The only problem is that the patients live longer than the doctors, and one generation of researchers has an obligation to pass on the baton of enquiry to the next in a well constructed format.

The fascination of the study of pregnancy is the ability to investigate inheritance. Molecular biology has allowed many new genetic models to be studied, for both type 1 and type 2 diabetes, and more information on the simple transfer of genetic information from mother to fetus accumulates, but the specific effect of the immunological changes in pregnancy in "setting up" the offspring to develop diabetes at some remote later time will need better characterization. Ultimately this will lead to attempts to identify those at risk and to try and prevent the onset of the disease in the next generation.

This chapter will concentrate on some of the more mundane clinical problems that still require clarification, but it is hoped that the next generation of researchers in this field will find themselves sufficiently well equipped to ask the larger and more fascinating questions.

Clinical research problems

Clinical research in diabetic pregnancy is usually carried out jointly between internists, obstetricians and paediatricians. Any one of this group may take the lead in any specific centre but none can function fully without the others. There is nevertheless surprisingly little scientific communication between these three professional groups at a day to day research level, and clinical skills and methodologies which are so well known and apparently basic to one may be totally unknown to another. Obstetricians talk largely to other obstetricians, at obstetrical meetings, and record their results in obstetrical journals. Neonatal paediatricians and adult diabetologists are equally self-selective. Fortunately there are now some groups where these three angles can come together such as the Diabetes Pregnancy Study Group of the European Association for the Study of Diabetes, or the Council on Pregnancy of the American Diabetes Association, but these are not always easily accessible.

At these meetings it becomes clear that there are quite considerable differences in pregnancy-related practices from one country to another, so that international comparisons are difficult. Clinical research experience in one country tends to be published within that country, and even if it appears in a general rather than a speciality journal, broad spectrum recognition is slow. Epidemiological and laboratory clinical research in this field does not necessarily suffer from the same compartmentalization, but does very much depend on the lead from the clinical front. For all these reasons the main problems in clinical research in diabetic pregnancy still exist in terms of definitions of what we mean. The main thrust of this chapter is to identify the solid ground where definitions are agreed between all the interested groups, and to point out the problem areas.

Glucose metabolism in pregnancy is studied by the same techniques as for the non-pregnant state. The oral glucose tolerance test remains the essential diagnostic tool; the changing metabolic environment of advancing pregnancy is superimposed on both the well known variability of the physiological response to oral glucose and the different stages of the pathological development of the diabetic state. Attempts to improve both specificity and sensitivity of this response to oral glucose as an accurate means of classification include the use of fasting or untimed studies only, an intravenous challenge, pre-loading with glucocorticoids, as well as different glucose loads. Progression to concepts of insulin resistance and insulin sensitivity, while useful in understanding the pathophysiological processes, does not improve diagnostic precision. There is still need for a standard assessment for disordered glucose metabolism in pregnancy which would be internationally acceptable in different ethnic groups and with different dietary and climatic backgrounds. It does not seem that studies of fat or protein metabolism in diabetic pregnancy have any more useful application at present.

Intrauterine fetal and placental studies are relevant both to the short term pregnancy outcome, and to the long-term development of the offspring. Studies of the fetal-maternal unit, and of the neonatal growth and development of the baby are becoming an important aspect of long-term epidemiological investigations relevant to the transgestational interactions of the diabetic process. The immunological, as well as the biochemical interface between mother and child may prove to be as necessary to document as the genetic transfer of information.

Definitions of diabetes in pregnancy

It is generally agreed that a high blood glucose in the mother is a serious problem in pregnancy, both for the developing fetus and for the well-being of the mother. This knowledge dates back to the original case report by Bennewitz [1], in Berlin 1824, and to the small compilation of obstetrical results by Matthews Duncan in 1882, although in those days only urinary sugar could be evaluated [2]. The detection of glycosuria is now recognised to be an unsatisfactory method of diagnosing either hyperglycaemia or impairment of carbohydrate metabolism in pregnancy [3].

Measurement of glucose in blood is now a simple and remarkably precise laboratory procedure, but some special precautions are necessary in pregnancy because of the haemodilution which will alter the relationship between plasma and whole blood concentrations. If diabetes is defined as a state of hyperglycaemia it should not be too difficult to define a 'high level of blood glucose'. The series of reports by expert committees of the World Health Organisation (WHO) [4, 5], advised by senior and respected diabetes physicians and biochemists, have consistently agreed that a blood glucose above 11.0 mmol/l is abnormal at any time and that a single isolated measurement at that level would mean that the patient had diabetes at that time. This simple fact is not in dispute, although the clinical biochemist will need careful definition of laboratory technique, as true blood glucose measured by a glucose oxidase enzymatic method is less than blood total sugars measured as reducing substances. Plasma contains more glucose than whole blood after haemolysis as there is less glucose inside the red cell; venous blood contains less glucose than arterial blood, and capillary glucose approximates more to the arterial level. Fortunately, the two most widely used methods, venous plasma glucose (generally measured by a hospital laboratory on a venous specimen) and capillary whole blood glucose (measured by a self-monitoring enzyme-impregnated test strip), are virtually equivalent. These potential differences may have some importance in pregnancy [6]. If the blood glucose is below 6.0 mmol/l at the time of testing in a patient not on hypoglycaemic treatment, it is normal regardless of previous meals, and the patient does not have diabetes mellitus (Table 1).

There are two important questions in relation to the special definition of hyperglycaemia in pregnancy: what is the effect of pregnancy, at different stages, on the levels of blood glucose, and what is the level of increased blood glucose which produces an abnormal effect on the maternal-fetal unit? There is general agreement that in the early stages of normal pregnancy there is a fall in the fasting blood glucose, associated with an increased degree of fluctuation of glucose levels which has been termed 'accelerated starvation' [7]; later in normal pregnancy both fasting and postprandial blood glucose rise a little, though still within the normal non-pregnant range, associated with increasing serum insulin levels in producing 'facilitated anabolism'. Both of

Table 1 Plasma glucose, fasting and 2 hours after 75 g glucose in pregnancy

Venous plasma glucose (mmol/l)	Normal	Impaired glucose Tolerance	Diabetes
Fasting	< 6.0	6.0– 7.9	> 8.0
	and	and/or	
2 hour	< 9.0	9.0–10.9	> 11.0

Interpretation of venous plasma glucose values in pregnancy based on the WHO Technical Report Series 646, Geneva (1980), adapted to the criteria of the Diabetes Pregnancy Study Group of the European Association for the Study of Diabetes. The only difference between the non-pregnant and the pregnant state is in the 2 hour value for the diagnosis of impaired glucose tolerance which is 9.0 mmol/l compared to 8.0 mmol/l in the non-pregnant state.

these metabolic changes in normal pregnancy could be considered adaptations to encourage the development and growth of the fetus, the first by allowing short-term release of maternal energy from fatty acid breakdown, the second by the increased anabolic effect of endogenous insulin production. The potentially toxic effect of a high level of glucose on embryogenesis, fetal growth and fetal metabolism is certainly established at a maternal blood glucose level of 11.0 mmol/l, which is a level at which other long-term complications of diabetes affecting the vascular tree, kidneys and retina also occur. The evidence that milder maternal hyperglycaemia has similar effects below 11.0 mmol/l is still indefinite, except for an increase in the proportion of babies born above the 95th centile for weight, which may also relate to the age and weight of the mother.

Untimed or fasting blood glucose

An untimed, or 'random' blood glucose [8] is the simplest screening test for hyperglycaemia in pregnancy and should always be carried out at the first obstetrical examination to exclude the possibility that the mother is an undiagnosed diabetic, in which case her blood glucose level will be greater than 11.0 mmol/l (Table 2). The prevalence of newly diagnosed insulin-dependent

Table 2 Distribution of untimed ("random") venous plasma glucose, usually mid-morning values, in 1247 consecutive pregnant mothers at first antenatal booking at the Royal Maternity Hospital, Belfast

Mean:	4.69 mmol/l
Standard deviation:	0.64
Mean + 2 SD	5.69 mmol/l
Mean + 3 SD	6.61 mmol/l

diabetes in northern European countries is about 1 per 1000 of the population aged 10–40 years without regard to special risk factors such as pregnancy or a family history of diabetes. A dipstick urine glucose measurement should also be carried out, a negative result (urine glucose less than 5 mmol/l) being suggestive evidence that the blood glucose level is not raised, although positive glycosuria by itself is much less specific.

The use of a glucose oxidase enzyme test strip and a reflectance meter is sufficiently accurate to measure capillary whole blood glucose, provided the operator has good experience, the strips are not outdated and a sufficiently large drop of blood is obtained. This should now be a usual office or consulting room procedure. In parts of the world where non-insulin-dependent diabetes is prevalent, unrecognized pre-existing diabetes at a first obstetrical consultation can be discovered in up to one in 100 or more of the female population. Differences in the background prevalence of insulin-dependent and non-insulin-dependent diabetes in the obstetrical population will determine the most appropriate screening procedures. Whether this unrecognized hyperglycaemia predated the pregnancy is difficult to establish.

Fasting blood glucose is a much more informative measurement as it is subject to the various homeostatic physiological control mechanisms and is usually held within a very restricted range. In early pregnancy there is often a slight fall in fasting blood glucose, and in later stages it returns to normal or shows a slight rise [9].

Glucose profiles

If a single high blood glucose (> 11.0 mmol/l) is found in a mother, the next logical step in the investigation is to determine if this remains high or is an intermittent occurrence. There is now increasing interest in the concept of blood glucose profiles, and these vary from experimental protocols measuring every 30 min for the whole 24 h [10, 11] to simplified schemes measuring blood glucose before and after a standard meal [12, 13]. In many centres, these profile investigations are carried out after an oral glucose tolerance test (OGTT) is judged to be abnormal, but if hyperglycaemia during the mother's normal eating pattern is to be the index of potential fetal problems, it is much more logical to identify abnormal profile responses as the primary diagnostic process.

In Aberdeen, Sutherland and his colleagues [12] have published data on a breakfast tolerance test, with a 450 calorie "meal" containing 61% carbohydrate by weight prepared as a commercial formula product. In paired meal and glucose tolerance tests the closest correlation was shown between summed post-challenge glucose values. The 97th centile capillary plasma glucose at 2 h in the 75 g OGTT was 8.2 mmol/l and in the breakfast test meal 6.1 mmol/l. There is still no useful clinical indication as to what level of blood glucose in a meal challenge test in pregnancy should be considered abnormal. It will clearly be lower than after 75 g glucose, although it must not be forgotten that a level of abnormality defined as an upper sector of a continuous skewed distribution may not coincide with the toxic level to the fetus. Most of the previous studies of gestational glucose levels during OGTT definitions have shown very little relationship between OGTT results and fetal outcome if maternal age and obesity are taken into account.

We have used an even more simple meal profile test in Belfast, with a 300 calorie meal of cereal and bread using locally produced foodstuffs (Table 3) [13]. Mothers come fasting to the clinic and take a simple meal at 0900 h and 1200 h; blood glucose is measured before and 2 h after each meal. We use an arbitrary cutoff of 8.0 mmol/l at any time as being 'abnormal' and take that figure as an index for careful dietary advice (restricted food intake to 1500–2000 calories). If the profile remains 'abnormal' after one week on this diet the mother would be carefully considered for insulin therapy. In practice this protocol has reduced greatly the number of mothers referred for this intensive dietary advice, compared to the numbers identified as having 'gestational impaired glucose tolerance' using the 75 OGTT and WHO criteria.

Table 3 The simplified Belfast meal profile for detection of hyperglycaemia in pregnancy. Venous plasma glucose values are measured before and two hours after breakfast (0900h) and lunch (1200h) usually at 28 weeks gestation. Breakfast contained 42 g carbohydrate (300 calories total) and lunch 32 g carbohydrate (320 calories total).

Time h	Venous plasma glucose mmol/l Mean	95th centile
0900	5.3	5.5
1100	6.5	6.9
1200	5.7	6.0
1400	5.6	5.8

Any value above 8.0 mmol/l indicated an "abnormal" profile.

Glucose intolerance

The alteration of the homeostatic mechanisms of the body would be expected to mirror more closely the metabolic changes due to the diabetic disease process. This can be demonstrated more precisely by considering glucose dynamics following a carbohydrate load. It was recognized that standardization of such a load would allow the establishment of diagnostic criteria to help distinguish between a normal and abnormal response.

Hyperglycaemia (defined by a high blood glucose) is not necessarily the same thing as glucose intolerance (defined by the result of a glucose tolerance test). This simple dualism has contributed to the present obstetrical uncertainty about the concept of 'gestational diabetes mellitus', even when this is defined by a 'gold standard' 100 g OGTT, and interpreted by criteria laid down by prestigious US and international committees of experts.

Some pregnant mothers are found to have glucose intolerance in pregnancy, either because of pre-existing but unrecognized pre-pregnancy hyperglycaemia or because of a pregnancy-specific effect on blood glucose. The number of such mothers varies widely in different parts of the world, being lowest in the northern-most parts of Western Europe, and highest in subtropical and tropical developing countries; these geographical differences reflect the differing prevalence of both insulin and non-insulin-dependent diabetes.

Obstetricians, or their diabetologist colleagues, who wish to try and identify these patients during pregnancy must be aware of two major critical reviews in this field. Naylor [14] showed that the 'gold standard' in North America, the 100 g OGTT interpreted by US National Diabetes Data Group criteria, is not without major problems. The criteria were derived in the 1950's from an unrepresentative sample of women tested predominantly in the later stages of pregnancy, threshold values were set on an arbitrary statistical basis, reproducibility was not determined, measurements were made with a now outdated blood glucose technique and there were errors of translation to modern figures. Unfortunately, these "O Sullivan criteria" are so well established that it may be difficult ethically or legally to embark on studies needed to quantify risks to mother or baby and to define treatment strategies across the full range of plasma glucose values. Naylor not unjustifiably criticizes the pioneering Boston data. "These studies served as important signposts in an uncharted field. The issue now is whether yesterday's useful signpost is subtly misdirecting today's thinking about gestational diabetes mellitus – the challenge lies in finding better diagnostic tests or criteria for the 1990's and beyond".

A critical epidemiological review from New York [15] also seriously questions whether all pregnant women need to be screened for glucose intolerance in pregnancy. They carefully review the important clinical questions in this field: is there an excess maternal morbidity during the index pregnancy, is there excess perinatal mortality, does treatment affect this mortality, is there an excess of heavy infants, should we worry about them, and can birth weight be reduced by treatment? They conclude that there is only limited scientific data supporting a universal screening programme for gestational diabetes, or showing that treatment of the condition defined as gestational diabetes is beneficial. They ask why there is such pressure to screen all pregnant women and to treat even milder degrees of glucose intolerance in the USA, and suggest a more restrained approach than universal screening with OGTT's in pregnancy.

An even more radical approach is suggested by Hunter and Kierse [16] who state that except for research purposes all forms of glucose tolerance testing should be stopped, and the diagnosis of hyperglycaemia in pregnancy reached by repeated random blood glucose measurements. Reassessment of such a basic concept is not confined to pregnancy. The whole category of 'impaired glucose tolerance', introduced by the WHO and the US National Diabetes Data Group in 1979 is now recognized to be heterogenous – whether it is really a risk factor for diabetes or a 'diagnostic ragbag' may depend on further subclassification [17, 18].

For any clinical test procedure there are certain desirable functions. These include reproducibility, sensitivity, specificity, low cost and patient acceptability [19]. The oral glucose tolerance test has unfortunately proved to be rather poorly reproducible. The concepts of sensitivity and specificity depend on what the process is trying to define. If it is to define blood glucose responses then it can be both sensitive and specific, for example, if compared with a second identical test. However, it is the outcome of the pregnancy that the test is trying to predict and there is a poor relationship between fetal outcome and carbohydrate intolerance such that the test must be considered relatively non-specific and insensitive. The long term outcome in the mother and her offspring is a different consideration but the same concerns of specificity and sensitivity probably remain.

The recognition that pregnancy was an additional stress phenomenon in producing impairment of glucose tolerance led to a series of additionally stressed oral GTTs being developed in the belief that this would improve sensitivity and specificity for fetal outcome. The cortisone GTT and prednisone GTT were studied in several centres but did not fulfil these speculations [20, 21].

A direct comparison between the 75 g OGTT and the 300 calorie breakfast tolerance test in unselected normal women at 30 weeks gestation showed poor correlation between the results of the two tests. The question is not which test is more specific for the diagnosis of either hyperglycaemia in pregnancy or of impaired glucose tolerance, but rather which test is more appropriate to detect an adverse pregnancy outcome [13].

In the hope of improving these rather variable aspects of the oral glucose tolerance test by circumventing the glucose absorption phase, the intravenous glucose tolerance test was introduced. One attraction of the intravenous test was the almost exponential fall in blood glucose during the first hour which allowed a mathematical calculation of the glucose disappearance rate as a single figure and thus overcame the difficulties of interpreting the more variable response to the oral glucose load. The largest study of the IV glucose tolerance test in pregnancy was carried out on 917 unselected pregnancies in Aberdeen [22] and showed that there was a statistically significant association with some fetal outcome measurements but with a disappointing degree of clinical usefulness. Computerized methods of assessing the glucose disappearance slope had also been developed but with no improvement in precision [23].

Glucose clamping

In order to standardize the responses to intravenous glucose as far as possible and thus allow measurement of the glucose-induced insulin release from the pancreatic β-cell, the technique of glucose 'clamping' was introduced [24]. This became technically possible following the development of the radioimmunoassay for insulin. By infusing insulin at a steady rate it was possible to determine how much glucose was needed to maintain or 'clamp' the plasma glucose at a predetermined level. This gave a direct measurement of the whole body resistance to insulin action. The concepts of insulin sensitivity (the reciprocal of insulin resistance) had first been introduced by Himsworth in 1937 [25] and it was recognized from that time that some diabetic patients were more insulin resistant (or less insulin sensitive) than others. These concepts were extended to the study of insulin resistance in pregnancy by Ryan and Skyler [26]. They have shown in a small number of pregnant women that there is increased insulin resistance in the later part of pregnancy which confirms the well recognized need for increased insulin to maintain normal blood glucose in the third trimester in a diabetic woman. The resistance was greater in gestational onset diabetic pregnant women than in non-diabetic pregnancy, and both of these groups had more resistance than non-pregnant, non-diabetic women (Fig. 1). It has been possible to use the same principles to demonstrate insulin resistance in the pregnant diabetic rat. However, the procedure of glucose clamping is rather formidable for use in pregnancy and it has not been widely practiced.

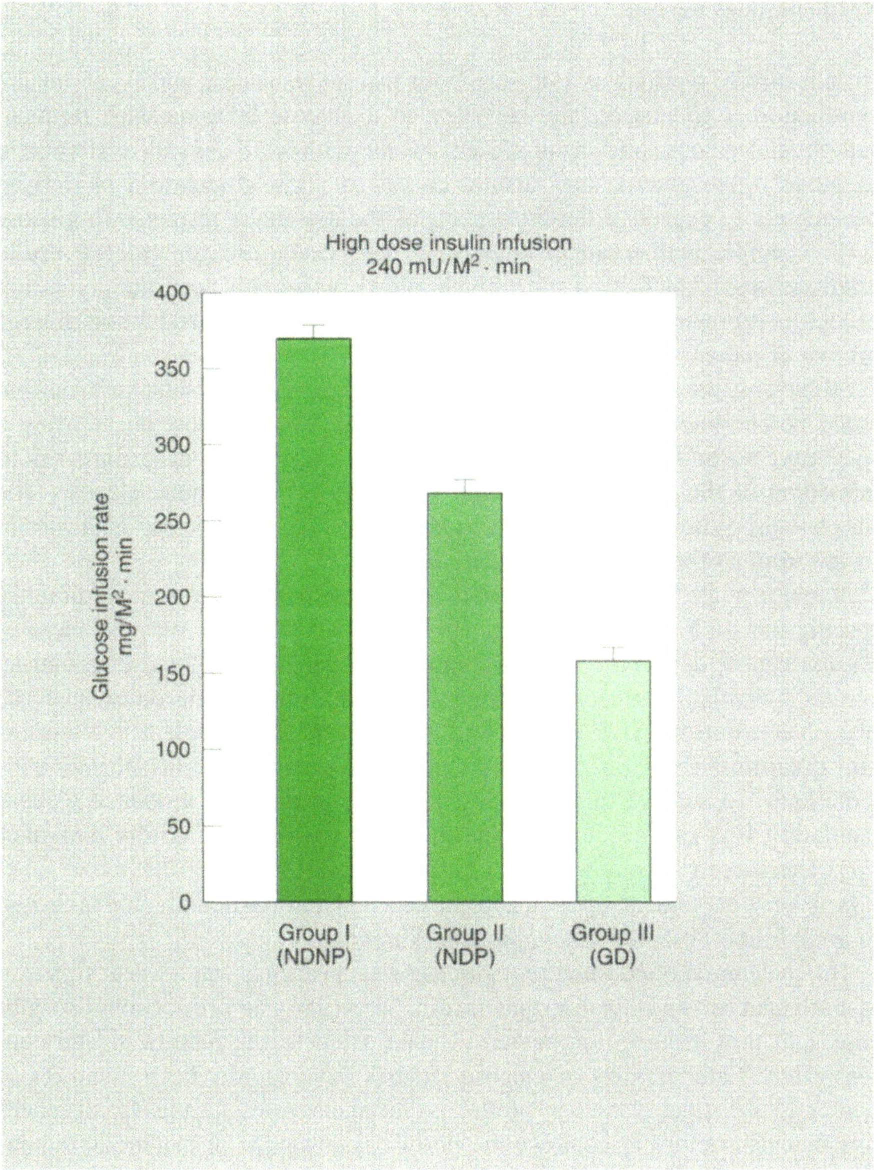

Fig. 1 Glucose clamping in pregnancy. Results of euglycaemic clamp studies (high-dose insulin infusion, 240 mU/M²/min) in three groups of subjects, designed to assess maximum insulin responsivity.
Group I: Non-diabetic non-pregnant
Group II: Non-diabetic pregnant
Group III: Gestational diabetes
From Ryan EA, O'Sullivan MJ, Skyler JS. Diabetes 1985; 34: 385 (reproduced by permission).

Mathematical models

An alternative method of assessing both insulin resistance and β-cell insulin production is to observe the response to a glucose infusion with frequent sampling of glucose and insulin levels. Many mathematicians have attempted to model these glucose and insulin curves to allow calculation of derived parameters to express different aspects of the metabolic response to glucose [27]. A simple mathematical model has been developed for glucose/insulin relationships in the fasting state which allows reasonably accurate derivation of factors representing insulin resistance and β-cell insulin production in large groups of patients – HOMA [28].

Studies on the oral glucose tolerance test showed that useful information could be extracted by assessment of the shape of the glucose curve using a sine wave formula [29]. The same desire to simplify the procedure led to modelling of the glucose and insulin responses to intravenous glucose. The simplest procedure is the CIGMA model which has shown close relationship to the results of glucose clamping studies [30].

A major goal of modelling carbohydrate metabolism has been to quantify specific metabolic processes when only the concentrations of substances in plasma can be determined. The dynamic responses of the glucose regulating system following a glucose challenge (in terms of the time courses of the plasma concentrations of glucose and insulin) can, in principle, reveal important quantitative information concerning endogenous substrate/hormone interactions. To achieve this goal it is necessary to define a model of glucose regulation that can account for the observed glucose and insulin dynamics [31]. The success of mathematical modelling in quantifying metabolic function is very dependent upon the complexity of the particular model chosen to analyse the observed glucose/insulin kinetics.

The early models assumed that glucose disappearance was a linear function of both glucose and insulin, that insulin secretion was proportional to glucose, and that insulin disappeared in proportion to the plasma insulin concentration. Later models of glucose kinetics have usually been members of one or two distinct classes of model, comprehensive or simple. Comprehensive models attempt to coalesce the body of knowledge of metabolic regulation into a generally large, non-linear model of high order, with a large number of model parameters: without extensive experimental investigation of a single individual it is not possible confidently to relate alterations in the dynamics of blood borne substances to specific changes in the derived parameters. Simple models do not attempt to encompass the physiology of metabolism, but to represent in the simplest terms the responses of plasma glucose and insulin to the oral or intravenous administration of glucose. The problem is that they may be so simple as to be inadequate representations of glucose and insulin kinetics. In particular the relationship between insulin secretion and glucose is not linear, and most simple models do not consider the complex interactive control of hepatic glucose production and uptake.

In the quest for the most suitable model Bergman and others felt that it was reasonable to assume that this would not be of the complex type. Not every known substrate/hormone interaction need be included because the response of the system must be relatively insensitive to many of the possible proposed relationships. In mathematical terms a "minimal model" describes a kinetic system by the least number of lowest order differential equations [32]. Bergman redefined the minimal model as that representation which is best able to simulate the dynamics of the system with the smallest number of identifiable parameters. In addition the minimal model would be physiologically based, it should have parameters that can be estimated with reasonable precision from a single dynamic response of the system; and these parameters must take on values that are reasonable in terms of the proposed system structure, and have a physiological interpretation.

Bergman evaluated seven mathematical models of glucose uptake to identify the one most capable of simulating glucose disappearance. They all involved frequent sampling of peripheral plasma after an intravenous glucose load. The measured time course of plasma insulin concentration was considered the input, and the plasma glucose concentration the output of the system regulating glucose disappearance. The chosen model was a three compartment non-linear model which could give an indirect measure of insulin sensitivity of the intact organisms. This has been extensively validated against clamping techniques [33], though the accuracy can be further increased by modifications such as artifically boosting the insulin response after complete mixing of the glucose load.

The intravenous glucose tolerance test is sampled at frequent intervals, and the glucose and insulin levels at each interval are determined. A computer programme analyses the data and provides the values for the parameters which represent insulin sensitivity (SI), glucose effectiveness (SG) and pancreatic responsiveness (first and second phase; phi 1 and phi 2). Using this model the increased insulin resistance (decreased sensitivity) of late pregnancy was confirmed [34] and reciprocal enhancements of the first and second phase insulin responses to the intravenous glucose demonstrated. In the gestational diabetic subjects studied there was not any greater degree of insulin resistance in late pregnancy, but the first phase insulin response was less in most cases, and the mean second phase response was probably also reduced (Fig. 2).

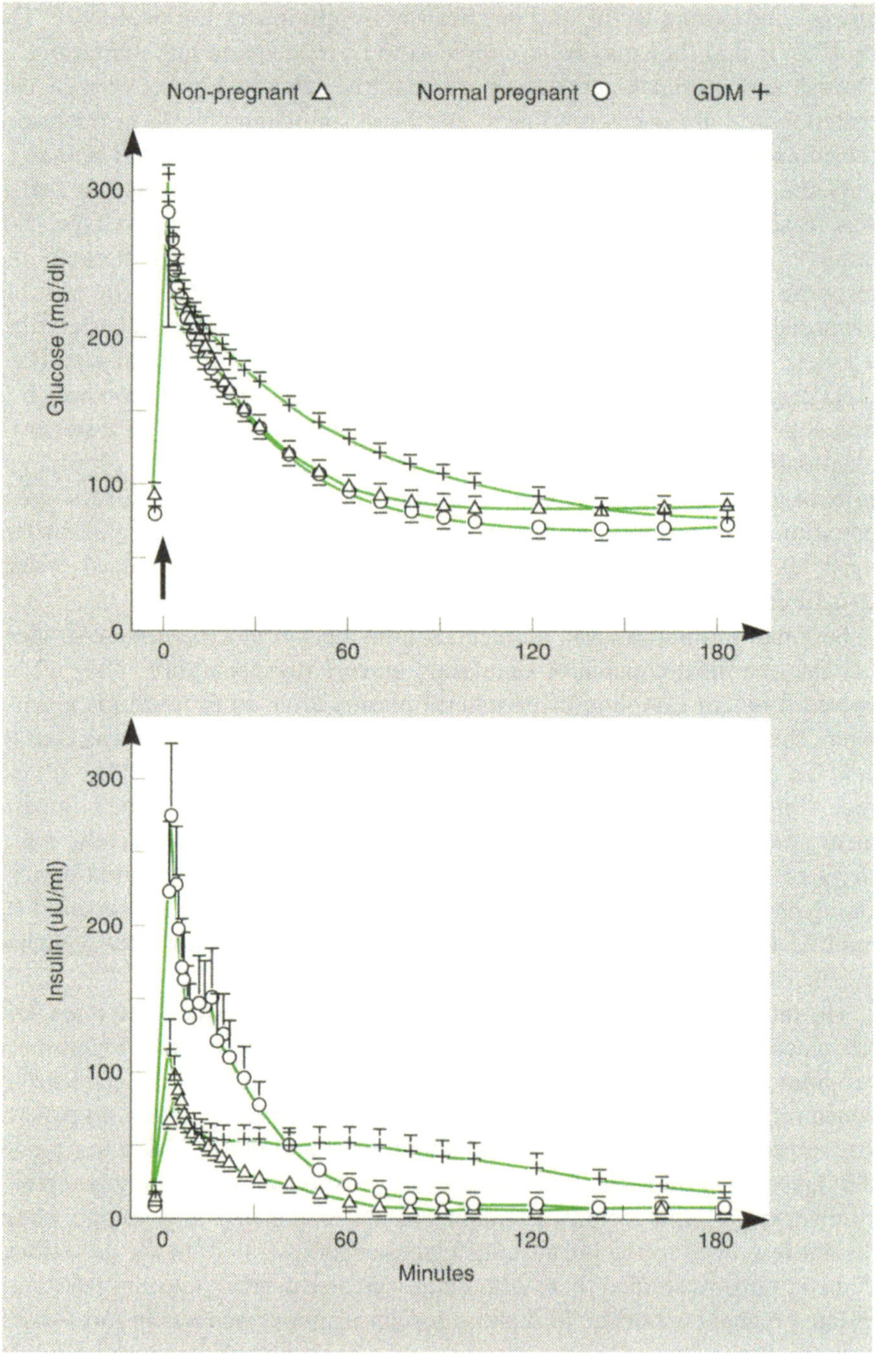
Non-pregnant △
Normal pregnant ○
GDM +
Glucose (mg/dl)
300
200
100
0
0
60
120
180
Insulin (uU/ml)
300
200
100
0
0
60
120
180
Minutes

These results were interpreted as showing that there is an impairment of pancreatic β-cell function in mild gestational diabetes which is superimposed on the normal insulin resistance of late pregnancy.

Fat metabolism in pregnancy

The changes in lipid metabolism which occur throughout normal pregnancy have been studied in terms of circulating levels of lipids in the mother, and transfer across the placenta to the fetus [35, 36]. The most striking change is an increase in plasma triglyceride which results primarily from an increase in very low density lipoprotein [37]. These changes may have a hormonal basis, related to the hormonal adaptations to the pregnant state. There is a positive correlation between plasma oestriol and triglyceride, and between VLDL triglyceride and insulin; these relations do not necessarily prove cause and effect, but are consistent with the known biochemical effects of these hormones on lipoprotein metabolism. The role of placental lipid transport still remains uncertain, but there is clinical evidence of enhanced delivery of lipoprotein lipids to the fetoplacental unit: for example, maternal free fatty acid concentration is associated with infant birth weight [38], and there may be a more important relationship to plasma triglyceride in diabetic pregnancy [39].

Pregnancy produces a metabolic stress that tends to exaggerate the already rather heterogenous characteristics of diabetic women, associated with insulin deficiency, insulin resistance, obesity or genetic factors as well as with varying degrees of hyperglycaemia. Although well controlled pregnant insulin-dependent diabetic women may not show any difference in lipoprotein

Fig. 2 The "minimal model" used to assess insulin sensitivity and β-cell responsiveness to glucose during late pregnancy in lean and moderately obese women with normal glucose tolerance or mild gestational diabetes.
Mean plasma glucose and insulin concentration during an intravenous glucose tolerance test in three study groups – non-pregnant, normal pregnant and gestational diabetic patients. Glucose (300 mg/kg) was injected intravenously at time zero.

	Insulin sensitivity	β-cell responsiveness first phase	second phase
Non-pregnant	3.0 ± 0.6	3.8 ± 1.1	39 ± 10
Normal pregnant	0.9 ± 0.3	11.0 ± 2.6	129 ± 32
Gestational diabetes	1.1 ± 0.2	2.4 ± 0.4	69 ± 9

From Buchanan TA, Metzger BE, Freinkel N et al Amer J Obstet Gynecol 1990; 162: 1011 (reproduced by permission).

levels from normal pregnancy, some non-insulin-dependent pregnant mothers with comparable glucose levels have higher triglyceride levels [39].

The major sources of fatty acid provided to the fetus and placenta have not yet been identified with certainty, and although fetal tissues can synthesize complex lipids the placenta may be more at risk if the maternal supply is impaired. Kinetic models with non-radioactive isotopes, or studies with cultured trophoblasts at a molecular level may help in the detailed understanding of these processes. From a simple clinical point of view a maternal lipid tolerance test might seem a useful indicator of potential hyperlipidaemia, and thus be a further way of exploring the concept of mixed nutrient effects on the feto-placental unit. A bolus infusion of a standard 10% fat emulsion did show that pregnancy was associated with decreased lipolysis of triglyceride but did not reveal any further difference in lipid metabolism between normal pregnant mothers and mothers found to have gestational diabetes by the criteria used in that study [40].

Protein metabolism in pregnancy

By comparison with studies of either carbohydrate or lipid metabolism in the pregnant diabetic there is probably more detailed analysis of the individual amino acid substrates but with rather less demonstrated abnormality. In the fasting state in an insulin-dependent diabetic there is evidence of increased gluconeogenesis and release of branched chain aminoacids, after a protein meal there is further gluconeogenesis and yet more branched chain aminoacid release. In pregnancy there is a generally lower level of plasma aminoacids, even after fasting [41], and the increase after a protein meal is smaller and more short-lived [9].

The phrase 'facilitated anabolism' was coined by Freinkel [7] to describe the metabolic response to feeding in diabetic pregnancy – characterized by hyperglycaemia, hyperinsulinaemia and hypertriglyceridaemia, with the teleological concept that these features would benefit the developing fetus. Likewise the term 'accelerated starvation' implicates the exaggerated but physiological metabolic response to short term fasting seen in the pregnant diabetic mother. The distinction between the physiological adaptations to the pregnant state and the pathological changes due to poorly controlled diabetes are sometimes confused. This distinction is more important in considering the metabolic state of the apparently well controlled diabetic mother, or the intermediate abnormalities found when the diabetic state starts during the pregnancy [9].

The long-term aspects of human development are throwing more concern on our understanding of fetal development but there is virtually no possibility of studying fetal protein turnover. Those interested in this field are confined to animal studies – in the sheep there is a higher rate of protein turnover in the fetus than in the adult. A mixed meal containing protein as well as glucose is usually thought of as representing a better indicator of normal living activities than a challenge of either glucose or aminoacids. Studies in diabetic pregnancy show smaller excursions of blood glucose from the fasting level than after an isocaloric glucose load.

Effect of the pregnancy on the subsequent development of diabetes and other disorders in either mother or child

For many years there had been a concept that pregnancy was in some way diabetogenic [42]. This became a complex epidemiological question linked to age and obesity as well as to diabetes, and in western countries with smaller family sizes it became of less clinical importance. Several recent developments have renewed the research interest in this area. It is now recognized there are very major differences in the age-standardized prevalence of both diabetes mellitus and impaired glucose tolerance in women of childbearing age in different ethnic populations in different parts of the world [43]. In recent studies using the 75 g OGTT the prevalence of diabetes in women aged 20–39 years was 1–3% in Italy and the USA, 7% in Fiji Indians, > 10% in Nauruan islanders and > 20% in Pima Indians. The prevalence of impaired glucose tolerance exceeded 10% in black and hispanic women in the USA, and much of this would go undetected in the absence of screening programmes. There is a major need for an agreed international standard in this area.

The maternal follow-up studies of O'Sullivan in Boston [44] have now continued for up to 30 years, with a cumulative incidence of diabetes of over 50% in these women originally diagnosed to have gestational diabetes. Other shorter term studies show the same trend, and despite the fundamental problems which arise in epidemiological and classification terms when attempting to compare diabetes incidence rates, there is broad general agreement on the predictive nature of gestational diabetes. The mechanism of the association has yet to be clarified, and genetic, immunological and nutritional hypotheses have all been proposed. The recognition that the incidence of childhood diabetes can vary as much as tenfold in western European countries [45] means that the complex interaction between genetic and environmental factors in the cause and pathogenesis of both insulin-dependent and non-insulin-dependent diabetes still requires much work.

The immunological aspects of the pathogenesis of diabetes involve the development of an antigenic potential in the cell membrane of the pancreatic β-cell (expression of a class 2 surface antigen). This may be a genetically determined feature, but must also in some degree be acquired, perhaps related to a viral, interferon or nutritional sensitization [46]. The altered humoral and cell mediated immunity processes which occur during pregnancy can be thought of as representing on the one hand a special clinical organ transplantation and on the other a sort of evolutionary mechanism not unlike that adopted by certain tumors for immuno-survival. The passage of islet cell antibodies and insulin antibodies across the placenta is likely to influence fetal pancreatic tissues and thus influence the ultimate development of diabetes either type 1 or type 2 in the offspring [47]. The work of Aerts and Van Assche has shown how these distinctions between inherited and acquired disease processes can become blurred in the maternal-fetal unit [48].

One easily quantified measurement is the weight of the baby. For years the birth of a big, or large for dates, baby has been recognized to be associated with some less well controlled diabetic pregnancies [49]. However, it is equally clear that many large for dates babies simply represent the extreme upper end of the normal range and can be thought of as showing the best normal growth pattern; the idea that supranormal growth *in utero* represented a very healthy pregnancy was recognized many years ago. It has been shown that mothers birth weight is an accurate predictor of macrosomia in her infant and knowledge of ones own birth weight is clearly an important prospective risk factor. This has become more topical due to the important demonstration from 50 year old birth records in the county of Hertfordshire in England that reduced growth in early life is strongly linked with impaired glucose tolerance and non-insulin-dependent diabetes 50 years later [51]. Reduced intrauterine growth is also linked to high blood pressure and possibly other features of the insulin resistance phenomenon. The concept of the "thrifty phenotype" [52], where poor fetal and early post-natal nutrition might impose mechanisms of nutritional thrift on the growing individual, will certainly become one of the major research areas in the next decade. This concept is linked to the earlier "thrifty genotype" hypothesis [53] where diabetogenic genes may persist at a high level in a population because they confer a survival advantage in times of nutritional deprivation, although in times of plenty they become detrimental. Clearly there are many questions raised by these ideas, and the main problem in addressing them will be the long gestation period and even longer life span of *homo sapiens*.

References

[1] Hadden DR. The first recorded case of diabetic pregnancy (Bennewitz HG, 1824, University of Berlin). Diabetologia 1989; 32: 625–628.
[2] Matthews Duncan. On puerperal diabetes. Trans Obstet Soc Lond 1882; 24: 256–285.
[3] Lind T, Hytten FE. The excretion of glucose during normal pregnancy. J Obstet Gynaecol Br Cwlth 1972; 79: 961–970.
[4] WHO Expert Committee on Diabetes Mellitus: Second Report. World Health Organization, Technical Report Series, 646. Geneva, 1980; 9–11.
[5] Diabetes Mellitus: Report of a WHO Study Group. World Health Organization, Technical Report Series, 727. Geneva, 1985; 10–14.
[6] Neely RGD, Kiwanuka JB, Hadden DR. Influence of sample type on the interpretation of the oral glucose tolerance test for gestational diabetes mellitus. Diabetic Med 1991; 8: 129–134.
[7] Freinkel N. The Banting Lecture 1980. Of pregnancy and progeny. Diabetes 1980; 29: 1023–1035.
[8] Hadden DR. Random plasma glucose as a screening tool for hyperglycaemia in pregnancy. In: HW Sutherland, JW Stowers, eds. Carbohydrate metabolism in pregnancy and the newborn 1984. Edinburgh: Churchill Livingstone, 1984; 203–205.
[9] Lind T, Aspillaga M. Metabolic changes during normal and diabetic pregnancies. In: Reece EA, Coustan DR, eds. Diabetes Mellitus in Pregnancy. New York: Churchill Livingstone, 1988; 75–102.
[10] Hollingsworth DR, Ney D, Stubblefield N et al. Heterogeneity of lean and obese women with gestational diabetes: metabolic assessment with isocaloric meal tolerance tests. Diabetes 1985; 34 (Suppl. 2): 81–87.
[11] Maresh MJA, Gillmer MGD, Beard RW et al. The effect of diet and insulin on metabolic profiles of women with gestational diabetes mellitus. Diabetes 1985; 34 (Suppl. 2): 88–93.
[12] Sutherland HW, Pearson DWM, Lean MEJ et al. Breakfast tolerance test in pregnancy. In: Sutherland HW, Stowers JM, Pearson DWM, eds. Carbohydrate metabolism in pregnancy and the newborn IV. London: Springer-Verlag, 1989; 267–275.
[13] McManus J, Roberts RN, Dobbs S et al. Comparison of 75 g oral glucose tolerance test (OGTT) and standardised breakfast tolerance test in the diagnosis of hyperglycaemic in pregnancy. First International Symposium on Diabetes and Pregnancy in the 90's. 1993 (in press).
[14] Naylor CD. Diagnosing gestational diabetes: is the gold standard valid? Diabetes Care 1989; 12: 565–572.
[15] Ales KL, Santini DL. Should all pregnant women be screened for gestational glucose intolerance? Lancet 1989; I: 1187–1191.
[16] Hunter DJS, Keirse MJNC. Gestational diabetes. In: Chalmers I, Enkin M, Kierse M eds. Effective Care in Pregnancy and Childbirth. Oxford University Press, 1989; 403–410.
[17] Yudkin JS, Alberti KGMM, McLarty DG et al. Impaired glucose tolerance: is it a fact or a diagnostic ragbag? Brit Med J 1990; 301: 397–402.
[18] Roberts RN, Moohan JM, Foo RLK et al. Fetal outcome in impaired glucose tolerance in pregnancy. Diabetic Medicine 1993; 162: 24–26.
[19] Hadden DR. Glucose tolerance tests in pregnancy. In: Sutherland HW, Stowers JM, eds. Carbohydrate metabolism in pregnancy and the newborn. Edinburgh: Churchill Livingstone, 1975; 19–41.
[20] Billis A, Rastogi GK. Studies in methods of investigating carbohydrate metabolism in pregnancy. Diabetologia 1966; 2: 169–177.
[21] Hadden DR, Harley JMG, Kajtar TJ et al. A prospective study of three tests of glucose tolerance in pregnant women selected for potential diabetes with reference to the fetal outcome. Diabetologia 1971; 7: 87–93.

[22] Farmer G, Russell G, Hamilton-Nichol DR et al. The influence of maternal glucose metabolism on fetal growth development and morbidity in 917 singleton pregnancies in nondiabetic women. Diabetologia 1988; 31: 134–141.
[23] Silcock DH, Hadden DR, Neill DW. Computer analysis of intravenous glucose tolerance tests. Diabetologia 1972; 8: 301–304.
[24] DeFronzo R, Tobin JD, Andres R. Glucose clamp technique. A method for quantifying insulin secretion and resistance. Am J Physiol 1979; 237: E214–223.
[25] Himsworth HP. Diabetes mellitus. Its differentiation into insulin-sensitive and insulin-insensitive type. Lancet 1936; I: 127–130.
[26] Ryan EA, O'Sullivan MJ, Skyler JS. Insulin action during pregnancy. Studies with the euglycaemic clamp technique. Diabetes 1985; 34: 380–389.
[27] Cerasi E, Efendic S, Luft R. Decreased sensitivity of the pancreatic beta cells to glucose in prediabetic and diabetic subjects. A glucose dose-response study. Diabetes 1972; 21: 224–234.
[28] Matthews DR, Hosker JP, Rudenski AS et al. Homeostasis model assessment: insulin resistance and beta cell function from fasting plasma glucose and insulin concentrations in man. Diabetologia 1985; 28: 412–419.
[29] McGarry RG. Modelling of insulin/glucose dynamics and application to the analysis of oral glucose tolerance tests. Thesis for the degree of PhD. The Queen's University of Belfast 1989.
[30] Hosker JP, Matthews DR, Rudenski AS et al. Continuous infusion of glucose with model assessment: measurement of insulin resistance and beta cell function in man. Diabetologia 1985; 28: 401–411.
[31] Bergman RN, Ider YZ, Bowden CR. Quantitative estimation of insulin sensitivity. Am J Physiol 1979; 236: E667–677.
[32] Tofollo GR, Bergman RN, Finegood DT et al. Quantitative estimation of β-cell sensitivity to glucose in the intact organism: a minimal model of insulin kinetics in the dog. Diabetes 1980; 29: 979–990.
[33] Bergman RN, Prager R, Volund A et al. Equivalence of the insulin sensitivity index in man derived by the minimal model and the euglycaemic glucose clamp. J Clin Invest 1987; 79: 790–800.
[34] Buchanan TA, Metzger BE, Freinkel N et al. Insulin sensitivity and β-cell responsiveness to glucose during late pregnancy in lean and moderately obese women with normal glucose tolerance or mild gestational diabetes. Am J Obstet Gynecol 1990; 162: 1008–1014.
[35] Knopp RH, Moutes A, Childs M et al. Metabolic adjustments in normal and diabetic pregnancy. Clin Obstet Gynecol 1981; 24: 21–49.
[36] Knopp RH, Magee MS, Bouet B et al. Lipid metabolism in pregnancy. In: Cowett RM ed. Principles of Perinatal-Neonatal Metabolism. New York: Springer-Verlag, 1991; 177–203.
[37] Warth MR, Arky AR, Knopp RH. Lipid metabolism in pregnancy III. Altered lipid composition in intermediate, very low, low and high density lipoprotein fractions. J Clin Endocrinol Metab 1975; 41: 649–655.
[38] Sheath J, Grimwade HJ, Waldron K et al. Arteriovenous nonesterified fatty acids and glycerol differences in the umbilical cord at term and their relationship to fetal metabolism. Am J Obstet Gynecol 1972; 113: 358–362.
[39] Hollingsworth DR, Grundy SM. Pregnancy-associated hypertriglyceridaemia in normal and diabetic women: differences in insulin-dependent, noninsulin-dependent and gestational diabetes. Diabetes 1982; 31: 1092–1097.
[40] Cowett RM, Carr SR, Ogburn PL. Lipid tolerance testing in pregnancy. Diabetes Care 1993; 16: 51–56.
[41] Felig P, Kim YJ, Lunch V et al. Aminoacid metabolism during starvation in human pregnancy. J Clin Invest 1972; 51: 1195–1201.
[42] Malins JM. Is pregnancy diabetogenic? Definition and aetiology of diabetes mellitus. Clinical Diabetes Mellitus. London: Eyre and Spottiswoode, 1968; 26–28.
[43] World Heath Organization Ad Hoc Diabetes Reporting Group. Diabetes and impaired glucose tolerance in women aged 20–39 years. Diabetes 1993.

[44] O'Sullivan JB. The Boston gestational diabetes studies: review and perspectives. In: Sutherland HW, Stowers JM, Pearson DWM, eds. Carbohydrate metabolism in pregnancy and the newborn IV. London: Springer-Verlag, 1989; 287–294.
[45] Green A, Gale EAM, Patterson CC, for the EURODIAB ACE group. Incidence of childhood-onset insulin-dependent diabetes mellitus: the Eurodiab-Ace study. Lancet 1992; 339: 905–909.
[46] Hoet JJ, Reusens-Billen B. The fetomaternal unit and the immune reactions associated with diabetes. In: Andreani D, Bompiani GD, Di Mario U et al. Immunobiology of normal and diabetic pregnancy. Chichester: John Wiley, 1990; 283–289.
[47] Di Mario U, Gargiulo P, Andreani D. Humoral immune aspects in diabetic pregnancy. In: Andreani D, Bompiani GD, Di Mario U et al, eds. Immunology of normal and diabetic pregnancy. Chichester: John Wiley, 1990; 263–272.
[48] Aerts L, Van Assche F. Is gestational diabetes an acquired condition? J Developmental Physiol 1979; 1: 219–225.
[49] McCance DR, Hadden DR, Harley JMG. Are all infants of diabetic mothers "macrosomic"? Brit Med J 1989; 298: 524–525.
[50] Klebanoff MA, Mills JL, Bevendes HW. Mothers birth weight as a predictor of macrosomia. Am J Obstet Gynecol 1985; 152: 253–257.
[51] Hales CN, Barker DJP, Clark PMS et al. Fetal and infant growth and impaired glucose tolerance at age 64. Br Med J 1991; 303: 1019–1022.
[52] Hales CN, Barker DJP. Type 2 (non-insulin-dependent) diabetes mellitus: the thrifty phenotype hypothesis. Diabetologia 1992; 35: 595–601.
[53] Neal JV. Diabetes mellitus: a thrifty genotype rendered detrimental by "progress". Am J Human Genet 1962; 14: 353–362.

Research methodologies in evaluation of fetal dysfunction

U. J. Eriksson

Introduction

Before the introduction of insulin in the treatment of diabetic pregnant women, the fetal and neonatal mortality was close to 50% [49, 109]. Improved knowledge of the pathogenic mechanisms involved in this type of high-rish pregnancy and improved clinical management of pregnant diabetic women have successfully decreased the mortality and morbidity rates to levels slightly above the normal range [25, 57, 73, 76, 128]. The single most important factor contributing to the decreased incidence of fetal malformation appears to be the improved metabolic control that the diabetic woman is now able to achieve, implying near-normalization of most maternal metabolic parameters and the obtaining of normoglycemia [93, 103]. It is generally assumed that if optimal metabolic control is achieved, the perinatal morbidity and mortality rate in diabetic pregnancy will be comparable to that observed in normal pregnancies [53, 60, 141], with the possible exception of the morbidity and mortality related to the congenital malformations [79, 93, 101].

In the early days of insulin treatment, the fetuses of the diabetic mother faced an increased risk of developing macrosomia and pulmonary immaturity (RDS), as well as a considerable risk of sudden (unexplained) intrauterine death (20%). These deaths occurred late in pregnancy, mainly after week 32 post-conception. Improved medical care of the mother in recent years has made all of these unwanted complications of the diabetic gestation less common, and, at the same time, the numbers of diabetic pregnant women with vascular disease, hydramnios, or pre-eclampsia have diminished in many centers. The most dramatic decrease has occurred in the incidence of sudden intrauterine death, supporting the view that this severe complication has possible etiologic factors including hypoxia, hyperinsulinemia, and/or hyperglycemia, all of which have now diminished in diabetic pregnancies treated in specialist centers [25, 61].

While the neonatal mortality due to other complications has decreased during the last decades, congenital malformations have emerged as the most important cause of the persistently above-average overall perinatal mortality in diabetic pregnancy [133]. Diabetic pregnancy has thereby become associated with a significantly increased risk for congenital malformation. The magnitude of the increased risk has been estimated to be 2–10 times the rate of malformations in non-diabetic pregnancy [6, 57, 61, 80, 99].

Several authors have addressed the issue of monitoring fetal development in order to detect malformations or other dysfunctions of the offspring and presented different suggestions for research strategies in diabetic pregnancy. This review will describe some current clinical methods, and aims to answer the question of which clinical procedures to assess fetal status are of greatest interest for use in diabetic pregnancy. In addition, some methodologies not currently used clinically to monitor fetal functions, as well as a few selected experimental procedures, will be discussed.

Methods of assessing fetal status

Ultrasonography

Ultrasonography is the method par preference in the evaluation of suspected embryo-fetal maldevelopment in diabetic pregnancy, because it can detect growth disturbances and several types of congenital malformations. Ultrasonography can be used as early as weeks 7–8 post-conception, and may be repeated every 4–6 weeks during pregnancy in order to closely monitor fetal development. Using ultrasound, Pedersen and Mølsted-Pedersen have reported an early growth retardation among the embryos of diabetic mothers. This early growth disturbance amounts to a mean delay of 5–6 days, although there is considerable individual variation [110]. This early growth retardation is also associated with an increased risk for congenital malformations [111], as well as potential psychological and motor dysfunction [114]. These studies have thus demonstrated a coupling between early growth disturbance and teratogenic susceptibility in diabetic pregnancy. This challenging data is currently being discussed with intensity. Some authors have not been able to confirm the early growth delay in diabetic pregnancy [62, 65], others find a growth retardation but no coupling to congenital malformations [15], and other investigators fail to demonstrate any long-term psychomotor or psychological effects on the infants of the diabetic mother [56, 113].

Somatic development of the embryo/fetus can be monitored throughout pregnancy with the aid of serial ultrasonographic determinations, where the estimations of abdominal circumference (AC), bi-parietal diameter (BPD), and the length of a specific long bone (femur) give precise information regarding intrauterine growth. Both the AC measurement and the AC/BPD ratio are estimated, and the method is able to identify macrosomic fetuses with high sensitivity in diabetic pregnancy [13, 83, 138]. It has been shown by consecutive ultrasonographic examination that macrosomia may be present in some fetuses of diabetic mothers as early as weeks 26–28 post-conception, and that the fetuses with accelerated intrauterine growth are also exposed to elevated amniotic fluid insulin concentration [106]. Sonographic evaluation of shoulder soft tissue in the third trimester may offer an accurate prediction of macrosomia [97].

Ultrasonography can also be used to detect growth retardation in late pregnancy with high accuracy. This condition is of great clinical interest, although retarded embryo-fetal growth has not been a particularly common feature of diabetic pregnancy, except in those diabetic women with vascular complications [109].

Fetal breathing movements, which are of importance in a more complete assessment of fetal intrauterine status, can be easily shown. Perhaps the most important of all clinical applications, ultrasonography is extremely valuable for determine fetal malformations in utero. The technique can actually diagnose neural tube defects (assisted by the measurement of serum α-fetoprotein concentration in the mother), and other gross structural abnormalities in the fetus [15].

Cardiotocography

When the embryo/fetus has developed a beating heart, it is possible to perform cardiotocography (CTG), by simultaneously registering the activity of the fetal heart and the contractions of the maternal uterine musculature. The clinically relevant CTG registrations are performed, however, when the fetus has started to obtain capacity for extrauterine survival, in post-conception weeks 24–25 and beyond. The CTG curve can be analyzed with respect to a number of parameters; the fetal basal heart rate and its variations, as well as the presence of periods with profound changes in heart rate – both accelerations and decelerations. If particular efforts are made to estimate the reactivity of the fetal heart in relation to the uterine contractions, this variant of ultrasound evaluation is called a non-stress test (NST). CTG and NST have proven to be reliable methods and very sensitive indicators of fetal distress after post-conception weeks 28–30 [153]. The CTG curve or NST, assessed once or twice weekly in diabetic pregnancy, provides a good understanding of fetal well-being, and a normal (non-pathological) result, such as a negative CTG or a reactive NST, has been shown to indicate a very low risk for intrauterine death [39, 48].

If there is clinical concern regarding the fetal status, such as a non-reactive NST, a contraction stress test (CST) can be performed. Oxytocin is then administered to the mother to provoke uterine contractions and a response in fetal heart rate, which can be subsequently evaluated. Late decelerations, or periods of markedly decreased heart rate which are initiated after the peak of the uterine contraction, indicate fetal hypoxia, and demand clinical actions [39]. A pathological CST in diabetiv pregnancy has been associated with an increased perinatal mortality rate, growth retardation, and increased risk for the respiratory distress syndrome [48].

In some centers a "biophysical profile" is compiled when the CTG or NST yields an abnormal result. It includes the registration of fetal breathing, movements and tonus, as well as estimating the amniotic fluid volume and performing a CST [88]. This relatively complex method has been reported to give a very high predictability for fetal dysfunction in high-risk pregnancy, including diabetic gestation [75, 89]. The precise value of the biophysical profile after a non-reactive NST, remaines uncertain [27, 51].

Fetal movements

Systematic registration of fetal movements is an easy method for the assessment of fetal well-being in pregnancies complicated by concurrent maternal disease. With the aid of ultrasonography, it has been found that the fetus performs about 30 movements per hour during the last 10 weeks of pregnancy [107]. Maternal hyperglycaemia (glucose levels in excess of 7.8 mmol/l) does not seem to alter the number of fetal movements, but maternal hypoglycemia (serum glucose concentration less than 3.3 mmol/l) doubles the number of fetal movements [69], which makes this straightforward test of fetal dysfunction of special importance in diabetic pregnancy.

Maternal samples

Traditionally, a considerable amount of information regarding the fetus has been obtained by analyzing metabolites and hormones present in maternal blood and urine. Some of these compounds warrant discussion with reference to diabetic pregnancy.

α-fetoprotein: Elevated maternal serum levels of α-fetoprotein signal increased concentration of this globulin in amniotic fluid. This may be a consequence of an increased leakage of α-fetoprotein to the amniotic cavity, or a disruption of the fetal removal of amniotic fluid [14], and is associated with increased risk for fetal neural tube malformation [95]. Determination of this serum compound is a useful tool for the estimation of possible fetal dysfunction in diabetic pregnancy, especially in conjunction with ultrasonographic evaluation of the morphology of the fetus.

Female steroid hormones: Urinary estriol assays were the first tests widely employed for fetal monitoring in pregnancies complicated by diabetes mellitus. Increasing estriol concentration with time were interpreted as a positive prognostic sign, signalling minimal risk of intrauterine death for the fetus. However, urinary estriol assays have a high false-positive rate and several studies have shown the limited predictive values of the urinary estriol assay in diabetic pregnancy [28, 42]. One particular steroid compound, however, may be of specific value as a predictive parameter. The serum concentration of unconjugated estriol has shown to be selectively low in women carrying a fetus with Down's syndrome [18]. Serum progesterone increases in both normal and diabetic pregnancy to the same extent [137], which diminishes the possible prognostic use of the maternal serum levels of this hormone in diabetic pregnancy.

Glycosylated hemoglobin (HbA_{1c}): Measurement of the concentration of glycosylated hemoglobin (HbA_{1c}) in the maternal blood, which reflects the degree of metabolic control during the preceding 6–8 weeks, has become of paramount interest for the estimation of the risk for congenital malformation in diabetic pregnancy [46]. It has repeatedly been shown that a high value in early gestation is a bad prognostic sign [54, 84, 91, 123, 151]. The predictive value of an elevated HbA_{1c} concentration is not completely clear with respect to the risk for spontaneous abortion [26, 94, 98, 150], and among women with only marginally increased HbA_{1c} values there appear to be other factors in addition to an unbalanced carbohydrate metabolism that determine the induction of malformations [93].

Insulin, C-peptide, insulin-like growth factors: Low maternal serum insulin and C-peptide concentrations were found to be associated with increased fetal skin-fold thickness and increased amniotic levels of C-peptide [135]. A correlation between maternal serum concentrations of insulin-like growth factors (IGF : s) and fetal growth has been suggested [58]. Other studies have, however, failed to demonstrate an increased IGF-I concentration in the serum of macrosomic infants of diabetic mothers [66].

Human chorionic gonadotropin and human placental lactogen: Human chorionic gonadotropin (hCG) is an excellent indicator of pregnancy. The hormone is produced exclusively by the syncytiotrophoblast and in amounts which can be detected in maternal serum by immunocytochemically based methods at 14 days post-conception, by the time of the first missed period. The serum concentration of hCG during pregnancy is increased in diabetic compared to non-diabetic women [137], but the physiological implications of this fact are unclear and hCG determinations are currently not used to assess fetal dysfunction in diabetic pregnancy. Human placental lactogen (hPL), which is responsible for the increased lipolysis in pregnancy, is also produced exclusively by the syncytiotrophoblast, but does not appear to be selectively increased in diabetic pregnant women [137].

Amniocentesis

The amniotic fluid, which is produced and recirculated by the fetus, can give particular information regarding the status of the fetus. The function of the fetal lung and pancreas are of particular interest to the diabetologist, and may be assessed by analysis of the amniotic fluid.

Phospholipids in amniotic fluid: The estimation of the lecithin/sphingomyelin ratio (L/S) in amniotic fluid has become a good method for excluding pulmonary immaturity, where a L/S ratio > 2.0 is associated with a significantly diminished risk for RDS [47, 142]. If the phosphatidylglycerol concentration is also determined, an added reassurance of fetal pulmonary maturation can be achieved [59, 143].

Insulin and other hormones in amniotic fluid: Measurement of insulin in amniotic fluid has been correlated with fetal growth status, and has in some clinical centers been used as an indicator of the effectiveness of the maternal insulin treatment [148]. In general, amniotic fluid insulin concentration seems to be increased in both early [124] and late diabetic pregnancy [40, 143]. Amniotic fluid concentrations of insulin, C-peptide, and pro-insulin were found to be increased in diabetic compared to non-diabetic pregnancy, and the C-peptide levels correlated positively with infant birth weight [40, 112]. Diabetic pregnancies with neonatal morbidity showed higher amniotic fluid concentrations of C-peptide and insulin than did diabetic pregnancies without neonatal morbidity [40, 112].

Increased values of hPL have been found in the amniotic fluid in some diabetic women, although without any statistical association to the birth weight of the fetus [16].

Cells in amniotic fluid: Cells obtained from the amniotic fluid and cultured for two weeks yield enough chromatin material to allow a chromosomal analysis and to identify aberrations. The isolation of DNA and the exposure of the genetic material to restriction fragment length polymorphism (RFLP) analysis also allow the detection of specific genetic diseases. At present no particular chromosomal aberration nor any monogenic disease has been associated with diabetes mellitus.

Amniotic fluid volume: The amount of amniotic fluid is of importance for assessing fetal status, and, in particular, an increased volume (polyhydramnios) may indicate an increased risk for fetal CNS aberration affecting the fetal ability to swallow. Less severe polyhydramnios may also be of specific interest, since this condition is present in a large proportion of diabetic pregnant women, and may signify a less than optimal maternal metabolic control. The reason for the increased volume of amniotic fluid in diabetic pregnancy is presumed to be fetal polyuria due to fetal hyperglycemia, the latter condition clearly dependent upon the degree of maternal metabolic control.

Chorionic villous biopsy

A biopsy of the chorionic villous may be performed during pregnancy as early as amniocentesis, and is of great value for obtaining fetal genetic information. The procedure can be performed with acceptable embryo-maternal risk by post-conception week 8. A culture of fast-growing trophoblast cells allows a genetic answer to be obtained in 1–2 days, which is markedly faster than that obtained from culture of the desquamated amniotic fluid cells.

Maternal glucose concentration and glucose tolerance test

In a recent multicenter study, it was found that maternal non-fasting serum glucose concentration in the third trimester was a strong predictor for fetal birth weight percentile [77]. The prognostic value of non-fasting serum glucose measurements was also reported by Combs et al. [22], who found that fetal macrosomia was statistically associated with maternal post-prandial glucose levels between gestational weeks 29 and 32. In other studies, the maternal glucose tolerance test (GTT) result (area under the curve) in the last trimester was found to correlate with fetal urinary C-peptide excretion and skin-fold thickness in offspring of gestational diabetic women [85]. Mild disturbances in GTT did not, however, correlate with fetal growth disturbances or morbidity [125].

Methods of estimating placental function

The placenta has been investigated using several different methods aimed at identifying a specific functional impairment of this organ in diabetes. One grim feature of the late diabetic pregnancy, the increased risk for fetal death, has spurred an interest in understanding the structure and monitoring of the function of the placenta. Placental changes causing diminished intervillous blood flow, thereby predisposing the fetus to fetal intrauterine hypoxia as a consequence of the altered maternal-fetal energy metabolism, is a favored etiologic explanation for the malformation of the fetus in late diabetic pregnancy [87].

Doppler blood flow measurements

If fetal dysfunction, manifested as growth retardation, is suspected as a consequence of placental dysfunction, a valuable test is to determine the blood flow in the umbilical vessels and uteroplacental unit. This is done by Doppler measurements of the blood flow in the umbilical artery and the myometrical arteries adjacent to the placenta [108]. This procedure yields Doppler waveforms for analysis, indicating the relative blood flow velocity from both the maternal and fetal circulation system. If both sets of waveforms are normal, the risk of fetal demise or dysfunction appears to be minimal [108]. One strong feature of the technique is the ability to detect pathological wave forms in arteria umbilicalis. These waveforms appear when the umbilical arterial flow is close to zero in diastole and the fetus is severely under-supplied with nutrients, and is considered a fetal indication for Caesarean section. Pathological waveforms on the maternal side are associated with increased vascular resistance in the uteroplacental circulation and increased risk for maternal hypertension, but if the fetal waveforms are normal, the risk for fetal dysfunction seems to be less pronounced, and conservative treatment is advised [108].

In diabetic pregnancy complicated by maternal vascular disease, the Doppler blood flow measurement may confirm a state of increased vascular placental resistance which could contribute to the fetal dysfunction [82]. If, however, the pregnant diabetic woman does not have hypertension, nephropathy, or preeclampsia, the Doppler test is of limited value for assessing fetal status.

Dynamic placental scintigraphy

Two analogous methods have been used in order to dynamically determine the maternal uteroplacental blood flow in diabetic pregnancy. Placental scintigraphy has been performed after the intravenous administration of the short-lived radio nucleotide indium 113 m [104, 131], or xenon 133 [81] to the pregnant woman. The emitted radiation was registered in a scintillation camera positioned over the placenta and the dynamic pattern of isotope accumulation was subsequently analyzed. The ratio between the maximum activity and the rise time (time between 5–95% of maximum activity) of indium 113 m (uteroplacental blood flow index) should conceivably be proportional to the maternal placental blood flow [105]. This relationship has been statistically confirmed in primate pregnancy by comparison of the uteroplacental blood flow index value with the actual blood flow measured with injected radioactive microspheres [134].

In all of the placental scintigraphy studies the result indicated decreased maternal uteroplacental blood flow [81, 104, 131], remarkably similar to measurements in pregnancies with intrauterine growth retardation. In addition, the uteroplacental blood flow index did not show any correlation with birth weight in the diabetic pregnancies [104], indicating that factors other than the decreased maternal blood supply to the intervillous space are of importance for fetal growth.

Placental histopathological morphometry

A logical strategy for studying the possible role played by placental (dys)-function in the developmental disturbances encountered in the fetus of the diabetic mother would be to evaluate the histological structure of the placenta. Such studies have been carried out, but so far they have not been able to identify any unique change present exclusively in the placenta of the diabetic woman [43]. Some histopathological findings, however, seem to describe a recurring pattern. The placenta of the diabetic woman frequently shows an immature microscopic villous morphology in relation to the length of gestation. Increased villous branching has been reported, and individual villi show numerous cytotrophoblastic cells on a diffusely-expanded basement membrane [9]. One consequence of these findings, an increased total maternal-fetal exchange area, has been demonstrated in stereological studies, both in the placenta of the gestational diabetic woman [139] and the insulin-dependent diabetic woman [140]. Furthermore the changes in placental morphology were shown to be proportional to the variability in maternal glucose concentration [12]. Ultrastructurally, the trophoblastic cells showed an increased number of microvilli and intracellular vesicles, which together with the enlarged surface area available for maternal-fetal exchange suggest increased, rather than decreased, transport capability [43].

In this context, it is pertinent to refer to a recent series of histological studies of fetal and maternal arterial morphology, which have shown endarteritis and an increased frequency of hypovascular villi in the placenta from diabetic pregnancies, as compared to normal placentae [10]. Increased number of spiral arterial lesions in the form of intramural fibrosis in the deciduous part of the vessels were also found in proportion to the degree of maternal metabolic control and C-peptide levels [11].

Methods of evaluating postnatal effects

The important question of whether the child of the diabetic mother shows any functional impairments in adult age has been investigated by long-term epidemiological follow-up studies performed at centers with large registers of diabetic patients.

Methods of assessing intellectual and psychomotor status in the fetus

A controversy exists regarding the intellectual development of the infant of the diabetic mother. A number of early reports have suggested that infants of diabetic mothers may show signs of impaired intellectual development [7, 20, 64, 136, 152]. There are also several negative reports. Cummins & Norrish [23], Hadden and collaborators [56], and Persson [113] failed to demonstrate any effect on the children of diabetic mothers in this respect, whereas the group at Northwestern University in Chicago found a relationship between the IQ of the child and maternal levels of ketone bodies in the two last trimesters [127, 132]. Changes in the psychomotor development of the offspring of diabetic mothers have also been demonstrated [114, 126, 132], and there have been a few negative reports from northern Europe [56, 113].

Methods of assessing weight and glucose homeostasis in the fetus

The question regarding a possible long-term effect of diabetic pregnancy on the future weight gain of the fetus has been answered affirmatively by several studies of the Pima Indians [115, 118], and by some reports from Europe and USA [41, 50, 90, 146], but such a relationship has been difficult to demonstrate in other studies [56, 113].

The risk for developing diabetes is increased in the children of diabetic Pima Indian mothers compared to children born to non-diabetic Indian mothers [116, 117, 118]. In other populations as well, the risk for incurring diabetes is increased in the children of diabetic mothers, however, the risk is three times greater when only the father is diabetic [147].

In a series of studies from southern England, adults with low birth weight have shown increased risk for developing impaired glucose tolerance [122], as well as having increased risk to develop adult-onset diabetes mellitus [5].

Non-clinical methods

In a survey of methodological procedures aimed at detecting fetal dysfunction in human diabetic pregnancy, there are a number of problems that do not seem possible to address when one is restricted to the methods currently used in clinical settings [38]. Indeed, some of the more fundamental questions with regard to fetal dysfunction and its detection are at present only approachable by experimental methods. A few of these will be briefly reviewed here. What types of malformations yield organ dysfunction [80]? Is there a general pattern for the development effects exerted by maternal diabetes on the offspring among various animal species – such as fetal endocrine B-cell-supermaturation, and retarded development of fetal lung cells? When do dysmorphogenic changes occur during embryonic development [29, 31, 92]? Are there genetically predisposing factors for the disturbed development of offspring in diabetic pregnancy [30, 33]? Which cellular and subcellular mechanisms are capable of causing fetal dysfunction as a consequence of maternal diabetes [17, 35, 37, 144]?

Experimental in vivo methods

Oxygenation of the fetus: In their expansion of the Pedersen hypothesis, MacFarlane & Tsakalakos [86] suggested that fetal hyperinsulinemia causes macrosomia with increased demand for oxygen, and increased risk for fetal hypoxia. In a clinical evaluation of perinatal asphyxia in diabetic pregnancy, poor maternal glycemic control emerged as one important risk factor [96].

The possibility of fetal hypoxia as a consequence of fetal hyperglycemia or hyperinsulinemia has been investigated in various experimental settings. Infusion of glucose [119], or insulin [19] to fetal sheep in utero yields decreased fetal oxygenation [121] and increased levels of fetal erythropoietin [120]. Similar findings are reported both from studies of newborn infants of diabetic mothers, and from hyperinsulinemic rhesus monkey fetuses [149].

Timing of the induction of congenital malformations: Evidence in favor of a very early induction of the congenital malformations is supplied by the theoretical considerations of Mills and collaborators [92], who designated the embryonic period up to the 7th gestational week as the teratologically susceptible time period. Strong indirect support for this notion was also obtained from studies where early preconception counseling and treatment of the mothers yielded markedly reduced malformation rates [45, 100]. The problem of the timing of the teratological induction, which is currently not scientifically accessible by clinical methods, has been studied experimentally in vivo. The outcome of pregnancy in animals with either spontaneous diabetes (BB rat), or chemically (streptozotocin) induced diabetes has been analyzed. The pregnant rats were treated so their offspring were exposed to a manifest maternal diabetic state only during a limited period of the gestation. The findings in these studies suggest the post-conception days 6–10 in the rat, which corresponds to human post-conception weeks 2–4, constitute the teratogenic period for skeletal malformations [3, 29, 31].

Long-term effects on the offspring: Several animal models have been used to assess the long term effects of a maternal diabetic state on the offspring, and in particular on the glucose homeostasis and function of the endocrine pancreas. The adult offspring of rats, made severely diabetic by a streptozotocin injection on the day of conception, were evaluated. These adult rats showed insulin resistance [70, 71], and slightly enhanced glucose-stimulated insulin secretion [145]. A similar pattern – insulin resistance concomitant with normal insulin secretion – was seen in the adult offspring of partly insulin-treated manifestly diabetic rats, made diabetic with streptozotocin one to three weeks before mating [55]. In the latter model, the male offspring showed more pronounced insulin resistance than the female offspring [55].

The adult offspring of mildly diabetic rats (streptozotocin injection on the day of conception) did not show signs of insulin resistance [1], but displayed decreased insulin secretory capacity [145]. A similar pattern of inhibited insulin secretion was also found in the adult offspring of rats subjected to two other diabetes-like conditions; maternal glucose infusions in late pregnancy [8], and maternal dietary protein deficiency during pregnancy and lactation [24]. In addition, rats with decreased insulin secretion due to consumption of a protein poor diet for 3 weeks after weaning were made pregnant and showed signs of a very mild glucose intolerance during gestation [36]. Compared to control newborns, these rats produced newborns with higher than normal body weight, as well as increased pancreatic insulin content and B-cell mass supporting the concept of mild disturbance of maternal glucose homeostasis [36].

Another suspected long-term effect of maternal diabetes, disturbed psychomotor behavior in the offspring, has been studied experimentally in a manifestly diabetic rat model. Diabetic rats were treated with insulin during the latter half of pregnancy, the offspring were reared by foster mothers and monitored regarding the development of basic behavioral patterns up to adult age. In the immediate postnatal period, the neonatal rats of the diabetic mothers emitted more ultrasound calls than the controls. At adult age, however, the offspring of the diabetic rats showed no difference in basic behavior compared to the offspring of normal mothers [74].

Experimental in vitro methods

Cellular and subcellular teratological mechanisms: Whole embryo culture [102] has been a useful method for delineating a number of teratogens with specific relevance to diabetic pregnancy (cf. Table 1). Thus, glucose, β-hydroxybutyrate, the leucine metabolite α-keto-isocaproate, and pyruvate in excess have been shown to exert teratogenic influence on early rodent embryo development [21, 35, 72]. Decreased glucose concentration in the culture medium has also shown to be teratogenic [2]. Furthermore, somatomedin inhibitor(s) [129] and mannose [44] in excess cause embryonic maldevelopment in vitro.

Table 1 Teratological compounds identified in the whole embryo culture system

Teratological compound	Reference
Excess glucose	[4, 17, 21, 30, 32, 34, 35, 37, 52, 63, 67, 68]
Deficiency of glucose	[2]
Excess β-hydroxybutyrate	[30, 35, 37, 72]
Excess α-ketoisocaproic acid	[35]
Excess mannose	[44]
Excess somatomedin inhibitor(s)	[129]

The culture method also allows the evaluation of various possible teratological mechanisms operating in diabetic pregnancy, such as arachidonic acid deficiency [52], prostaglandin imbalance [4], myoinositol deficiency [63, 68], sorbitol accumulation [32, 67], and free oxygen radical generation [34, 35, 37].

Evidently, several of these teratological pathways may interact very closely, and, in fact, be identical in the sense that they represent different aspects of one process. It will the challenge of future research in this field to clarify the interrelationships between these, and other, teratological pathways in diabetic pregnancy, as well as their exact mode of interaction with embryonic gene expression [17, 78, 130, 144] (cf. Table 2).

Table 2 Teratological mechanisms induced by increased glucose concentration in vitro

Teratological mechanisms induced by excess glucose	Reference
Accumulation of sorbitol	[32, 63, 67]
Deficiency of myo-inositol	[4, 63, 67, 68]
Deficiency of arachidonic acid	[52]
Alteration of prostaglandins	[4]
Free oxygen radical generation	[34, 35, 37]

Concluding remarks

Diabetic pregnancy is an exciting field of research, in which a dramatic improvement in the previously serious prognosis for the offspring has occurred in recent years. It is widely recognized that an interdisciplinary approach is necessary for a full understanding of the basic pathogenic and teratogenic mechanisms in this field.

The exact (cellular) changes in embryonic/fetal development provoked by maternal diabetes are not known. A number of teratogens and possible teratological mechanisms have been identified, and their interrelationships and physiological relevance for human diabetic pregnancy will be investigated in the future studies.

Acknowledgements

The author is grateful to Dr. David R. Hadden, Belfast, Northern Ireland, for his very helpful comments on this chapter. He is also indebted to Dr. Ove Axelsson, Uppsala, and Dr. Ulf Hanson, Örebro, Sweden, whose comments provided valuable insight into several clinical research fields. With regard to the work from the Department of Medical Cell Biology at Uppsala University referred to in this review, grateful acknowledgement is made to support from The Swedish Medical Research Council (Grant no 12X−7475), The Family Ernfors Fund, The Novo Nordisk Insulin Foundation Committee, The Swedish Diabetes Association, The Juvenile Diabetes Foundation International, and The Bank of Sweden Tercentenary Foundation.

References

[1] Aerts L, Sodoyez-Goffaux F, Sodoyez JC et al. The diabetic intrauterine milieu has a long-lasting effect on insulin secretion by the B cells and on insulin uptake by target tissue. Am J Obstet Gynecol 1988; 159: 1287–1292.

[2] Akazawa S, Akazawa M, Hashimoto M et al. Effects of hypoglycaemia on early embryogenesis in rat embryo organ culture. Diabetologia 1987; 30: 791–796.

[3] Baker L, Egler JM, Klein SM et al. Metculous control of diabetes during organogenesis prevents congenital lumbosacral defects in rats. Diabetes 1981; 30: 955–959.

[4] Baker L, Piddington R, Goldman A et al. Myo-inositol and prostaglandins reverse the glucose inhibition of neural tube fusion in cultured mouse embryos. Diabetologia 1990; 6: 593–596.

[5] Barker DJ, Hales CN, Fall CH et al. Type 2 (non-insulin-dependent) diabetes mellitus, hypertension and hyperlipidaemia (syndrome X): relation to reduced fetal growth. Diabetologia 1993; 36: 62–67.

[6] Becerra JE, Khoury MJ, Cordero JF et al. Diabetes mellitus during pregnancy and the risks for specific birth defects: A population-based case-control study. Pediatrics 1990; 85: 1–9.

[7] Bibergeil H, Gödel E, Amendt P. Diabetes and pregnancy: early and late prognosis of children of diabetic mothers. In: Camerini-Davalos RA, Cole HS, eds. Early diabetes in early life. New York: Academic Press 1975, 427–434.

[8] Bihoreau MT, Ktorza A, Kinebanyan MF et al. Impaired glucose homeostasis in adult rats from hyperglycemic mothers. Diabetes 1986; 35: 979–984.

[9] Björk O, Persson B. Placental changes in relation to the degree of metabolic control in diabetes mellitus. Placenta 1982; 3: 367–378.

[10] Björk O, Persson B. The fetal arterial vasculature in placentas of insulin-dependent diabetic mothers. Acta Pathol Microbiol Immunol Scand 1982; 90: 289–294.

[11] Björk O, Persson B, Stangenberg M et al. Spiral artery lesions in relation to metabolic control in diabetes mellitus. Acta Obstet Gynecol Scand 1984; 63: 123–127.

[12] Björk O, Persson B. Villous structure in different parts of the cotyledon in placentas of insulin-dependent diabetic women. A morphometric study. Acta Obstet Gynecol Scand 1984; 63: 37–43.

[13] Bochner, CJ, Medearis AL, Williams J et al. Early third-trimester screening in gestational diabetes to determine the risk of macrosomia and labour dystocia at term. Am J Obstet Gynecol 1987; 157: 703–708.

[14] Brock DJH. Mechanisms by which amniotic fluid alpha-fetoprotein may be increased in fetal abnormalities. Lancet 1976; II: 345–346.

[15] Brown ZA, Mills JL, Metzger BE et al. Early sonographic evaluation for fetal growth delay and congenital malformations in pregnancies complicated by insulin-requiring diabetes. Diabetes Care 1992; 15: 613–619.

[16] Bybee DE, Metzger BE, Freinkel N et al. Amniotic fluid prolactin in the third trimester of pregnancies complicated by gestational or pregestational diabetes mellitus. Metabolism 1990; 39: 714–718.

[17] Cagliero E, Forsberg H, Sala et al. Maternal diabetes induces increased expression of extracellular matrix components in rat embryos. Diabetes 1993; 42: 975–980.

[18] Canick JA, Knight GJ, Palomaki GE et al. Low second trimester maternal serum unconjugated oestriol in pregnancies with Down's syndrome. Br J Obstet Gynecol 1988; 95: 330–333.

[19] Carson BS, Philipps AF, Simmons MA et al. Effects of a sustained insulin infusion upon glucose uptake and oxygenation of the ovine fetus. Pediatr Res 1980; 14: 147–152.

[20] Churchill JA, Berendes HW, Nemore J. Neuro-psychological deficit in children of diabetic mothers. Am J Obstet Gynecol 1969; 105: 257–268.

[21] Cockroft DL, Coppola PT. Teratogenic effects of excess glucose on head-fold rat embryos in culture. Teratology 1977; 16: 141–146.

[22] Combs CA, Gunderson E, Kitzmüller JL et al. Relationship of fetal macrosomia to maternal postprandial glucose control during pregnancy. Diabetes Care 1992; 15: 1251–1257.
[23] Cummins M, Norrish M. Follow-up of children of diabetic mothers. Arch Dis Child 1980; 55: 259–264.
[24] Dahri S, Snoeck A, Reusens-Billen B et al. Islet function in offspring of mothers on low-protein diet during gestation. Diabetes 1991; 40 (Suppl. 2): 115–120.
[25] Damm P, Mølsted Pedersen L. Significant decrease in congenital malformations in newborn infants of an unselected population of diabetic women. Am J Obstet Gynecol 1989; 161: 1163–1167.
[26] Dicker D, Feldberg D, Samuel N et al. Spontaneous abortion in patients with insulin-dependent diabetes mellitus: the effect of preconceptional diabetic control. Am J Obstet Gynecol 1988; 158: 1161–1164.
[27] Dicker D, Feldberg D, Yeshaya A et al. Fetal surveillance in insulin-dependent diabetic pregnancy: predictive value of the biophysical profile. Am J Obstet Gynecol 1988; 159: 800–804.
[28] Dooley SL, Depp R, Socol ML et al. Urinary estriols in diabetic pregnancy: a reappraisal. Obstet Gynecol 1984; 64: 469–475.
[29] Eriksson RSM, Thunberg L, Eriksson UJ. Effects of interrupted insulin treatment on fetal outcome of pregnant diabetic rats. Diabetes 1989; 38: 764–772.
[30] Eriksson UJ. Importance of genetic predisposition and maternal environment for the occurrence of congenital malformations in offspring in diabetic rats. Teratology 1988; 37: 365–374.
[31] Eriksson UJ, Bone AJ, Turnbull DM et al. Timed interruption of insulin therapy in diabetic BB/E rat pregnancy: Effect on maternal metabolism and fetal outcome. Acta Endocrinol (Copenh) 1989; 120: 800–810.
[32] Eriksson UJ, Brolin SE, Naeser P. Influence of sorbitol accumulation on growth and development of embryos cultured in elevated levels of glucose and fructose. Diabetes Res 1989; 11: 27–32.
[33] Eriksson UJ, den Bieman M, Prins JB et al. Differences in susceptibility for diabetes induced malformations in separated rat colonies of common origin. In: Proc 4th FELASA Symp. Lyon, France: 1990; 53–57.
[34] Eriksson UJ, Borg LAH. Protection by free oxygen radical scavenging enzymes against glucose-induced embryonic malformations in vitro. Diabetologia 1991; 34: 325–331.
[35] Eriksson UJ, Borg LAH. Diabetes and embryonic malformations. Role of substrate-induced free-oxygen radical production for dysmorphogenesis in cultured rat embryos. Diabetes 1993; 42: 411–419.
[36] Eriksson UJ, Swenne I. Diabetes in pregnancy: fetal macrosomia, hyper-insulinism, and islet hyperplasia in the offspring of rats subjected to temporary protein-energy malnutrition early in life. Pediatr Res 1993; 34: 791–795.
[37] Eriksson UJ, Borg LAH, Cagliero E et al. Increased activity of superoxide dismutase in transgenic mouse embryos protects from diabetes-induced dysmorphogenesis. Submitted for publication, 1994.
[38] Eriksson UJ. Teratological mechanisms associated with maternal metabolic imbalance. In: Diamond MP, Naftolin F, eds. Metabolism in the female life cycle. Rome: Areno Symp 1993; 215–226.
[39] Evertson LR, Gauthier RJ, Collea JV. Fetal demise following negative contraction stress tests. Obstet Gynecol 1978; 51: 671–673.
[40] Fallucca F, Gargiulo P, Troili F et al. Amniotic fluid insulin, C-peptide concentrations, and fetal morbidity in infants of diabetic mothers. Am J Obstet Gynecol 1985; 153: 534–540.
[41] Farquhar JW. Prognosis for babies born to diabetic mothers in Edinburgh. Arch Dis Child 1960; 44: 36–47.
[42] Fern PE, Grunert GM, Lewis SB. Urinary estriols: are they of value in normoglycemic diabetic pregnancy? Diabetes Care 1982; 5: 316–318.

[43] Fox H. The placenta in diabetes mellitus. In: Sutherland HW, Stowers JM, Pearson DWM, eds. Carbohydrate metabolism in pregnancy and the newborn. New York: IV. Springer Verlag, 1989; 109–117.
[44] Freinkel N, Lewis NJ, Akazawa S et al. The honeybee syndrome – implications of the teratogenicity of mannose in rat embryo culture. N Engl J Med 1984; 310: 223–230.
[45] Fuhrmann K, Reiher H, Semmler K et al. The effect of intensified conventional insulin therapy before and during pregnancy on the malformation rate in offspring of diabetic mothers. Exp Clin Endocrinol 1984; 83: 173–177.
[46] Gabbay KH, Hastry K, Breslow JL et al. Long term blood glucose control in diabetes mellitus. J Clin Endocrinol Metab 1977; 44: 859–864.
[47] Gabbe SG, Lowensohn RI, Mestman JH et al. Lecithin/sphingomyelin ratio in pregnancies complicated by diabetes mellitus. Am J Obstet Gynecol 1977; 128: 757–760.
[48] Gabbe SG, Mestman JH, Freeman RK et al. Management and outcome of pregnancy in diabetes mellitus classes B to R. Am J Obstet Gynecol 1977; 129: 723–732.
[49] Gabbe SG. Management of diabetes in pregnancy: six decades of experience. In: Pitkin RM, Zlatnik F, eds. The Yearbook of Obstetrics and Gynaecology. Chicago: Year Book Medical Publishers, 1980; 37–49.
[50] Gerlini G, Arachi S, Gori MG et al. Developmental aspects of the offspring of diabetic mothers. Acta Endocrinol (Copenh) 1986; (Suppl. 277): 150–155.
[51] Golde SH, Montoro M, Good-Anderson B et al. The role of non-stress tests, fetal biophysical profile, and contraction stress tests in the outpatient management of insulin-requiring diabetic pregnancies. AmJ Obstet Gynecol 1984; 148: 269–273.
[52] Goldman AS, Baker L, Piddington R et al. Hyperglycemia-induced teratogenesis is mediated by a functional deficiency of arachidonic acid. Proc Natl Acad Sci USA 1985; 82: 8227–8231.
[53] Greene MF, Hare JW, Krache M et al. Prematurity among insulin-requiring diabetic gravid women. Am J Obstet Gynecol 1989; 161: 106–111.
[54] Greene MF, Hare JW, Cloherty JP et al. First-trimester hemoglobin A1 and risk for major malformation and spontaneous abortion in diabetic pregnancy. Teratology 1989; 39: 225–231.
[55] Grill V, Johansson B, Jalkanen et al. Influence of severe diabetes mellitus early in pregnancy in the rat: effects on insulin sensitivity and insulin secretion in the offspring. Diabetologia 1991; 34: 373–378.
[56] Hadden DR, Byrne E, Trotter I et al. Physical and psychological health of children of Type 1 (insulin-dependent) diabetic mothers. Diabetologia 1984; 26: 250–254.
[57] Hadden DR, Traub AI, Harley JM. Diabetes-related perinatal mortality and congenital fetal abnormality: a problem of audit. Diabetic Med 1988; 5: 321–323.
[58] Hall K, Hansson U, Lundin G et al. Serum levels of somatomedins and somatomedin-binding protein in pregnant women with type I or gestational diabetes and their infants. J Clin Endocrinol Metab 1986; 63: 1300–1306.
[59] Hallmann M, Teramo K. Amniotic fluid phospholipid profile as a prediction of fetal maturity in diabetic pregnancies. Obstet Gynecol 1979; 54: 703–707.
[60] Hanson U, Persson B, Stangenberg M. Factors influencing neonatal morbidity in diabetic pregnancy. Diabetes Res 1986; 3: 71–76.
[61] Hanson U, Persson B, Thunell S. Relationship between haemoglobin. A1c in early type 1 (insulin-dependent) diabetic pregnancy and the occurrence of spontaneous abortion and fetal malformation in Sweden. Diabetologia 1990; 33: 100–104.
[62] Harper MA, Morrow RJ. Early growth delay in diabetic pregnancy. BMJ 1988; 296: 1005–1006.
[63] Hashimoto M, Akazawa S, Akazawa M et al. Effects of hyperglycemia on sorbitol and myo-inositol contents of cultured embryos: treatment with aldose reductase inhibitor and myo-inositol supplementation. Diabetologia 1990; 33: 597–602.
[64] Haworth JC, McRae KN, Dilling LA. Prognosis of infants of diabetic mothers in relation to neonatal hypoglycemia. Dev Med Child Neurol 1976; 18: 471–479.

[65] Heita-Heikurainen H, Teramo K. Comparison of menstrual history and basal body temperature with early fetal growth by ultrasound in diabetic pregnancy. Acta Obstet Gynecol Scand 1989; 68: 457–459.
[66] Hill WC, Pelle-Day G, Kitzmiller JL et al. Insulin-like growth factors in fetal macrosomia with and without maternal diabetes. Horm Res 1989; 32: 178–182.
[67] Hod M, Star S, Passonneau JV et al. Effect of hyperglycemia on sorbitol and myo-inositol content of cultured rat conceptus: failure of aldose reductase inhibitors to modify myo-inositol depletion and dysmorphogenesis. Biochem Biophys Res Comm 1986; 140: 974–980.
[68] Hod M, Star S, Passonneau JV et al. Glucose-induced dysmorphogenesis in the cultured rat conceptus: Prevention by supplementation with myo-inositol. Isr J Med Sci 1990; 26: 541–544.
[69] Holden KP, Jovanovic L, Druzin ML et al. Increased fetal activity with low maternal blood glucose levels in pregnancies complicated by diabetes. Am J Perinatol 1984; 1: 161–164.
[70] Holemans K, Aerts L, Van Assche FA. Evidence for an insulin resistance in adult offspring of pregnant streptozotocin-diabetic rats. Diabetologia 1991; 34: 81–85.
[71] Holemans K, Van Bree Rm Verhaeghe J et al. In vivo glucose utilization by individual tissues in virgin and pregnant offspring of severely diabetic rats. Diabetes 1993; 42: 530–536.
[72] Horton WE, Sadler TW. Effects of maternal diabetes on early embryogenesis. Alterations in morphogenesis produced by the ketone body, B-hydroxybutyrate. Diabetes 1983; 32: 610–616.
[73] Jerwell J, Bjerkedal T, Moe N. Outcome of pregnancies in diabetic mothers in Norway 1967–1976. Diabetologia 1980; 18: 131–134.
[74] Johansson B, Meyerson B, Eriksson UJ. Behavioural effects of an intrauterine or neonatal diabetic environment in the rat. Biol Neonate 1991; 59: 226–235.
[75] Johnson JM, Lange IR, Harman CR et al. Biophysical profile scoring in the management of the diabetic pregnancy. Obstet Gynecol 1988; 72: 841–846.
[76] Jovanovic L, Druzin M, Peterson CM. Effects of euglycemia on the outcome of pregnancy in insulin-dependent diabetic women as compared with normal control subjects. Am J Med 1980; 68: 105–112.
[77] Jovanovic-Peterson L, Peterson CM, Reed GF et al. Maternal postprandial glucose levels and infant birth weight: the Diabetes in Early Pregnancy Study. Am J Obstet Gynecol 1991; 164: 103–111.
[78] Kashihara N, Watanabe Y, Makino H et al. Selective decreased de novo synthesis of glomerular proteoglycans under the influence of reactive oxygen species. Proc Natl Acad Sci USA 1992; 89: 6309–6313.
[79] Kitzmiller JL, Gavin LA, Gin GD et al. Preconception care of diabetes. Glycemic control prevents congenital anomalies. JAMA 1991; 265: 731–736.
[80] Kucera J. Rate and type of congenital anomalies among offspring of diabetic women. J Reprod Med 1971; 7: 61–70.
[81] Käär K, Jouppila P, Kuikka et al. Intervillous blood flow in normal and complicated late pregnancy measured by means of an intravenous 133Xe method. Acta Obstet Gynecol Scand 1980; 59: 7–10.
[82] Landon MB, Gabbe SG, Bruner JP et al. Doppler umbilical artery velocimetry in pregnancy complicated by insulin dependent diabetes mellitus. Obstet Gynecol 1989; 73: 961–965.
[83] Landon MB, Mintz MG, Gabbe SG. Sonographic evaluation of fetal abdominal growth: predictor of the large-for-gestational age infants in pregnancies complicated by diabetes mellitus. Am J Obstet Gynecol 1989; 160: 115–121.
[84] Leslie RDG, Pyke DA, John PN et al. Hemoglobin A1 in diabetic pregnancy. Lancet 1978; II: 958–959.
[85] Lunell NO, Persson B, Devarajan LV et al. Urinary C-peptide in the neonate correlates both to maternal glucose tolerance and the fetal size at birth. Am J Perinatol 1988; 5: 144–145.

[86] MacFarlane CM, Tsakalakos N. The extended Pedersen hypothesis. Clin Physiol Biochem 1988; 6: 68–73.
[87] Madsen H. Fetal oxygenation in diabetic pregnancy. With special reference to maternal blood oxygen affinity and its effectors. Dan Med Bull 1986; 33: 64–74.
[88] Manning FA, Platt LD, Sipos L. Antepartum fetal evaluation: development of a fetal biophysical profile. Am J Obstet Gynecol 1980; 136: 787–795.
[89] Manning FA, Morrison I, Lange IR et al. Fetal assessment based on fetal biophysical profile scoring: experience in 12.620 referred high-risk pregnancies. I. Perinatal mortality by frequency and etiology. Am J Obstet Gynecol 1985; 151: 343–350.
[90] Metzger BE, Silverman BL, Freinkel N et al. Amniotic fluid insulin concentration as a predictor of obesity. Arch Dis Child 1990; 65: 1050–1052.
[91] Miller EM, Hare JW, Cloherty JR et al. Major congenital anomalies and elevated hemoglobin A1c in early weeks of diabetic pregnancy. N Engl J Med 1981; 304: 1331–1334.
[92] Mills J, Baker L, Goldman AS. Malformations in infants of diabetic mothers occur before the seventh gestational week. Diabetes 1979; 28: 292–293.
[93] Mills JL, Knopp RH, Simpson JL et al. and The National Institute of Child Health and Human Development-Diabetes in Early Pregnancy Study. Lack of relation of increased malformation rates in infants of diabetic mothers to glycemic control during organogenesis. N Engl J Med 1988; 318: 671–676.
[94] Mills J, Simpson J, Driscoll SG et al. and The National Institute of Child Health and Human Development-Diabetes in Early Pregnancy Study. Incidence of spontaneous abortion among normal women and insulin dependent diabetic women whose pregnancies were identified within 21 days of conception. N Engl J Med 1988; 319: 1617–1623.
[95] Milunsky A, Alpert E, Kitzmiller JL et al. Prenatal diagnosis of neural tube defects. VIII. The importance of serum alfa-fetoprotein screening in diabetic pregnant women. Am J Obstet Gynecol 1982; 142: 1030–1032.
[96] Mimouni F, Miodovnik M, Siddiqi TA et al. Perinatal asphyxia in infants of insulin dependent diabetic mothers. J Pediatr 1988; 113: 345–353.
[97] Mintz MC, Landon MB, Gabbe SG et al. Shoulder soft tissue width as a predictor of macrosomia in diabetic pregnancies. Am J Perinatol 1989; 6: 240–243.
[98] Miodovnik M, Lavin JP, Knowles HC et al. Spontaneous abortion among insulin-dependent diabetic women. Am J Obstet Gynecol 1984; 150: 372–376.
[99] Mølsted-Pedersen L, Tygstrup I, Pedersen J. Congenital malformations in newborn infants of diabetic women. Correlation with maternal diabetic vascular complications. Lancet 1964; I: 1124–1126.
[100] Mølsted-Pedersen L. Pregnancy and diabetes, a survey. Acta Endocrinol (Copenh) 1980; 94 (Suppl. 238): 13–19.
[101] Mølsted-Pedersen L, Kühl C. Obstetrical management in diabetic pregnancy: the Copenhagen experience. Diabetologia 1986; 29: 13–16.
[102] New DAT. Whole-embryo culture and the study of mammalian embryos during organogenesis. Biol Rev 1978; 53: 81–122.
[103] Nordlander E, Hanson U, Persson B. Factors influencing neonatal morbidity in gestational diabetic pregnancy. Br J Obstet Gynecol 1989; 96: 671–678.
[104] Nylund L, Lunell NO, Lewander R et al. Uteroplacental blood flow in diabetic pregnancy: measurements with indium 113m and a computer linked gramma camera. Am J Obstet Gynecol 1982; 144: 298–302.
[105] Nylund L, Lunell NO, Sarby B et al. Functional placental scintigraphy: A methodological and clinical investigation. Acta Radiol [Diagn] (Stockh) 1983; 24: 165–170.
[106] Ogata ES, Sabbagha R, Metzger BE et al. Serial ultrasonography to assess evolving fetal macrosomia. JAMA 1980; 243: 2405–2408.
[107] Patrick J, Campbell K, Charmichael L et al. Patterns of gross fetal body movements over 24-hour observation intervals during the last 10 weeks of pregnancy. Am J Obstet Gynecol 1982; 142: 363–371.

[108] Pearce JM. The application of uteroplacental waveforms to complicated pregnancies. In: Pearce JM, ed. Doppler ultrasound in perinatal medicine. Oxford: Oxford University Press, 1992; 159–177.
[109] Pedersen J. The pregnant diabetic and her newborn. Problems and management. 2nd ed. Copenhagen: Munksgaard, 1977.
[110] Pedersen JF, Mølsted-Pedersen L. Early growth retardation in diabetic pregnancy. BMJ 1979; 1: 18–19.
[111] Pedersen JF, Mølsted-Pedersen L. Early growth delay detected by ultrasound marks increased risk for congenital malformation in diabetic pregnancy. BMJ 1981; 283: 269–271.
[112] Persson B, Heding LG, Lunell NO et al. Fetal beta cell function in diabetic pregnancy. Amniotic fluid concentrations of proinsulin, insulin, and C-peptide during the last trimester of pregnancy. Am J Obstet Gynecol 1982; 144: 455–459.
[113] Persson B. Longterm morbidity in infants of diabetic mothers. Acta Endocrinol (Copenh) 1986; (Suppl. 277): 156–158.
[114] Petersen MB, Pedersen SA, Greisen G et al. Early growth delay in diabetic pregnancy: relation to psychomotor development at age 4. BMJ 1988; 296: 298–600.
[115] Pettitt DJ, Baird HR, Aleck KA et al. Excessive obesity in offspring of Pima Indian women with diabetes during pregnancy. N Engl J Med 1983; 308: 242–245.
[116] Pettitt DJ, Aleck KA, Baird HR et al. Congenital susceptibility to NIDDM. Role of intrauterine environment. Diabetes 1988; 37: 622–628.
[117] Pettitt DJ, Bennett PH, Saad MF et al. Abnormal glucose tolerance during pregnancy in Pima Indian women. Long-term effects on offspring. Diabetes 1991; 40 (Suppl. 2): 126–130.
[118] Pettitt DJ, Nelson RG, Saad MF et al. Diabetes and obesity in the offspring of Pima Indian women with diabetes during pregnancy. Diabetes Care 1993; 16: 310–314.
[119] Philipps AF, Dubin JW, Matty PJ et al. Arterial hypoxemia and hyperinsulinemia in the chronically hyperglycemic fetal lamb. Pediatr Res 1982; 16: 653–658.
[120] Philipps AF, Widness JA, Garcia JF et al. Erythropoietin elevation in the chronically hyperglycemic fetal lamb. Proc Soc Exp Biol Med 1982; 170: 42–47.
[121] Philipps AF, Porte PJ, Stabinsky S et al. Effects of chronic fetal hyperglycemia upon oxygen consumption in the ovine uterus and conceptus. J Clin Invest 1984; 74: 279–286.
[122] Phipps K, Barker DJ, Hales CN et al. Fetal growth and impaired glucose tolerance in men and women. Diabetologia 1993; 36: 225–228.
[123] Reid M, Hadden DR, Harley JMG et al. Fetal malformations in diabetics with high haemoglobin A1c in early pregnancy. BMJ 1984; 289: 1001.
[124] Reiher H, Fuhrmann K, Noack S et al. Age-dependent insulin secretion of the endocrine pancreas in vitro from fetuses of diabetic and non diabetic patients. Diabetes Care 1983; 6: 446–451.
[125] Roberts RN, Moohan JM, Foo RL et al. Fetal outcome in mothers with impaired glucose tolerance in pregnancy. Diabetes Med 1993; 10: 438–443.
[126] Rizzo T, Freinkel N, Metzger BE et al. Correlations between antepartum maternal metabolism and newborn behaviour. Am J Obstet Gynecol 1990; 163: 1458–1464.
[127] Rizzo T, Metzger BE, Burns et al. Correlations between antepartum maternal metabolism and child intelligence. N Engl J Med 1991; 325: 911–916.
[128] Roberts AB, Pattison NS. Pregnancy in women with diabetes mellitus, twenty-years experience: 1968–1987. N Z Med J 1990; 103: 211–213.
[129] Sadler TW, Phillips LS, Balkan W et al. Somatomedin inhibitors from diabetic rat serum alter growth and development of mouse embryos in culture. Diabetes 1986; 35: 861–865.
[130] Schreck R, Rieber P, Baeuerle PA. Reactive oxygen intermediates as apparently widely used messengers in the activation of the NF-$_{\kappa}$B transcription factor and HIV-1. EMBO J 1991; 10: 2247–2258.
[131] Semmler K, Kirsch G, Zöllner P et al. Die Messung der uteroplazentaren Durchblutung mit Indium-113m in der diabetischen Schwangerschaft. Zentralbl Gynakol 1985; 107: 793–802.
[132] Silverman BL, Rizzo T, Green OC et al. Long-term prospective evaluation of offspring of diabetic mothers. Diabetes 1991; 40 (Suppl. 2): 121–125.

[133] Simpson JL, Elias S, Martin AO et al. Diabetes in pregnancy, Northwestern University series (1977–1981). I. Prospective study of anomalies in offspring of mothers with diabetes mellitus. Am J Obstet Gynecol 1983; 146: 263–270.
[134] Skjöldebrand A, Jansson T, Kjellmer I et al. Comparison between measurements of maternal placental blood flow with dynamic placental scintigraphy and radioactive microspheres. Placenta 1989; 10: 95–102.
[135] Stangenberg M, Persson B, Fredholm BB et al. Profiles of intermediary metabolites in insulin-dependent pregnant diabetic women with or without endogenous insulin production. Diabetes Care 1982; 5: 409–413.
[136] Stehbens JA, Baker GL, Kitchell M. Outcome at ages 1, 3, and 5 years of children born to diabetic women. Am J Obstet Gynecol 1977; 127: 408–413.
[137] Stewart MO, Whittaker PG, Persson B et al. A longitudinal study of circulating progesterone, oestradiol, hCG, and hPL during pregnancy in type 1 diabetic mothers. Br J Obstet Gynecol 1989; 96: 415–423.
[138] Tamura RK, Sabbagha RE, Depp R et al. Diabetic macrosomia: accuracy of third trimester ultrasound. Obstet Gynecol 1986; 67: 828–832.
[139] Teasdale F. Histomorphometry of the placenta of the diabetic women: class A diabetes mellitus. Placenta 1981; 2: 241–251.
[140] Teasdale F. Histomorphometry of the human placenta in class B diabetes mellitus. Placenta 1983; 4: 1–12.
[141) Teramo K, Kuusisto AN, Raivio KO. Perinatal outcome of insulin-dependent diabetic pregnancies. Ann Clin Res 1979; 11: 146–155.
[142] Tydén O, Berne C, Eriksson UJ et al. Fetal maturation in strictly controlled diabetic pregnancy. Diab Res 1984; 1: 131–134.
[143] Tydén O, Berne C, Eriksson UJ et al. Amniotic fluid C-peptide and phosphatidylglycerol in diabetic pregnancy. J Perinat Med 1984; 12: 69–73.
[144] Unger E, Eriksson UJ. Regionally disturbed production of cartilage proteoglycans in malformed fetuses from diabetic rats. Diabetologia 1992; 35: 517–521.
[145] Van Assche FA, Aerts L. Long term effects of diabetes and pregnancy in the rat. Is acquired insulin resistance responsible? Diabetes 1985; 34: 590–597.
[146] Vohr BR, Lipsitt LP, Oh W. Somatic growth of children of diabetic mothers with reference to birth size. J Pediatr 1980; 97: 196–199.
[147] Warram JH, Krolewski AS, Kahn CR. Determinants of IDM and perinatal mortality in children of diabetic mothers. Diabetes 1988; 37: 1328–1334.
[148] Weiss PAM, Hofmann HMH, Winter R et al. Diagnosis and treatment of gestational diabetes according to amniotic fluid insulin levels. Arch Gynecol 1986; 239: 81–90.
[149] Widness JA, Susa JB, Garcia JF et al. Increased erythropoiesis and elevated erythropoietin in infants born to diabetic mothers and in hyperinsulinemic rhesus fetuses. J Clin Invest 1981; 67: 637–642.
[150] Wright AD, Nicholson HO, Pollack A et al. Spontaneous abortion and diabetes mellitus. Postgrad Med J 1983; 59: 295–298.
[151] Ylinen K, Aula P, Stenman U-H et al. Risk of minor and major fetal malformations in diabetics with high hemoglobin A1c values in early pregnancy. BMJ 1984; 289: 345–346.
[152] Yssing M. Long-term prognosis of children born to mothers diabetic when pregnant. In: Camerini-Davalos RA, Cole HS, eds. Early diabetes in early life. New York: Academic Press, 1975; 575–586.
[153] Östlund E, Hanson U. Antenatal nonstress test in complicated and uncomplicated pregnancies in type-1-diabetic women. Eur J Obstet Gynecol Reprod Biol 1991; 39: 13–18.

Exercise protocols in diabetes

H. Galbo

Why study exercise?

A certain minimum of skeletal muscle activity is necessary for all people for everyday activities such as smiling, dressing, cooking and eating. House work and walking and bicycling for the purpose of transportation represent heavier exercise, and severe physical activity may be required in occupational activities in agriculture, forestry, fishing, industry and, obviously, professional sports and ballet. In addition to such obligatory exercise, many people also engage in sports to increase their physical, psychological and social well-being.

Since exercise is an essential part of life, it is important to know the inherent risks and to know how it influences the body with regard to organ function, dietary needs, and interaction with medicine and environment. Exercise studies in people with diabetes are of particular interest since many of the characteristics and manifestations of this disease would be expected to interfere with work performance and vice versa.

Until quite recently, physical activity had been recommended in the metabolic control of diabetes, equivalent to diet and insulin or oral antidiabetic drugs. However, as a result of extensive scientific evidence, it is now assumed that exercise accelerates the rate at which both hyper- and hypoglycemia develop and thus renders difficult the regulation of diabetes, particularly the insulin-dependent type [1–5]. In type 1 diabetes, metabolic control is not improved by exercise [1, 4–6]. In type II diabetes, the lowering of plasma glucose concentrations induced by acute exercise is closely related to the exercise-induced increase in overall energy expenditure. It is likely that a reduction in energy intake would have the same net effect as a corresponding increase in energy expenditure. In fact, it seems that behavioral changes improve long-term glycemic control in type II diabetics only if the patients achieve a considerable weight loss [1, 2, 7].

In addition to effecting glucose homeostasis, regular exercise has a beneficial effect on many organ systems in healthy subjects. Like normal individuals, diabetics respond to endurance training with a decrease in blood pressure and an increase in maximal oxygen uptake and in oxidative enzymatic potential in the muscles [1]. In response to strength training, both groups show an increase in muscle mass and force [1]. However, it cannot be taken for granted that diabetics react the same as healthy subjects. For instance, in physically active diabetics, in contrast to normal subjects, the capillary density may not increase during endurance training, and changes in plasma lipids are not a consistent finding [1, 5]. This indicates that the effects of training have to be explored in diabetics. Interestingly, physical activity probably reduces the occurrence of non-insulin-dependent diabetes [8, 9]. This observation calls for future studies on the effect of exercise on people who are predisposed to develop diabetes.

Finally, exercise can be used in diabetics as in other people to reveal the dysfunction of organs, the capacity of which is taxed during physical activity [10, 11]. Exercise stress testing of skeletal muscles, the myocardium, coronary and leg circulation, respiration and GH secretion is common. Particularly in diabetics, exercise is used to reveal glomerular protein leakage, which may reflect general microvascular dysfunction [12].

Exercise equipment

Clearly, it is important to study diabetics in ordinary living conditions, carrying out their habitual physical activities. A few such field studies have been carried out [13]. However, due to the lack of standardization of the activities and experimental conditions it is difficult to draw very precise general conclusions valid for bigger populations of diabetics from these field studies. The value of these studies is also restricted by methodological limitations.

Portable devices for blood sampling and recording heart rates, arterial blood pressure and oxygen uptake (V_{O2}) are now available. This equipment can be used in ordinary living conditions and in the future will allow a more sophisticated description of the physiology of the exercising diabetic than hitherto possible. The interpretation of results will thus also be improved by the decreased uncertainty regarding the kinetics of the measured variables.

In the laboratory, it is possible to use optimum methodology and to study different subjects, or the same subject at different times, with near-identical conditions. In comparison to real life, however, laboratory experiments mostly represent a simplification. In real life, physical activity is characterized by the use of different muscle groups at different times (e. g. arm and leg muscles), and by varying modes (concentric-muscle shortening vs eccentric-muscle lengthening) and intensity of contractions. In contrast, in the laboratory the various aspects of muscle activity are generally studied separately and a steady-state is aimed at. This makes interpretation and generalization easier, and a steady-state is a prerequisite for the application of many physiological methods. Still, all kinds of activities can be imitated in the laboratory, and protocols with intermittent exercise are frequently used as an obvious simulator of natural activity patterns [14].

During dynamic (isotonic) exercise, muscles alternately contract and relax, and metabolism is predominantly aerobic at most loads, i. e. energy is delivered by oxygen-requiring processes. At high dynamic exercise intensities, energy is also delivered to a considerable extent by anaerobic chemical processes which do not use oxygen. Anaerobic processes are predominant in maintained static (isometric) contractions of more than mild intensity. It is essential for laboratory studies of both dynamic and static exercises that the activity is reproducible and that its intensity can be varied. Dynamic exercise is mostly studied using bicycle ergometers or treadmills, the speed and inclination of which can be varied. Ergometers allow quantitation of the external work produced and, accordingly, of work efficiency, if the metabolic rate is also determined by direct or indirect calorimetry. In addition to bicycle ergometers, ergometers have also been developed for various other activities, e. g. rowing and canoeing. Swimming can be studied in swimming flumes in which the subject swims against a current, the speed of which can be varied [14]. Muscle force can be measured by simple dynamometers during static contractions. A more complete description of mechanical muscle performance is achieved by use of isokinetic dynamometers allowing determination of the relationship between force and velocity of muscle shortening [14].

Standardization of exercise protocols

There are several factors known to have an extensive influence on response to acute exercise. If the influence of another factor, i. e. one which serves to distinguish between two groups of patients, is studied, it is necessary to standardize the experimental conditions so that effects resulting from differences in these major exercise determinants do not make the interpretation difficult. Exemplified by catecholamine, lactate and heart rate response, the general determinants for responses to dynamic exercise are given below. These factors should always be carefully controlled and described:

Intensity of exercise

Heart rate and epinephrine and lactate concentrations in the plasma increase with exercise intensity [15–19]. If possible the external work should be given in watts, however, it may not be possible or easy to calculate the work performed (e. g., in swimming). Furthermore, work efficiency differs between activities (e. g. higher during the crawl than the breast stroke). Accordingly, it is useful to characterize work intensity by V_{O2}, the two parameters being directly related (Fig. 1).

In addition to describing work intensity in absolute terms, it should also be described relative to work capacity. The latter depends on body size and degree of training, and many variables (e. g. epinephrine, lactate and heart

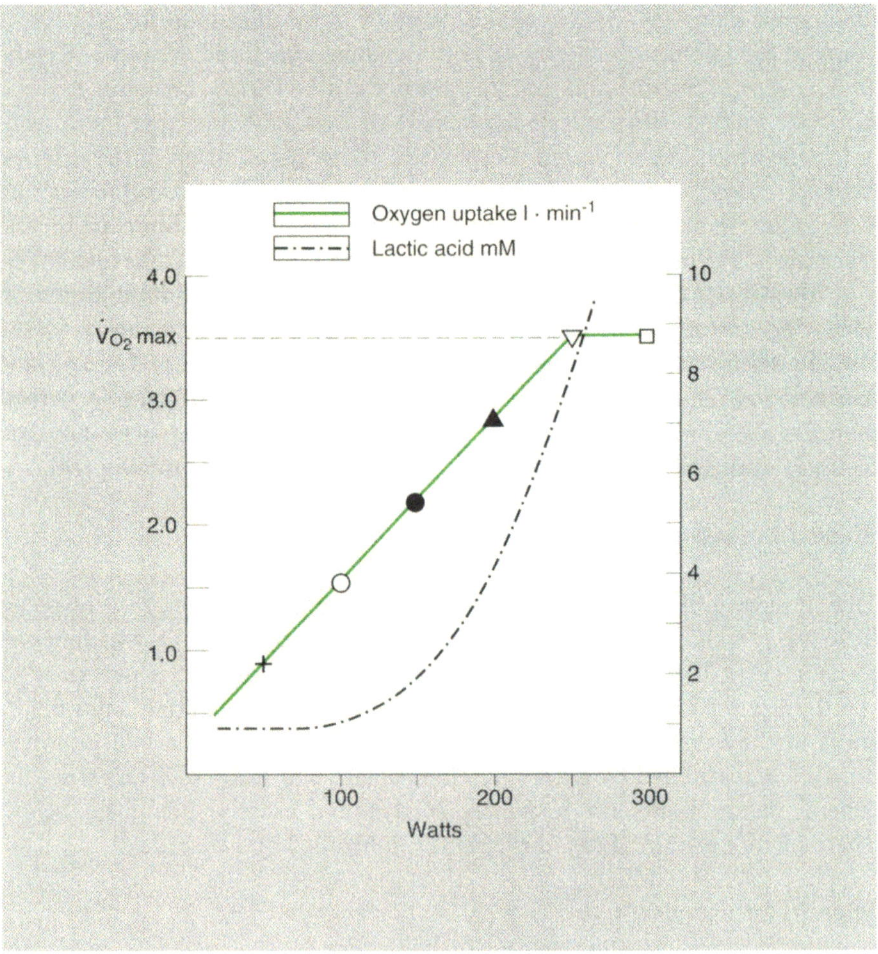

Fig. 1 Relationships between oxygen uptake ($\dot{V}_{O2}$), blood lactic acid, and work load in a subject, whose $\dot{V}_{O2max}$ is indicated

rate [14, 16] are more closely correlated with work intensity expressed in relative than in absolute terms. Work capacity is usually measured as the maximally achievable oxygen uptake (V_{O2max}) during the actual activity (see below). Accordingly, the relative work intensity, i. e. the work load normalized for body size and physical fitness, is $V_{O2} \cdot V_{O2max}^{-1} \cdot 100\%$. Generally, for a given individual, V_{O2max} determined during different activities engaging major muscle groups (e. g. running, bicycling, swimming) varies only slightly [14]. Figure 2 illustrates the relative work concept. It shows that the stress of

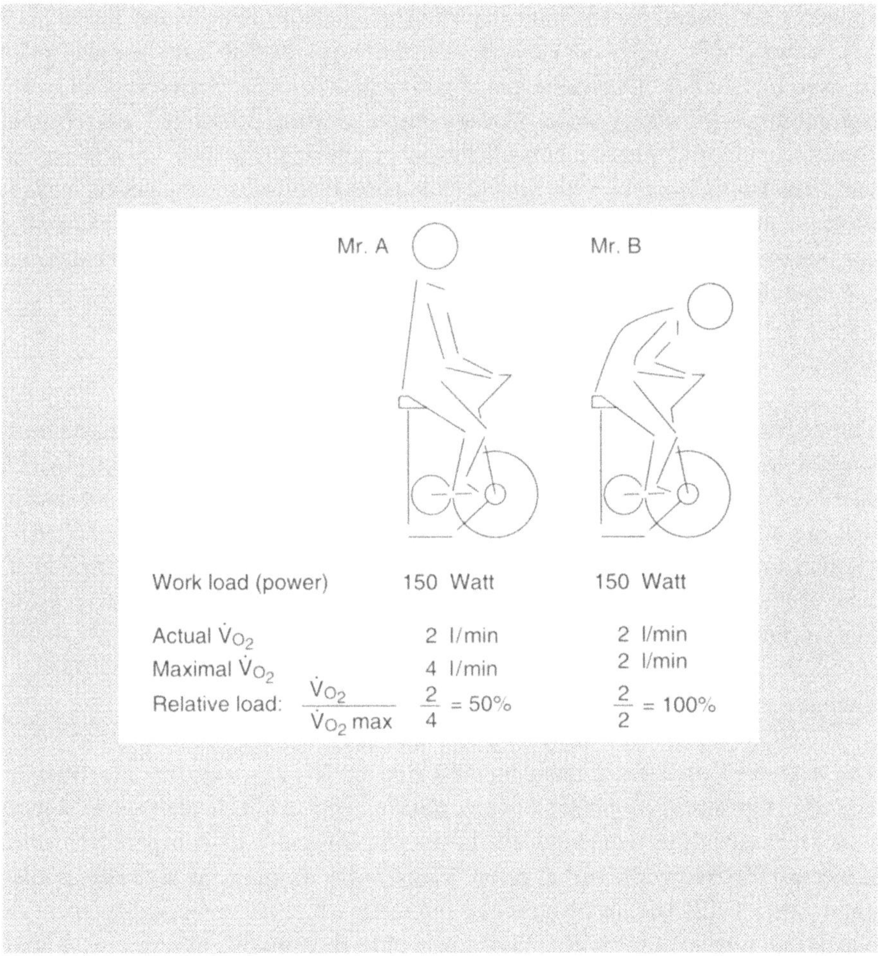

Fig. 2 Two persons with different $\dot{V}_{O2max}$ are differently stressed at a given absolute work load and $\dot{V}_{O2}$, because the relative work load differs

a given absolute work load is higher in an individual with a low work capacity than in an individual with a high work capacity. As heart rate generally varies linearly with V_{O2}, relative work intensity can also be estimated as $(HR_{actual}-HR_{rest}) \cdot (HR_{max}-HR_{rest})^{-1} \cdot 100\%$. HR_{max} can be roughly estimated as 220 – the patients age [14, 20]. However, HR_{max} varies considerably between individuals and should preferably be measured directly.

Previous exercise and exercise duration

Previous exercise influences the response to subsequent exercise bouts, with recovery dependent on the intensity and duration of the previous activity [14, 15]. Accordingly, extensive exercise is usually avoided at least one day prior to exercise studies. During a given prolonged exercise many variables will not maintain a steady-state. For example, during prolonged exercise the secretion rate and plasma concentration of epinephrine and, to a lesser extent, heart rate increase with time [21]. Plasma lactate concentrations initially increase and then decrease towards basal levels [14]. Sometimes exercise is continued to "exhaustion". If so, the criterion should be precisely defined, e. g. inability to maintain a given pedal frequency.

Diet

The nutritional state influences response to exercise. Subjects are generally studied in the post-absorptive state after having fasted overnight [14, 15, 22–24]. Meals taken immediately prior to exercise will influence response as will the administration of nutrients and fluids during exercise [25, 26]. Also the diet in the days prior to exercise is important. For example, during exercise, epinephrine and heart rate increase more and lactate less after a diet high in fat than after a diet high in carbohydrate [26].

Training

The degree of physical fitness, as indicated by $V_{O2max} \cdot kg\ BW^{-1}$, influences exercise response. For example, epinephrine, lactate and heart rate responses to a given absolute workload are lower in physically fit compared to unfit subjects [16]. However, at a given V_{O2max} the amount of training is also important. Thus, the absolute work intensity which is necessary to increase plasma lactate to 4 mM, i. e. "the anaerobic threshold", may increase with the amount of training, even if V_{O2max} does not change. So, in order to characterize physical fitness and state of training it is important to report

V_{O2max} (see below), BW and training schedule. This information may be supplemented by percentage of body fat, the concentration of mitochondrial enzymes in muscle (e. g. cytochrome oxidase) and the anaerobic threshold.

Muscle mass

The responses of many variables (e. g. epinephrine, lactate and heart rate [14, 15, 27] are inversely related to the amount of muscle involved in a given absolute work load (e. g. higher responses in arm than in leg exercise at a given watt and V_{O2}).

Environment

Signals from both skin and core temperature receptors may influence neuroendocrine activity (e. g. higher norepinephrine concentrations during exercise in hot or cold compared to a thermo-neutral environment [28, 29]. In diabetics it should be remembered that both warm temperatures and exercise increase insulin absorption [30]. The ambient pressure influences arterial oxygen tension and, in turn, V_{O2max} and relative work intensity, and with that many variables (see above). Other environmental factors (e. g. noise and pollution [14]) are also important for performance.

Time of day

Circadian rhythms exist which influence exercise performance [14].

Drugs and diseases

Caffeine, tobacco and alcohol influence various exercise responses, and so may other drugs and the diseases for which they are taken [14, 15]. In diabetics, the metabolic response to exercise depends critically on the actual plasma insulin level and, accordingly, on the time and dose of the last administration of insulin or oral antidiabetic drug stimulating insulin secretion [1, 2, 4]. The metabolic control in the weeks prior to exercise is also important [1, 4] probably in part due its effects on hydration. Long-term diabetic complications may also influence exercise responses. Increases in heart rate, cardiac output, splanchnic vascular resistance, catecholamines and blood pressure are impaired in diabetics with autonomic neuropathy [17–19, 24]. Furthermore, diabetics with incipient nephropathy have an impaired V_{O2max} [31].

Age, sex, race and psychological stress

Heart rate and sympathoadrenal response to given relative work loads diminish with ageing [32]. The influence of race and sex per se on exercise responses has not been studied much. However, even the menstrual phase may be of importance for responses to exercise [14, 15]. If subjects are made familiar with the applied procedures and good emotional contact is established between them and the staff then the influence of psychological factors on response to non-competitive exercise is probably minimal [15].

In general, responses to isometric exercise depend on the same factors listed above. Therefore, developed force should be given in absolute terms, as well as relative to individual maximal force, for the studied muscle group.

Determination of maximal oxygen uptake, V_{O2max}

The most reliable way of determining V_{O2max} is based on the fact that V_{O2} increases linearly with work intensity until it levels off at high intensities [14] (Fig. 1). When V_{O2} plateaus in spite of increasing exercise intensity, the extra energy required is delivered by anaerobic processes and, accordingly, blood lactate concentrations increase sharply (Fig. 1). It appears that V_{O2max} is elicited at a work load which is not maximal. One can be sure that V_{O2max} has been achieved, when an increase in exercise intensity is not accompanied by any significant increase in V_{O2}. Less reliable criteria are: an increase in blood lactate above 9 mM, peaking five minutes after exercise; heart rate attaining a value corresponding to the average maximum for the subjects age; the respiratory exchange ratio ($R = V_{CO2} \cdot V_{O2}^{-1}$) is above one; the highest exercise intensity is tolerated for less than 5 minutes; and that the subject feels exhausted. A visual analog scale can be used to rate the subject's perceived exertion [33]. It should be remembered that due to autonomic neuropathy diabetics may reach V_{O2max} at a relatively low heart rate [17].

In practice, the subject is exposed to a series of increasing loads [23, 31]. Short rest periods can be inserted, the number depending on the subject's fitness and experience [17]. After rest periods, subjects should always warm up at low exercise intensities. Oxygen uptake is measured by collecting expiratory air in Douglas bags and subsequent volume and gas analysis [17, 31] or by on-line analysis using air flow and gas meters. In order for a V_{O2} measurement to be representative of a certain exercise intensity this must have lasted one to 5 minutes, the shorter the time, the heavier the exercise.

Activities engaging large muscle groups should be used to determine individual V_{O2max}. Ergometer bicycling or treadmill running is most often applied, and these procedures give similar values [14]. During bicycling, optimum pedal frequency is 50–60 revolutions/min^{-1}. During treadmill running, both inclination and speed can be increased to increase exercise intensity. If a fixed inclination of 7% is used, speeds promoting accidents can be avoided. Testing should be performed in a thermo-neutral room with good ventilation [14]. Subjects should be without acute illnesses and should be studied in the post-absorptive state, having avoided heavy exercise and stimulants for 24 hours. Type 1 diabetics may be studied three hours after breakfast. The total exercise duration will often be less than 45 minutes and a reduction in insulin dose not necessary [17]. However, a reduction by 50–100% of any short-acting morning insulin will mimic the normal physiological response. The exercise will justify an extra energy intake of about 400 KJ which can be accompanied by the omitted insulin, if any.

Finally, it may be mentioned that it is possible to obtain an indirect estimate of V_{O2max} from determinations of V_{O2} and heart rate at sub-maximum exercise intensities (see above) and also from heart rate at a known ergometer bicycle load with standard tables or nomograms [14]. However, such estimates are very imprecise.

Training protocols

Cross-sectional studies, comparing individuals who are very physically active and/or have a high $V_{O2max} \cdot kg^{-1}$ with sedentary individuals, are often used to evaluate the long-term effects of regularly repeated exercise, i. e. physical training. The disadvantage of such studies is that differences between groups, rather than reflecting the effects of training as such, may reflect constitutional dissimilarities, as people who choose to train and/or have a high V_{O2max} may possess special genetic endowments. This reservation is not inherent in longitudinal studies, in which the same individuals are compared before and after a period of training [34–36]. Still, it should be remembered that subjects who volunteer in such studies may not be representative of the population as a whole. Ideally, subject selection should be strictly random.

Another problem is that changes observed during a period of training may not be elicited by the increased physical activity per se, but by other changes more or less directly related to the training regimen (e. g. increase in food intake or stop of smoking). In long-lasting training studies it is necessary to include a non-training control group to allow for changes reflecting seasonal variation, aging and progression of disease. An interesting possibility for studying local effects on muscle is to train only one leg and let the other serve as a non-training control [37, 38]. Diabetics in good metabolic control and without long-term complications can train on equal terms with healthy subjects. If whether they have completely normal responses to training is to be studied, it is also necessary to train a healthy control group. In addition to serving research purposes, longitudinal training protocols are used in the treatment of patients.

The adaptations induced by regularly repeated exercise are very intimately defined by the characteristics of the training program [14]. Accordingly, it is of vital importance to fully realize the aim of training before designing the program. Strength is achieved by bursts of intense activity lasting only a few seconds. Intense dynamic activity lasting about one minute and repeated after at least four minutes develops anaerobic power in particular. Central cardiovascular adaptations and increases in aerobic power (V_{O2max}) are developed if heavy, not necessarily exhausting, dynamic exercise is performed with major muscle groups for periods of at least four minutes. Dynamic or static endurance is enhanced if dynamic or static exercise bouts, respectively, are prolonged.

The specificity of training effects is illustrated by the fact that – after a period of training – enhanced endurance and diminished heart rate are observed during work with the trained (e. g. leg) but not with the untrained (e. g. arm) muscles. Also, for a given muscle group, increases in isometric and dynamic strength do not vary in parallel but reflect the mode of training [14]. Increases in dynamic strength and endurance for a particular muscle group even vary with the movement tested. The magnitude of a training effect depends on the training effort in terms of intensity and time spent, the exact relationship depending on the studied variable.

The effects of aerobic training with major muscle groups (e. g. bicycling and running) are often studied ("endurance training"). If such exercise is carried out for 30 minutes at an intensity of 70% V_{O2max}, three times a week for six weeks, cardiovascular fitness, endurance and – at least in healthy individuals – coronary risk factors will improve. Some improvement may also be seen at lower exercise intensities with accordingly lower risks, and the decrease in intensity may to some extent be compensated for by a longer time spent on exercise. An increase in strength can be achieved by isometric contractions at 70% of maximal force maintained for five seconds and repeated five times a day. Alternatively, strength can be increased by short bouts of dynamic contractions. If 10 RM ("repetitions maximum") designates the maximum load, which a muscle group can lift ten times, then an effective training protocol could consist in three bouts of ten contractions at 0.5 10 RM, 0.75 10 RM and 10 RM, respectively, performed three times a week.

For all kinds of training, it is advisable to begin with short training periods and then gradually increase the duration. The effect of training should be frequently determined. This will allow adjustment of loads according to improvement, so that the relative training intensity (e. g. % maximum force or % V_{O2max}) can be maintained and further gain achieved. Low compliance is a major problem in training programs [14]. Prevention of drop out may include motivation of participants, monitoring of training effects, supervision during training and training in groups [34, 35]. If possible training should be made enjoyable, e. g. by including ball games and mixing different activities [34, 35]. Sometimes, training can be facilitated by supplementing patients with ergometer bicycles in their private residences [2, 36]. As the detailed design of training protocols may differ tremendously (even though their aim is the same), and as compliance is a matter of concern, expected effects (e. g. increase in V_{O2max} or maximum force, see above) should be thoroughly documented at the end. This makes it possible to exclude insufficient training effort as a reason for a lack of effect on a studied variable and to compare different training protocols.

During training, each exercise bout has effects on the body, which wane rather rapidly post-exercise (e. g. decrease in muscle glycogen; increase in appetite and insulin sensitivity). In addition, repeated exercise induces more long-lived adaptations (e. g. increases in myocardial mass and in GLUT 4 glucose transporters and insulin responsiveness in muscle) reflecting accumulated effects of the repeated stimulus and often requiring protein synthesis. However, even the latter effects disappear gradually if training is discontinued. It follows that the "trained state" is characterized by a mixture of effects from the last exercise bout and genuine adaptations. Furthermore, this state has to be maintained, and thus requires a permanent behavioral "life style" change. Accordingly, in studies of the effect of training it is interesting to study trained subjects in their "habitual state". This can be in the laboratory between two regular training sessions [37–39] or in ordinary living conditions [40].

It is, however, also important to differentiate between residual effects of the last exercise bout and more profound adaptations to training. One way to achieve this is to compare the trained state with the untrained state, measured before as well as after a single exercise session. In this way it may be concluded, whether a difference between the trained and untrained state can be explained as an effect of acute exercise or if it reflects a training-induced adaptation [37, 39]. Still, training enhances exercise capacity and, accordingly, each exercise bout in the trained state may be more strenuous and, thus have more marked effects than exercise bouts in the untrained state. If such differences exist between trained and untrained states, then one might expect that an extra exercise bout between two training sessions in the "habitual trained state" would only have a modest influence as compared to exercise in the untrained state, because the residual effects of the preceding exercise bout would be marked. Thus, the comparison between trained and untrained states may also benefit from evaluation of responses to acute exercise in the trained state [41].

An addditional approach is to study abstinence from training, i. e. detraining. Training is discontinued for a period during which, in the untrained state, any effect on the studied variable of a single exercise session would disappear. If then the variable nevertheless still differes between the detrained and the untrained state, it may be concluded that a training-induced adaptation has taken place [37, 41]. For example, the conclusion that training induces adaptations in maximal insulin action on glucose metabolism that cannot be ascribed to effects of the last exercise bout, is based on the findings that maximum insulin mediated glucose disposal is higher in the trained state than in the untrained state studied both before and after a single exercise bout, and also higher after five days of detraining than in the untrained state [37, 39, 41].

Limitations, risks and precautions

For everyone, exercise is associated with an increased risk of various illnesses, particularly musculoskeletal injuries, and even of death, e. g. from myocardial infarction. Diabetics have additional problems due to abnormal metabolic responses to exercise and to the interaction of exercise with diabetic long-term complications [1, 4, 5, 20, 42, 43]. Therefore, diabetics who want to exercise should have regular medical examinations [1, 4, 5]. The doctor can teach the diabetic to self-monitor blood glucose and to adjust insulin dose and diet in relation to exercise [4]; he can detect and treat secondary diabetic complications and point out appropriate exercise options [42]; and he can treat and give advice regarding other medical disorders limiting exercise performance. If the diabetic is older than 35 years, or has had the disease for more than 10 years, or has documented complications, or has experienced symptoms of cardiac disease, he should – prior to embarking on an exercise program – be subjected to a proper graded exercise test (see above) including ECG and blood pressure measurements [4, 20]. For ethical and legal reasons all diabetics recruited for exercise research should have such a test before participation. Subsequent exercise must be limited to levels below which anginal symptoms, ST depression, ventricular arrhythmia or fall in blood pressure occur.

Diabetics should not exercise if blood glucose is lower than 6 mM or higher than 16 mM, or if they have ketonuria [4, 5]. Furthermore, in the incubation and fever phases of infectious diseases exercise which markedly increases V_{O2} and cardiac output should be avoided. Caution as regards physical exercise should also be exerted in other acute as well as unstable chronic medical disorders. However, if patients are in optimal medical treatment few absolute contraindications to any kind of exercise exist. From analysis of the patients condition and the requirements during exercise it is possible to tell what kind of exercise he can tolerate. The load is then adjusted to his capacity, and further safety is obtained if critical variables are monitored during the exercise. In order to prevent injuries, during all kinds of training progression in exercise intensity and duration should be slow, and each training bout should begin and end with muscle stretching and contractions at low intensities. Optimum equipment (e. g. shoes) should be used and exercise should be interrupted in case of unusual sensations (e. g. chest pain).

Patients with retinopathy should be cautious with exercise that may greatly increase blood pressure (e. g. static exercise and arm exercise), elicit hypoglycemia (e. g. prolonged endurance exercise) or be accompanied by abrupt head movements. Following retinal photo-coagulation, exercise should be avoided for six weeks. Even diabetics with normal resting blood pressure may show an exaggerated blood pressure response to exercise [44], and particular attention should be given to high increases in pressure in hypertensive patients and in patients with kidney disease. In contrast, diabetics with autonomic neuropathy may respond to exercise with a decrease in blood pressure [24]. It should also be remembered that in these patients the exercise stress is underestimated when evaluated from heart rate measurements [17, 24]. Patients with sensorimotor neuropathy or leg atherosclerosis are prone to develop wounds on the feet during running and may, like overly obese diabetics and diabetics with renal osteodystrophy, be advised to bicycle or swim instead [42].

In the laboratory, subjects should always be carefully watched during exercise experiments. Measures should be taken to avoid accidents, e. g. during fast running subjects can wear slings to avoid falling. Concentrated glucose solutions and glucagon should be available to treat hypoglycemia. An electrocardiograph, a cardiac defibrillator, epinephrine, bicarbonate, and, for artificial ventilation, a Ruben balloon and pure oxygen should be available in case need for resuscitation arises. Whether a medical doctor has to be present during exercise experiments depends on the patient, the exercise and the other experimental conditions.

Variables to be studied

Only technology and ethics fix limits to what variables can be studied. In exercise experiments, diabetics have been subjected to the same non-invasive and invasive procedures as healthy individuals, e. g. cardiac and hepatic venous catheterization [22] and muscle biopsy [35]. It may be remembered that an experiment which will not be able to answer the posed question, e. g. due to insufficient methods, is unethical. Finally, attention should be drawn to the fact that during phases which are far from steady-state, e. g. early exercise and postexercise periods, the timing of measurements should be quite exact.

References

[1] Galbo H. Exercise and diabetes. Scand J Sports Sci 1988; 10: 89–95.
[2] Galbo H, Linstow M, Dela F et al. Exercise and diabetes. Med Sport Sci 1992; 37: 227–236.
[3] Galbo H. Integrated endocrine responses and exercise. In: De Groot. Endocrinology, 3rf edn., chapter 146, WB Saunders, 1995; 2692–2701.
[4] Gudat U, Berger M. Diabetes and exercise. In: Mogensen CE, Standl E, eds. Concepts for the ideal diabetes clinic. Diabetes Forum Series. Berlin–New York: Walter de Gruyter, 1993; 171–185.
[5] Wallberg-Henriksson H. Exercise and diabetes mellitus. Exercise Sport Sci Rev 1992; 20: 339–368.
[6] Position statement. Diabetes mellitus and exercise. Diabetes Care 1991; 14 (Suppl. 2): 36–37.
[7] Cahill GF, Buskirk ER, Delahanty LM et al. Consensus development conference on diet and exercise in non-insulin-dependent diabetes mellitus. Diabetes Care 1987; 10: 639–644.
[8] Manson JE, Rimm EB, Stampfer MJ et al. Physical activity and incidence of non-insulin-dependent diabetes mellitus in women. Lancet 1991; 338: 774–778.
[9] Helmrich SP, Ragland DR, Leung RW et al. Physical activity and reduced occurrence of non-insulin-dependent diabetes mellitus. N Engl J Med 1991; 325: 147–152.
[10] Karlefors T. Circulatory studies during exercise with particular reference to diabetics. Acta Med Scand 1976; 180 (Suppl.): 4–49.
[11] Peerson G. Exercise tests in male diabetics. Acta Med Scand 1977; 605: 7–23.
[12] Dahlquist G, Aperia A, Carlsson L et al. Effect of metabolic control and duration on exercise-induced albuminuria in diabetic teen-agers. Acta Pædiatr Scand 1983; 72: 895–902.
[13] Sane T, Helve E, Pelkonen R et al. The adjustment of diet and insulin dose during long-term endurance exercise in Type 1 (insulin-dependent) diabetic men. Diabetologia 1988; 31: 35–40.
[14] Aastrand P-O, Rodahl K. Textbook of Work Physiology. New York: McGraw-Hill Book Company, 1986; 756 pp.
[15] Galbo H. Hormonal and metabolic adaptation to exercise. Stuttgart–New York: Thieme-Stratton, 1983; 116 pp.
[16] Kjær M, Bangsbo J, Lortie G et al. Hormonal response to exercise in humans: influence of hypoxia and physical training. Am J Physiol 1988; 254: R197–R203.
[17] Hilsted J, Galbo H, Christensen NJ. Impaired cardiovascular responses to graded exercise in diabetic autonomic neuropathy. Diabetes 1979; 28: 313–319.

[18] Hilsted J, Galbo H, Christensen NJ. Impaired responses of catecholamines, growth hormone, and cortisol to graded exercise in diabetic autonomic neuropathy. Diabetes 1980; 29: 257–262.
[19] Hilsted J, Galbo H, Tronier B et al. Hormonal and metabolic responses to exercise in insulin-dependent diabetics with and without autonomic neuropathy and in normal subjects. Int J Sports Med 1981; 2: 216–219.
[20] Schneider SH, Ruderman NB. Exercise and NIDDM. Diabetes Care 1991; 14 (Suppl.): 52–56.
[21] Kjær M, Christensen NJ, Sonne B et al. Effect of exercise on epinephrine turnover in trained and untrained male subjects. J Appl Physiol 1985; 59: 1061–1067.
[22] Wahren J, Sato Y, Ostman J et al. Turnover and splanchnic metabolism of free fatty acids and ketones in insulin-dependent diabetics at rest and in response to exercise. J Clin Invest 1984; 73: 1367–1376.
[23] Kjær M, Hollenbeck CB, Frey-Hewitt B et al. Glucoregulation and hormonal responses to maximal exercise in non-insulin-dependent diabetes. J Appl Physiol 1990; 68: 2067–2074.
[24] Hilsted J, Galbo H, Christensen NJ et al. Haemodynamic changes during graded exercise in patients with diabetic autonomic neuropathy. Diabetologia 1982; 22: 318–323.
[25] Galbo H. Autonomic neuroendocrine responses to exercise. Scand J Sports Sci 1986; 8: 3–17.
[26] Galbo H, Holst JJ, Christensen NJ. The effect of different diets and of insulin on the hormonal response to prolonged exercise. Acta Physiol Scand 1979; 107: 19–32.
[27] Lewis SF, Taylor WF, Graham RM et al. Cardiovascular responses to exercise as functions of absolute and relative work load. J Appl Physiol 1983; 54: 1314–1323.
[28] Galbo H, Houston ME, Christensen NJ et al. The effect of water temperature on the hormonal response to prolonged swimming. Acta Physiol Scand 1979; 105: 326–337.
[29] Rönnemaa T, Marniemi J, Leino A et al. Hormone response of diabetic patients to exercise at cool and warm temperatures. Eur J Appl Physiol 1991; 62: 109–115.
[30] Rönnemaa T, Koivisto VA. Combined effect of exercise and ambient temperature on insulin absorption and postprandial glycemia in type 1 patients. Diabetes Care 1988; 11: 769–773.
[31] Jensen T, Richter EA, Feldt-Rasmussen B et al. Impaired aerobic work capacity in insulin dependent diabetics with increased urinary albumin excretion. Brit Med J 1988; 296: 1352–1354.
[32] Jensen EW, Espersen K, Kanstrup I-L et al. Age-related changes of exercise-induced plasma catecholamines and neuropeptide Y responses in normal human subjects. Acta Physiol Scand 1992; 144: 129–133.
[33] Borg G. Perceived exertion as an indicator of somatic stress. Scand J Rehab Med 1970; 2–3: 92–98.
[34] Krotkiewski M, Lönnroth P, Mandroukas K et al. The effects of physical training on insulin secretion and effectiveness and on glucose metabolism in obesity and Type 2 (non-insulin-dependent) diabetes mellitus. Diabetologia 1985; 28: 881–890.
[35] Wallberg-Henriksson H, Gunnarsson R, Henriksson J et al. Increased peripheral insulin sensitivity and muscle mitochondrial enzymes but unchanged blood glucose control in Type 1 diabetics after physical training. Diabetes 1982; 31: 1044–1050.
[36] Wallberg-Henriksson H, Gunnarsson R, Rössner S et al. Long-term physical training in female Type 1 (insulin-dependent) diabetic patients: absence of significant effect on glycaemic control and lipoprotein levels. Diabetologia 1986; 29: 53–57.
[37] Dela F, Mikines KJ, Linstow M et al. Effect of training on insulin-mediated glucose uptake in human muscle. Am J Physiol 1992; 263: E1134-–E1143.
[38] Galbo H, Linstow M, Dela F et al. The effect of physical training on secretion and effect of insulin in middle aged men. In: Beregi E, Gergely IA, Rajczi K, eds. Recent advances in aging science. Bologna: Monduzzi Editore, 1993; 817–821.
[39] Mikines KJ, Sonne B, Farrell PA et al. Effect of training on the dose-response relationship for insulin action in men. J Appl Physiol 1989; 66: 695–703.

[40] Dela F, Mikines KJ, Linstow M et al. Twenty-four-hour profile of plasma glucose and glucoregulatory hormones during normal living conditions in trained and untrained men. J Clin Endocrinol Metab 1991; 73: 982–989.
[41] Mikines KJ, Sonne B, Tronier B et al. Effects of acute exercise and detraining on insulin action in trained men. J Appl Physiol 1989; 66: 704–711.
[42] Graham C, Lasko-McCarthey P. Exercise options for persons with diabetic complications. Diabetes Educator 1990; 16: 212–220.
[43] Stein R, Goldberg N, Kalman F et al. Exercise and the patient with Type 1 diabetes mellitus. Pediatric Clinics North America 1984; 31: 665–673.
[44] Blake GA, Levin SR, Koyal SN. Exercise-induced hypertension in normotensive patients with NIDDM. Diabetes Care 1990; 13: 799–801.

Assessment of stress hormone responses in diabetes: secretion, circulating levels and action in vivo

N. Møller, L. Ørskov, O. Schmitz, H. Ørskov

Introduction

Insulin deficiency, whether relative or absolute, is a distinct feature of diabetes. Other hormones with metabolic activity may, however, contribute to the metabolic set-up of the disease. These include catecholamines, glucagon, cortisol, growth hormone (GH), collectively termed "counterregulatory" or "stress" hormones [1–4]. Furthermore, there is mounting evidence that insulin-like growth factors and glucagon-like peptide 1 [7–36] should be added to the group of hormones with insulin-like actions [5, 6].

Release of stress hormones is augmented under a variety of circumstances, demanding and/or potentially noxious to the individual. In normal persons, stress hormones thus serve to maintain an optimal supply of fuel substrates under conditions of fasting, exercise and acute and chronic illness. In patients with diabetes, the spectrum is extended to cover states of both acute insulin deficiency (e. g. ketoacidosis and hyperosmolar coma) and acute insulin excess (hyperglycaemia). It has additionally been suggested that inappropriately increased secretion of glucagon [7, 8] and GH [9] may play key roles in the development and maintenance of insulin resistance in diabetes. Finally, it remains possible that chronic hypersecretion of GH and pertubed secretion of IGF I may be involved in the pathogenesis of long-term diabetic complications [10].

Given the vastness of the field being dealt with, this review can only be kaleidoscopic, and will merely seek to outline some assets and some limitations of methods currently available for assessment of stress hormone release and action in human diabetes mellitus.

Measurements of hormone secretion and circulating levels of hormones

With the advent of radioimmunoassays, the 1960s and 70s saw a virtual burst of studies identifying "specific" hormonal aberrations in patients with diabetes. In this prolific period it was shown that type I diabetic patients under conditions of ordinary metabolic control had raised levels of GH [11] and glucagon [12] and that both acute insulin deficiency and hypoglycaemia were associated with increased concentrations of all stress hormones [11–21]. Hyperglucagonaemia has also been noted in type II diabetic patients and may possibly contribute to the increased endogenous glucose production observed [22, 23]. The scenery is, however, entangled by a variety of complicating factors. In general the aforementioned investigations employed straightforward measurements of blood hormone concentrations over an extended period of time. Frequently, measurements were performed at hourly intervals. Bearing in mind that the plasma half-life of stress hormones ranges from a few minutes to perhaps 60 min and that secretion is pulsatile, it becomes apparent that useful information and potential differences may readily escape detection with this crude approach. It therefore seems wise to interpret these results with caution.

Hormone secretion

Secretion of a hormone may be estimated either through simultaneous measurements of blood flow and hormone concentrations in efferent blood or indirectly, based on deconvolution of peripheral measurements. As the former method is, for most purposes, unfeasible in humans, the latter has gained a strong foothold. The deconvolution model requires valid estimates of circulating half-lives (often obtained from the literature), precise, accurate and specific hormone assays, condensed sampling over an appropriate time span (depending on pulse frequency and half-life) and access to an accepted mathematical model incorporating these variables [24]. The major problems relating to such modelling are that clearance may vary between groups as well as intraindividually (with time), and that the radioimmunoassays employed often lack sensitivity and specificity and therefore pick up molecular mixtures with varying receptor affinity and bioactivity. A specific problem pertains to estimation of peptide secretion from the endocrine pancreas into the portal bed. As regards insulin, additional estimation of C-peptide secretion may be valuable, but quantification of glucagon release is severely impeded by insufficient information on initial hepatic extraction. Nevertheless, the introduction of the deconvolution technique generally represents a major advance, since it allows for more detailed analysis of hormone secretion in terms of pulse amplitude and periodicity, tonic interpulse activity, as well as estimation of secretory rates on, for example, a diurnal basis.

In the case of GH, Hartman et al. [25] have estimated that normal humans secrete 0.25 mg/m2 body surface of GH per 24 h (corresponding roughly to between 0.4 and 0.5 mg/24 h in any one subject) and that GH is almost exclusively released in major "pulses within pulses" episodes. They detected 12 such "macro"-episodes/24 h, during each of which an estimated average of 45 μg of GH with a half-life of 17 min was distributed into the circulation. Though it has been reported that the hypersecretion of GH tends to normalize with appropriate metabolic control [26, 27], there is little doubt that type I diabetic patients, in general, are exposed to excessive amounts of circulating GH [11, 28]. A recent study has estimated that type I diabetic subjects under conditions of poor control (Hgb A1c above 12%) are characterized by integrated 24 h GH concentrations 2–3 fold higher than those of normal control subjects; the GH excess is due to augmentation of both pulse and interpulse secretion, in a manner very similar to patterns observed in fasting normal man [29]. Allowing for the reported delay in clearance of GH in diabetic subjects and for the suppression of GH secretion with improved control, the GH excess of more-ordinary-controlled type I diabetic patients would plausibly extrapolate to a diurnal secretion rate between 0.5 and 1 mg [25, 30].

As discussed below, optimal quantitative assessment of the perturbed stress hormone release in diabetes is crucial for the understanding of the relative contribution of these hormones to metabolic disarray.

Circulating hormone concentrations

This chapter deals with methodological approaches to assess the hormonal and metabolic characteristics in diabetes (IDDM and NIDDM), when it is particularly well or poorly controlled, and when it is in a state moving between these extremes. Some of the features has been dealt with in other chapters, and we have tried to refrain from overlapping. However, some of the inherent problems are common to the tasks the editors haven given us, the various authors.

During the past decades it has become increasingly clear that peptide hormone concentrations measured with conventional immunoassays do not reflect the abundance of a single unique protein, but rather the sum of peptides with different molecular nature and common immunoactivity. The heterogeneity arises from both pre- and post-secretory events. The term "isohormones" usually describes peptides with different primary (amino acid sequence) structure, whereas "variants" refers to molecular forms derived from the same primary structure. The picture is in many cases further blurred by the existence of circulating hormone binding proteins, which may additionally modify hormone activity.

For example, glucagon is a 29-aminoacid peptide synthesized in pancreatic alpha cells. The initial gene product, pre-proglucagon, is a 179-aminoacid peptide, with several split products, including: 1. Glicentin (enteroglucagon) (1–69), 2. Oxyntomodulin (33–69), 3. Glucagon (33–61), 4. Glucagon-like peptide 1 (72–108), 5. Glucagon-like peptide 1 (78–108 or 7–37) and 6. Glucagon-like peptide 2 (126–158). Of these glicentin and oxyntomodulin are of interest, since they may share immunoactivity with glucagon in some assays, whereas their biological activity is in general far weaker – often only 1/10th of that of glucagon [31, 32]. In addition, glucagon-like peptide 1 (7–37) is attracting considerable interest because of its potential as insulin secretagogue and insulin agonist [6].

GH is a 191-aminoacid 22kD peptide secreted from the pituitary gland. Two genes serve as a code for GH, namely the hGH-N gene (for normal) and the hGH-V gene (for variant). Both produce 22kD GH, but the latter is probably only expressed in the placenta, where distinct GH forms may additionally be generated. In the circulation, various molecular forms of growth hormone may be detected, including the 20kD variant and a variety of di- and polymers. Most of these are bound to carrier proteins [33]; notably, Bauman has assessed that free monomeric 22kD GH averages a mere 20% of total immunoreactivity in plasma [6].

One of the confounding aspects is immunoassay of the hormones that participate in the complex diabetic states of metabolism, which are plagued by several paradoxical or vicious responses to the metabolic aberrations. Hales et al. (in Volume 5 A) have dealt with the advantages of new superspecific assays of insulin, which exclude coestimation of several pro- or split products. This important effort is also relevant for most other hormones and has been applied in several assays. In brief, the assays exploit the possibilities of identifying solely the intact hormone or peptide by utilizing 2 monoclonal antibodies directed at different sites, which may be hidden or non-existent in the previously competing prohormones/polymers/degradation products that, to an often unpredictable degree, "interfere" in the assays. At the same time, high sensitivity has changed into supersensitivity, so minute amounts of the "true" immunoreactivity may now be detected, and the applicable assay range has increased by several fold.

The glorious days of Berson and Yalow's revolutionary discovery have changed with the realization that not just any polyclonal antibody can be used to detect the true levels of "immunoreactive" hormone. Nowadays, part of the scientific competition is, again, directed at identifying one substance, the "one and only", but on the basis of vastly enlarged knowledge and sophisticated techniques.

The new superspecificity and supersensitivity have made many of us believe that we have now approached the truth about serum and tissue concentrations of hormones and peptides. And there is no doubt that the renaissance will offer new information on, for example, minute variations, which were previously hidden because of the insufficient specificity and sensitivity of previous assays. On the other hand, what will we lose with the new technology? Are we closer to the truth about the biological activity of the substances, we wish to estimate? Will we exclude determination of relevant moieties, which have full/fractional biological activity after discrete differences have occurred from the true antigen during its passage from glands or intestinal or subcutaneous/intramuscular depots to plasma and tissue? These alterations may include formation of dimers/polymers and removal of small immunoreactive epitopes, which are relatively/totally irrelevant for the biological effects.

These reservations are probably applicable to some of the very recent estimates of immunoreactivity reported in this volume. However, the data on hormone analyses used in many of the reviews on insulin and counterregulatory mechanism in diabetes were reached using old-fashioned RIAs, employing "robust" polyclonal antibodies, which are not superspecific or supersensitive. Most of us believe that the conclusions reached using various polyclonal antibodies in several centres are very dependable! They should, however, obviously not be regarded as absolutely quantitative.

Assessment of hormone action

The vast majority of studies aimed at assessing hormone action are designed to create or study an experimental situation in which the hormone in focus is either clearly in excess or clearly deficient. Depending on the extremes to which this is pursued, the outcome may be relevant to physiology, pathophysiology or – at times – pharmacology. This often leaves the investigator in a dilemma, since carrying matters to extremes may admittedly improve the prospects of "seeing something", but may at the same time impair the relevance and validity of the study.

The specific methods employed within assessment of the action of stress hormones are in general similar to those discussed elsewhere in this book, and will only briefly be touched on.

Chronic hormone deficiency and excess

Disease states characterized by specific chronic hormone abnormalities are obvious targets for metabolic studies and a large body of knowledge stems from such studies.

Patients with acromegaly and Cushing's disease are markedly insulin resistant, in terms of fasting hyperinsulinaemia, impaired insulin-stimulated glucose disposal and relatively increased levels of free fatty acids [34–37]. In contrast, patients with GH-deficiency are hypersensitive to insulin [38]. Intermediary metabolism in patients with pheochromocytoma and glucagonoma is less well characterized.

Needless to say, extrapolation from these studies to everyday life of diabetic subjects should only be made with great caution.

Hormone administration studies and hormone sensitivity

The administration of hormones to normal or diabetic subjects has been widely used to obtain knowledge about their metabolic impact. In particular, investigations in which hormones have been perfused locally across a vascular bed (e. g. the forearm), have proven valuable, since this approach allows "uncontaminated" observation of direct hormone effects [39–41]. Some studies have employed simultaneous administration of selected hormones, often in combination with hormone clamps (see below), to dissect the relative importance of each individual hormone [42–44]. With these approaches it has become clear that epinephrine and glucagon have swift and potent actions to oppose insulin, whereas GH and cortisol have more delayed, but also more protracted effects.

One methodological aspect does, however, warrant comment, namely the hormone dosages employed. In the case of GH, it is well substantiated that large increments in circulating levels may in the course of several hours perturb metabolic control in diabetic subjects [45]. From this finding, it has been surmised that nocturnal GH surges may be responsible for the so-called dawn-phenomenon (i. e. an increase in insulin requirements in the early morning hours) in diabetic subjects. In support of this view, an array of studies has shown that administration of large amounts of GH at night may increase insulin requirements [46, 47]. During these experiments, GH doses of 6–800 µg were employed, i. e. doses that are close to or above 24 h secretion rates. When more modest amounts of GH were administered, however, no "dawn-like" phenomena were recorded [48]. As pointed out by Blackard et al. it therefore remains a distinct possibility that the dawn-phenomenon relates primarily to the period of arousal, and that the role of GH may merely be that of a permissive factor [49]. Evidently, the question of whether an appropriate hormone dosage has been employed is decisive to the interpretation of such studies.

Considering the multitude of efforts that has been put into the characterization of insulin sensitivity, strikingly little is known about sensitivity to stress hormones in diabetes. Only a few studies have addressd this issue [50, 51], and they coherently recorded disproportionate sensitivity to stress hormones, thus providing fresh evidence of the central pathogenic role these agents play in diabetes.

Stress models

Since the turn of the century, it has been known that severe infections are often accompanied by glucose intolerance or "stress diabetes" [52] and later surveys have estimated that acute infections precipitate more than 50% of all cases of diabetc ketoacidosis [53]. Acute infections generate a full blown stress hormone response, which accounts for the bulk of insulin resistance observed [54, 55]. Still, it is also likely that bed rest and the sedentary life associated with infection may contribute. A problem inherent to the study of naturally occurring infections is that they differ markedly in severity and duration, ranging from mild viral illness to fulminant sepsis. This may explain why one recent study failed to detect aberrations in basal intermediary metabolism in 9 infected patients several weeks after the onset of symptoms, whereas insulin sensitivity was visibly impaired [56]. Alternatively healthy volunteers may be inoculated with microorganisms of low virulence such as sand-fly fever virus [57], or, taking one step further, purified bacterial endotoxin may be administered [54]. Considerable valuable information has been gained from such studies, where one benefits from a higher degree of standardization and predictability, but exposing normal volunteers to the discomfort and hazards of this approach can be difficult to endorse from an ethical point of view. A third avenue of exploring the metabolic consequences of infection has been opened with the appearance of biosynthetically manufactured cytokines, in particular tumor necrosis factor-α and interleukin-1. These agents, formerly known as "endogenous pyrogens", induce hyperthermia and hormonal and metabolic responses indistinguishable from genuine infections and have been administered to humans [58]. Ethical hesitations are, however, again likely to restrain experimental usage. Other possible stress models include external heating [59, 60] and surgical stress [61]. Exercise also generates a general stress hormone response, but ultimately results in increased insulin sensitivity, as discussed elsewhere in this book.

Whenever one specifically wants to study the mechanisms leading to diabetic ketoacidosis, several approaches are possible. Insulin deprivation, when inflected for a sufficient period of time, generates overt ketosis [62, 63]. It may, however, be argued that this model does not adequately mirror reality and probably understates the importance of stress hormones, inasmuch as isolated insulin deficiency triggers the cascade. Studying patients with "spontaneous" occurring ketoacidosis or type I diabetic patients exposed to one of the stress models discussed above, therefore seems to hold some advantages over the insulin withdrawal model.

Hormone clamp studies

Since the report that somatostatin suppresses insulin secretion in humans [64], the peptide has gained wide experimental use. In order to segregate direct metabolic events from effects secondary to changes in hormone levels, somatostatin may be infused alone – to clamp insulin, glucagon and growth hormone levels – or together with adrenergic blockers and glucocorticoid synthesis inhibitors to further control catecholamine and cortisol action [65, 66].

The interpretation of metabolic studies employing somatostatin is, however, complicated by a variety of factors. Firstly, somatostatin may act to decrease splanchnic blood flow, suppress release of gut hormones (of which the metabolic significance is largely unknown) and delay gastrointestinal absorption [67, 68]. Secondly, studies in which hormones such as insulin, glucagon or growth hormone are co-infused to recreate a desired hormonal profile invariably fail to reproduce the anatomical site of hormone release (e. g. the portal bed) and the intricate pattern of pulsatile hormone secretion and fail to imitate the molecular mixture of variously sequenced peptides released in this pattern. Finally, the question of whether somatostatin *per se* acts to potentiate the actions of insulin on glucose metabolism remains unanswered. Employing a systematic infusion of somatostatin, some studies have reported such an insulin augmenting effect on the peripheral disposal of glucose [69–73], whereas others have not [74, 75].

Cholinergic blockers have also been used to clamp GH levels, and the observation that such a nocturnal blockade abolishes the dawn phenomenon [76, 77], has been unequivocally interpreted in favour of a crucial pathogenic role for GH; it is, however, possible that an anticholinergic blockade *per se* may improve insulin action [78].

These are only some examples of the complexities that may arise with the use of hormone blockers. Still, bearing in mind the above limitations, hormone clamp techniques offer many advantages for experimental manipulation.

Conclusions

The present brief review has sought to expose some of the interpretative problems that may arise with the use of complex modern techniques for quantification of factors critical to diabetic stress syndromes. They include some limitations in the assessment of both hormone secretion and resultant concentrations and the drawbacks of the various hormone deprivation/saturation models. As a consequence, new questions and possibilities are emerging continuously.

References

[1] Newsholme EA, Leech AR. Biochemistry for the medical sciences. John Wiley & Sons, 1983, ISBN 0471 90056 7.
[2] Bratusch-Marrain PR. Insulin-counteracting hormones: Their impact on glucose metabolism. Diabetologia 1983; 24: 74−79.
[3] Cryer PE, White NH, Santiago JV. The relevance of glucose counterregulatory systems to patients with insulin-dependent diabetes mellitus. Endocrine Reviews 1986; 7: 132−139.
[4] Gerich JE, Campell PJ. Overview of counterregulation and its abnormalities in diabetes mellitus and other conditions. Diabetes/Metabolism Reviews 1988; 4: 93−111.
[5] Guler HP, Zapf J, Froesch ER. Short-term metabolic effects of recombinant human insulin-like growth factor 1 in healthy adults. N Engl J Med 1987; 317: 137−140.
[6] Gutniak M, Ørskov, Holst JJ et al. Antidiabetogenic effect of glucagon-like peptide-1 (7−36) in normal subjects and patients with diabetes mellitus. N Engl J Med 1992; 326: 1316−1322.
[7] Unger RH, Foster DW. Diabetes Mellitus, pp 1255−1333. In: Wilson JD, Foster DW, eds. Williams Textbook of Endocrinology. WB Saunders Company, 1992.
[8] Dinneen S, Gerich J, Rizza R. Carbohydrate metabolism in non-insulin-dependent diabetes mellitus. N Engl J Med 1992; 327: 707−713.
[9] Ørskov H. Growth hormone hyperproduction inducing some of the vicious circles in diabetes mellitus. Acta Med Scand 1985; 217: 343−346.
[10] Lundbæk K, Jensen VA, Olsen TS et al. Diabetes, diabetic angiopathy and growth hormone. Lancet 1970; II: 131 ff.
[11] Hansen AP, Johansen K. Diurnal patterns of blood glucose, serum free fatty acids, insulin, glucagon and growth hormone in normals and juvenile diabetics. Diabetologia 1970; 6: 27−38.
[12] Unger RH, Aguilar-Parada E, Muller WA. Studies of pancreatic alpha-cell function in normal and diabetic subjects. J Clin Invest 1970; 49: 837−848.
[13] Christensen NJ. Plasma norepinephrine and epinephrine in untreated diabetics, during fasting and after insulin administration. Diabetes 1973; 23: 1−8.
[14] Muller WA, Faloona GR, Unger RH. Hyperglucagonaemia in diabetic ketoacidosis. Am J Med 1973; 54: 52−57.
[15] Alberti KGMM, Christensen NJ. Iversen J et al. Role of glucagon and other hormones in development of diabetic ketoacidosis. Lancet 1975; I: 1307−1311.
[16] Rayfield EJ, Curnow RT, Reinhard D et al. Effects of acute endotoxiemia on glucoregulation in normal and diabetic subjects. J Clin Endocrinol Metab 1977; 45: 513−521.
[17] Schade DS, Eaton RP. The temporal relationship between endogenously secreted stress hormones and metabolic decompensation in diabetic man. J Clin Endocrinol Metab 1980; 50: 131−136.
[18] Gerich JE, Schneider V, Dippe SE et al. Characterization of the glucagon response to hypoglycemia in man. J Cin Endocrinol Metab 1974; 38: 77−82.

[19] Vendsalau A. Studies on adrenaline and noradrenaline in plasma. Acta Physiol Scand 1960; Suppl. 49, 173: 1−123.

[20] Roth J, Glick GM, Yalow RS et al. Hypoglycemia: A powerful stimulus to secretion of growth hormone. Science 140: 987−991.

[21] Greenwood FC, Landon J, Stamp TCB. The plasma sugar, free fatty acid, cortisol, and growth hormone response to insulin. J Clin Invest 1966; 45: 429−436.

[22] Baron AD, Schaeffer L, Shragg P et al. Role of hyperglugagonemia in maintenance of increased rates of hepatic glucose output in type II diabetics. Diabetes 1987; 36: 274−283.

[23] Reaven GM, Chen Y-DI, Golay A et al. Documentation of hyperglucagonaemia throughout the day in nonobese and obese patients with noninsulin-dependent diabetes mellitus. J Clin Endocrinol Metab 1987; 64: 106−110.

[24] Veldhuis JD, Iranmanesh A, Johnson ML et al. Twenty-four-hour-rhythms in plasma concentrations of adenohypophyseal hormones are generated by distinct amplitude and/or frequency modulation of underlying pituirary secretory bursts. J Clin Endocrinol Metab 1990; 71: 1616−1623.

[25] Hartmann ML, Faria ACS, Vance ML et al. Temporal structure of in vivo growth hormone secretory events in humans. Am J Physiol 1991; 260: E101−110.

[26] Tamborlane Wv, Sherwin RS, Koivisto V et al. Normalization of the growth hormone and catecholamine response to exercise in juvenile-onset diabetic subjects treated with a portable insulin infusion pump. Diabetes 1979; 28: 785−788.

[27] Wurzburger MI, Prelevic GM, Sonksen PH et al. The effects of improved blood glucose control on growth hormone and cortisol secretion in insulin-dependent diabetes mellitus. Clin Endocrinol 1990; 32: 787−797.

[28] Schaper NC. Growth hormone secretion in type 1 diabetes: A review. Acta Endocrinol 1990; 122: 7−12.

[29] Asplin CM, Faria ACS, Carlsen EC et al. Alterations in the pulsatile mode of growth hormone release in men and women with insulin-dependent diabetes mellitus. J Clin Endocrinol Metab 1989; 69: 239−245.

[30] Boucher BJ, Butterfield WJH, Whichelow MJ. The disappearance of labelled human growth hormone from the forearm circulation in normal and diabetic subjects. Clin Sci 1969; 37: 721−730.

[31] Unger RH. Glucagon in diabetes. In: Alberti KGMM, Krall LP, eds. The diabetes annual/ 1. Elsevier Science Publishers B. V. 1985; 480−491.

[32] Conlon JM. Proglucagon-derived peptides: nomenclature, biosynthetic relationships and physiologic roles. Diabetologia 1988; 31: 563−566.

[33] Baumann G. Growth hormone heterogeneity: Genes, Isohormones, Variants, and Binding Proteins. Endocrine Reviews 1991; 12: 424−449.

[34] Hansen I, Tsalikian E, Beaufrere B et al. Insulin resistance in acromegaly; defects in both hepatic and extrahepatic insulin action. Am J Physiol 1986; 250: E269−273.

[35] Møller N, Schmitz O, Jørgensen JOL et al. Basal and insulin stimulated substrate metabolism in patients with active acromegaly before and after adenomectomy. J Clin Endocrinol Metab 1992; 74: 1012−1019.

[36] Nosadini R, Del Prato S, Tiengo A et al. Insulin resistance in Cushing's syndrome. J Clin Endocrinol Metab 1983; 57: 529−536.

[37] Page R, Boolell M, Kalfas A et al. Insulin secretion, insulin sensitivity, and glucose mediated glucose disposal in Cushing's disease: a minimal model analysis. Clin Endocrinol 1991; 35: 509−517.

[38] Jørgensen JOL, Møller J, Alberti KGMM et al. Effects of a low basal growth hormone (GH) elevation on day-to-day fuel metabolism: Studies in GH deficient patients and healthy untreated subjects. Journal of Clinical Endocrinology and Metabolism, in press.

[39] Baltzan MA, Andres R, Cader G et al. Effects of epinephrine on forearm blood flow and metabolism in man. J Clin Invest 1965; 44: 80−92.

[40] Rabinowitz D, Klassen DA, Zierler KL. Effects of human growth hormone on muscle and adipose tissue metabolism in the forearm of man. J Clin Invest 1965; 44: 51−61.

[41] Posefsky T, Tancredi RG, Mopley RT et al. Metabolism of forearm tissues with glucagon. Diabetes 1976; 25: 128–135.
[42] Gerich JE, Lorenzi M, Bier DM et al. Effects of physiologic levels of glucagon and growth hormone on human carbohydrate and lipid metabolism. J Clin Invest 1976; 57: 875–884.
[43] Gerich J, Cryer P, Rizza R. Hormonal mechanisms in acute glucose counterregulation: The relative roles of glucagon, epinephrine, norepinephrine, growth hormone and cortisol. Metabolism 1980; 29: 1164–1175.
[44] Gelfand RA, Matthews DE, Bier DM et al. Role of counterregulatory hormones in the catabolic response to stress. J Clin Invest 1984; 74: 2238–2248.
[45] Press M, Tamborlane WV, Sherwin RS. Importance of raised growth hormone levels in mediating the metabolic derangements of diabetes. N Engl J Med 1984; 310: 810–815.
[46] Campell PJ, Bolli GB, Cryer PE et al. Pathogenesis of the dawn phenomenon in patients with insulin dependent diabetes mellitus. N Engl J Med 1985; 312: 1473–1479.
[47] Periello G, De Feo P, Torlone E et al. Nocturnal spikes of growth hormone secretion cause the dawn phenomenon in type 1 (insulin-dependent) diabetes mellitus by decreasing hepatic (and extrahepatic) sensitivity to insulin in the absence of insulin waning. Diabetologia 1990; 33: 52–59.
[48] Møller N, Schmitz O, Møller J et al. Effects of a growth hormone pulse on fuel metabolism in insulin dependent diabetic subjects. Journal of Clinical Endocrinology and Metabolism 1992; 75: 432–436.
[49] Blackard WG, Barlascini CO, Clore JN et al. Morning insulin requirements. Critique of dawn and meal phenomena. Diabetes 1989; 38: 273–277.
[50] Shamoon H, Hendler R, Sherwin RS. Altered responsiveness to cortisol, epinephrine and glucagon in insulin infused juvenile-omset diabetics. Diabetes 1980; 29: 284–291.
[51] Ørskov L, Alberti KGMM, Mengel A et al. Decreased hepatic glucagon responses in type 1 (insulin dependent) diabetes mellitus. Diabetologia 1991; 34: 521–526.
[52] Hibbard CM, Morrissey MJ. Glycusuria in diphteria. J Exp Med 1899; 4: 137–145.
[53] Keller U. Diabetic ketoacidosis: Current views on pathogenesis and treatment. Diabetologia 1986; 29: 71–77.
[54] Rayfield E, Curnow RT, Reinhard D et al. Effects of acute endotoxiemia on glucoregulation in normal and diabetic subjects. J Clin Endocrinol Metab 1977; 45: 513–521.
[55] Beisel WR. Metabolic response to infection. In: Annual Review of Medicine. Palo Alto, California: Annual Reviews Inc, 1975; 9–20.
[56] Virkamaki A, Puhakainen I, Koivisto VA et al. Mechanisms of hepatic and peripheral insulin resistance during acute infections in humans. J Clin Endocrinol Metab 1992; 74: 673–679.
[58] Van der Poll T, Romijn JA, Endert E et al. Tumor necrosis factor mimicks the metabolic response to acute infection in humans. Am J Physiol 1991; 261: E457–465.
[59] Christensen SE, Jørgensen JOL, Møller N et al. Characterization of growth hormone release in response to external heating. Comparison to exercise induced release. Acta Endocrinologica 1984; 107: 295–301.
[60] Møller N, Beckwick R, Butler PC et al. Metabolic and hormonal responses to exogenous hyperthermia in man. Clinical Endocrinology 1989; 30: 651–660.
[61] Frayn KN. Hormonal control of metabolism in trauma and sepsis. Clin Endocrinol 1986; 24: 577–599.
[62] Alberti KGMM, Christensen NJ, Iversen J et al. Role of glucagon and other hormones in development of diabetic ketoacidosis. Lancet 1975; I: 1307–1311.
[63] Barnes AJ, Kohner EM, Bloom SR et al. Importance of pituitary hormones in aetiology of diabetic ketoacidosis. Lancet 1978; I: 1171–1174.
[64] Alberti KGMM, Christensen SE, Christensen NJ et al. Inhibition of insulin secretion by somatostatin. Lancet 1973; II: 1299–1301.
[65] Bolli G, De Feo P, Periello G et al. Role of hepatic autoregulation in defense against hypoglycemia in humans. J Clin Invest 1985; 75: 1623–1631.
[66] De Feo P, Periello G, Ventura MM et al. The pancreatic-adrenocortical-pituitary clamp technique for study of counterregulation in humans. Am J Physiol 1987; 252: E565–570.

[67] Wahren J, Felig P. Influence of somatostatin on carbohydrate disposal and absorption in diabetes mellitus. Lancet 1976; II: 1213–1216.
[68] Reichlin S. Somatostatin. N Engl J Med 1983; 309: 1495–1501, 1556–1563.
[69] Bergman RN, Ader M, Finegood DT et al. Extrapancreatic effect of somatostatin infusion to increase glucose clearance. Am J Physiol 1984; 47: E370–E379.
[70] Wu MS, Ho LT, Chen JJ et al. Somatostatin potentiation of insulin-induced glucose uptake in normal individuals. Am J Physiol 1986; 251: E674–679.
[71] Stevenson RW, Steiner KE, Hendrick GK et al. Effect of somatostatin on glucose homeostasis in conscious long-fasted dogs. Am J Physiol 1987; 253: E435–442.
[72] Hendrick GK, Frizzell RT, Cherrington AD. Effect of somatostatin on nonesterified fatty acid levels modifies glucose homeostasis during fasting. Am J Physiol 1987; 253: E443–452.
[73] Meneilly GS, Elahi D, Minaker KL et al. Somatostatin enhances insulin-mediated glucose disposal in the elderly. J Clin Endocrinol Metab 1988; 67: 407–410.
[74] Baron AD, Wallace P, Brechtel G et al. Somatostatin does not increase insulin stimulated glucose uptake in humans. Diabetes 1987; 36: 33–36.
[75] Meneilly GS, Elahi D, Minaker KL et al. Somatostatin does not alter insulin-mediated glucose disposal. J Clin Endocrinol Metab 1987; 65: 364–367.
[76] Davidson MB, Harris MD, Ziel FH et al. Suppression of sleep-induced growth hormone secretion by antocholinergic agents abolishes dawn phenomenon. Diabetes 1988; 37: 166–171.
[76] Atiea JA, Creagh F, Page M et al. Early morning hyperglycemia in insulin-dependent diabetes; acute and sustained effects of cholinergic blockade. J Clin Endocrinol Metab 1989; 69: 390–395.
[77] Bevan JS, Ara J, Page MD et al. Cholinergic blockade with piperenzine induces a dose-related reduction in glucose and insulin responses to a mixed meal in normal subjects and non-insulin dependent diabetics. Clin Endocrinol 1991; 35: 85–91.

Exploring diabetic heart disease

L. Thuesen

Introduction

Investigation of the diabetic heart may include visualization of the coronary arteries, assessment of the systolic and the diastolic function of the myocardium, description of the thickness and motion of the left ventricular wall and pathological examination of biopsies from the myocardium.

Investigations of the diabetic heart include both invasive and non-invasive techniques. The invasive investigations, most commonly used, are coronary arteriography, left heart catherization and endomyocardial biopsy. These investigations are associated with a definite, but low risk. Therefore, they can only be applied in patients with symptoms or clinical signs of cardiac disease. The non-invasive techniques include echocardiography, radionuclide techniques and systolic time intervals. These non-invasive methods are not associated with risk or significant inconvenience and can be used in larger numbers of symptomatic or asymptomatic patients.

Invasive studies of the diabetic heart

Coronary arteriography, ventriculography of the left ventricle, catherization of the left ventricle and endomyocardial biopsy

Ventriculography is performed by injection of radiopaque contrast media into the cavity of the left ventricle, and the ejection fraction is calculated from the systolic and diastolic ventriculograms. Intracavitary and intraluminal pressures are measured continuously in the aorta and in the left ventricle before and after the ventriculography. The end-diastolic left ventricular pressure, the ejection fraction and description of the regional wall motion are important parameters in the assessment of left ventricular function.

By selective injection of small volumes of radiopaque contrast media in the right and the left coronary artery while performing cineangiography in a number of projections, intraluminal abnormalities of the coronary arteries can be detected.

These invasive techniques have been used in diabetics with clinical signs of congestive cardiomyopathy [1, 2] and in diabetics with end-stage renal disease, candidates for renal transplantation [3]. In these studies it has been demonstrated, that diabetics may present with normal or near-normal coronary angiograms, while the ejection fraction was decreased indicating an impaired left ventricular function. The impairment of the left ventricular function in combination with normal coronary arteries has been interpreted as a result of a diabetic cardiopathy [3]. The coexistence of a diabetic cardiopathy and coronary atherosclerosis has also been documented.

Endomyocardial biopsy can be performed from the right or the left ventricle. Endomyocardial biopsies have been investigated in patients with clinical signs of congestive cardiomyopathy and in diabetics with an abnormal stress radionuclide ventriculography [4]. In these studies signs of interstitial fibrosis and basement membrane thickening were thought to represent a diabetic cardiopathy [4].

Coronary arteriography, left heart catheterization and endomyocardial biopsy do not seem to be associated with increased risk in diabetic patients as compared to non-diabetic subjects.We recommend invasive investigations to be carried out in the morning after a 6-hour fast. The patients are kept normo-glycaemic by administration of subcutaneous long-acting insulin and intravenous glucose infusion. If there are signs of impaired renal function, the use of x-ray contrast media should be kept at a minimum to reduce the risk of temporary reduction of the renal function. Problems with the renal function after coronary arteriography seem to be especially prevalent in diabetic patients.

Non-invasive studies of the diabetic heart

The most commonly used non-invasive methods for assessment of cardiac function are and have been, echocardiography, scintigraphy techniques and systolic time intervals. These methods of investigation gave valuable direct or indirect information of the systolic and diastolic function and the structure of the diabetic heart.

The left ventricular systolic function

Ejection phase indices: The left ventricular ejection fraction (EF), the left ventricular fractional shortening (FS) and the mean velocity of circumferential fibre shortening (VcF) are ejection phase indices, parameters which are extensively used in the assessment of cardiac function. The ejection fraction is calculated from the systolic (SV) and the diastolic (DV) left ventricular volumes ([DV-SV]/DV). The ejection fraction can be assessed planimetrically by two dimensional echocardiography, contrast ventriculography, or by radionuclide ventriculography. The fractional shortening (FS) and the mean circumferential shortening velocity (VcF) are similar ejection phase indices, which can be assessed by M-mode echocardiography. The FS is calculated from the short diastolic (LVIDd) and systolic (LVIDs) diameters as [(LVIDd-LVIDs) × 100]/LVIDd (%) and Vcf as FS/(left ventricular ejection time) (circumferences/sec) [5, 6].

There are limitations to the use of the above-mentioned ejection phase indices in the evaluation of cardiac function.

FS, Vcf and EF are inaccurate measurements of the cardiac function in asymmetrically contracting hearts, as seen in ischaemic heart disease, because focal hypofunction of diseased myocardium is often followed by compensatory hyperfunction of normal myocardium. Furthermore, apical wall motion abnormalities may not be detected by the assessment of the left ventricular short diameters, which are used in the calculation of FS and Vcf [7].

The EF, FS and Vcf are sensitive to changes in after-load. An acute increase of the after-load reduces the EF, FS and Vcf, and an acute after-load reduction enhances the same parameters [7]. The pre-load also influences the ejection phase indices, but to a lesser degree. Here an acute increase of pre-load tends to increase and an acute reduction of pre-load to reduce EF, FS and Vcf [7].

A change of loading conditions of the heart may be a significant problem in studying cardiac function in diabetic patients, as acute changes in blood glucose seem to influence pre-load [8]. Thus, acute hyperglycaemia have been shown to increase the left ventricular diastolic diameter (increasing pre-load) [8], while an insulin induced acute decrease of blood glucose has been shown to have the opposite effects [9].

During normal loading conditions, EF, FS and Vcf are reliable indices of myocardial contractility [7]. The same parameters are also useful during conditions of chronic volume or pressure overload, provided the left ventricle has had sufficient time to develop compensatory hypertrophy [7].

Concerning heart rate, the ejection phase indices EF and FS are independent of heart rate. In contrast, Vcf is related to the heart rate [10], because the left ventricular ejection time is closely related to heart rate. The increased heart rate, which is seen in diabetics, implies a decreased LVET and an increased Vcf. Therefore, Vcf may be a poor indicator of myocardial contractility in diabetic patients with abnormalities of heart rate.

Cardiac output: Cardiac output is likely to be an important parameter in the evaluation of possible haemodynamic disturbances in IDDM [11]. Unfortunately, cardiac output is difficult to measure, and the best methods, Fick oximetry, dye dilution and thermodilution, involve rather invasive techniques. Cardiac output have been assessed by means of M-mode echocardiography, where ventricular volumes were calculated from the systolic and diastolic internal diameters. This method is, however, rather imprecise. Some improvement may be seen when planimetry of a two-dimensional echocardiogram or a Doppler measurement of the aortic or the pulmonary blood flow velocities are used. Coefficient of variation in measurement of cardiac output usually varies between 15 and 20%. Therefore, data in cardiac output must be used with caution.

Echocardiographic investigations: The earliest echocardiographic studies included both IDDM and NIDDM patients, without detailed information on the type of diabetes and the presence of microvascular complications [12, 13]. Furthermore, presence of coronary artery disease probably influenced the results. In these studies, the fractional shortening and the mean velocity of circumferential fibre shortening were found to be within normal limits in the diabetic patients. Decreased values of fractional shortening were only seen in hypertensive diabetics [14].

In later studies, patients with clinical signs of coronary artery disease have been excluded from the study populations and the diabetic patients have been divided into subgroups according to type of diabetes and to the presence of microvascular complications [14, 15, 16]. We investigated fractional shortening and mean velocity of circumferential fibre shortening in IDDM patients in 2 studies [17, 18]. In the first study, these parameters were found to be increased as compared to normal control subjects. In this study, only 3 of the patients had minor signs of microvascular disease and the patients had a short duration of disease (8 years). In the second study [18], the mean duration of disease was 18 years. Also, in this study, the fractional shortening in the diabetic patients was increased as compared to control subjects. The diabetics were grouped according to their status of microvascular complications. The fractional shortening was increased in all the diabetic groups, except in the groups of proliferative retinopathy or clinical nephropathy, as the diabetics with the lowest values of the fractional shortening were found in these groups.

Results are diverging concerning patients with microvascular complications. In the study by Sampson et al. [15], the fractional shortening was significantly increased in diabetics with clinical nephropathy, while the fractional shortening was found to be within normal limits in the two other studies on similar patients [14, 18].

Scintigraphic techniques: The cardiac function during a stress test may reveal functional disturbances in spite of a normal resting state examination [19]. Echocardiographic studies have been performed following physical exercise, but there are considerable methodological problems in these studies [20, 21]. The left ventricular ejection fraction (EF) during rest and exercise can be assessed reliably by multigated radionuclide ventriculography accompanied by electrocardiographic tracing [22].

Radionuclide ventriculography is usually carried out with the patient in supine position. The best separation of the left and right ventricles are usually obtained in the left anterior oblique position with an angle of 30–45° and with a cranio-caudal tilt of 15° to separate the atria from the ventricles. The left ventricular ejection fraction is calculated using the formula: (end diastolic counts – end systolic counts)/(end diastolic counts – background counts). Also the regional wall motion can be described.

By this method the diastolic left ventricular function can also be evaluated from the filling rate or the time to peak filling rate [23].

Scintigraphic investigations: A number of scintigraphic investigations have shown that the left ventricular ejection fraction at rest is either within the normal range or increased in IDDM patients. However, the patients were rather inhomogeneous in most of these studies. A considerable number of patients had microvascular complications [24–26], and in some of the studies both IDDM and NIDDM patients were investigated. None of the studies gave specific information on the ejection fraction in IDDM patients without microvascular disease.

The function of the diabetic heart during a stress test: Changes of ejection fraction during an exercise test have been widely used in detecting subclinical abnormalities of cardiac function. The normal cardiac response to physical exercise is an increase of the ejection fraction, while unchanged or decreasing ejection fraction is a sign of impaired contractile reserve [22]. A number of studies in diabetic patients have shown a smaller increase of ejection fraction during exercise than in control subjects [4, 27], but one study showed a normal increase of ejection fraction during exercise in young IDDM patients with no clinical signs of heart disease [26]. Two studies [27, 28] have shown that the left ventricular contractile reserve was related to the presence of microvascular disease, but in other studies such a relationship has not been found [4, 25].

The aetiology of the reduced increase of ejection fraction during an exercise test in diabetic patients has not been established so far. Coronary arteriography or thallium scintigraphy [4] in patients with impaired contractile reserve have shown no signs of ischaemic heart disease, and therefore the cardiac abnormalities were attributed to a diabetic cardiomyopathy in these patients. This conclusion was questioned in a study by Borow et al. [28]. They found a normal baseline contractility by echocardiography and showed that a decreased ejection fraction with exercise was found in patients with a high resting state ejection fraction. By retrospective revaluation of two similar studies, the same relation between ejection fraction at rest and during exercise was found. It has previously been shown that one of the most important determinants of ejection fraction during exercise is ejection fraction at rest, and that reduced increase of ejection fraction is a common finding in normal subjects with a resting state fraction of $\geq 70\%$ [29, 30]. Thus, there is evidence that the increase of ejection fraction plays a role in the reduced myocardial response to a stress test described in many diabetic patients.

Systolic time intervals: Systolic time intervals can be measured by echocardiography [5], but were traditionally measured by simultaneous registration of electrocardiogram, phonocardiogram and the carotid pulse wave [31]. In cases of impaired left ventricular function the pre-ejection period (PEP) is prolonged at the expense of the ejection period [LVET). Therefore, PEP/LVET has been widely used as an index of cardiac function and seems to be most closely related to the left ventricular function. Because PEP is only slightly influenced by heart rate and LVET considerably influenced by heart rate, these intervals are corrected for heart rate by different constants [31]. However, the ratio PEP/LVET is usually not corrected for heart rate, although the heart rate independency of PEP/LVET has been questioned [32]. In IDDM patients, cardiac function, as assessed by systolic time intervals, has been found within normal limits in patients without microvascular complications [33], and impaired in patients with long-term, complicated disease [12, 34]. However, there may be problems in the interpretation of systolic time intervals in diabetic patients, because the increased heart rate in these patients tends to increase the PEP/LVET. It is possible that the abnormalities of PEP/LVET in some of the studies are a consequence of increased heart rate rather than an expression of impaired cardiac function [32]. These indirect estimations of cardiac function have now been replaced by echocardiographic and radionuclide techniques.

The left ventricular diastolic function

Diastolic time intervals can be measured by combining phonocardiography and echocardiography [35]. The isovolumetric relaxation period is the interval from the closure of the aortic valve to the opening of the mitral valve. Another parameter is the interval from the minimal left ventricular cavity dimension to the opening of the mitral valve. The prolongation of these intervals is a non-specific sign of disturbed myocardial function [36].

Changes in the cavity shape and the wall thickness can be inferred from the echocardiogram by digitisation. These changes give information about co-ordination of the wall motion and the wall thinning rates [37]. While incoordination usually is a sign of coronary artery disease, a decreased wall thinning rate is a sign of impaired diastolic function and probably due to increased stiffness of the myocardium [37].

Pulsed Doppler echocardiography is another method for evaluation of left ventricular filling. Here the transmitral early (passive) flow and the late (atrial) flow are assessed. The ratio between the early and the late diastolic flow velocity (E/A), is reproducible, and it correlates well with flow profiles measured by cineangiography and radionuclide techniques [38].

However, the heart rate has been reported to influence the E/A ratio in such a way that an increase of heart rate is associated with a reduction of the E/A ratio [39], therefore, abnormalities of the E/A ratio in diabetics may be a result of heart rate abnormalities rather than an expression of impaired diastolic function.

Studies on the diastolic function of the diabetic heart: In insulin-dependent diabetics with short-term, uncomplicated disease and non clinical signs of heart disease, the isovolumetric relaxation period, the wall thinning rate, the filling rate and time to peak filling rate of the left ventricle have been found to be normal, suggesting a normal diastolic function in these patients [13, 34]. In patients with clinical nephrophaty, autonomic neuropathy and proliferative retinopathy, the diastolic function has been found to be impaired [13, 14, 34, 40, 41]. Shapiro et al. found significant correlation between an index of microvascular complications and variables of the diastolic function in IDDM and NIDDM patients with no clinical signs of heart disease [42]. In the same study, uncoordinated left ventricular relaxation was found in 22% of the patients, which suggests a high frequency of subclinical coronary heart disease in these patients.

The left ventricular filling, as assessed by Doppler echocardiography, has been investigated in IDDM patients with a high prevalence of microvascular complications and in IDDM patients with uncomplicated disease [15, 43, 44]. In these studies, the atrial contribution to the left ventricular filling was found to be increased as compared to non-diabetic controls, indicating impairment of the diastolic function. The left ventricular filling abnormalities did not correlate with duration of disease, retinopathy, nephropathy or peripheral neuropathy in one study [43], but were related to the level of albuminuria and to the blood pressure in the other study on patients with complicated disease [15].

In the above-mentioned studies, the left ventricular systolic function, as assessed by the fractional shortening or the ejection fraction, was either normal [13, 14, 34, 44] or increased [15, 16]. Thus, impairment of the diastolic function seems to be an early sign of diabetic heart muscle disease and seems to precede a detectable abnormality of the systolic function in IDDM patients.

The reason for the impaired diastolic function in diabetic patients cannot be deduced from the above-mentioned studies. The diastolic function abnormalities have been suggested to be an early marker of a diabetic cardiomyopathy [44]. However, increased heart rate [39], elevated blood pressure [45], increased thickness of the left ventricular wall [46] or myocardial ischaemia [47] will influence the diastolic function and may contribute to the abnormalities of the diastolic function described in diabetic patients.

Left ventricular thickness and wall mass: The thickness of the lect ventricular septum and posterior wall in diastole are measured at the level just below the mitral valve and at the peak of the electrocardiographic R wave [6]. From the septal thickness (IVT), the posterior wall thickness (PWT) and the left ventricular diastolic diameter (LVIDd) the left ventricular wall mass can be estimated by the following formula: $1.04 \times [(IVT + LVIDd + PWT)^3 - (LVIDd)^3] - 13.6\,(g)$ [48].

Early echocardiographic studies showed increased left ventricular wall thickness in hypertensive diabetes with a high prevalence of microvascular complications [13]. Later studies have shown normal wall thickness and wall mass in short-term uncomplicated diabetes [49], but increased wall thickness seems to be an early and prevalent finding in hypertensive microalbuminuric and proteinuric diabetic patients [50].

Conclusions

The diabetic heart can be studied by invasive and non-invasive techniques. Because invasive investigations are associated with a risk of cardiovascular complications, invasive investigations can only be performed in patients with symptoms or clinical signs of heart disease.

In asymptomatic diabetics, cardiac function and structure can be assessed reliably by non-invasive techniques. At present scintigraphic techniques and Doppler echocardiography are valuable instruments in the description of the diabetic heart and in the evaluation of different interventions in diabetic patients. Furthermore, these methods have a great potential for monitoring and describing development of diabetic abnormalities of cardiac function and structure in longitudinal studies.

References

[1] Hamby RI, Zoneraich S, Sherman L. Diabetic cardiomyopathy. JAMA 1974; 229: 1749–1754.

[2] Dash H, Johnson RA, Dinsmore RE et al. Cardiomyopathic syndrome due to coronary artery disease. II: Increased prevalence in atients with diabetes mellitus: a matched pair analysis. Br Heart J 1977; 39: 740–747.

[3] D'elia JA, Weinrauch LA, Healy RW et al. Myocardial dysfunction without coronary artery disease in diabetic renal failure. Am J Cardiol 1979; 43: 193–199.

[4] Fisher BM, Gillen G, Lindop GBM et al. Cardiac function and coronary arteriography in asymptomatic type 1 (insulin-dependent) diabetic patients: evidence for a specific diabetic heart disease. Diabetologia 1986; 29: 706–712.

[5] Feigenbaum H. Echocardiographic evaluation of cardiac chambers. In: Feigenbaum H, ed. Echocardiography, 3rd ed. Philadelphia: Lea and Febiger, 1981; 119–221.

[6] Sahn DJ, DeMaria A, Kisslo J et al. The committee on M-mode standardization of the American Society of Echocardiography. Recommendations regarding quantitation in M-mode echocardiography: results of a survey of echocardiography measurements. Circulation 1978; 58: 1072–1083.

[7] Braunwald E. Assessment of cardiac function. In: Braunwald E, ed. Heart disease. A text book of cardiovascular medicine. 3rd ed. Philadelphia: W. B. Saunders Company, 1988; 449–470.

[8] Thuesen L, Christiansen JS, Schmitz O et al. Increased myocardial performance following acute hyperglycaemia in insulin-dependent diabetic patients. A consequence of increased peripheral blood flow. Scand J Clin Lab Invest 1987; 47: 571–579.

[9] Thuesen L, Christiansen JS, Schmitz O et al. Increased myocardial contractility during intravenous insulin infusion in type 1 (insulin-dependent) diabetic patients: an echocardiographic study. Scand J Clin Lab Invest 1988; 48: 275–284.

[10] DeMaria AN, Neumann A, Schubart PJ et al. Systematic correlation of cardiac chamber size and ventricular performance determined with echocardiography and alterations in heart rate in normal persons. Am J Cardiol 1979; 43: 1–9.

[11] Zatz R, Brenner BM. Pathogenesis of diabetic microangiopathy. The hemodynamic view. Am J Med 1986; 80: 443–453.

[12] Shapiro LM, Howat AP, Calter MM. Left ventricular function in diabetes mellitus I: Methodology, and prevalence and spectrum of abnormalities. Br Heart J 1981; 45: 122–128.

[13] Shapiro LM. A prospective study of heart disease in diabetes mellitus. Quart J Med 1984; 209: 55–68.

[14] Danielsen R, Nordrehaug JE, Lien E et al. Subclinical left ventricular abnormalities in young subjects with long-term type 1 diabetes mellitus detected by digitized M-mode echocardiography. Am J Cardiol 1987; 60: 143–146.

[15] Sampson MJ, Chambers JB, Sprigins DC et al. Abnormal diastolic function in patients with type 1 diabetes and early nephropathy. Br Heart J 1990; 64: 266–271.
[16] Uusitupa M, Mustunen J, Laakso M et al. Impairment of diastolic function in midle-aged insulin-dependent (type 1) and non-insulin-dependent (type 2) diabetic patients free of cardiovascular disease. Diabetologia 1988; 31: 783–791.
[17] Thuesen L, Christiansen JS, Falstie-Jensen N et al. Increased myocardial contractility in short-term type 1 diabetic patients: an echocardiographic study. Diabetologia 1985; 28: 822–826.
[18] Thuesen L, Christiansen JS, Mogensen CE et al. Cardiac hyperfunction in insulin-dependent diabetic patients developing microvascular complications. Diabetes 1988; 37: 851–856.
[19] Borer JS, Bacharach SL, Green MV et al. Real-time radionuclide cineangiography in the non-invasive evaluation of global and regional left ventricular function at rest and during exercise in patients with coronary-artery disease. N Engl J Med 1977; 296: 839–844.
[20] Feigenbaum H. The echocardiographic examination. In: Feigenbaum H, ed. Echocardiography. 3rd ed. Philadelphia: Lea and Febiger, 1981; 51–118.
[21] Thuesen L, Christiansen JS, Sørensen KE et al. Exercise capacity and cardiac function in type 1 diabetic patients tested with continuous subcutaneous insulin infusion. A controlled study. Scand J Clin Lab Invest 1986; 46: 779–784.
[22] Borer JS, Kent KM, Bacharach SL et al. Sensitivity, specificity and predictive accuracy of radionuclide cineangiography during exercise in patients with coronary artery disease. Comparison with exercise electrocardiography. Circulation 1979; 60: 572–580.
[23] Poliner LR, Farber SH, Glaeser DH et al. Alteration of diastolic filling rate during exercise radionuclide angiography: a highly sensitive technique for defection of coronary artery disease. Circulation 1984; 70: 942–950.
[24] Arvan S, Singal K, Knapp R et al. Subclinical left ventricular abnormalities in young diabetics. Chest 1988; 93: 1031–1034.
[25] Fisher BM, Gillen G, Ong-Tone et al. Cardiac function and insulin-dependent diabetes: radionuclide ventriculography in young diabetics. Diabetic Medicine 1985; 2: 251–256.
[26] Margonato A, Gerundini P, Vicedomini G et al. Abnormal cardiovascular response to exercise in young asymptomatic diabetic patients with retinopathy. Am Heart J 1986; 112: 554–560.
[27] Zola B, Kahn JK, Juni E et al. Abnormal cardiac function in diabetic patients with autonomic neuropathy in the absence of ischemic heart disease. J Clin Endocrinol Metab 1986; 63: 208–214.
[28] Borow KM, Jaspan JB, Williams KA et al. Myocardial mechanics in young adult patients with diabetes mellitus: effects of altered load, inotropic state and dynamic exercise. JACC 1990, 15: 1508–1517.
[29] Gibbons RJ, Lee KL, Cobb F et al. Ejection fraction response to exercise in patients with chest pain and normal coronary arteriograms. Circulation 1981; 64: 952–957.
[30] Rozanski A, Diamond GA, Jones R et al. A format for integrating the interpretation of exercise ejection fraction and wall motion and its application in identifying equivocal responses. J Am Coll Cardiol 1985; 5: 238–248.
[31] Weissler AM, Harris WS, Schoenfeld CD. Bedside technics for the evaluation of ventricular function in man. Am J Cardiol 1969; 23: 577–583.
[32] Cokkinos DV, Heimonas ET, Demopoulos JN et al. Influence of heart rate increase in uncorrected pre-ejection period/left ventricular ejection time (PEP/LVET) ratio in normal individuals. Br Heart J 1976; 38: 683–688.
[33] Posner J, Ilya R, Wanderman K et al. Systolic time intervals in diabetes. Diabetologia 1983; 24: 249–252.
[34] Shapiro LM, Leatherdale BA, Mackinnon J et al. Left ventricular function in diabetes mellitus II: Relation between clinical features and left ventricular function. Br Heart J 1981; 45: 129–132.
[35] Chen W, Gibson D. Relation of isovolumic relaxion to left ventricular wall movement in man. Br Heart J 1979; 42: 51–56.

[36] Gibson DG, Brown D. Measurement of instantaneous left ventricular dimension and filling rate in man, using echocardiography. Br Heart J 1973; 35: 1141–1149.
[37] Traill TA, Gibson DG, Brown DJ. Study of left ventricular wall thickness and dimension changes using echocardiography. Br Heart J 1978; 40: 162–169.
[38] Rokey R, Kuo Lc, Zoghbi WA et al. Determination of parameters of left ventricular diastolic filling with pulsed doppler echocardiography: comparison with cineangiography. Circulation 1985; 71: 543–550.
[39] Smith SA, Stoner JE, Russell AE et al. Transmitral velocities measured by pulsed Doppler in healthy volunteers: effects of acute changes in blood pressure and heart rate. Br Heart J 1989; 61: 344–347.
[40] Sanderson JE, Brown DJ, Rivellese A et al. Diabetic cardiomyopathy? An echocardiographic study of young diabetics. Br Med J 1978; 1: 404–407.
[41] Kahn JK, Zola B, Juni JE et al. Radionuclide assessment of left ventricular diastolic filling in diabetes mellitus with and without cardiac autonomic neuropathy. JACC 1986; 7: 1303–1309.
[42] Shapiro LM. Echocardiographic features of impaired ventricular function in diabetes mellitus. Br Heart J 1982; 47: 439–444.
[43] Zarich SW, Arbuckle BE, Cohen LR et al. Diatolic abnormalities in young asymptomatic diabetic patients assessed by pulsed Doppler echocardiography. JACC 1988; 12: 114–120.
[44] Paillole C, Dahan M, Paycha F et al. Prevalence and significance of left ventricular filling abnormalities determined by Doppler echocardiography in young type I (insulin diabetic) diabetic patients. Am J Cardiol 1989; 64: 1010–1016.
[45] Phillips RA, Coplan NL, Krakoff LR et al. Doppler echocardiographic analysis og left ventricular filling in treated hypertensive patients. J Am Coll Cardiol 1987; 9: 317–322.
[46] Pearson AC, Labovitz AJ, Mrosek D et al. Assessment of diastolic function in normal and hypertrophied hearts: comparison of Doppler echocardiography and M-mode echocardiography. Am Heart J 1987; 113: 1417–1425.
[47] Aroesty JM, McKay RG, Heller GV et al. Simultaneous assessment of left ventricular systolic and diastolic function during pacing induced ischaemia. Circulation 1985; 71: 889–900.
[48] Devereux RB, Reicheck N. Echocardiographic determination of left ventricular mass in man. Anatomic validation of the method. Circulation 1977; 55: 613–618.
[49] Thuesen L, Christiansen JS, Mogensen CE et al. Echocardiographic-determined left ventricular wall characteristics in insulin dependent diabetic patients. Acta Med Scand 1988; 224: 343–348.
[50] Sampsom MJ, Chambers JB, Sprigings DC et al. Interventricular septal hypertrophy in type 1 diabetic patients with microalbuminuria or early proteinuria. Diabetic Med 1990; 7: 126–132.

Electrophysiological methods in the evaluation of diabetic neuropathy

P. K. Thomas

Introduction

In discussing the use of electrophysiological methods for the investigation of diabetic neuropathy it is first necessary to consider the nature of the disturbances of peripheral nerve function that occur in association with diabetes mellitus. A wide variety of abnormalities are encountered that are likely to have different causations and significance. In general, these can be subdivided into rapidly reversible phenomena and more persistent abnormalities [1]. Phenomena that are encountered in patients with newly diagnosed or poorly controlled diabetes and which are rapidly corrected by establishing euglycaemia include distal lower limb sensory symptoms ('hyperglycaemic neuropathy'), reduced nerve conduction velocity and increased resistance to ischaemic conduction failure. More persistent disturbances can be subdivided into symmetric polyneuropathies, on the one hand, and focal and multifocal neuropathies, on the other. The symmetric polyneuropathies comprise the distal sensory polyneuropathy, which may include minor motor manifestations, and autonomic neuropathy. These are the characteristic neuropathies of insulin-dependent diabetes mellitus (IDDM) but also develop in non-insulin-dependent diabetes mellitus (NIDDM). The syndrome of acute painful diabetic neuropathy appears to constitute a distinct syndrome. It may be associated with precipitous weight loss [2] or be triggered by the initiation of treatment or the establishment of tight glycaemic control [3]. Focal and multifocal neuropathies are typically seen in older patients with NIDDM or longstanding IDDM. They include focal cranial and limb neuropathies, thoracoabdominal neuropathy and asymmetric lower limb motor neuropathy (diabetic amyotrophy). Focal limb neuropathies often occur at common sites of entrapment or external compression, reflecting the increased susceptibility of diabetic nerve to compression injury. Finally, there is evidence that chronic inflammatory demyelinating polyneuropathy (CIDP) may be superimposed on diabetic neuropathy as a secondary immune-mediated event [4].

This chapter will address the electrophysiological techniques available for examining peripheral nerve function in diabetes in relation to these various syndromes. The main techniques available are the assessment of motor nerve conduction, including F wave latency and evoked muscle action potential amplitudes, electromyography (EMG), the recording of sensory and mixed nerve action potentials, and the recording of spinal and cerebral somatosensory evoked potentials. The broad principles of the techniques will be emphasized. Details concerning their neurophysiological basis and detailed methodology are available in standard textbooks, such as those by Brown [5], Kimura [6] and Brown and Bolton [7].

Motor nerve conduction

Motor nerve conduction is most commonly examined in the peroneal and tibial nerves in the lower limbs and the median and ulnar nerves in the upper limbs. Other motor nerves may be investigated depending upon the clinical situation. Thus in patients with diabetic amyotrophy, assessment of conduction in the femoral nerve may be useful.

Examination of motor conduction in nerves to distal limb muscles

This is usually undertaken with surface recording electrodes, although if the muscle is severely denervated, an intramuscular needle electrode recording may be required. With surface recording, an active electrode is placed over the muscle belly with an indifferent electrode over its tendon (belly-tendon recording) and an earth (ground) electrode distally on the limb. If the active electrode is over the motor point of the muscle, a biphasic compound muscle action potential is obtained on nerve stimulation with an initial negative deflection and a later positive deflection. If the potential is preceded by a negative wave, it is preferable to adjust the position of the electrode to obtain initial negativity. The electrodes are placed over extensor digitorum brevis, abductor hallucis, abductor pollicis brevis and abductor digiti minimi for the peroneal, tibial, median and ulnar nerves, respectively.

The motor nerve is stimulated with a bipolar probe electrode at two or more points along its course, at the ankle and the neck of the fibula for the peroneal nerve, at the ankle and in the popliteal fossa for the tibial, and at the wrist, elbow and possibly in the axilla for the median and ulnar nerves. The nerve is activated under the cathode, which is placed distally. The position of the stimulating electrode is adjusted using a submaximal stimulus to define the site at which a maximal response is obtained. The stimulus intensity is then increased until the maximal amplitude of the evoked muscle action potential is achieved. It is usual to record the response with a stimulus that is about 20 per cent supramaximal to ensure that the full amplitude of the potential is obtained.

The latency of the evoked muscle response is taken from the stimulus to the onset of the negative deflection (Fig. 1). With a stimulus at the wrist or ankle, the latency includes both conduction time in the segment of nerve to the muscle and neuromuscular transmission time. Together they are referred to as the terminal or distal motor latency (DML). The distance between the proximal and distal stimulating electrodes is obtained using a tape measure placed on the skin along the course of the nerve. This is used to calculate motor nerve conduction velocity (MNCV) between the two sites. It represents the velocity of the fastest conducting motor fibres in the nerve. Procedures are available for estimating the distribution of conduction velocities over the range of extrafusal muscle fibres and have been applied to diabetic neuropathy [8]. For routine studies, most current EMG machines have a cursor that can be adjusted by the operator to measure latency or possess computer programs that automatically identify the onset of the potentials. This may have to be adjusted on the screen by the operator. The machine will provide a printout of the recording for documentation.

As nerve conduction velocity is highly temperature dependent, skin temperature over the distal part of the limb must be measured at the time of the recording and the limb warmed so that it is at or above 32 °C. If below, the limb must be warmed. Heating devices are available with skin sensors that provide an automatic cutout if skin temperature reaches too high a level. This is important, so as to avoid burning in patients with loss of thermal pain sensibility.

Control values for MNCV and terminal latency are given in Kimura [6] and other texts. Conduction velocity in children reaches the adult range by about 5 years of age. During later childhood, velocity increases slightly in the upper limbs and falls slightly in the lower limbs [9]. It then remains relatively stable but begins to diminish after 30 or 40 years of age and falls by less than 10 m/s by the 60th year, or even the 80th [6]. Accurate estimates for the average rate of decline per year for normal subjects with ageing are not available.

Peripheral nerve fibres are unresponsive to activation for a period following conduction of an impulse. This refractory period can be determined by using paired stimuli at varying intervals. This may be useful in detecting subclinical neuropathy. Refractory periods have been shown to be increased in diabetic patients not only with clinical and electrophysiological evidence of neuropathy but in patients with normal nerve conduction [10, 11]. The ability of nerve to conduct impulses at a high frequency, which depends upon the refractory period, is also impaired in diabetics [10].

Examination of motor conduction in nerves to proximal muscles

This has greatest relevance for the investigation of patients with proximal lower limb motor neuropathy (diabetic amyotrophy). Conduction time can be measured in the femoral nerve on recording from the anterior compartment thigh mucles. A recording is made with a needle electrode in rectus femoris or vastus intermedius and the femoral nerve is stimulated supramaximally in the groin. The latency to the onset of the evoked muscle action potential is obtained. A nomogram is available for relating conduction time to conduction distance [12]. Prolonged latency may be related to loss of the larger and faster conducting fibres or to demyelination/remyelination.

Acute facial palsy is more frequent in patients with diabetes and is stated more frequently to involve axonal degeneration than idiopathic Bell's palsy. It has been suggested that this may be related to ischaemic changes in the nerve. In the presence of total paralysis of the facial muscles the existence of conduction block in the nerve fibres in the facial canal with preservation of axonal continuity can be demonstrated by showing a mechanical response in the muscles on stimulation of the nerve at the stylomastoid foramen, but not before 4 days after the onset of paralysis. Conduction time to the facial muscles can be measured but is of little diagnostic value. It has been found to be increased in patients with diabetic neuropathy [13]. In patients with a generalized demyelinating polyneuropathy, severe prolongation may be found.

Measurement of compound muscle action potential amplitude

The amplitude of the evoked compound muscle action potential (CMAP) is an important measure. It can be taken either as the height of the negative peak from baseline or the peak-to-peak amplitude measured between the tips of the negative and succeeding components (Fig. 1). The duration of the potential, taken from the onset of the negative wave to the final return to baseline is also important. The total area under the waveform can be obtained by point counting or other methods or by electrical averaging if available.

The amplitude of the CMAP reflects the number of conducting motor axons and the size of their motor units. It will be reduced by temporal disper-

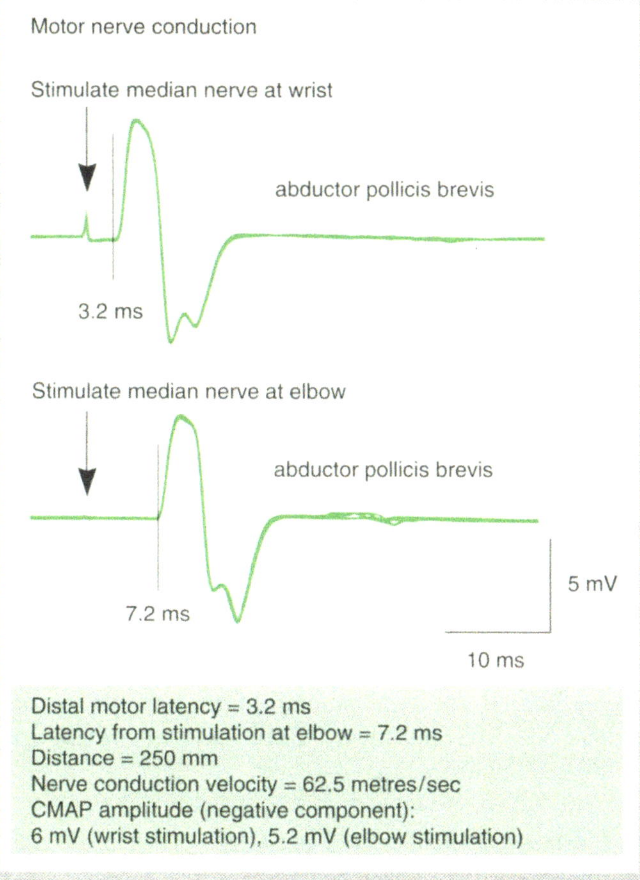

Fig. 1 Motor conduction in the median nerve on recording from abductor pollicis brevis with stimulation at the wrist and elbow. Figure kindly provided by Dr Philip Thompson

sion of conduction related to unequal degrees of slowing between motor axons. This will increase the duration of the potential and can also result in reduction in amplitude of the compound action potential because of phase cancellations between the potentials derived from individual motor units.

Attempts have been made to estimate the number of motor units contributing to the CMAP [14, 15]. This is done by measuring the amplitude of the initial increments in the CMAP, each increment representing the addition of a further motor unit, when the stimulus strength is slowly increased from the time of the first detectable response. An average value for motor unit amplitude is thus obtained and, when divided into the total CMAP amplitude with supramaximal stimulation, gives an estimate of the total number of motor units (and hence motor axons) contributing to the potential. This technique may give an inaccurate estimate of the numbers if the size of the initial units to be activated is not representative of the later ones, if two motor axons have identical thresholds for electrical stimulation, or if motor units have too small an amplitude to be reliable detected.

In single fibre electromyography (SFEMG) a special needle electrode is employed with a small leading-off surface and a restricted pick-up distance. Recordings can therefore be made from individual muscle fibres within a motor unit. By this means the density of fibres innervated by a single motor axon can be examined and also the latency difference for the activation of different fibres within the unit (jitter) can be assessed. In macro EMG a different type of needle is used which, from one surface, records from a wider zone within the muscle. It also has a side port with a restricted leading-off surface for SFEMG amplified through a separate channel. The larger pick-up surface will record from several motor units but using the SFEMG and an averaging technique, the total potential from a single motor unit can be collected. So far SFEMG and macro EMG have not found applications in the study of diabetic neuropathy.

Recording of 'late' potentials

The direct response in the muscle produced by stimulation of the motor nerve ('M' response) may be followed by 'late' waves. The most useful of these are the F waves (Fig. 2). These are potentials of considerably smaller amplitude than the M waves and tend to be variable in their size, configuration and latency, although the range between the earliest and latest F waves in the normal subject (chronodispersion) is small. They are the result of antidromic conduction proximally along motor axons which then leads to 'backfiring' of the anterior horn cells and orthodromic conduction out to the muscle.

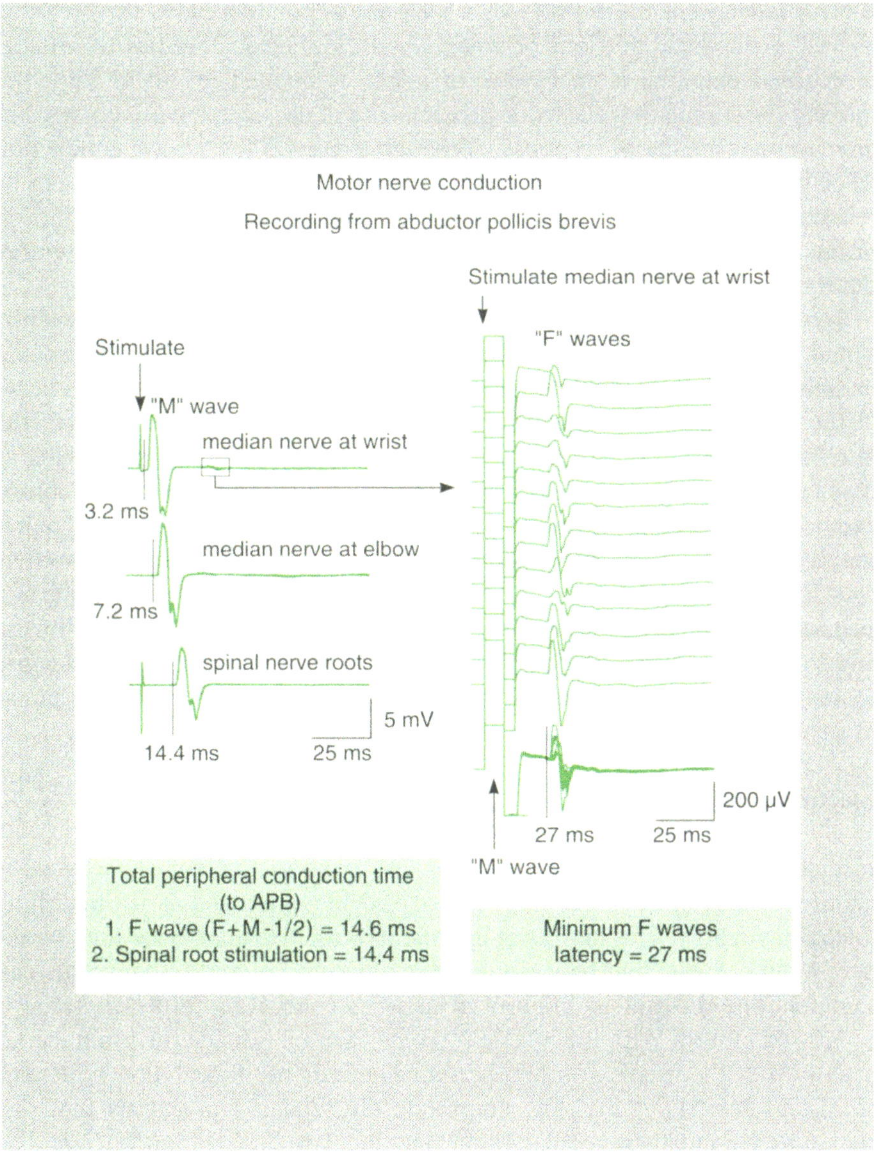

Fig. 2 Recordings from abductor pollicis brevis (APB) with stimulation, in the 3 traces to the left of the figure, at the wrist and elbow and over the spinal nerve roots. Calculation of total conduction time from the spinal roots to the muscle using F wave latency gives a value (14.6 ms) that is closely similar to that obtained with stimulation paraspinally over the spinal roots (14.4 ms). Recordings of F wave responses are seen in the traces shown on the right of the figure which are at higher amplification than with stimulation at the wrist. The superimposed traces in the lowermost part of the figure indicate that, in the normal subject, F wave latency varies little, although the amplitude in successive sweeps differs. Figure kindly provided by Dr Philip Thompson

F wave latency therefore provides a measure of conduction to the proximal as well as the distal portions of motor axons. If there is doubt as to whether a recorded potential is an F wave or a late component of an M response, moving the stimulating electrode proximally will decrease F wave latency but increase that for the M response. Although estimates for F wave conduction velocity can be obtained, it is usual to express them as a latency that can be related to the height of the individual. Conduction in the proximal portion of the motor fibres can also be examined directly by stimulation percutaneously over the spinal roots with a high voltage stimulator (Fig. 2).

Recordings of the H (Hoffmann) reflex are less useful. This monosynaptic spinal reflex is only obtainable from certain muscles such as the gastrocnemius on stimulation of the tibial nerve. With weak stimulation of this nerve in the popliteal fossa, the earliest evoked potential is a 'late response', the H reflex, which is the result of the activation of muscle spindle afferents as they have a slightly lower threshold for stimulation than the extrafusal motor axons. With increasing stimulus strength an earlier M wave appears, representing the orthodromic response for activation of the extrafusal motor efferents. This is accompanied by a corresponding reduction in the amplitude and eventually disappearance of the H response because of the collision of the antidromic impulses in the motor axons with those descending in response to activation of the spinal afferents. Not surprisingly, loss of the H response in gastrocnemius is correlated with loss of the ankle reflex.

Electromyography (EMG)

In diabetes, sampling the spontaneous and volitional activity in muscles is mainly of value in detecting the presence of denervation and in distinguishing it from myopathy. This may arise in patients with proximal lower limb weakness when a distinction between diabetic amyotrophy and polymyositis can sometimes be difficult on clinical grounds. A concentric needle electrode is usually employed. With the muscle relaxed, a search is made for spontaneous activity with the needle at a number of different sites. Fibrillation potentials consist of brief (1–2 ms) low amplitude (50–200 μV) potentials that discharge at a completely regular rate. They indicate denervation but are also seen in polymyositis and other myopathic disorders where there is segmental necrosis of fibres so that portions of individual muscle fibres become isolated from their innervation. 'Positive sharp waves' have the same significance, as does increased fibrillary insertion activity seen on needle movement. This may take the form of high frequency pseudomyotonic discharges. Spontaneous motor unit activity (fasciculation potentials) is most often encountered in anterior horn cell disease but may occur in peripheral neuropathies both of demyelinating type and in axonopathies. It is occasionally seen in diabetic neuropathy.

On slight volitional contraction, the amplitude, duration and morphology of the motor unit potentials are examined. Their size varies between muscles but in most limb muscles they have an amplitude of 0.5–2 mV, sometimes reaching 4 mV, and a duration of 5–10 ms. They are usually triphasic with a small proportion of polyphasic potentials. With denervation, motor unit recruitment is reduced so that the normal interference pattern on maximal volition, in which the potentials from the motor units in the neighbourhood of the needle electrode run into each other, is reduced, sometimes to a discrete pattern in which individual motor unit potentials are seen firing in isolation. With chronic partial denervation, collateral reinnervation of denervated muscle fibres may occur. The resulting expanded motor units have potentials of increased amplitude and duration and they may be polyphasic. In myopathies, individual motor unit potentials are of lower amplitude, are brief and are frequently polyphasic. On maximal volition the recruitment pattern is preserved unless the disease is very severe.

Apart from confirming denervation in distal limb muscles, as already stated, needle electrode EMG studies are particularly valuable for distinguishing between diabetic amyotrophy and conditions such as polymyositis in patients with proximal lower limb weakness. In diabetic truncal neuropathy, EMG sampling of abdominal and paraspinal muscles may be useful.

Sensory conduction

In the upper limbs, conduction in sensory fibres can be examined by stimulating the digital nerves of the thumb, index or middle finger and recording over the median nerve at the wrist, or stimulating the fifth finger and recording over the ulnar nerve. Surface recording electrodes are usually employed and the digital nerves are stimulated through ring electrodes. The potential obtained is triphasic, a small positive wave being followed by a larger negative component and then a smaller positive wave (Fig. 3). The latency of the response is measured to the onset of the negative deflection. A low amplitude potential, usually about half that obtained at the wrist, can be recorded over the median and ulnar nerves at the elbow. Conduction velocity in the fastest conducting sensory fibres can be calculated between the fingers and wrist and between the wrist and elbow. Normal values are given by Kimura [6]. Conduction velocities are similar to those for the fastest conducting motor fibres to the small hand muscles. Some laboratories prefer to record from the digital nerves and to stimulate the median and ulnar nerves at the wrist. A larger potential is obtained. Sensory conduction can be examined in the radial nerve by recording over the course of the nerve at midforearm level and stimulating at the base of the thumb.

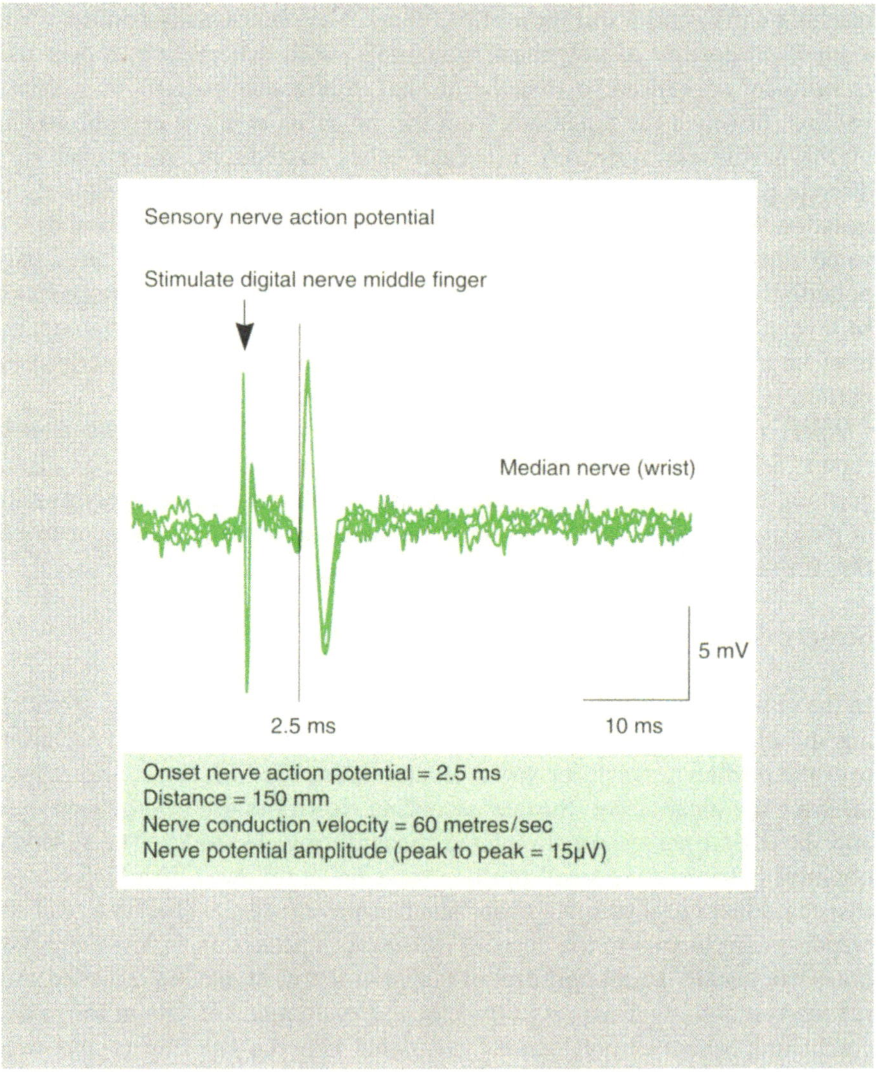

Fig. 3 Median sensory nerve action potential with stimulation of the digital nerves of the middle finger and recording with surface electrodes at the wrist; 5 traces have been superimposed. Figure kindly provided by Dr Philip Thompson

In the lower limbs, the nerve most commonly examined is the sural, either orthodromically, recording over the nerve in the calf and stimulating at the ankle or antidromically, with recording at the ankle and stimulating in the calf. A potential of larger amplitude can be obtained by near-nerve needle recording. A superficial peroneal sensory nerve action potential is obtained by stimulating over the nerve in the lower leg and recording from the common peroneal nerve at the neck of the fibula. It is sometimes useful to record a saphenous sensory action potential. The medial plantar sensory action potential represents a very sensitive measure of a distal sensory polyneuropathy. The hallux is stimulated with ring electrodes and a recording made from the tibial nerve posteroinferior to the medial malleolus, usually with needle electrodes. Lower limb sensory action potentials may be of reduced amplitude or undetectable in subjects over the age of 65–70 years. This applies particularly to the medial plantar sensory action potential.

Sensory conduction can be examined in the trigeminal nerve (together with facial nerve motor fibres) by means of the blink reflex. This has been studied in diabetic neuropathy by Kimura [16].

Somatosensory evoked potentials (SEPs)

On electrical stimulation of peripheral nerve, evoked potentials can be recorded over the spinal cord or from the scalp. Commonly employed sites for stimulation are the median and ulnar nerves at the wrist, the peroneal nerve at the neck of the fibula and the tibial nerve at the ankle. A stimulus strength sufficient to cause a small muscle twitch is adequate to activate the larger myelinated fibres that result in the SEP. The potentials are of small amplitude and averaging of a large number of responses is necessary. Details of the techniques involved are given in Kimura [6] and other texts. Abnormalities of spinal SEPs in diabetic neuropathy suggesting altered spinal cord conduction have been obtained in some studies [17, 18]. Cortical evoked potentials with a long latency can be obtained on CO_2 laser stimulation of the skin [19]. They are the consequence of stimulation of small fibres. Their potential usefulness for examining patients with diabetic "small fibre neuropathy" is limited by problems in recording these potentials in older subjects (A. M. Purves, personal communication).

Autonomic function

Autonomic function is not readily assessed by neurophysiological procedures (if electrocardiography is excluded). The sympathetic skin response, the slow potential change related to changes in skin conductance following a stimulus that evokes a response in sympathetic fibres, has been examined in diabetic neuropathy [20] but has not been adequately standardized. Recordings from sympathetic fibres with intraneural microelectrodes are possible [21] and have been employed in patients with diabetic neuropathy [22]. This is an exacting procedure but may be applicable for some research studies. For the examination of diabetic patients with impotence, spinal and cortical pudendal evoked potentials, the bulbocavernous reflex and nerve conduction velocity in the dorsal nerve of the penis have been studies [23–26] but these tests examine conduction in somatic fibres.

Research applications

Identification, characterization and staging of neuropathy

In epidemiological surveys or in the selection of patients for trials it is necessary to identify the presence of neuropathy and to characterize its nature and severity. On the one hand, patients may experience sensory symptoms that suggest neuropathy but which are due to other causes and, on the other, subclinical neuropathy, detectable electrophysiologically, may be present in the absence of symptoms or abnormalities on clinical examination. The presence of neuropathy can be established electrophysiologically, although normal findings do not necessarily exclude mild abnormality of peripheral nerve function. The range of normal variation is high and significant deterioration may occur without the results for nerve conduction transgressing the limits of normality.

The highly diverse manifestations of diabetic neuropathy are reflected in correspondingly varied electrophysiological changes. A discussion of these is beyond the scope of the present survey. Recent comprehensive descriptions of these have been provided by Daube [27] and Wilbourn [28].

The commonest form of diabetic neuropathy is the distal symmetric sensory polyneuropathy and it is on this form that most treatment trials are conducted. For the electrophysiological assessment of such patients it is important to identify and exclude superimposed focal peripheral nerve lesions such as the carpal tunnel syndrome or ulnar nerve lesions at the elbow which would otherwise complicate the evaluation. For the distal symmetric polyneuropathy, Dyck [29, 30] has proposed minimal criteria for diagnosis and a series of criteria for the staging of neuropathy based on (1) nerve conduction studies, (2) neurological examination, (3) quantitative motor, sensory and autonomic testing and (4) neuropathic symptoms. Neuropathy was divided into 4 stages, stage 0 being no neuropathy, stage 1 asymptomatic neuropathy, stage 2 symptomatic neuropathy and stage 3 disabling neuropathy. Dyck et al [30] compared scored symptoms, neurological deficit, quantitative sensory testing and nerve conduction studies with an Index of Pathology obtained from the findings on sural nerve biopsy. They showed that symptoms, neurological deficits and abnormalities of nerve conduction were statistically associated but were not precisely correlated with the Index of Pathology. Abnormalities of nerve conduction were found to be both sensitive and reliable for detection of neuropathy. Median and peroneal motor conduction velocity, distal latency and CMAP amplitude and median and sural SAP velocity and amplitude were assessed. Peroneal motor velocity was found to be the variable that was most frequently abnormal, followed closely by sural SAP amplitude, peroneal F wave latency and median SAP amplitude. A consensus group of the American Diabetic Association [31] recommended that, for research purposes, symptoms, neurological deficits, nerve conduction studies, quantitative sensory examination and quantitative autonomic examination should be used, but such an evaluation is highly time consuming.

Monitoring therapy

For treatment studies in which observations have to be repeated throughout the duration of trials that may extend over periods of 2 or more years, it is important that the maximum information is obtained from observations that are not too exacting either for the subject or the investigator. As diabetic polyneuropathy is a distal length-related disorder, the changes will be maximal in the lower limbs. On the other hand, the changes there may be too severe, such that they are not helpful for assessing treatment response. Sural SAPs may be absent and the small foot muscles may be completely denervated. Therefore observations both on the lower and upper limbs are desirable. MNCV has the lowest coefficient of variation amongst the electrophysiological variables that are available for assessment and the same is true when it is compared with clinical assessments. It has therefore been widely applied in treatment trials. The study by Dyck [29] showed that it is statistically correlated with the severity of pathology in the normal nerve. On the other hand, it is likely that changes in MNCV within the range of a few metres per second may reflect metabolic effects on peripheral nerve and not structural repair or deterioration. More important indices of neuropathy are SAP and CMAP amplitude as they will reflect the number of conducting nerve fibres. Both of these measures, however, as already stated, have a high coefficient of variation and are correspondingly less discriminating. Although in terms of assessing the severity of neuropathy they are of paramount importance, it is thus justifiable to use MNCV as a surrogate measure in view of its correlation with clinical variables providing the limitations of this approach are appreciated. It should not replace clinical evaluation. With these considerations in mind, it is therefore advisable to study both motor and sensory conduction in the lower and upper limbs. Motor conduction can be assessed in the median or ulnar nerves in the upper limb and peroneal or tibial in the lower limb. For the lower limb the peroneal nerve is easier to examine but has the disadvantage that it is more liable to be exposed to compression injury at the neck of the fibula. For sensory conduction, the sural nerve is most often employed in the lower limb and the median in the upper. In view of the frequency of occurrence of the carpal tunnel syndrome in diabetic subjects, the radial SAP might be more suitable although recording is slightly more difficult.

When using nerve conduction to assess the degree of improvement in clinical trials, Dyck and O'Brien [32] suggested that a mean change of 2 points on the neurological disability scale would be clinically meaningful. They found that this would correspond to a mean change of 2.2 $m.s^{-1}$ for motor conduction velocity in the peroneal nerve and 2.9 $m.s^{-1}$ for the median, ulnar and peroneal nerves combined. The corresponding changes in CMAP amplitude were 1.2 and 0.7 mV, respectively. Smaller changes were found if patients with IDDM were assessed alone. These results were based on cross-sectional data. It is likely that for longitudinal data, smaller changes would be meaningful.

References

[1] Thomas PK, Tomlinson DR. Diabetic and hypoglycemic neuropathy. In: Dyck PJ, Thomas PK, Griffin JW et al, eds. Peripheral Neuropathy, 3rd edn. Philadelphia: W. B. Saunders, 1993; 1219–1250.

[2] Archer AG, Watkins PJ, Thomas PK et al. The natural history of acute painful neuropathy in diabetes mellitus. J Neurol Neurosurg Psychiatry 1983; 46: 491–499.

[3] Llewelyn JG, Thomas PK, Fonseca V et al. Acute painful diabetic neuropathy precipitated by strict glycaemic control. Acta Neuropathol. (Berl) 1986; 72: 157–163.

[4] Cornblath DR, Drachman DB, Griffin JW. Demyelinating motor neuropathy in patients with diabetic polyneuropathy. Ann Neurol 1987; 22: 126.

[5] Brown WF. The Physiological and Technical Basis of Electromyography. Stoneham, MA: Butterworths, 1984.

[6] Kimura J. Electrodiagnosis in Diseases of Nerve and Muscle. Principles and Practice, 2nd edn. Philadelphia: F. A. Davis, 1989.

[7] Brown WF, Bolton CF. Clinical Electromyography, 2nd edn. Boston: Butterworth–Heinemann, 1993.

[8] Dorfman LJ, Cummins KL. Nerve-fiber conduction velocity distributions in normal and diabetic human nerves. Neurology 1980; 30: 415.

[9] Lang HA, Puusa A, Hynninen P et al. Evolution of nerve conduction velocity in later childhood and adolescence. Muscle Nerve 1985; 8: 38–43.
[10] Tackmann W, Lehmann HJ. Conduction of electrically elicited impulses in peripheral nerves of diabetic patients. Eur Neurol 1980; 19: 20–31.
[11] Schutt P, Muche H, Lehmann HJ. Refractory period impairment in sural nerve of diabetics. J Neurol 1983; 229: 113–120.
[12] Gassel MM. A study of femoral nerve conduction time. Arch Neurol 1963; 9: 607–614.
[13] Johnson EW, Waylonis GW. Facial nerve conduction delay in patients with diabetes mellitus. Arch Phys Med 1964; 45: 131–142.
[14] Hansen S, Ballantyne JP. Axonal dysfunction in the neuropathy of diabetes mellitus: a quantitative electrophysiological study. J Neurol Neurosurg Psychiatry 1977; 40: 555–563.
[15] Brown WF, Feasby T. Estimation of motor axon loss in diabetics. J Neurol Sci 1974; 23: 275–281.
[16] Kimura J. An evaluation of the facial and trigeminal nerves in polyneuropathy: electrodiagnostic study in Charcot-Marie-Tooth disease, Guillain-Barré syndrome, and diabetic neuropathy. Neurology 1971; 21: 745–752.
[17] Gupta PR, Dorfman LJ. Spinal somatosensory conduction in diabetes. Neurology 1981; 31: 841–850.
[18] Cracco J, Castells S, Mark C. Spinal somatosensory evoked potentials in juvenile diabetics. Ann Neurol 1984; 15: 55–63.
[19] Kakigi R, Shibasaki H, Ikeda A. Pain-related somatosensory evoked potentials following CO_2 laser stimulation in man. EEG Clin Neurophysiol 1989; 74: 139–146.
[20] Knezevic WV, Bajada S. Peripheral autonomic surface potential. A quantitative technique for recording sympathetic conduction in man. J Neurol Sci 1985; 67: 239–251.
[21] Fagius J, Wallin BG. Sympathetic reflex latencies and conduction velocity in normal man. J Neurol Sci 1980; 47: 433–444.
[22] Fagius J, Wallin BG. Sympathetic reflex latencies and conduction velocities in patients with polyneuropathies. J Neurol Sci 1980; 47: 499–507.
[23] Haldeman S, Bradley WE, Bhatia NN et al. Neurogenic evaluation of bladder, bowel and sexual disturbance in diabetic men. In: Goto Y, Horiuchi A, Kogure E, eds. Diabetic Neuropathy. Amsterdam: Excerpta Medica, 1982; 298–301.
[24] Haldeman S, Bradley WE, Bhatia NN. Pudendal evoked responses. Arch Neurol 1982; 92: 280–283.
[25] Bradley WE, Lin JT. Assessment of diabetic sexual dysfunction and cystopathy. In: Dyck PJ, Thomas PK, Asbury AK et al, eds. Diabetic Neuropathy. Philadelphia: W. B. Saunders, 1987; 146–154.
[26] Ertekin C, Reel F. Bulbocavernosus reflex in normal men and in patients with neurogenic bladder and/or impotence. J Neurol Sci 1987; 28: 1–15.
[27] Daube JR. Electrophysiologic testing in diabetic neuropathy. In: Dyck PJ, Thomas PK, Asbury AK et al, eds. Diabetic Neuropathy. Philadelphia: W. B. Saunders, 1987; 162–176.
[28] Wilbourn AJ. Diabetic neuropathies. In: Brown WF, Bolton CF, eds. Clinical Electromyography, 2nd edn. Boston: Butterworth–Heinemann, 1993; 477–515.
[29] Dyck PJ. Detection, characterization and staging of polyneuropathy: assessed in diabetics. Muscle Nerve 1988; 11: 21–32.
[30] Dyck PJ, Karnes JL, Daube J et al. Clinical and neuropathological criteria for the diagnosis and staging of diabetic polyneuropathy. Brain 1985; 108: 861–880.
[31] American Diabetes Association Consensus Statement. Diabetes Care 1988; 11: 592.
[32] Dyck PJ, O'Brien PC. Meaningful degrees of prevention or improvement of nerve conduction in controlled clinical trials of diabetic neuropathy. Diabetes Care 1989; 12: 649–652.

Clinical assessment of neuropathy, vascular disease and the leg in diabetes

T. S. Purewal, M. E. Edmonds, P. J. Watkins

The leg in diabetes can be affected by neuropathies and circulatory changes with or without additional problems from trauma and infection, causing potentially serious foot problems. The clinical abnormalities affecting the lower limb are thus diverse, ranging from permanent abnormalities and symptoms in the feet, to the crippling but reversible disorders due to mononeuropathy (proximal motor neuropathy), causing a painful wasting disease of the thigh. A summary of potential disorders affecting the leg is shown in Table 1.

Before considering technical methods of assessment of neuropathies, it is necessary to present a brief description of these conditions, so that relevant diagnostic techniques can be applied.

Table 1 Potential disorders of the diabetic leg

	Neuropathy	Ischaemia
Symptoms	None Paraesthesiae Pain Oedema Painful wasted thigh Foot drop	None Claudication Rest pain
Structural Damage	Ulcer Sepsis Abscess Osteomyelitis Digital gangrene	Ulcer Sepsis Gangrene
	Charcot joints	

The diabetic neuropathies

Peripheral nerves are prone to several different types of damage in diabetes, and there are thus highly distinctive syndromes which include: the common symmetrical sensory neuropathy associated with autonomic neuropathy which slowly progresses; and acutely painful neuropathies and mononeuropathies which have a relatively acute presentation and normally recover [1]. Pressure palsies (especially carpal tunnel syndrome, ulnar nerve compression, and those causing foot drop) are commoner but not distinctive in diabetes and are not considered further here. A classification of diabetic neuropathies are summarised in Table 2.

Table 2 Classification of diabetic neuropathies

I Progressive:	Symmetrical sensory polyneuropathy and autonomic neuropathy.
II Reversible:	Acute painful neuropathies, radiculopathies and mononeuropathies (including proximal motor neuropathy/femoral neuropathy/diabetic amyotrophy).
III Pressure palsies:	Carpal tunnel syndrome Ulnar nerve compression Foot drops

Symmetrical sensory and autonomic neuropathy

This is a very common condition affecting 11 to 50% of diabetic patients, depending on the criteria used or the population selected. Neuropathy is always diffuse and symmetrical (stocking distribution) probably starting with involvement of the smallest fibres (pain, temperature, autonomic) and sometimes but not always progressing to involve all nerve fibre types. Yet definition and characterization of diabetic neuropathy present considerable problems. Dyck [2] has described many of the pitfalls, and both he and the San Antonio Conference (1988) [3] made complex recommendations difficult to apply in routine clinical practice. Thomas [4] suggested that diabetic neuropathy "behaves as a systems degeneration in which particular sets of neurons are primarily affected because of differential vulnerability", and emphasized the importance of distinguishing diabetic neuropathy from neuropathies of various causes co-existing with diabetes.

Lawrence believed that "small non-medullated nerve fibres" were the first to be affected and that this gave rise to some of the characteristic features of diabetic neuropathy. This small fibre degeneration leads or loss of pain and temperature sensory modalities, with associated autonomic features, and in these early stages, other sensory modalities can remain intact, notably light touch sensation [5]. Early neuropathy is frequently not detected in the clinic because temperature and pain sensation are difficult to assess. Sympathetic failure causes loss of sweating and denervation of peripheral vessels, leading to vascular rigidity and calcification, with a very high peripheral blood flow, chiefly from opening of arteriovenous anastomoses. These blood flow changes can occur quite early in the course of diabetes, but need sophisticated techniques for their detection.

Small fibre neuropathies sometimes progress as a selective entity in some patients leading to symptomatic autonomic neuropathy (causing diarrhoea, gastroparesis, orthostatic hypotension, impotence, neurogenic bladder, gustatory sweating and other problems), often associated with Charcot joints. These patients sometimes develop iritis as well, and there is some evidence that immune mechanisms may be involved. On the other hand, in some patients, neuropathy progresses to involve all nerve fibre types and in the worst cases the feet and lower legs become anaesthetic. Major motor involvement is surprisingly uncommon even in the severest cases.

Neuropathy also causes abnormalities of vascular response to heat and trauma, and altered flare responses, as decribed below.

The evolution of sensory and autonomic diabetic neuropathy is extremely slow and very variable, occurring over many years, with the increasing age of the patient and duration of diabetes. It never remits. Study is further complicated by differential rate of progression of different fibre types and there are only a few observations over periods of 5–10 years.

Neuropathies which recover mononeuropathies, radiculopathies and acute painful neuropathies [1]

Painful neuropathies in diabetes have highly characteristic features which include constant 'burning', paraesthesiae and shooting pains, together with exquisite contact discomfort caused by clothes and bedclothes [6–9]. The pains are continuous day and night and cause severe insomnia. They are accompanied by profound weight loss. They occur either in a symmetrical sensory stocking distribution affecting both feet; they may be confined to a single or adjacent group of nerve roots affecting feet and/or legs; or they may be confined to one or both thighs, often but not always accompanied by wasting, and sometimes debilitating weakness, causing falls. The latter syndrome is known as proximal motor neuropathy, femoral neuropathy or diabetic amyotrophy and is due either to radiculopathy or femoral neuropathy [8, 9]. All of these conditions normally recover in 6 to 18 months.

Neurological examination of the feet in cases of symmetrical painful neuropathy can confuse the physician since abnormalities range from severe sensory neuropathy with major deficits in all modalities (the "painless painful foot"), to an almost complete lack of neurological abnormalities, including almost normal EMG findings. This makes assessment and diagnosis of this condition very complex. EMG findings in proximal motor neuropathy show clear evidence of damage, normally in the distribution of L2, 3, 4 nerve roots, and these changes are not discussed further in this chapter.

Diagnostic techniques

Conclusions: The disease nature of diabetic neuropathies with their very slow and yet variable progression over many years and the frequent dissociation of symptoms and signs altogether make measurement for both diagnosis and assessment of change extremely difficult. At the very least, several different modalities of sensation need to be assessed, motor nerve conduction used as a reliable 'gold standard', and some attempt made to assess effects of neuropathy on circulatory changes. When new treatments are to be evaluated, sufficient time must elapse for meaningful results to be obtained, and two years is probably the minimum period for worthwhile results.

The purposes for which diagnostic techniques are required must be clearly defined. They can be summarized as follows:

1. Detection of abnormalities causing foot disorders to establish a diagnosis and institute preventive measures.
1.1. Observation of foot deformities
1.2. Detection of peripheral vascular disease
1.3. Detection of sensory loss due to neuropathy
2. Assessment of neuropathy to study the natural history of the disease and evaluate new treatments.

These two chief aims require different approaches. In particular, the techniques needed to observe progression of the disease and assess the effects of new treatments, need to be much more sophisticated and precise.

Detection of abnormalities causing foot disorders

Techniques are needed to establish the presence of neuropathy and/or vascular disease both for diagnostic purposes and to institute preventive measures.

Observations of foot abnormalities: Clinical examination of the foot is simple, cheap and highly effective in preventing the development of problems, providing that the correct measures are taken and accompanied by clear advice. Points to look for are:

1. Foot deformities e.g. clawed toes, high arched foot, bunions, hammer toes, overlapping toes, hallux rigidus; or major bone deformities of the Charcot foot with rocker sole.
2. Callus formation at any site, especially over bony prominences or in between the toes.
3. Sites of cracked skin or any other blisters, abrasions or ulcers which might act as a portal for entry of infection.
4. Evidence of fungal infection which can predispose to entry of bacterial infection.
5. Nail abnormalities.
6. Skin colour – see under ischaemia below.

All of the above are crucial in assessing the lower limb, and their presence or absence will, in part, determine which investigations will be needed.

Detection of peripheral vascular disease (PVD): Examination of skin colour and integrity provide information regarding the presence of peripheral vascular disease. Pulses must be palpated, and if dorsalis pedis and posterior tibial pulses are absent, then popliteal and femoral pulses should also be palpated and femoral bruits detected. Where PVD is suspected, assessment is aided by simple Doppler measurements which can be performed at the bedside. The technique is described below.

Severe ischaemia may cause a painful foot syndrome, with continuous and especially severe nocturnal pain associated with pink discolouration of the foot, which worsens to a deep purplish discolouration on dependence. Gangrene may *follow.* These are features of critical ischaemia which always requires urgent attention, and where possible, intervention.

Critical ischaemia is defined by the following two criteria: Persistently recurring ischaemic rest pain requiring regular adequate analgesia for ≥ 2 weeks, with an ankle systolic pressure ≤ 50 mmHg and or a toe systolic pressure of ≤ 30 mmHg or ulceration or gangrene of the foot or toes, with an ankle systolic pressure of ≤ 50 mmHg or a toe systolic pressure of ≤ 30 mmHg [10].

Techniques used in assessment of PVD are described below.

Detection of sensory loss due to neuropathy: Clinical diagnosis of neuropathy in diabetes is normally performed by routine clinical neurological examination; a sensory level in a stocking distribution is readily established using a finger, or with cotton wool. Neuropathy is unlikely if ankle reflexes are intact. If more precision is required, an EMG is performed as well. Sophisticated sensory measurements are not generally required, although quantitative measurement of vibration perception (VPT) threshold is useful and simple: it demonstrates the presence of neuropathy to patient and physician, and can be used both to encourage the patient to take proper preventive measures, and for the physician to follow the progression of the disease. Foot ulcers are unlikely to occur unless the VPT exceeds 25 volts (biothesiometer) or a score of 4 using the graduated tuning fork.

Techniques for measuring vibration perception thresholds are described below. The calibrated tuning fork is recommended as a simple, cheap and relatively reliable technique, while electrically operated systems (biothesiometer, vibrameter) are also of value.

Assessment of neuropathy to study the natural history of the disease and evaluate new treatments

The requirements for assessing neuropathy need to take account of (1.) the need for precision, and (2.) the differential vulnerability of nerve fibre types, which makes it essential to study several different sensory modalities. The gold standard and most reproducible observations are based on EMG examination, but since the neuropathy is predominantly sensory, a variety of techniques are needed.

The following presentation examines critically, both clinical and mechanical techniques used to establish and quantify the presence of diabetic neuropathy. They should all be accompanied by a full clinical neurological examination.

Clinical methods

San Antonio Consensus Statement (1988) [3] on the diagnosis of diabetic neuropathy concluded that "at least one parameter from five categories be measured to classify DN: symptom profiles, neurological examination, quantitative sensory testing, nerve conduction studies, and autonomic function testing". The recommendations are complex, time consuming and not always clinically relevant. They have not been widely accepted or applied.

Scoring systems

Dyck and colleagues have developed three scoring systems to aid in the diagnosis and assessment of severity of neuropathy [11–13]. The neurological symptom score (NSS) assesses symptoms of muscle weakness, sensory disturbances and autonomic symptoms. One point is scored if a symptom is present in each of 17 categories. The neurological disability score (NDS) is produced from clinical examination of cranial nerves, muscle strength, reflexes and sensation. Scoring is from 0 for no deficit, 1 for mild deficit, 2 for moderate deficit, 3 for severe deficit, and 4 for complete absence of function or severest deficit. In each scoring system the total score is proportional to the severity of neuropathy. In pilot studies using quantitative sural nerve morphometry as the indicator of presence of neuropathy, Dyck et al. found that NDS was a good indicator of the presence of neuropathy, as were sensory and motor nerve conduction velocities, and vibration sense. NSS in comparison was a poor test [11]. These findings were further substantiated by the 5 year Rochester Diabetic Neuropathy study [14].

More recently the same group has developed a true/false questionnaire called the neuropathy symptom profile (NSP) [13]. In the pilot study of 72 patients with known diabetic neuropathy, 46 had total scores above the 97.5 percentile and 31 had levels above this for sensory symptoms. However, of 34 subjects without clinical neuropathy, 5 had total scores above the 97.5 percentile and 2 sensory scores above this level.

Quantitative neurological tests

Quantitative neurological testing presents numerous problems on account of the obvious subjective nature of sensory tests; the decline of sensory function with age; and the variability of the results when different sites are used. There is not usually a sex difference, although induction of sweating shows it to be more profuse in men than in women [15]. The lower limbs are always more severely affected than the upper limbs. Selection of appropriate tests needs

Table 3 Methods of assessment of different sizes of nerve fibres

Nerve fibre size	Sensory functions and sensory function tests in order of clinical usefulness and availability
Aα	Light touch sensation (Semmes Weinstein monofilaments)
Aβ	Vibration perception threshold
Aδ	Cold sensory threshold
C	Warm sensory thresholds
C	Sweat tests (sympathetic)
C	Flare responses (histamine-axon reflex)
C	Galvanic skin resistance
C	Pain threshold assessment
Various	Electric current (sine wave) Stimulator (large and small fibres)

to take account of speed and cost, especially when serial investigations have to be performed. Many quantitative tests are available and are summarized in Table 3 in relation to nerve fibre size.

Sensory tests

General description

Somatic sensation is not a uniform sensory experience, but has several qualities. Each sensory episode has a quality or modality (e. g. heat or cold) and intensity. Modality is carried on different nerve fibres (e. g. vibration on large myelinated, and thermal on small myelinated and unmyelinated fibres), whilst intensity is pattern coded and depends on the patterns of firing of sensory receptors [16]. The localization of the stimulus is dependent on the density of cutaneous receptors, and the segmental organisation of sensory input into the posterior roots of the spinal cord and of the sensory cortex. Most sensations evoke affective responses e. g. warm is pleasant and hot is painful. Lesions interrupting connections between the prefrontal cortex and subcortical centres result in the patient sensing pain, but it no longer disturbs him. This is important to appreciate because although in diabetes we are concerned with peripheral neuropathy, the measurement of neuropathy is a psychophysical test. All tests should be performed with a fully alert and informed patient to achieve optimal results. Variation in thresholds is mainly due to psychological reasons and can be as high as 90 to 256% on a single test, but reduces to 8–18% if the average of several readings is taken [17].

The ideal system for measurement should be quick, simple, reliable and reproducible. However, the minute stimuli required and the psychophysical nature of testing make it difficult to use simple apparatus. Some research workers in the field of sensory testing feel that hand held and commercially available instruments are not adequate [2]. They have developed Computer Assisted Sensory Examination. This is a purpose built laboratory, devoted to sensory testing. It assesses touch-pressure, vibration and thermal sensory modalities, using forced choice testing. These methods are probably the best available, but because of both cost and time taken to perform them, they are unlikely to become routine clinical tools of measurement.

Using this system, Dyck concluded that sensory thresholds in diabetic patients are most commonly elevated in the feet followed by the hand, and least affected in the face; and that vibration sensation was more commonly abnormal than touch-pressure; and touch pressure than cooling thresholds; and that sensory testing was less sensitive than demonstration of nerve conduction abnormalities [2].

Diabetic neuropathy and sweating defects [15, 18–21]

Diminished or absent sweating in the feet and legs commonly occurs in patients with diabetic neuropathy as a manifestation of peripheral sympathetic denervation. Indeed, anhidrosis of the feet may be responsible for cracking of the skin, resulting in a portal of entry for infections. The sweating loss normally occurs in a stocking distribution, which can extend into the trunk and above which there may be excessive sweating. Patchy sweating loss sometimes occurs.

Sweating defects assessed by Quantitative sudomotor axon reflex test (QSART) and silastic imprint methods show a relationship with abnormalities of autonomic function, assessed by heart rate variability and the Valsalva manoeuvre. Most patients with postural hypotension have absent foot sweating, indicative of their common cause, namely, sympathetic denervation; 75% of those with neuropathic foot ulcers and 36% with Charcot joints also show absence of sweating in their feet [16]. Loss of pain sensation is correlated with diminished sweating.

Sweating responses [19–21]

Acetylcholine mediated stimulation of sweating depends on an intact sympathetic nerve supply to the sweat glands; tests involving stimulation of sweating can therefore be used to test peripheral sympathetic function. None of the four available tests are simple to perform at the bedside, and all of them require special equipment.

The quantitative sudomotor axon reflex test (QSART) [21]

This test depends on the integrity of the axon reflex mediated by C fibres. Acetylcholine is used to stimulate an antidromic nerve impulse by binding to nicotinic receptors of the postganglionic sympathetic axon. The nerve impulse changes direction at a branch point and then travels to the sweat gland, which is stimulated by release of acetylcholine.

The apparatus to achieve this comprises three concentric rings: the outer ring is filled with acetylcholine, which is iontophoresed using a constant current generator; the middle ring merely establishes a gap between the outer ring and the centre ring, from which the sweat volume is recorded, by passing nitrogen gas over the area. Abnormal sweating patterns include those where sweating is reduced or absent or occasionally increased, and sometimes latencies are shortened.

Silastic imprint method [15]

Direct stimulation of sweat glands in this method is achieved by iontophoresis of pilocarpine which binds to the muscarinic receptor. A silastic impression material is spread over the relevant area, and when this hardens, each sweat droplet leaves an impression so that both its size can be measured, and total droplets (sweat glands) can be counted. Sweat glands stimulated directly in this way require intact sympathetic nerves and do not respond when denervated.

Thermoregulatory sweat test [15]

Stimulation of sweating in this test is achieved by total body warming, in which the oral temperature must rise to 38 °C or increase by 1.0 °C. Areas of sweating are identified by indicator powder mixture. The stimulus to sweating is mediated by pre-ganglionic centres and postganglionic pathways, including the sympathetic chain and postganglionic sudomotor nerves. Using this technique, it is possible to map the areas of defective sweating.

Bioelectric skin potentials (galvanic skin response) [15]

Sympathetic activation by stimuli, such as a loud noise or a cough causes the skin potential to change by activation of sweat glands. Latency rather than amplitude of the response is more constant, and gives some indication of conduction velocities of between 0.8 and 1.5 m/s (lower and upper limbs respectively). Recording electrodes are placed in pairs on the dorsal and vertical surfaces of foot, thigh or hand. Abnormalities are found in patients with diabetic neuropathy, and when it is severe, there is a correlation with the QSART test for sweating described above; but it is prone to great variability and not, in reality, a very valuable clinical test.

Flare response

Histamine, substance P and capsaicin can activate the afferent branch of the axon reflex (small (c) nerve fibres) and cause a flare response. This can be examined if these substances are administered by iontophoresis. The flare response is not normally diminished in diabetes per se, while in diabetic neuropathy patients it may or may not be reduced.

Skin biopsy [22, 23]

Epidermal and sweat gland nerves can be visualized on skin biopsy samples taken from the calf region: neuropeptide content of nerve endings is then identified by immunohistochemical staining and can be quantitated. In this way, the neuronal marker, protein gene product (PGP 9.5) and calcitonin gene related peptide (CGRP) are found to be reduced in diabetic patients and in those with neuropathy, although correlation with nerve function tests has not been demonstrated. Sweat gland PGP 9.5 and vasoactive intestinal polypeptide are not apparently reduced in diabetes. These observations are interesting but non-specific, and not helpful as diagnostic tests. Progression or remission of the disease could, in theory, be followed by performing serial biopsies, but this seems impracticable.

Forced choice (FC) and method of limits (MOL)

The method of limits is that most often used clinically: by this technique the stimulus intensity is increased progressively until it is felt by the patient, and repeated several times to find a stable minimal threshold. Forced choice testing uses timed periods when a stimulus is either applied or not. The periods are switched randomly, the subject is asked to say if a stimulus is applied during each period and answers yes, no, or don't know. The intensity of the stimulus is decreased until 50% responses are correct and this is called the threshold.

The method of limits is criticized by research workers but favoured by clinicians. It is much more rapid than forced choice testing but reputed to be less accurate. In a study on 87 subjects Claus et al used a Marstock stimulator to compare the two protocols [24]. The time taken to perform the tests was up to six times longer for FC than MOL (normal subjects MOL 6.2 ± 2.2 min vs FC 37.5 ± 9.3 min, and diabetic patients MOL 7.0 ± 3.0 vs FC 40.9 ± 13.7 min). The thresholds achieved were slightly higher for MOL than FC, but the differences were not statistically significant.

General principles of testing

To obtain optimal results perform the test with the patient fully alert and cooperative, and demonstrate the stimulus at a non-affected site at a supramaximal threshold after explaining the test to the patient.

The majority of devices are either totally hand held or the "probe" used to apply the stimulus is hand held. The advantages of this are that the devices are cheap, easy to use, and transportable. The disadvantages are that the impact is variable, and the wave form of deformation is variable and not defined [2].

Light touch

This modality is served by large myelinated Aα and Aβ fibres [25]. Examination with cotton wool is impossible to quantify and poorly reproducible. Original attempts at quantitating measurements were made with horsehairs of different thicknesses and lengths by von Frey. The modern counterparts are nylon monofilaments (e. g. Semmes Weinstein). These come in standardized thicknesses so that the pressure applied to buckle the shaft is known. The 10 g filament may distinguish those prone to foot ulceration [5]. The filaments have been compared to the biothesiometer in 182 subjects [26]. Filaments of 1 g, 10 g, and 75 g corresponded to VPT of 10.6 ± 6.7 (mean $\pm$ SD), 22.8 ± 12.7, and 32 ± 14.3 (p 0.001) at the great toe. The filaments were more specific (90.6%) but less sensitive (81%) at identifying patients with foot ulcers compared to the biothesiometer.

Using nylon filaments to examine light touch sensation we have been able to demonstrate remarkable preservation of this sensory modality in patients with Charcot joints and autonomic neuropathy who are otherwise devastated by loss of thermal and pain sensation (i. e. small fibre neuropathy with preservation of larger fibres) [5]. Observations of this type emphasize the importance of testing more than one sensory modality before excluding the presence of neuropathy.
(Semmes Weinstein filaments, Gillis W Long, Hansen's Disease Center, Hansen's Disease Foundation, Inc., Filament Project – Building 18, Carville, Louisiana, 70721, USA).

More recent methods that have failed to achieve widespread use include: jets of air as stimuli; mechanical forms for placing monofilaments; electric sparks; and the depth sense aesthiometer. The latter is an instrument where the pulp of the finger is run along a ridge which becomes higher from 0 to 1 mm until it is felt [2].

Vibration perception threshold (VPT)

This modality is also carried on large myelinated Aα and Aβ fibres [25]. Pacinian corpuscles have been shown to respond to stimuli in range 85–1000 Hz [27]. However this is not a physiological stimulus and a tuning fork applied to a bony prominence which reverberates may amplify the stimulus. The test however, yields clinically useful information.

This is the most commonly used quantitative test. Loss of vibration sense in the feet is a more sensitive indicator of neuropathy than loss of light touch [28]. Motor and sensory nerve compound action potentials and motor nerve conduction velocity remain the as gold standards for the presence of neuropathy. Compared to these VPT is less reproducible but correlates adequately with neuropathy. Symptom scores have the worst reproducibility and correlate least with the presence of neuropathy [14].

Tuning forks: VPT is clinically tested with tuning forks. A series of observations has shown that frequencies of 64, 128, 256, and 512 Hz have approximately similar thresholds [2]. The 128 Hz tuning fork is the one most commonly recommended to assess the presence of neuropathy. However, quantitation is not possible.

Graduated tuning fork: This was described at the beginning of the century but has not achieved widespread acceptance. The base of the vibrating fork is applied to either the tip of the great toe or the lateral malleolus. The prongs are weighted with calibrated adjustable cursors. When these are at the extremities of the prongs the fork vibrates at 64 Hz. The frequency can be increased by moving the cursors towards the base of the fork. The cursors

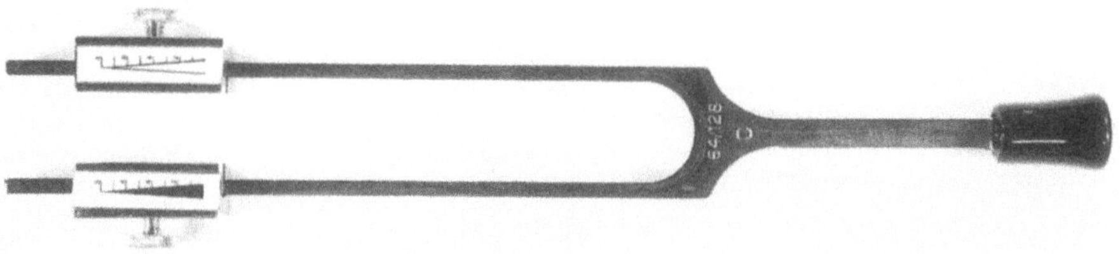

Fig. 1 Photograph of Reidell Seiffer Graduated Tuning Fork

are marked with a triangle graduated from 0 to 8 (Fig. 1). When the fork vibrates each triangle appears double. The number nearest to the apparent point of intersection of the long sides of the "two" vibrating triangles at the moment when the subject ceases to perceive the vibration constitutes the threshold [29, 30] (Fig. 2). It should be noted that different suppliers have the scale on the cursor running from 0−8 base to apex or 8−0 base to apex, in either case the closer vibrating intersection is to the base of the triangle when the subject loses the perception of vibration, the greater the degree of neuropathy.

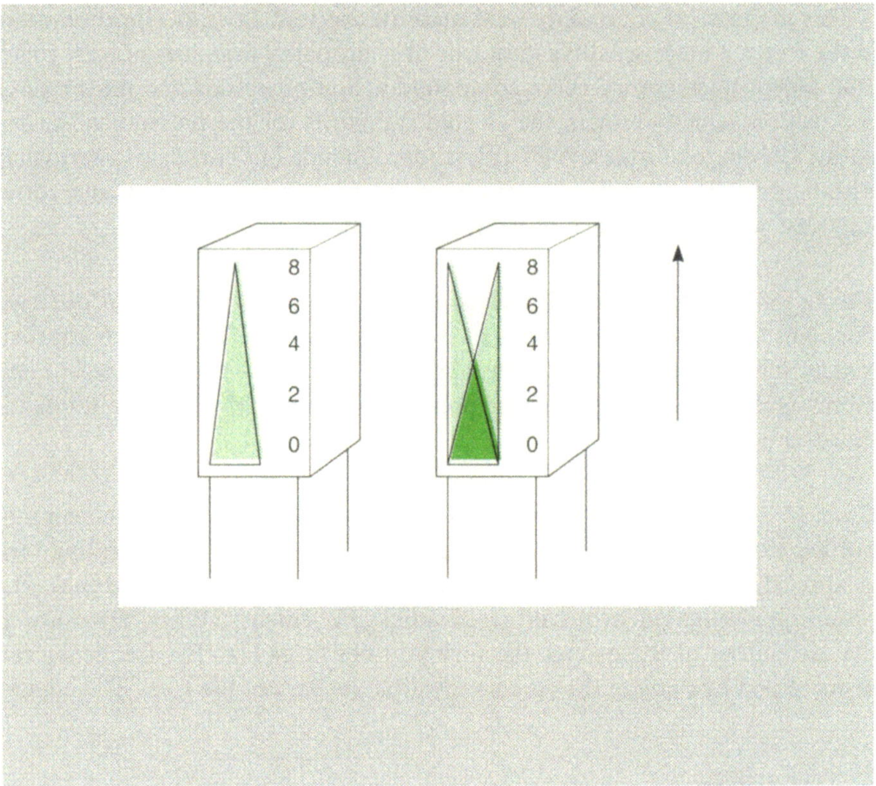

Fig. 2 The diagram on the left shows the triangle on the cursor of the Reidell Seiffer Fork. When the fork vibrates, the triangle appears double, as illustrated on the right. The intersection of the "two" triangles moves from 0 to 8. The point at which the vibration is no longer perceived is the threshold. (Hence abnormal thresholds are numerically lower than normal thresholds)

Recently, Liniger et al have produced normal ranges in 214 normal subjects aged 20–90 years [31]. They also compared it to the vibrameter (Somedic, Stockholm, Sweden). Intra-individual subject variation for two tests was 6%, and the median inter-examiner variation was also 6%. Normal values are given in Table 4. In diabetic patients intra-individual subject variation was 24%. These compare with figures for the vibrameter of 25% median intra-subject variation in normal and 48% in diabetic subjects. Vibration threshold assessed by the Reidell–Seiffer graduated tuning fork correlated well with that assessed by the vibrameter ($r - 0.90$, $p < 0.001$). A tuning fork threshold < 4.0 was found in 95% of ulcerated diabetic feet, suggesting that thresholds in this range are predictive of the risk of foot ulceration.

Table 4 Published normal ranges of vibration thresholds

Site	Threshold*	SD	Mean age	Reference
Biothesiometer				
Carpal	0.3 micrometres	0.02	35.2 ± 1.4 (SEM)	47
Malleolar	0.45	0.03		
Dorsum carpals	0.21 micrometres	0.02 micrometres	10–19 years	17
	0.65	0.09	60–74 years	
Dorsum tarsals	0.25	0.02	10–19 years	
	0.86	1.14	60–74 years	
Wrist	0.78 mic (9 volts)		Young	Biothesiometer
Hallux	0.78 mic (9 volts)		adults	handbook
Fingertips	0.37 mic (2 volts)			
	mean (volts)	range		
Index finger	3.9	2.4– 6.3	< 55 years	43
Hallux	5.6	3.1–10.3	< 55 years	
	97.5% centiles			
Thumb	9.6 volts		10 years	35
Hallux	14.7		50 years	
Medial malleoli	11.3		10 years	
	28		50 years	
	15		10 years	
	33.9		50 years	
Vibrameter	99% centile	SD		
Index finger	0.86 micrometres	0.19 micrometres	21–45 years	3
	mean	SEM		
Tarsal	0.35	0.07	20–29 years	37
	1.78	1.03	50–59 years	
Carpal	0.2	0.02	20–29 years	
	0.27	0.03	50–59 years	
Graduated tuning				
fork First metatarsal	8		20 years	31
	7.5		50 years	
	6.4		90 years	

* 99th percentile unless otherwise stated

The slight drawback of presenting results as arbitrary numbers rather than continuous readings of the biothesiometer and vibrameter is more than overcome by its clinical usefulness. It is quick, cheap and reasonably reproducible. (Reidell–Seiffer graduated tuning fork, Firma Martin, Tuttlingen, FRG).

Biothesiometer: The biothesiometer uses an electromagnet to activate a spring loaded stimulator. It reads from 0–50 volts but the vertical probe displacement for a given voltage is different for each instrument, hence each machine is calibrated separately before it leaves the factory and provided with a chart for conversion of volts to micrometres of probe movement. The instrument has the disadvantages of a hand held instrument; thus a decrease in vibration amplitude occurs with increasing pressure of application of the probe. The rate of increase of voltage is operator dependent, and the probe can move in more than one plane. A dummy switch is incorporated which allows an increase in voltage to be shown on the display, while the probe remains still to aid detection of non-compliant patients. The vibrator moves at twice the frequency of alternating current, which in the UK is 50 Hz, giving a stimulus frequency of 100 Hz.
The biothesiometer uses the method of limits to define the threshold.

1. Explain the procedure to the patient (warm quiet room).
2. Demonstrate the stimulus on the hand or sternum with an amplitude well above the threshold.
3. Use the weight of the machine to provide a standard pressure of application of the probe (hold lightly by handle only) over the medial malleolus or the tip of the great toe.
4. Increase the voltage at a uniform rate until the stimulus is perceived as definitely present by the patient.
5. Repeat three times discounting first reading and then use average result.
6. If desired convert voltage threshold into microns of displacement from chart.

Adipose tissue, fatigue, increasing age and poor concentration produce elevated thresholds. The odds ratio for foot ulceration occurring with a VPT over 25 has been calculated as 3.5, and this increases dramatically to 22.7 with a VPT of more than 42 [32].

The coefficient of variation varies according to the care with which the test is performed – a single operator is best. In 120 healthy subjects the variation was 30% at the medial malleolus and 21% at the hallux [33]. Normal results from different studies are given in Table 4 and age, sex, and site centile charts have been produced from a study of 1365 normal subjects [34] and 348 subjects [35].
(Biothesiometer, Biomedical Instrument Co., Newbury, Ohio).

Vibrameter: This instrument is similar to the biothesiometer in that a plastic probe vibrates at 100 Hz, and the instrument is hand held. However, the result is given directly in micrometres of probe displacement, and facility exists to calibrate the pressure exerted by the vibrating rod and visually check that it remains at this level during the test [36, 37]. Intra-individual variation for repeat tests was 25% [31].
(Vibrameter, Somedic, Stockholm, Sweden).

Thermal thresholds

Warm sensation receptors are innervated by unmyelinated C fibres, whilst cold sensation receptors are innervated by small myelinated Aδ fibres. Single fibre studies have shown that different receptors are responsible for perception of warm and cold stimuli and these receptors have a different cutaneous distribution [2].

The best clinical method of using metal tubes (glass is a poor conductor) filled with hot/cold water is unreliable and only severe loss of sensation is detected reproducibly. Thermal thresholds are important as small nerve fibres are thought to be involved first in diabetic neuropathy [38], and thermal thresholds can be abnormal when even nerve conduction studies which reflect mainly large myelinated fibre pathology are still normal [39]. Defects of peripheral thermal sensation may occur in isolation from vibration sensation in cases of small fibre neuropathy [40, 41].

Most studies show higher thresholds for warm than cold in normal subjects (Table 5) and this is also true for diabetic patients [42]. This difference is probably due to the warm receptors being innervated by unmyelinated C fibres, and cold receptors by Aδ fibres.

Several instruments for testing thermal thresholds are now available. They all use the Peltier principle by which metal elements are heated or cooled, depending on direction of flow of electric current. They take a minimum of 10 minutes per site tested and are relatively expensive. They use the forced choice method protocol in their design but can also perform tests much more rapidly by the method of limits protocol. Three commonly used machines include the Marstock (Somedic, Stockholm, Sweden), the Medelec (Medelec Ltd, Vickers Healthcare, Surrey, UK), and the Sensortek (TST, Sensortek Inc., Clifton, New Jersey) thermal threshold testers.

*Table 5 Published normal ranges of thermal thresholds (*99th percentile unless otherwise stated)*

Site	Hot *	SD	Cold *	SD	Mean age years ± SD	Method	Reference
Wrist	0.37°C	0.08°C	0.32°C	0.07°C	34 ± 13.5	Medelec	Medelec handbook
Foot	0.86°C	0.72°C	0.62°C	0.12°C	33.7 ± 10.9	Medelec	
Hand	0.24°C	0.05°C	0.3°C	0.06°C	25–34 years	Medelec	57
	0.41°C	0.08°C	0.37°C	0.08°C	55–64 years		
Foot	8.24°C	1.93°C	1.03°C	0.24°C	25–34 years		
	11.77°C	2.33°C	1.88°C	0.44°C	55–64 years		
Dorsum hand	0.15 to 0.30°C				< 70 years		58
Dorsum foot	0.15 to 0.50°C				< 70 years		
Volar wrist	0.4°C	0.06°C	0.27°C	0.05°C	33 ± 17	Medelec	44
Below medial malleolus	3.28°C	0.73°C	0.32°C	0.06°C			
Index finger	1.6°C	0.31°C			18–65 years	Sensortek	45
Hallux	2.84°C	0.61°C					
	Thermal difference 96% interval						
Thenar	4°C				18–39 years	Marstock	59
Lateral foot	3°C						
Face	2.5°C						
Thenar	2°C	0.1°C			35.2 ± 1.4 (SEM)	Marstock	47
Foot	3.9°C	0.1°C					
	Thermal difference						
Thenar	0.9°C	0.15°C			21–30 years	Marstock	17
	1.3°C	0.25°C			61–70 years		
Lateral foot	4.3°C	1.1°C			21–30 years		
	12°C	3.6°C			61–70 years		
	Thermal difference						
	mean	range					
Thenar	2.6°C	1.5–4.0°C			< 55 years	Marstock	43
Lateral foot	6°C	3.6–9.8°C			< 55 years		
Pain	mean	SEM	mean	SEM			
Thenar	44.5°C	0.4°C	14.7°C	0.5°C	35.2 ± 1.4 (SEM)	Marstock	47
Foot	44.2°C	0.3°C	14.7°C	0.7°C			

Marstock stimulator: This uses a plate of 25 by 50 mm which has its posterior surface buffered by water circulating at 30 °C. The temperature of the probe is measured by a thermocouple and can be displayed on a chart recorder [43]. The rate of change of temperature over the range 15–45 °C is 1 °C/second. The plate is placed on the site to be tested and heated or cooled. The subject is asked to press a switch as soon as the plate is felt to be either warm or cool. Once the switch is pressed the direction of the current alters and the switch is pressed again when the opposite sensation is felt (Fig. 3). This is continued for 5–6 cycles and the peak to peak difference taken as the ther-

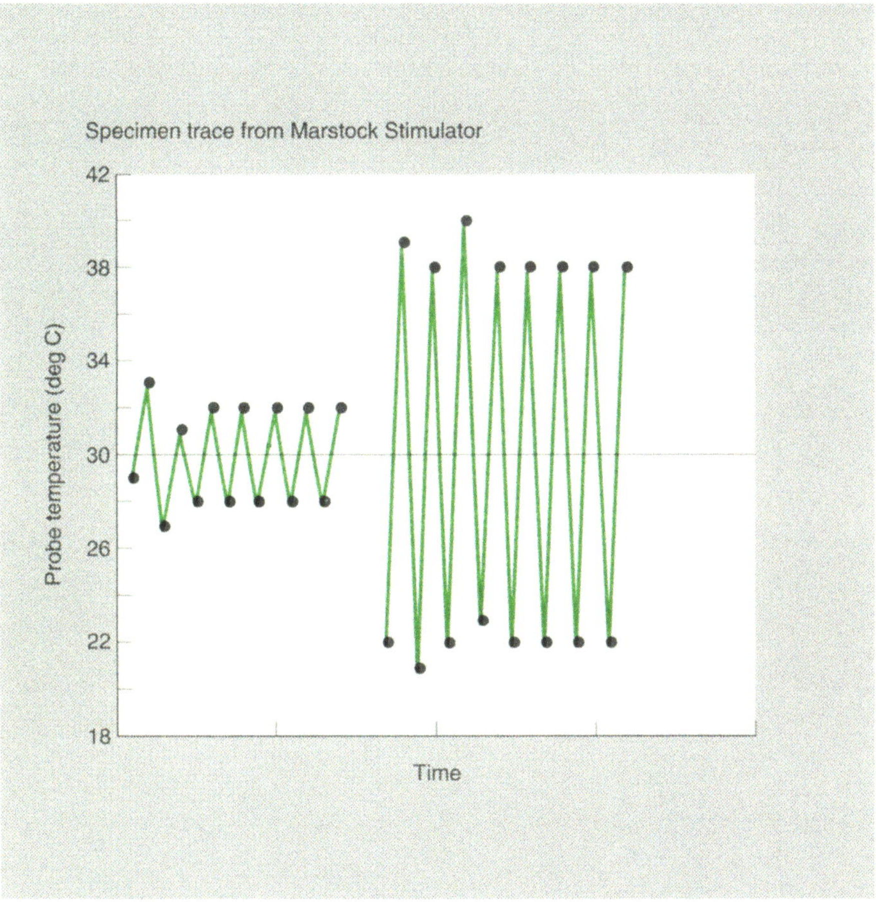

Fig. 3 Specimen trace from a Marstock Stimulator. The temperature sensation threshold of a control is shown on the left and for a diabetic neuropathic subject on right. As soon as warmth (above 37 °C) or cold (below 30 °C) is perceived, the subject presses a switch reversing the temperature. The thresholds shown are 4 °C in the control and 16 °C in the diabetic subject

mal difference. This method does not give an absolute threshold for hot or cold, but the information is valuable, rapidly obtained, and quantitatively establishes thermal sensory loss.

Medelec thermal tester: This is a microprocessor controlled unit. A 450 g 13.5 cm^2 thermode in contact with the skin is held at constant temperature (this is automatically calibrated to the skin temperature at each site), and during one of two time slots the temperature is increased or decreased. The

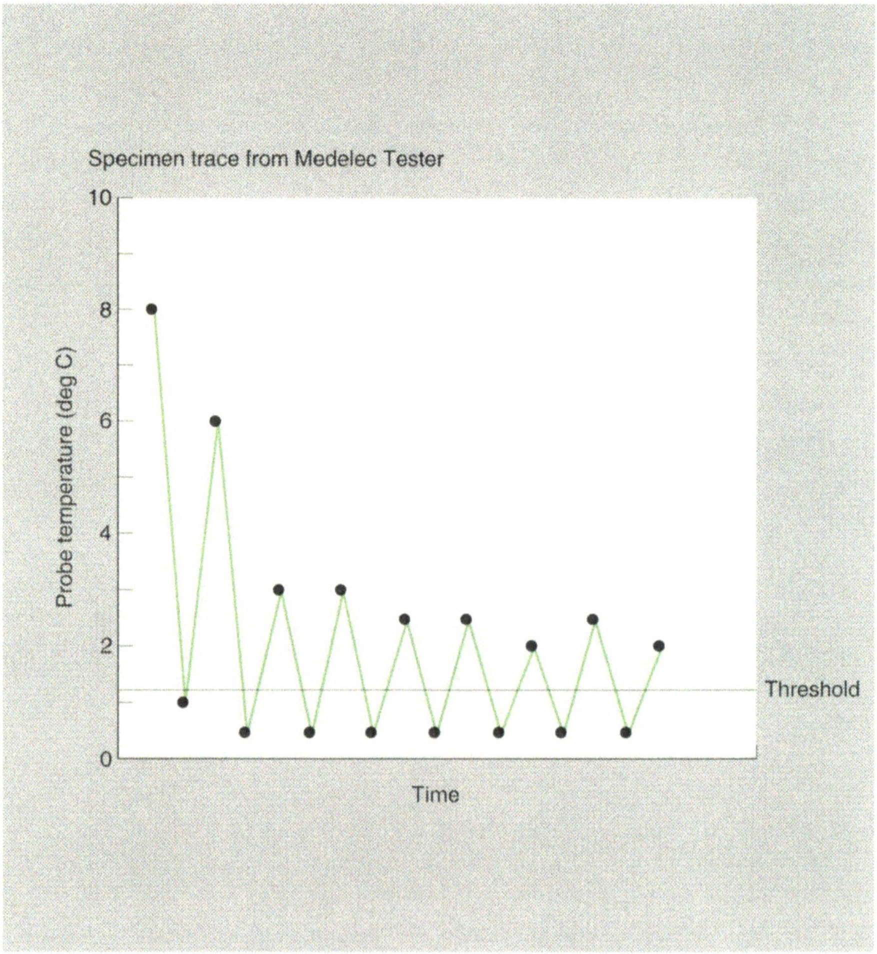

Fig. 4 Specimen trace from the Medelec Tester. The amplitude of the temperature change is decreased from supramaximal to the threshold value which is a mean of the turning points (1.2 °C in the case shown)

patient is asked to indicate by means of a hand held control unit if the temperature is altered in time slot A or B, i. e. forced choice. The amplitude of the stimulus is decreased until a threshold is determined (this is a mean of the turning points, see Fig. 4). During the stimulus the temperature changes at 1 °C per second. Normal values from different studies are given in Table 2. Intra-individual variation was 5% [39, 44]. This test can be very slow to perform when the neuropathy and therefore the sensory loss is advanced.

Sensortek: The third type of unit in common use is typified by the Sensortek thermal sensitivity tester (TST, Sensortek Inc., Clifton, New Jersey) [45]. This uses 2 identical nickel coated copper plates connected to separate power units and perfused with water. Heating or cooling is by the Peltier principle. One plate is maintained at 25 °C and the other heated or cooled. The temperature of each plate and the difference is displayed constantly. The patient is asked to state which plate is hotter or cooler. Subjects place a digit on each plate for 2 seconds with sufficient pressure to blanch a nail. The difference between the plates is decreased until 50% correct responses are achieved. The coefficient of variation varies from 8.3% for fingers of a 22 year old to 47.1% for the great toe in a 66 year old. The overall mean for the fingers was 19% and for the hallux 26.6% [45].

Thermal disks: These were designed by Dyck and Curtis for their ease of use and are cheap [2]. Copper, stainless steel, glass and PVC probes act as recipients of heat from the skin. Copper conducts away heat most easily and so feels coldest. The others feel less cold in the order listed. Each probe is the same weight and surface area. They are placed on the skin of a blindfolded subject one at a time. Copper and PVC are used initially in random order as they have the largest temperature difference. The probes contact skin for 2 seconds with an 8 second interval. Patient answers *warmer*, *colder*, or *don't know.* Since 50% responses will be correct by chance, 75% correct answers is taken as the threshold. The method is reproducible and easy to perform. However, the result is only semi-quantitative and the threshold is not given in degrees of temperature change.

Nociceptive stimuli

Pain thresholds are extremely difficult to measure reproducibly, not least because of the individual differences as to what constitutes pain. It is traditionally assessed by pinprick sensation for superficial, and tendon compression for deep pain. It is not proven that either test represents the modality it is used for, and both tests are poorly reproducible and not quantitative. The majority of afferent nonmyelinated C fibres in skin innervate polymodal C nociceptors, and additional information can therefore be obtained from thermal pain thresholds [46]. It is possible to perform this on thermal threshold testers such as the Marstock. On the Marstock hot and cold thresholds are performed by separate procedures. The patient presses the hand held switch reversing the temperature change as soon as pain is felt. The temperature returns to 30 °C and the test is repeated to get a stable threshold. Maximal levels are set at 50 °C and 0 °C when the temperature is automatically reversed to avoid tissue damage. Normal values are given in Table 2. Although foot thermal thresholds increase with age, this was not found for pain threshold in normal subjects. In diabetic patients both pain and thermal thresholds increase with age [47, 48].

Pinchometer: Pain threshold can also be measured with the "pinchometer" developed at the University of London [47, 49]. Skin folds are pinched between the flat plates of a pair of forceps (area 16 mm^2). Force is transmitted by a spring to a pair of silicon strain gauges. The skinfold is lifted and pinched at a uniform rate until pain is felt. The peak force is registered on the dial. It is usual to take the mean of several readings in the same area. In control subjects mean pain threshold at eight sites on the dorsum of the foot was 0.84 kg (SD 0.24), which was significantly different from a group of diabetic patients (1.22 ± 0.40 kg, p 0.001) [44]. The mean standard deviation of the eight individual observations in each normal subject was 0.21 kg.

Other tests

Other methods of assessing unmyelinated and C nerve fibre function include the quantitative sudomotor axon reflex (QSART), and use of the laser doppler to measure blood flux changes induced by acetylcholine iontophoresis or electrical stimuli [21, 50, 51]. The responses are reduced to both stimuli in diabetic neuropathy, and using the combination of the two methods it may be possible to diagnose early neuropathy. Patients with neuropathy also initially show a paradoxical fall in laser flux when the skin is heated from 35 °C to 44 °C, and have a reduced maximal hyperaemia [41]. An interesting method of producing reproducible stimuli for assessment of warm and pain thresholds involves the use of Argon and CO_2 lasers, but this requires further evaluation [52]. These methods all involve expensive equipment and as yet are not suitable for routine clinical use.

Current perception threshold: This is a relatively new device that uses an unusual stimulus. An electric sine wave of up to 10 mA is produced by a portable battery powered current generator. The current output is maintained by a feedback circuit to ensure that changes in skin resistance are automatically compensated for. The receptors stimulated are unknown, although it is possible that nerves are stimulated directly. The device is the Neurometer (Minimed Technologies, Sylmar, California, USA) which uses small electrodes taped to the skin. There are no problems of applied pressure of probes or standardization of site. Patients are rested in a warm environment, the procedure explained and the current perception thresholds (CPT) determined for 5 Hz, 250 Hz, 2000 Hz at the index finger and hallux. The stimulus is initially increased until it is easily felt and then decreased with short applications of 2–5 seconds until a minimal threshold is reached. A dummy switch is provided to allow a forced choice protocol if desired. The method has been tested by several workers [53–55]. Masson et al [53] tested the machine in 31 healthy and 90 diabetic subjects. The device was compared with the biothesiometer, warm thresholds by the thermoaesthiometer (Free University Hospital, Amsterdam, The Netherlands) and peroneal nerve motor conduction velocity. The device was quick and easy to use. It can discriminate on average between neuropathic and non-neuropathic subjects ($p < 0.001$). The 2000 Hz frequency correlated weakly with large nerve fibre function tests (biothesiometer and conduction velocity, r 0.42–0.69, $p < 0.001$), whilst the lower frequencies (5 and 250 Hz) correlated weakly with tests for small nerve fibres (thermoaesthiometer, r 0.34–0.46, $p < 0.005$). The coefficient of variation was 8–11% at 2000 Hz. Other workers have found CPT correlates better with physical examination and symptom scores than sensory and motor nerve conduction velocities [54, 55].

We found thresholds in patients with neuropathy were on average different from controls at all three frequencies in both hands and feet, but again the correlation with the biothesiometer were weak (2000 Hz: r 0.49, 250 Hz: r 0.31, and 5 Hz: r 0.29), and with the thermal thresholds assessed with the Medelec thermal tester were very weak [56]. There were very wide discrepancies in some of the diabetic subjects. An interesting feature of this machine is that we found the thresholds tended to be lower than normal in patients with painful diabetic neuropathy (unpublished observations).

Although simple to use, this method is not suitable for use as a sole test for neuropathy, for either research or diagnostic purposes, and use of the different frequencies does not reliably discriminate between different nerve fibre types.

Vascular disease in the diabetic leg

In addition to neuropathy, peripheral vascular disease leading to ischaemia is crucially important in affecting lower limb function in the diabetic leg. Measurements of the circulation can be divided into indirect and direct methods [60]. Indirect methods include the use of ultrasound to measure segmental pressures including ankle pressure and also to examine the blood flow pattern by analysis of the Doppler waveform. Other indirect methods are plethysmography, including strain gauge plethysmography, volume plethysmography and photoplethysmography. These are most commonly used to measure toe pressure. Finally, indirect methods include measurement of regional tissue perfusion by the measurement of laser Doppler flux, transcutaneous oxygen and isotope clearance of perfusion. Direct methods allow visualization of the anatomy of the arteries of the diabetic leg and consist of Duplex scanning, magnetic resonance imaging (MRI) and the gold standard of angiography (including digital subtraction angiography).

Techniques to measure blood flow

Indirect methods

Ultrasound: A variety of devices are available, ranging from simple hand held machines to complex equipment, which gives anatomical and physiological information regarding vessels [60]. In the most conventional apparatus, ultrasound is transmitted as a continuous beam and the output may be transferred to a chart recorder or as an audio signal. The Doppler probe contains two piezo electric crystals, one of which transmits the crystals, and the other is the receiving crystal which vibrates in response to reflected waves and produces an output which is measured. The output may be presented as an audio signal, or converted to a chart recorder as an analogue display of the wave form. In the basic hand held equipment, the output does not usually distinguish between flow towards and flow away from the probe. However, most laboratory instruments now have a zero crossing detector to determine the directionality of blood movement.

The recorded Doppler signal is used in two ways:

1. to measure segmental systolic pressure, in particular, ankle pressure,
2. to produce flow velocity waveforms for analysis.

Segmental pressures: Pressure cuffs 12 cm wide are placed at high thigh level above the knee, below the knee and at ankle level. By listening to the Doppler probe over one of the pedal vessels, it is possible to obtain pressure at the level of the inflated cuffs. The pressure index is obtained by dividing the segmental systolic pressure by the brachial systolic pressure. The most frequently measured index in the diabetic is the ankle systolic pressure which should be slightly higher than the brachial systolic pressure. However, between 5 to 10% of diabetic patients have stiff, non compressible peripheral vessels, giving a falsely elevated systolic pressure. Furthermore, the ankle pressure takes no account of the effect of disease of the arteries of the foot.

Toe pressure [61]: Measurement of toe pressure is not affected by the objections raised for ankle systolic pressure. The reproducibility of measurement is stated to be similar to that of ankle measurements. However, the measurement is technically more demanding and the end point may be difficult to determine, partly at low levels of pressure in digital arteries. Furthermore, special equipment is needed to measure the return of flow after inflation of the toe cuff and this equipment is described below.

If the level of ankle blood pressure is borderline, then it is possible to perform an exercise test, although this is not often carried out in diabetic patients with ulceration or gangrene. It is useful in patients with claudication. Exercise results in peripheral vasodilatation, resulting in a fall in pressure, if there is a significant arterial disease. The patients are exercised on a treadmill at a speed of 4 km per hour and at a gradient of 10%, up to 10 minutes or less, until the patient develops claudication. It is important to measure the walking time, the lowest level of ankle pressure after exercise and the time for ankle pressure to return to normal. A fall of 20% or more indicates the presence of significant arterial disease.

Analysis of waveform [62]: In the analogue display of the waveform, the height of tracing is proportional to the blood flow velocity. However, by itself the velocity profile conveys limited information and more useful data can be collected by spectral analysis, which analyses the frequency of emitted sounds against time. Analysis of the signal in this way provides the most accurate information about the blood flow velocity because the method is free of the errors which are present in the production of the analogue output.

Essentially, spectral analysis examines the complete spectrum of frequencies formed in the arterial waveform during a cardiac cycle. It is most usually carried out using Real Time Fast Fourier Transform Spectrum Analysis. In a normal artery, the range or spectral width is narrow during systole, when the majority of blood cells are moving at constant velocity. However, this widens out during diastole, when there is more variation in the cell velocities. The spectral waveform also widens considerably in the presence of haemodynamically significant stenoses, so called spectral broadening.

Several methods of signal analysis have been proposed to quantify changes in spectral waveform and provide an index of severity of arterial disease. These include the pulsatility index, pulse waveform, transit ratios and principal component analysis, but none of these methods have become well established.

Plethysmography [61, 62]: Plethysmography is based on the principle that short term changes in the volume of a limb are mainly due to changes in amount of blood present. The change in blood content following transient circulatory arrest by tourniquet against time represents blood flow. Various types of plethysmograph are available including mercury strain gauge, volume plethysmograph and photoplethysmography.

Strain gauge plethysmography: This works on the principle that the electrical resistance of a conductor (such as a column of mercury in a thin Silastic tube) through which a current is passed varies with length and cross sectional area of the gauge. The gauge is placed around the limb and changes in its resistance are specifically related to changes in volume. This technique is most often used to measure toe blood pressure when the gauge is used as a pulse detector to indicate return of flow when pressure in the cuff falls below systolic pressure.

Volume plethysmography: In actual practice, this is known as the pulse volume recorder. Cuffs are placed around the limbs at several levels and closely applied to the skin to produce a pressure of 65 mmHg. Changes in the pressure of the cuff caused by arterial pulsations are recorded via a pressure transducer and an analogue recorder. Proximal arterial disease will produce changes in the contour and amplitude of the pulse, such as decrease in the rate of rise of wave forms, reduced amplitude and absence of reflected diastole wave with marked decrease in the amplitude of the waveform. The distal cuffs can also be used as pulse detectors in the measurement of ankle systolic pressure. Reproducibility is less than that for ankle pressure measurement [62].

Photoplethysmography: This studies blood flow in the skin and consists of a light emitting diode and a photodetector. The light is reflected back from the blood in the cutaneous microcirculation. The intensity of the reflected light depends on the amount of blood in the microcirculation which is related to the degree of ischaemia. Its main role is in the measurement of toe pressure. The photo transducer is taped to the end of the toe with a double faced cellophane tape and a cuff attached to the base of the digit. The pressure which the wave form returns corresponds to the digital systolic pressure. The photoplethysmograph can also be used to measure skin perfusion pressure. The probe is placed under the cuff to detect the pressure that allows blood pressure of the skin directly under the cuff to return after occlusion. In this situation it is important that the electrode is embedded in a case of plastic material so that artefacts from the pressure effect at the edge of the transducer may be controlled.

Measurement of regional tissue perfusion [63]: Techniques that essentially measure regional tissue perfusion have been used to assess the degree of ischaemia in the diabetic foot. These include the measurement of transcutaneous oxygen, laser Doppler frowmetry and radioisotope clearance and perfusion.

Transcutaneous oxygen: The transcutaneous oxygen technique uses a Clarke type oxygen electrode to measure the partial pressure of oxygen that diffuses through heated skin. The skin should be prepared by swabbing with alcohol and removing hairs. The electrode is positioned by means of a fixation ring which is attached to the skin. An electrolyte solution is then placed within the ring facilitating contact between the electrode and the skin. Many factors affect the level of transcutaneous oxygen ($TcpO_2$) in normal subjects. They include age, arterial oxygen tension, room temperature, consumption of oxygen by the epidermis, the barrier to diffusion produced by keratin in the skin and the amount of blood flow to the area examined. At normal skin temperature, oxygen tension of the skin is low, but if the skin is heated to 43–44 °C, there is hyperaemia of the underlying tissues, oxygen is in excess of demand and the $TcpO_2$ indicates arterial oxygen tension.

The wide variability and overlap of resting $TcpO_2$ values have been a significant problem for the applicability of the method. In patients with marked oedema, hyperkeratosis or cellulitis, $TcpO_2$ readings are unreliable as a result of reduced oxygen transmission. Furthermore, transcutaneous oxygen measurements may be unreliable with very low oxygen partial pressure associated with very low blood flow. This is due to the oxygen requirement of the measuring electrode itself and the diffusion field generated by it. This results in a so called 'flow blind range' in which oxygen can not be detected in the capillary loops on the surface even though blood is flowing [66]. Several modifications have been introduced, including a regional perfusion index which measures the ratio of trunk to limb $TcpO_2$, and the measurement of $TcpO_2$ responses to certain physiological stimuli, such as elevation of limb position and response to 100% oxygen breathing [64, 65]. Hauser et al compared the diagnostic values of $TcpO_2$ with other non-invasive diagnostic tests that are currently used in patients with diabetes and peripheral vascular disease [66, 67]. They found a significantly higher diagnostic accuracy with $TcpO_2$ expressed as a regional perfusion index than for Doppler ankle blood flow ratio and pulse volume recording.

Laser Doppler flowmetry [63]: Laser Doppler flux assess microvascular perfusion by measuring the flux of red blood cells near the surface of the skin. Laser flowmetry has been shown to correlate in a more linear fashion to a progressive reduction in limb blood flow compared to photoplethysomography or transcutaneous oxygen measurement [67]. Since the speed of movement of erythrocytes is dependent on local vasomotion (period vasoconstriction vs dilatation) it is possible to distinguish between various vasomotor patterns and determine which of these reflect healthy or insufficient microcirculation [63].

Isotope methods: Radio isotopes are used in two ways to assess blood flow, first by measurement of isotope clearance from the skin and second by isotope perfusion scanning when the rate of accumulation of isotope is measured following systemic administration. Isotope clearance involves the intradermal injection of a small dose of radio isotope mixed with a vasodilator drug in order to eliminate the effect of local nervous or humoral factors. External counter pressure is applied over the isotope depot until the clearance of the isotope is finished. The pressure required to obliterate the clearance is called the skin perfusion pressure and in normal subjects is due to mean arterial pressure and probably represents the local arterial perfusion pressure. The most commonly used isotope is Xenon, a gas isotope, that when injected into tissue is removed by crossing the capillary cell membrane by a diffusion down a concentration gradient.

In isotope perfusion scanning, the radioactive tracer is administered by intraarterial injection and the accumulation of isotope in the ulcer and the surrounding skin is measured. The ratio of activity around the ulcer to the activity in the floor of the ulcer is measured, the critical level being 3.5 [62]. Furthermore, blood flow velocity in the leg can be studied with this technique by following the activity of Technetium which has been injected intraarterially [69].

Direct methods of assessing the circulation

Duplex scanning: Duplex scanning employs a combination of a real time B mode sonography and a pulse Doppler. This design allows two dimensional visualization of the blood vessel. The B mode positions the sample volume in the centre of the blood stream and gives an anatomical description of the arterial wall, including calcified plaques, ulcers, thrombi and aneurysmal dilations. When the sample volume has been positioned in the centre of the blood stream, real time spectral analysis of the pulse Doppler waveform can then be derived with measurement of flow velocities. Spectral analysis from the centre of the artery shows a narrow band of frequencies. However, in turbulent flow, such as seen just beyond an arterial stenosis, a much wider band of frequencies is seen. Recently, colour mapping has been added to Duplex scanning, aiding the interrogation of the vessels. Duplex scanning has been compared to angiography in the assessment of the peripheral vascular system [70]. Duplex visualized 99% of arterial segments proximal to the tibial vessels with overall sensitivities for detecting a 50% or greater lesion, ranging from 89% in the iliac vessels to 67% at the popliteal artery. In the tibial vessels, Duplex was better at visualizing anterior tibial and posterior tibial segments, 94% and 96% respectively, and peroneal arteries segments – 83%. However, Duplex scanning is operator dependent, requiring a considerable amount of experience. Nevertheless, it has been an important advance in providing non invasively new information as to the degree of severity of arterial occlusive disease.

Magnetic resonance imaging (MRI): Magnetic resonance imaging is still being evaluated, but is likely that it will be useful in diabetic patients to visualize calf and foot vessels. It can be used to detect atherosclerotic disease with markedly thickened wall and lesions protruding into the lumen of the artery, lumen narrowing and calcifying plaques. MRI is also capable of measuring and displaying intraarterial blood flow velocity and three dimensional reconstruction of blood vessels using special techniques [62]. Using MRI gated subtraction of a systolic from a diastolic image, leaves only the signal from the pulsatile arteries. This allows the representation of arteries in a two dimensional image resembling angiography [71]. Furthermore, by using various strategies to enhance phase contrast magnetic resonance angiography, the visualization of lower extremity vasculature including popliteal, tibial and peroneal vessels has been achieved [72].

Angiography including digital subtraction angiography: Angiography remains the gold standard for assessing vascular supply in the leg and foot [73]. Indications for angiography are disabling claudication, ischaemic rest pain, ischaemic ulceration and gangrene. Angiography provides anatomical information on which decisions for both angioplasty and surgery are made as well as for assessing the efficacy of interventional measures including both medical and surgical treatments.

Diabetic patients should be kept well hydrated and if the serum creatinine is above 120 mmols/L, a renal dose of dopamine (2.5 µgs/ml/min) should be infused at the time of angiography. The risk of contrast medium induced renal failure can be reduced by using low osmolality contrast agents. Classically the transfemoral approach is carried out, but it is important to visualize the popliteal and tibial arteries in the diabetic leg, and this can be done by passing the catheter from the contralateral common femoral artery across the aortic bifurcation and passing it down the ipsilateral common femoral artery. Alternatively, an antegrade puncture can be made to the ipsilateral common femoral artery and the catheter passed into the superficial femoral artery or popliteal artery. Digital subtraction angiography is a computer assisted technique, in which an area of interest obtained before injection of radio contrast is electronically subtracted from one obtained after injection of radiographic contrast. It is particularly useful for evaluating the circulation of the lower leg, ankle and foot [74].

Assessment of the biomechanical function of the foot

The function of the foot is essentially mechanical. The mechanics of the foot can be studied in two ways: the first is called kinetics, which is concerned with the analysis of forces exerted on the foot for the purposes of weight bearing and locomotion, and the second is kinematics, and deals with the relative movements of the lower limb elements during various activities [75].

Kinetics of the foot

A number of methods are available for the measurement of external forces on the foot. Most work is concentrated on the measurement of the vertical reaction between the sole of the foot and its supporting surface, namely, plantar pressure measurements.

Devices that measure plantar pressure are of three types:

1. those that measure total pressure under the foot,
2. those that measure the distribution of total pressure across the entire sole, and
3. those that measure pressure at a few discrete locations.

As well as vertical forces, the foot is subjected to forces or stress applied at right angles to the normal load, that is horizontal forces, and these are called shear forces. These have proved difficult to measure, but recent work has developed new techniques.

The interface at which the measurement of vertical forces is made varies with different devices. Some measure pressure between the base of the foot and ground, so called platform measurements, whilst others measure pressures between the foot and the shoe. For bare foot measurement, the patient walks onto the platform and the information from a single foot contact is collected. For insole measurement, pressure transducers are manufactured into a thin pliable insole which is placed in the shoe in direct contact with the foot. Information from multiple steps can be obtained [76].

The choice to make measurements at local sites or under the entire plantar surface will depend on the purpose of the investigation. For localizing pressure peaks as a means of screening the foot, a pressure map which good spatial resolution is needed. On the other hand, direct transducers can be employed to determine pressures under specific anatomical sites, and even for observing functional characteristics of the foot such as pronation or supination.

Furthermore, for each technique, plantar pressure may be measured by two different methods; statistically when measurements are made during standing, and dynamically when measurements of foot to floor contact are made while walking. The choice of the method will again depend on the purpose of the investigation. Static measurements present plantar pressure distribution based on the subject's foot form and weight shift. Deformities resulting in high pressure areas can be identified, but foot loading during function cannot be established. Dynamic measurements allow foot function and gait to be observed. Most researchers have stressed the importance of making dynamic measurements. However, Duckworth et al stressed both static and dynamic recordings were important for a complete picture of plantar loading [77].

Methods of plantar pressure measurement between barefoot and ground

Measurement of total pressure with force plate: Force plates are capable of measuring total body forces acting through the foot. The force plate consists of a load sensitive surface set on a walkway which measures the changing forces opposed upon it during the period of foot contact. A typical force plate in modern use consists of a rigid rectangular plate about 50 cm by

30 cm set into the floor of the walkway and supported near each corner by load cells. Total vertical, longitudinal and transverse forces can be measured separately, and it is possible to derive the centre of load, the point under force plate at which the forces exerted beneath the foot and the ground can be considered to act [78].

An important feature in the design of a force plate is the frequency response of the system. This reflects how fast and with what accuracy the system will respond to abrupt changes in load. Thus, a load measuring system must have a lowest natural frequency which is substantially higher than any of the applied frequencies. Most modern load cells and force plates are electronic and they use a variety of piezo-metric transduction systems to convert force to pressure to an equivalent electronic variable. A technique which combines the potential of accuracy of good dynamic response and high sensitivity is offered by piezo electric crystals. These substances generate electric charge which defuse along central consisting of 128 cells each 40 mm square and each supplied by a strain gauged ring [85]. Peak forces on each cell for the entire step, instantaneous distributions at different support phases, and the progression of the centre of pressure are examples of the types of display that are almost immediately available after recording.

Matrix mat systems: Several pressure mat systems have been used to measure the distribution of plantar pressure; these include:

1. EMED System
2. Musgrave foot print
3. Piezo electric pressure distribution mat (Penn. State)
4. Electroposturgraph and the electropodograph of clinical interactive research
5. Tek scan system – Bigmat system

EMED systems: This uses capacitance transducers as the sensory element [86]. The EMED system consists of a matrix mat in which individual series are formed electronically at the intersection of row and columns of conductive material. Initially, a rectangular device with 40 rows and 40 columns each 1 by 48 cm, it appeared functionally to be a 1600 element mat with a 1 by 1 cm element separated by a gap of 2 mm [87]. Currently, the EMED system is marketed with several sizes of platform available. Between 2 and 9 sensors per cm^2 are manufactured in platforms ranging in sizes from 48 cm by 31 cm down to 10 cm by 10 cm. Small flexible units can be made for in shoe measurements. The principle of operation is the same for either a platform or an in shoe device. Recently Hughes et al have demonstrated the reliability of pressure measurements using the EMED system [88].

Musgrave foot print: This uses a polymer film as the sensing element. It is a force sensitive resistive technique in which a polymer thick film device exhibits a decreasing resistance with increasing force applied vertical to its surface. The film can be made in small squares (5 × 5 mm) giving good spatial resolution. A recent version [89] based on this force sensitive resistive technology consists of 2048 transducers. The dimensions of this version are 63 cm by 32.5 cm and 3. 2cm thick. The software developed and supplied as standard with the system provides comprehensive foot pressure analysis.

The piezo electric pressure distribution mat (Penn State): [87] This is a 1000 element system used at the Centre for Locomotion Studies at Penn State University and is based on small piezoelectric squares made of lead zirconate titanate, each 5 mm by 5 mm, arranged to form a load-sensitive area.

Electroposturgraph and electropodograph: The electroposturgraph allows analysis of postural sway while the electropodograph allows analysis of static and dynamic foot loading.

Tek scan Bigmat system: This uses force sensitive resistive technology and sensing cells are placed 1 cm apart in a matrix less than 4 mm thick and 500 cm by 500 cm. Comprehensive software provides analysis of entire plantar pressure or force, discrete area analysis of pressure or force, graphical representation of the data against time with playback facility of the recording and centre of load display.

Direct visualization techniques: The instrument which embraces this technique is the pedobarograph [90]. The apparatus consists of a glass plate illuminated from the sides, producing total internal reflection. A thin plastic material which has tiny dimples on the surface covers the plate. When pressure is applied, light is scattered and reflected out of the glass. As more pressure is exerted more light is scattered which produces a grey scale image and is picked up by video camera. The image is captured by a monochrome television camera and translated into a colour contour map using an interface microprocessor system. A commercial version of this device is now available (Biokinetics). The spatial resolution of the system is very high (pixel size approximately 1 mm by 1.5 mm) and the material used for covering the glass plate allows pressures up to 30 kg/cm^2 to be measured accurately [91]. Efficient and accurate data capture is possible at high frequency. The pressure measuring device is built into a walkway of sufficient length to enable the subject's gait to become established [90]. The subject is told to disregard the pressure plate and look straight ahead and walk at a normal speed. Those recordings where the patient has failed to step on the centre of the plate are discarded. Reproducible results are said to be relatively easy to obtain.

The video output is processed by a video digitizer which converts every alternate frame of the analogue signal into a digital form and the digital information can then be used to provide video images comprising a matrix of 128 by 64 elements, giving a resolution of the order of 25 mm for the average adult foot. Specific areas of interest can be selected using an electronic joystick and the computer analysis information within the area of interest.

Methods of plantar pressure measurement in shoes [92]

The major disadvantage of barefoot techniques is that the data obtained is removed from typical every day shoe wearing environment. As most patients wear shoes and often sustain injury while wearing them, the ability to measure pressures inside the shoe is an important extension of techniques. One advance of in shoe transducers compared to pressure platforms is that multiple steps can be collected more easily. However, in shoe measurement is technically much more demanding than pressure measurement on the flat walking surface. The transducer cables often bend as they emerge from the shoe and there is repeated local compression of the same areas of the transducer. The inside of the shoe can be regarded as a hostile environment as it is warm, deep and contoured. These factors can lead to measurement error and device failure. However, in shoe measurements probably provide useful data to understand the effects of shoe design and modification on the mechanics of the foot.

The techniques can be divided into two categories: one employing a number of discrete transducers that are attached to the specific areas of the plantar surface and the other using a series of transducers in a matrix of elements that are incorporated in the insoles.

The advantage of discrete transducers are small size, affordability and ease of crystallographic axes. The charge between the two faces of a crystal is proportional to the compressive force with a suitable selected material. This method is used in the highly accurate transducer system of the Kistler force plate [79].

Plantar pressure distribution: The simplest method available is the Harris mat [80]. The underside of a multilayered inked rubber mat makes contact with a piece of paper. As the patient walks across the mat, a variable density impression is left on the paper, with local density depending on plantar pressure. Small mats are also available that can be placed inside the shoe. However, the mat has only an approximate four point scale and saturates at a pressure well within the normal range and thus, all values above this level, result in the same reading [81]. Thus, the Harris mat can only give a general indication of plantar pressure distribution.

Two other commercial systems for obtaining direct foot pressures are available, Shutrak is presented as a perforated units of continuous stationery, with a carbonated layer between two outer sheets. After impression, the top sheet is removed to reveal an ink density proportional to pressure [82]. The pressure range is adequate to define gross patterns of standing pressure. Another method is called Prescale which has a similar structure of colour encapsulated between two sheets [83].

There are three main systems to assess plantar pressure patterns quantitatively. These consist of:

1. The modified force plate
2. Matrix mat systems
3. Direct visualization techniques

Modified force plate: The force plate has been modified to record force distribution by subdividing the force plate into 12 independent strips, each recording against a base of time, the vertical component of load. The strips can be orientated either transverse or longitudinal to the direction of walking, and their output used to generate the longitudinal and transverse load profiles [84]. A further development has been the construction of a full matrix force plate manufacture. The main disadvantage is that the transducer may act as a foreign body in the shoe and alter the mechanical condition of the foot shoe interface. Capacitance transducers are disadvantaged as they are at least 3–4 mm deep. Strain gauge transducers can also be quite bulky when encapsulated and are extremely sensitive to temperature. Discrete methods are also liable to inaccuracies due to imprecise positioning of the sensors. Furthermore, the sensors may also migrate, due to shear stress. To overcome this, sensors have been recessed into insoles. An objection to measurements using the discrete system is that assumptions about the pattern of plantar pressure must be made when placing sensors on the foot. Not all regions can be studied.

The following systems are in use to measure in shoe pressures. Two capacitance systems insole systems are currently available and comprise Computer Dyno Graphy (CDG) system and the EMED system. Two systems based on force sensitive resistive technology include the Electrodynogram and the Tekscan F-Scan system.

Computer Dyno Graphy (CDG): This system places eight sensors at predetermined sites in special slippers which are stated to give a satisfactory gait pattern representation. Computer analysis includes plots of force against time graphs and centre of pressure readings.

EMED system: This system uses sensors based on those in the capacitive pressure mat. Seventy two sensors are incorporated in the insoles which are supplied in standard sizes 6 and 8. Software allows data to be represented as a pressure map which can be analysed in particular areas.

Electrodynagram: The device has a waist pack worn by the patient and 7 very thin sensors are applied to areas thought to be at risk under the forfoot and heel of each foot. There is some doubt about the properties and calibration of sensors on the foot [87].

The Tekscan F-scan system: This system consists of two conductive polymer layers deposited on a mylar substrate. The conductive polymer is deposited in tracks which essentially run along and across the insole shaped sensor. The two layers are glued together and where two perpendicular tracks cross a load cell is created. The novelty of the system, which comes complete with hardware and software interfacing, is in the flexibility of the insoles which allows them to be trimmed to size with scissors before insertion into a shoe. The software allows the centre of force to be plotted, plantar force or pressure movies to be played back in either 2-D or 3-D, analysis of forces or pressures under discrete sites and graphs of force or pressure to be plotted. One research group has recently published work conducted with the first version of the system in a study of the effects of heel wedges on plantar pressure distribution and centre of force [93].

Measurement of shear forces: Shear forces are difficult to measure, and there are no commercially available instruments to measure shear force. However, recent interest has resulted in several groups attempting to measure this. The underlying principle is to use magneto-resistive elements attached to the sole and by this means horizontal and longitudinal shearing forces can be measured. Tappin et al [94] were the first to describe the use of this technique for measuring discrete plantar stresses with a uniaxial shear transducer. Laing et al [95] have further developed Tappin's device by making it smaller in diameter and thickness (10 mm & 1 mm respectively). A triaxial transducer incorporating a biaxial shear stress section has been described by Lord et al [96] based on the same magneto-resistive principle. This measures shear in two orthogonal directions and also as a direct pressure measurement stage. The transducer is mounted in an inlay which can directly replace the normal deep inlay of an extra depth shoe.

Kinematics of gait

Gait analysis: A number of techniques are available to track the spatial position of targets attached to segments of the lower limb during gait. Reflective markers are used and are tracked by high speed video [97, 98]. This allows joint motion in the foot to be quantitatively measured during normal function. Very few such measurements of foot movement have been made in diabetes although the techniques have been widely used in orthopedic biomechanics [99].

Range of motion of joints: The kinematics of gait may also be assessed by measuring the range of motion of the joints of the foot. The two crucial movements in the diabetic foot are dorsiflexion of the talocrural joint and of the first metatarsal-phalangeal joint. Limitations in these motions will cause an increase in plantar pressure during gait [100].

The measurement of joint motion can take two basic forms, measurement of the stiffness of the joint and measurement of the range of motion. For stiffness measurements, it is necessary that the motion and force required to cause the given movement of the joint be simultaneously recorded so that a force per unit of angular displacement can be calculated. Examples of this approach are the first-ray mobility device of Rodgers and Cavanagh [101] and the hallux extension measurements of Birke [102] and associates. There are no commercially available devices of this type for routine clinical use. Range of motion is much easier to measure and is thus more commonly performed.

In range of motion measurement, a goniometer is used to assess the end point of the range in both directions either with the patient moving the joint to its voluntary end point or with the clinician applying a force to achieve the end point [103, 104]. The goniometer is fixed across the joint in such a way that its axis of rotation is aligned with that of the joint. Although most goniometric measurements are made with the subject non-weight bearing, Fromherz [105] has suggested that increased reliability of digital measurements can be obtained when made during weight bearing. An association has been demonstrated between limited joint mobility and foot ulceration in the diabetic foot [106, 107].

References

[1] Watkins PJ. Clinical observations and experiments in diabetic neuropathy. Diabetologia 1992; 35: 2–11.

[2] Dyck PJ, Karnes J, O'Brien PC. Detection of thresholds of cutaneous sensation. In: Dyck PJ, Thomas PK, Asbury AK, Porte D, eds. Diabetic Neuropathy. Philadelphia: WB Saunders Co., 1987; 107–121, 140–145.

[3] San Antonio Conference on Diabetic Neuropathy: report and recommendations. Neurology 1988; 38: 1161–1165.

[4] Thomas PK. Diabetic neuropathy: a neurologist's view. In: Treatment of diabetic neuropathy: a new approach. Edinburgh: Churchill Livingstone, 1992, 11–20.

[5] Stevens MJ, Edmonds ME, Foster AVM et al. Selective neuropathy and preserved vascular responses in the diabetic Charcot foot. Diabetologia 1992; 35: 148–154.

[6] Boulton AJM, Ward JD. Diabetic neuropathies and pain. In: Watkins PJ, ed. Long term complications of diabetes. Clinics in endocrinology and metabolism. London: Saunders, 1986; 917–931.

[7] Young RJ, Ewing DJ, Clark BF. Chronic and remitting painful diabetic polyneuropathy. Diab Care 1988; 11: 34–40.

[8] Archer AG, Watkins PJ, Thomas PK et al. The natural history of acute painful neuropathy in diabetes mellitus. J Neurol Neurosurg Psychiat 1983; 46: 491–499.

[9] Coppack SW, Watkins PJ. The natural history of diabetic femoral neuropathy. Quart J Med 1991; 79: 307–313.

[10] Bell P, London N. Surgical treatment of critical ischaemia. Critical Ischaemia 1992; 2 (1): 15–23.

[11] Swanson CJ. Human diabetic endoneurial sorbitol, fructose, and myo-inositol related to sural nerve morphometry. Ann Neurol 1980; 8: 590–596.

[12] Dyck PJ, Karnes JL, Daube J et al. Clinical and neuropathological criteria for the diagnosis and staging of diabetic polyneuropathy. Brain 1985; 108: 861–880.

[13] Dyck PJ, Karnes J, O'Brien PC et al. Neuropathy symptom profile in health, motor neuron disease, diabetic neuropathy, and amyloidosis. Neurology 1986; 36: 1300–1308.

[14] Dyck PJ, Kratz KM, Lehman K et al. The Rochester Diabetic Neuropathy Study: Design, criteria for types of neuropathy, selection bias, and reproducibility of neuropathic tests. Neurology 1991; 41: 799–807.

[15] Low PA, Fealey RD. Sudomotor neuropathy. In: Dyck PJ, Thomas PK, Asbury AK et al, eds. Diabetic neuropathy. Philadelphia: WB Saunders Co., 1987, 140–145.

[16] Disorders of function in the light of anatomy and physiology. In: Brain's Diseases of the Nervous System. 9th ed. Sir John Walton. Oxford: Oxford University Press, 1985; 37.

[17] Fagius J, Wahren LK. Variability of sensory determination in clinical use. J Neurol Sci 1981; 51: 11–27.

[18] Ahmed ME, Le Quesne P. Quantitative sweat test in diabetics with neuropathic foot lesions. J Neurol Neurosurg Psychiatry 1986; 49 (9): 1059–1062.

[19] Kennedy WR, Sakuta M, Sutherland D et al. The sweating deficiency in diabetes mellitus: methods of quantitation and clinical correlation. Neurology 1984; 34: 758–763.

[20] Parkhouse N, LeQuesne PM. Impaired neurogenic vascular responses in patients with diabetes and neuropathic foot lesions. New Eng J Med 1988; 318: 1306–1309.

[21] Low PA, Caskey PE, Tuck RR et al. Quantitative sudomotor axon reflex test in normal and neuropathic subjects. Ann Neurol 1983; 14 (5): 573–580.

[22] Levy DM, Reid G, Abraham RR et al. Assessment of basal and stimulated sweating in diabetes using a direct-reading computerised sudorometer. Diab Med 1991; (S78).

[23] Levy DM, Terenghi G, Gu XH et al. Immunohistochemical measurements of nerves and neuropeptides in diabetic skin: relationship to tests of neurological function. Diabetologia 1992; 35: 889–897.

[24] Claus D, Hilz MJ, Neundorfer B. Thermal discrimination thresholds: a comparison of different methods. Acta Neurol Scand 1990; 81: 533–540.

[25] Dyck PJ, Thomas PK, Lambert EH et al, eds. Peripheral Neuropathy. Vol. 1. 2nd ed. Philadelphia: WB Saunders, 1984; 210–230.

[26] Kumar S, Fernando DJS, Veves A et al. Semmes–Weinstein monofilaments – a simple screening device to identify diabetic patients at risk of foot ulceration. Abstract. Diab Med 1990; Suppl 7: 4A.

[27] Hunt CC. On the nature of vibration receptors in the hind limb of the cat. J Physiol (London) 1961; 155: 175.

[28] Dyck PJ, Zimmerman IR, O'Brien PC et al. Introduction of automated systems to evaluate touch pressure, vibration and thermal cutaneous sensation in man. Ann Neurol 1978; 4: 502–510.

[29] Crausaz FM, Clavel S, Liniger C et al. Additional factors associated with plantar ulcers in diabetic neuropathy. Diabetic Med 1988; 5 (8): 771–775.

[30] Thivolet C, El Farkh J, Petiot A et al. Measuring vibration sensations with graduated tuning fork. Simple and reliable means to detect diabetic patients at risk of neuropathic foot ulceration. Diabetes Care 1990; 13 (10): 1077–1080.

[31] Liniger C, Albeanu D, Bloise D et al. The tuning fork revisited. Diabetic Med 1990; 7: 859–864.

[32] Boulton AJ, Kubrusly DB, Bowker JH et al. Impaired vibratory perception and diabetic foot ulceration. Diabetic Med 1986; 3 (4): 335–337.

[33] Armstrong FM, Bradbury JE, Ellis SH et al. A study of peripheral diabetic neuropathy. The application of age-related reference values. Diabetic Med 1991; 8 Symposium: S94–S99.

[34] Wiles PG, Pearce SM, Rice PJS et al. Vibration perception threshold: Influence of age, height, sex, and smoking, and calculation of accurate centile values. Diabetic Med 1991; 8: 157–161.

[35] Bloom S, Till S, Sonksen P et al. Use of a biothesiometer to measure individual vibration thresholds and their variation in 519 non-diabetic subjects. Br Med J 1984; 288 (6433): 1793–1795.

[36] van Dijk J, Huyser W, Stijl-Pek M. Vibration disappearance threshold may be raised by measuring it. Clin Neurol Neurosurg 1991; 93 (4): 289–291.

[37] Goldberg J, Lindblom U. Standardised method of determining vibratory perception thresholds for diagnosis and screening in neurological investigation. J Neurol Neurosurg Psychiatry 1979; 42: 793–803.

[38] Watkins PJ, Edmonds ME. Sympathetic nerve failure in diabetes. Diabetologia 1983; 25: 73–77.

[39] Jamal GA, Hansen S, Weir Al et al. An improved automated method for measurement of thermal thresholds in normal subjects. J Neurol Neurosurg Psychiatry 1985; 48: 54–60.

[40] Guy RJ, Gilbey SG, Sheehy M et al. Diabetic neuropathy in the upper limb and the effect of twelve months sorbinil treatment. Diabetologia 1988; 31 (4): 214–220.

[41] Stevens MJ, Edmonds ME, Douglas SLE et al. Influence of neuropathy on the microvascular response to local heating in the human diabetic foot. Clinical Science 1991; 80: 249–256.

[42] Ali Z, Carroll M, Robertson KP et al. The extent of small fibre sensory neuropathy in diabetics with plantar ulceration. J Neurol Neurosurg Psychiatry 1989: 94–98.

[43] Guy RJC, Clark CA, Malcolm PN et al. Evaluation of thermal and vibration sensation in diabetic neuropathy. Diabetologia 1985; 28: 131–137.

[44] Jamal GA, Weir AL, Hansen S et al. An improved automated method for the measurement of thermal thresholds. 2. Patients with peripheral neuropathy. J Neurol Neurosurg Psychiatry 1985; 48 (4): 361–366.

[45] Arezzo JC, Schaumburg HH, Laudadio C. Thermal sensitivity tester. Device for quantitative assessment of thermal sense in diabetic neuropathy. Diabetes 1986; 35 (5): 590–592.
[46] Hallis R, Torebjork H, Wiesenfeld Z. Nociceptors and warm receptors innervated by C fibres in human skin. J Neurol Neurosurg Psychiatry 1981; 44: 313–319.
[47] Le Quesne P, Fowler CJ. A study of pain threshold in diabetics with neuropathic foot lesions. J Neurol Neurosurg Psychiatry 1986; 49 (10): 1191–1194.
[48] Ziegler D, Mayer P, Wiefels K et al. Assessment of small and large fibre function in long-term type 1 (insulin dependent) diabetic patients with and without painful neuropathy [Published erratum in: Pain 1988 Sept.; 34 (3): 322]. Pain 1988; 34 (1): 1–10.
[49] Lynn B, Perl E. A comparison of four tests for assessing the pain sensitivity of different subjects and test areas. Pain 1977; 3: 353–365.
[50] Parkhouse N, Le Quesne P. Impaired neurogenic vascular response in patients with diabetes and neuropathic foot lesions. N Engl J Med 1988; 318 (20): 1306–1309.
[51] Westerman R, Widdor R, Hannaford J et al. Laser doppler velocimetry in the measurement of neurovascular function. Australasion Physical and Engineering Sciences in Medicine 1988; 1 (2): 53–66.
[52] Arendt-Nielsen L, Bjering P. Sensory and pain threshold characteristics to laser stimuli. J Neurol Neurosurg Psychiatry 1988; 51: 35–42.
[53] Masson EA, Veves A, Fernando D et al. Current perception thresholds: a new, quick, and reproducible method for the assessment of peripheral neuropathy in diabetes mellitus. Diabetologia 1989; 32 (10): 724–728.
[54] Rendell MS, Dovgan DJ, Bergman TF et al. Mapping diabetic sensory neuropathy by current perception threshold testing. Diabetes Care 1989; 12 (9): 636–640.
[55] Rendell MS, Katims JJ, Richter R et al. A comparison of nerve conduction velocities and current perception thresholds as correlates of clinical severity of diabetic sensory neuropathy. J Neurol Neurosurg Psychiatry 1989; 52 (4): 502–511.
[56] Pitei D, Edmonds ME, Watkins PJ. The Neurometer: evaluation of a new technique for electrical sensory perception thresholds in neuropathy. Abstract. Diabetic Med 1992; Supplement.
[57] Bravenboer B, van Dam PS, Hop J et al. Thermal threshold testing for the assessment of small fibre dysfunction: normal values and reproducibility. Diabetic Med 1992; 9: 546–549.
[58] Bertelsmann FW, Heimans JJ, Weber EJM et al. Thermal discrimination thresholds in normal subjects and in patients with diabetic neuropathy. J Neurol Neurosurg Psych 1985; 48: 686–690.
[59] Fruhstorfer H, Lindblom U, Schmidt WG. Method for quantitative estimation of thermal thresholds in patients. N Neurol Neurosurg Psych 1976; 39: 1071–1075.
[60] Sidawy AN, Curry KM. Non invasive evaluation of the lower extremity arterial system. In: Frykberg RG, ed. The High Risk Foot in Diabetes Mellitus. New York: Churchill Livingstone, 1991; 241–245.
[61] Hurley, JJ, Woods JJ, Hershey FB. Non invasive testing: practical knowledge for evaluating diabetic patients. In: Levin MF, O'Neal LW, Bowker JH, eds. The Diabetic Foot. St Louis: Mosby Year Book, 1993; 321–340.
[62] Faris IB, McCollum P, Mantese V et al. Investigation of the patient with atheroma. In: Bell PRF, Jamieson CW, Ruckley CV, eds. Surgical management of Vascular Disease. London: WB Saunders Co. Ltd. 1992; 131–196.
[63] Rieger H, Scheffler A. Diagnosis of advanced stages of peripheral arterial occlusive disease. Critica Ischaemia 1990; 1: 15–21.
[64] McCollum PT, Spence VA, Walker WF. Oxygen inhalation induced changes in the skin as measured by transcutaneous oximetry. Br J Surg 1986; 73: 862–885.
[65] Hauser CJ, Shoemaker WC. Use of transcutaneous pO_2 regional perfusion index to quantify tissue perfusion in peripheral vascular disease. Ann Surg 1983; 197: 337–343.
[66] Hauser CJ, Appel P, Shoemaker WC. Pathophysiologic classification of peripheral vascular disease by positional changes in regional transcutaneous oxygen tension. Surgery 1984; 95: 689–693.

[67] Hauser CJ, Klien SR, Mehringer CM et al. Superiority of transcutaneous oxymetry in non invasive vascular diagnosis in patients with diabetes. Arch Surg 1984; 119: 690–694.
[68] Kverndo K, Megerman J, Hamilton G et al. Response of skin plethysmography, laser Doppler flowmetry and transcutaneous oxygen tensionometry to stenosis induced reductions in limb blood flow. Eur J Vas Surg 1989; 3: 113.
[69] Shionoya S, Hirae M, Kawai S et al. Haemodynamic study of ischaemic limb by velocity measurement in foot. Surgery 1981; 90: 10.
[70] Moneta GL, Yeager RA, Antonovic R et al. Accuracy of lower extremity arterial duplex mapping. J Vas Surg 1991; 5: 275.
[71] Meuli RA, Wedeen VJ, Gellit SC et al. MR gated subtraction angiography: evaluation of lower extremities. Radiology 1986; 159: 411.
[72] Wesley GE, Higgins CB, Amparo EG et al. Peripheral vascular disease: a correlation of MR imaging and angiography. Radiology 1985; 156: 733.
[73] Stokes KR, Pomposelli FB, Longmaid HEIII. Lower extremity arteriography in the diabetic patient. In: Frykbery RG. New York: Churchill Livingstone, 1991; 255–272.
[74] Welling RE, Baldridge ED, Frey RT. Vascular disease of the diabetic foot. In: Sammarco GJ, ed. The Foot in Diabetes. Philadelphia 1991: Lea and Febiger, 71–91.
[75] Hutton WC, Stokes IAF. Mechanics of the foot. In: Klenerman L, ed. The Foot and its Disorders. London: Blackwell Scientific Publications, 1991, 11–25.
[76] Cavanagh PR, Ulbrecht JS. Biomechanics of the foot in diabetes mellitus. In: Levin MF, O'Neal LW, Bowker JH, eds. The Diabetic Foot. St Louis: Mosby Year Book, 1993, 199–232.
[77] Duckworth T, Boulton AJM, Betts RP et al. Plantar pressure measurements and the prevention of ulceration in the diabetic foot. J Bone Jt Surg 1985; 67B: 79–85.
[78] Grundy M, Blackburn TPA, McLeish RD et al. An investigation of the centres of pressure under the foot whilst walking. J Bone Surg 1975; 57B: 98–103.
[79] Lord M. Foot pressure measurement: a review of methodology. J Biomed Engineering 1981; 3: 91–99.
[80] Harris RI, Beath T. Army foot survey. An investigation of foot ailments in Canadian soldiers. Ottowa, Canada: National Research Council, 1947; No 1574.
[81] Silvino N, Evanski PM, Waugh TR. The Harris Beath footprinting mat: diagnostic validity and clinical use. Clin Orthop Rel Res 1980, 151: 265–269.
[82] Minns RJ. Two simple plantar pressure recording devices in clinical use: evaluation using a pedobaragraph. Eng in Med 1982; 11: 117–120.
[83] Aritomi H, Morita M, Yonemoto K. A simple method of measuring the footsole pressure of normal subjects using prescale pressure-detecting sheets. J Biomech 1983; 16: 157–165.
[84] Stokes IAF, Stott JRR, Hutton WC. Force distributions under the foot – a dynamic measuring system. Biomechanical Engineering 1976; 9: 140–143.
[85] Dhanendran M, Hutton WC, Parker Y. The distribution of forces under the human foot – an on line measuring system. Measurement and Control 1978; 11: 261–264.
[86] Nicol K, Hennig EM. Measurement of pressure distribution by means of a flexible large surface mat. Biomechanics VI A. Baltimore: Univ Park Press, 1978; 374–380.
[87] Cavanagh PR, Ulbrecht JS. Plantar pressure in the diabetic foot. In: Sammarco GJ, ed. The Foot in Diabetes. Philadelphia: Lea & Febiger, 1991; 54–70.
[88] Hughes J, Pratt L, Linge K et al. Reliability of pressure measurements: the EMED-F system. Clinical Biomechanics 1991; 6: 14–18.
[89] Van der Meer D, Weir D. The Musgrave footprint. ACTUK Journal (Association of Chiropody Teachers in the United Kingdom) 1988; Autumn 2–3.
[90] Duckworth T, Betts RP, Franks J et al. The measurement of pressures under the foot. Foot Ankle 1982; 3: 130–141.
[91] Masson EA, Boulton AJM. Pressure assessment methods in the foot. In: Frykberg RG, ed. The High Risk Foot in Diabetes Mellitus. New York: Churchill Livingstone, 1991; 139–149.
[92] Cavanagh PR, Hewitt FG Jr., Perry JE. In shoe plantar pressure measurement: a review. The Foot 1992, 2: 185–194.

[93] Rose NE, Feiwell L, Cracchiolo A. A method for measuring foot pressures using a high resolution, computerised insole sensor: the effect of heel wedges on plantar pressure distribution and centre of force. Foot & Ankle 1992; 13 (5): 263–270.
[94] Tappin JW, Pollard J, Bechett EA. Method of measuring shear forces on the sole of the foot. Clin Phys Physiol Meas 1980; (1): 83–85.
[95] Laing P, Deogan H, Cogley D et al. The development of the low profile Liverpool shear transducer. Clin Phys Physiol Meas 1992; 13: 115–124.
[96] Lord M, Hosein R, Williams RB. Method for in shoe shear stress measurement. J Biomed Eng 1992; 14: 181–186.
[97] Krag MH. Quantitative techniques for analysis of gait. Automedica 1985; 6: 85–97.
[98] McBride ID, Wyss VP, Cooke TDV et al. First metatarsophalangeal joint reaction forces during high heel gait. Foot Ankle 1971; 11: 282–288.
[99] Andriaceli TP. Biomechanics and gait analysis in total kee replacement. Orthop Rev 1988; 17: 470–473.
[100] Cavanagh PR, Ulbrecht JS. The diabetic foot: a quantitative approach to the assessment of neuropathy, deformity and plantar pressure. In: Jahss M, ed. Disorders of the Foot. 2nd Ed. 1990.
[101] Rogers MM, Cavanagh PR. A device for the measurement of first ray mobility. In: Proceedings of the North American Congress on Biomechanics 1986. Montreal, Canada, 205–206.
[102] Birke JA, Cornwall MA, Jackson M. Relationship between hallux limitus and ulceration of the great toe. J of Orthop Sports Phys Ther 1988; 10: 172–176.
[103] Root ML, Orien WP, Weed JH et al. Biomechanical examination of the foot. Vol 1. Los Angeles Clinical Biomechanics Corp. 1971.
[104] Smith LS, Clarke TE, Hamill CL. The effects of soft and semirigid orthoses upon the rear foot movement in running. Podiatr Sports Med 1986, 76: 227–233.
[105] Fromberg WA. Examination. In: Hunt GC, ed. Physical Therapy of the Foot and Ankle. New York: Churchill Livingstone, 1988; 59–90.
[106] Delbridge L, Perry P, Marr S et al. Limited joint mobility and the diabetic foot: relationship to neuropathic ulceration. Diab Med 1988; 5: 333–337.
[107] Fernando DJS, Hutchinson A, Veves A et al. Relationship of limited joint mobility to abnormal foot pressures and diabetic foot ulceration. Diabetes Care 1991; 14: 8–11.

Research methodologies related to renal complications: structural changes

R. Østerby

Quantitative morphology

The introductory sections deal with general considerations concerning the objectives of quantitative structural studies, requirements that must be fulfilled, practical performance and categories of data. The following sections present examples of the applications within the area of renal problems in diabetes along with methodological considerations relevant to the individual measurements.

Objectives of quantitative structural studies

At the end of a quantitative morphological study, the results comprise a list of numbers, in which each structure is represented as a mean value. An evaluation of the accuracy of individual data is important for the interpretation of these results. Were the requirements for obtaining the data fulfilled; were the estimates heavily influenced by tissue preparation; how precise are the estimates? The mean values may reflect completely different conditions, i. e., if the parameter in question shows a marked variation between different areas, or if the kidney is homogeneous in that respect.

Assuming that a reasonable validity of the parameters exists, they may be useful for the description of the kidney. Such numerical – rather than verbal – descriptions are necessary for comparisons among clinically defined groups of cases, for the determination of a time course, and for the study of relationships between structural changes and clinical variables, e. g., some aspects of renal function or presumed risk factors.

Categories of structural quantities

Many structural parameters are estimated as densities within a defined reference space. The estimation may concern volume (ℓ^3), area of interfaces (ℓ^2), length of tubular structures (ℓ^1) and number of isolated particles (ℓ^0). With decreasing dimension the requirements and the necessary efforts increase: "for area and length estimates concern about the orientation distribution between structure and the plane of sectioning is needed" [1, 2]; to obtain number of isolated particles sampling of known volumes is required [3], which is more elaborate than sampling areas. The densities provide information about the composition of the space under study. Total quantities (total volume, area, length, number) can be derived from the densities when the total volume of the reference space is known. This last step may provide useful insights into the actual changes to individual structures.

A calculation of matrix volume per glomerulus is an example, which uses series of magnifications and two sequential levels having one reference space in common:

$$V(\text{matrix}) = V_V(\text{matrix/mesang}) \cdot V_V(\text{mesang/glom}) \cdot V(\text{glom})$$

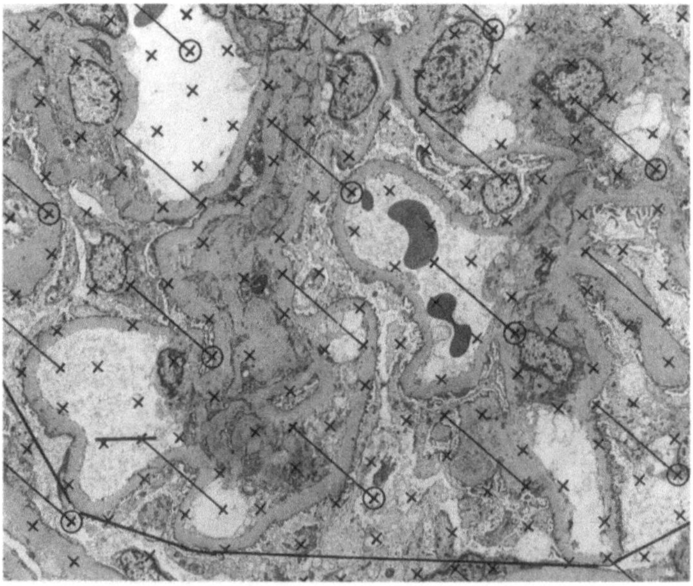

Fig. 1 Section of glomerular profile with the circumscribed, minimal, convex polygon indicated. The polygon is the reference space common to this level and light microscopy. The integral point and line grid is superposed in an independent position, since the placing of the micrograph with respect to the glomerulus was not independent. The magnification ~ 2,300x is used for the point-counting of polygon, tuft, and mesangium (ratio of points 1 : 1 : 8), and for counting intersections between test lines and three subsets of interfaces: PBM/urinary space, mesangium/capillary space and mesangium/urinary space

The first factor is estimated at ~ 10,000 ×, the second at 2–3,000 ×, the third at light microscopy (2–300 × magnification). The reference space common to first and second factor is the mesangial region, to second and third the circumscribed polygon (Fig. 1). Composition data and data on total quantities give different types of information, and it is important to realize which question is relevant in the clinical context.

The size of individual structures may also be of interest, and may be obtainable: renal and glomerular volume, membrane thickness, epithelial foot process width, and filtration slit width. Here not only mean values, but also the distribution of sizes are obtainable [2, 4–7].

Requirements for obtaining valid data

The fundamental requirements for obtaining valid data pertain to the sampling process, which is the most important step of the whole study. Sampling must be unbiased and sufficient, and preferably efficient as well. Unbiased and sufficient sampling is important at all levels: in the composition of patient groups, sampling from the kidney (a biopsy), sampling of blocks, levels, individual structures, visual fields, and points of measurements. When kidney biopsies are studied, we are not always free to design the optimal study concerning patient groups, and due respect should be paid to it when drawing conclusions. The use of data obtained in a kidney biopsy assumes that this small fraction of the kidney is representative of the whole [8]. Unbiased sampling of visual fields with a light microscope can be obtained with step-motors connected to the specimen stage. In the electron microscope micrographs can be sampled by moving the specimen stage in predetermined steps, marked on the handles. New options are available, for example, in the Philips microscope the stage controls can be directed by a programme which chooses fields within a specified area, either random or systematic random.

For sufficient sampling the requirements are different depending on which structure is estimated, and on the stage of disease. Obviously, less extensive sampling is needed with a low variation.

In cost-benefit terms, the advantages of performing efficient sampling are obvious. The general rule says that a large part of the effort should never be invested in a small area [7, 9], i. e., very precise measurement of individual micrographs is waste of effort. Instead, counting should be divided between many micrographs, or visual fields, representing a larger fraction of the total area. Therefore, the lowest magnification at which the structures are reasonably easy to identify should be chosen.

The influence of tissue preparation

The measurements are made from tissue in its processed form. How these data relate to the in vivo conditions is not known. Often it is not possible to check, and at best such a study would be very tedious.

A poor quality of fixation implies changes before the embedding, and the identification of structures may be hampered. For instance, capillary collapse would influence the structural composition. In the embedding procedure itself swelling or shrinkage of the whole tissue or parts thereof may also occur. It is therefore important to have a study design which minimizes the influence of tissue processing.

In most studies, the main questions concern comparisons between groups, e. g. diabetic patients vs. controls, or diabetic patients in different stages of disease. Ideally, the groups should be investigated concomitantly, and in random order, so that the laboratory procedures, fixation, embedding, batch of plastic polymers etc., are comparable. Hopefully, the structural modifications are thereby similar among groups. Admittedly, for biopsy series, this is not always possible in practice, such as in follow-up biopsies, where data from one patient is compared with that from the same patient some time later. What can be done is to keep the protocol as constant throughout as possible, and to use prescriptions and materials which prove to be reliable.

Definition of structures

An important condition in quantitative morphology is that the structures in question are precisely defined and described, e. g. profiles of mesangial regions, peripheral BM vs. mesangial matrix, and the areas used for reference space. Within the setting of one study an effort should be made to have one person do all measurements of the different groups for one structure category, and in random order, in order to produce the best possible consistency of morphological definitions.

The tools for obtaining structural data

The stereological methods: Stereological methods enable us to achieve data valid for 3-dimensional organs based on the observations of 2-dimensional cross-sections [2, 7, 10]. A set of formulas exists for this purpose. Their background and derivation are available in original papers referred to in text books and reviews [2, 3]. Their application depends on correct sampling. Therefore, it is necessary for the user to know the requirements which must be fulfilled for the individual formulas to be valid, requirements which usually need to be fulfilled during the sampling procedures.

Practical collection of data: The simple way of obtaining data is to use test probes, and to count the number of events. Counting is faster than measuring. For estimation of volume the probe is 0-dimensional points. The number of points hitting the structure of interest (a) relative to number of hits on the reference space (r) directly supplies the estimate of volume fraction, $V_V(a/r)$, which is dimensionless. Since the reference space is the larger of the two, it is advantageous to use a grid with two sets of points. Fewer points are needed for larger, more regular and coherent spaces. The ratio of 'coarse' and 'fine' (closer) points enters as a factor in the denominator. Grids with several sets of points (Figs. 1–2) are advantageous when several compartments are estimated.

The estimation of surface area density within the reference space is obtained by counting the intersections of the trace of surface and (1-D) test lines. The number of intersections increases with increasing surface density and with testline length within the reference space. The relationship is simple: $S_V = 2 \cdot I_L$, where I is the number of intersections and L the total line length within the reference space. The latter is estimated by point counting, using an integral test system with known ratio of points and line length (Fig. 1). The formula is correct, provided there is a uniform orientation distribution between test lines and the surface [1], i.e. any orientation is equally likely. This is fulfilled in random sections, if the structure itself has a uniform orientation distribution (isotropy), otherwise special precautions must be taken in preparing the sections to provide isotropy, or else the more special application of vertical sections is used [3]. Length of tubular structures (e.g. capillaries, filtration slits) is estimated by counting number of profiles (Q) within the (2-D) reference area (A). Counting profiles requires sampling independent of size and shape, which is easily obtained with an unbiased sampling frame [3]. The estimate of length density in the reference space is $L_V = 2 \cdot Q_A$, provided uniform orientation distribution between the tubular structure and the sampling areas [11].

The estimation of the number density (e.g. of glomeruli or cells) is done by sampling volumes, using the so-called disector: two parallel sections a known (measured) distance apart, one section with a sampling frame. The number of new-appearing objects (e.g. glomeruli) within the sampled volumes is the unbiased estimate of number per volume [12].

Test grids on visual fields or micrographs must be placed independently of the structures. If the field was obtained with a random position within the tissue, the grid may be placed systematically, e. g. aligned with the sides of the field (Fig. 2).

Advanced technical equipment with image analysis may lead to the same estimates. The drawback of this expensive machinery is that relatively great effort is made to get very detailed information about individual fields, which, however, provides only small amounts of information.

For each study, a protocol, which dictates exactly where to make sections, micrographs, measurements, and gives concise structural definitions must be worked out in advance. Afterwards there are no choices to be made during the course of the study.

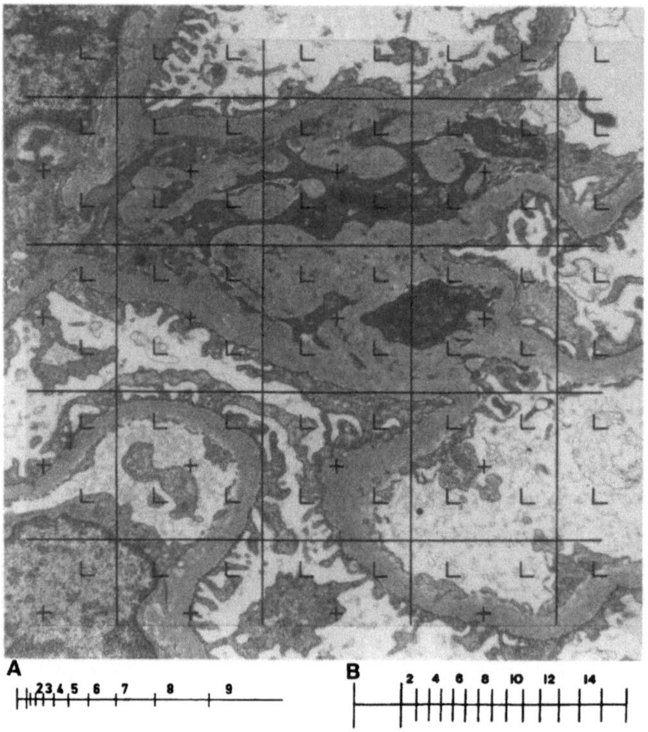

Fig. 2 The micrograph (magnification ~ 10,000x) was made with an independent position with respect to the glomerulus. The grid may then be placed systematically, as shown. This setting was used for the point-counting of tuft, mesangium (reference space common to this level and the low magnification, Fig. 1), matrix and PBM, using ratio of points = 1 : 2 : 4 : 4. The grid lines are used for the sampling of measuring points for PBM thickness (ruler A). Intercepts for matrix star volume are classified (ruler B) through ∟-hits, parallel to the horizontal grid lines

Among these measures mentioned above, only volume fractions are dimensionless. In all other cases the magnification must be known. In electron microscopy, a grating replica is photographed and prints made along with the micrographs for the calculation of actual magnification.

The following sections provide examples of the application in the diabetic kidney, as subdivided by the renal compartments. Most studies have concerned glomerular changes.

The quantitative estimation of glomerular changes in diabetes

Diabetic glomerulopathy

The sampling of glomeruli must be done independently of glomerular appearance. Ideal sampling [5] in order to be independent of glomerular size – requires exclusion of the glomerular profiles present on a random section, e. g. the first in the block (over-representation of large glomeruli), and exclusion of complete profiles with centres within the periphery of blocks, (over-representation of small glomeruli) [13]. However, in dealing with kidney biopsies it is not acceptable to sacrifice precious glomerular tissue for a theoretically optimal sampling.

A random level within glomeruli is represented e. g. in the first section in a block. If glomerular profiles are not present the next sampling level must be at least one glomerular radius deeper to avoid preferential sampling of peripheral segments [14]. Sampling of equidistantly spaced levels, with random position within glomeruli is done at predetermined distances from the baseline sections [15, 16]. Thin sections covering the entire extent of the block can be cut with diamond knives, thus avoiding trimming away any glomerular structures.

The description of the changes characterizing diabetic glomerulopathy is based on the thickness of the peripheral basement membrane (PBM) and estimates of the mesangial regions and the mesangial matrix.

Basement membrane thickness: There are two possible procedures for determining basement membrane thickness. In the first, thickness is estimated only where the section is perpendicular to the membrane surface, i. e. what appears on the section is the true thickness [16, 17]. Perpendicularity can be determined for the glomerular basement membrane (BM) [18]. Measuring points are sampled with a test-line grid. The probability of hitting the endothelial aspect with a test line is independent of BM thickness. At points of intersection between lines and the endothelial–BM interface the thickness is classified, provided the epithelial cell membrane is distinct at this point.

The second procedure is to estimate apparent thickness at any sectioning angle, and apply stereology for calculation of true thickness [4, 19]. The distance from the endothelial cell membrane perpendicular to the opposite epithelial cell membrane is termed the orthogonal intercept. The use of harmonic mean thickness, calculated from reciprocal intercept lengths, has some theoretical advantages to the arithmetic mean [19], and may be used for the measurements of true thickness as well.

With both methods a ruler is used for classification rather than exact measurements (Fig. 2). A ruler with narrow divisions in the low end is most efficient. Approximately 100–200 'true' thickness observations, (~ 50% more for orthogonal intercepts) are required per biopsy, provided an efficient distribution, i.e. at a reasonably low magnification (~ 10,000 × for normal thickness, mean ~ 3–4 mm on the micrographs), so that a large number of capillary loops are sampled. This is decisive in the orthogonal intercept method, since each loop often represents only one orientation. The class distributions are totalled from ~ 3 glomerular profiles before the calculation of the harmonic mean, i.e. the same class limits (same magnification) should pertain to all glomeruli studied in each biopsy. If desired, calculations can be done using the true thickness, for individual glomerular profiles and individual loops.

An increased thickness of the PBM is the first detectable sign of diabetic glomerulopathy [17]. The detection of minor increases in small groups of patients depends on the low variation in this measure among normal individuals. This is true even if BM thickness within any one glomerular cross section shows a very wide distribution. The inter-glomerular variation within biopsies in IDDM patients with early glomerulopathy showed a CV (coefficient of variation = SD/mean) of 7.4% [16]. Comparison of two separate biopsies, obtained from either kidney in cadaveric kidney donors, showed a CE of the double estimate of 1%, with a mean number of orthogonal intercepts per biopsy of 270 [8].

Mesangial and matrix volume fractions: For estimates of volume fractions, the main points to discuss concern sufficient and efficient sampling, assuming that unbiased sampling is always ensured.

The volume fraction of mesangium per glomerulus, V_V(mes/glom), tends to show a large variation within groups, also in normal subjects [20–22]. The demonstration of minor changes therefore requires improved precision. The question is whether this measure really has such a large biological variation among individuals, or whether the problem is imprecision in the estimation. Part of the variation in published data is likely to derive from a sparse sampling at a high magnification [21]. A methodological study addressed the question of distribution of variance of the V_V(mes/glom), the data from wich are shown in Tables 1–2. A sampling of sets of thin sections, spaced 30 μm apart, at a random position within glomeruli was performed, sectioning glomeruli exhaustively (Fig. 3). Photomontages, covering the entire profiles were prepared at each level at 1540 × magnification and the V_V(mes/glom) was

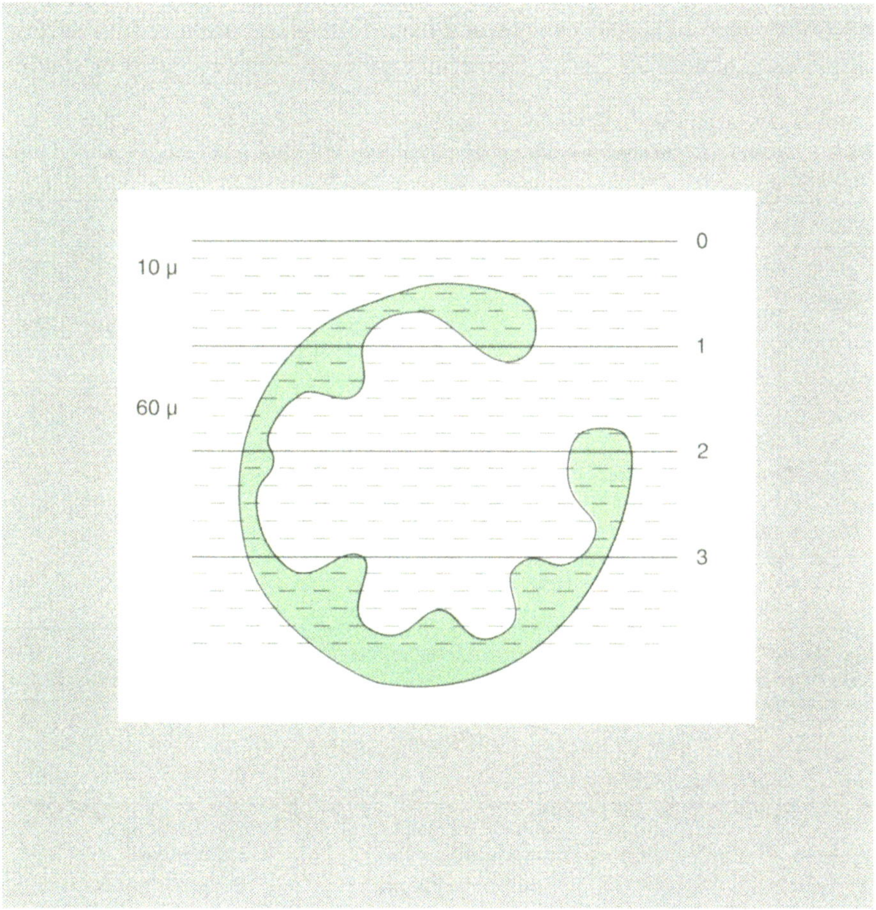

Fig. 3 The sampling of sections at random levels through glomeruli: the first 3 levels within a new-appearing glomerulus, with distance from the baseline section of 60 μm or multiples thereof, are sampled. The complete three levels are photographed at the low magnification (Fig. 1); within the largest of the three a systematic random sample ~ 25% of the area, is photographed at higher magnification (Fig. 2). All levels of the glomerulus, with 10 μm intervals are used for light microscopy, for the estimation of Cavalieri volume. For the analysis of variance of mesangial volume fraction, all levels of the glomerulus, with 30 μm intervals are used

estimated with an 8 : 1-grid. The V_V(mes/glom) estimates were calculated for each level, and for the glomerulus as a whole $\Sigma P(mes)/(\Sigma P(glom) \cdot 8)$ over all levels. The estimate for individual biopsies was derived from the ratio of points, summed over sections and over glomeruli. This is the standard procedure to obtain any ratio estimator for a given specimen. Particularly in the non-diabetic group, the intra- and interbiopsy variation was very low (Table 1).

The distribution of variance was studied in a nested analysis of variance. ANOVAs were balanced with results from four glomeruli and four sections within each glomerulus, extra glomeruli and levels being excluded by random

Table 1 Inter- and intrabiopsy variation in mesangial volume fraction with extensive intra-glomerular sampling

	IDDM	ND
n	4	4
Age	25	25
	(20–29)	(20–29)
Diabetes duration	9.5	
Years	(6–13)	
No. of glomeruli per biopsy	5.5	5.8
	(4–6)	(4–8)
No. of levels per glomerulus	5.3	5.2
	(4–9)	(3–7)
V_V(mes/glom), mean	0.21	0.19
V_V(mes/glom), CV among cases	0.18	0.08
V_V(mes/glom), CV among glomeruli	0.15	0.09
	(0.10–0.18)	(0.05–0.11)

The IDDM patients had normal albumin excretion, creatinine clearance, and blood pressure. Ranges are given in parentheses

Table 2 A balanced, nested analysis of variance

	Volume fraction mesang/glomerulus variance component, %	Surface density PBM/glomerulus variance component, %
Cases	6	13
Glomeruli	4	4
Levels within glomeruli	80	23
Repeat measures		60

For the S_V estimate a double counting was done on each profile. This was not done for volume fraction estimate numbers. The results showed no significant differences between the normo-albuminuric diabetic patients and controls. The variation between the glomeruli within each case was not a significant factor to the total variation, whereas the contributions from individual cases and from sections within glomeruli were significant. Estimates of variance components are shown in Table 2: 80% of the total lay among sections within glomeruli, indicating that as long as the near-normal conditions are under study, more extensive sampling within glomeruli is a good investment of effort. Systematic level-sectioning and estimation of V_V(mesang/glom) in 3 levels in each of 3 glomeruli has been used in recent studies of normo- and micro-albuminuric diabetic patients [15, 16].

Matrix star volume: Star volume is the average of volumes that can be 'seen' from random points within the structure [3]. It is an absolute measure which increases with increasing size and convexity of individual subunits. Matrix star volume is estimated in a set of micrographs, sampled with an independent position and orientation with respect to the matrix and at a suitable magnification (~ 10,000 ×). A point grid is superimposed, and through all points hitting matrix an intercept is classified (example of ruler, Fig. 2) in a predetermined direction. The star volume is calculated from observations totalled over a number (~ 3) of profiles: $\bar{V} = \pi/3 \cdot \ell^3$. In advanced stages of diabetic glomerulopathy the confluence and convexity of matrix branches is remarkable. Recent measurements concerned earlier stages of glomerulopathy (Table 3). A large intra-group variation was found. Analysis of variance

Table 3 Mesangial matrix star volume

Group	n	No. of intercepts per biopsy	Star volume μm^3	CV	Variance components		
					Cases %	Glomeruli %	Intercepts %
ND	12	169 (81–264)	14 (8–21)	0.32	−36	92	44
D_{NA}	9	152 (75–284)	22 (14–46)	0.43	70	12	18
D_{MI}	29	284 (111–693)	34 (15–100)	0.52	30	59	12
D_P	11	314 (121–456)	195 (29–559)	0.90	63	34	4

The groups are non-diabetic cases (ND); insulin-dependent diabetic (D) patients with normal albumin excretion (NA), microalbuminuria (MI) or proteinuria (P)

showed a heavy contribution from glomeruli. Whether this is attributable to the small sampling fraction, ~ 25–30% out of 3 glomerular profiles per case, or to the fact that glomeruli are different, is not known (a problem analogous to the estimates of mesangial volume fraction). However, even with the large variation between glomeruli, and the large intra-group variation, the abnormality of this parameter in early stages of diabetic glomerulopathy is clearly detectable; thus, for this particular purpose, an increase in sensitivity is not needed.

Matrix derived thickness, T: An arbitrary matrix thickness can be calculated as the volume-to-surface ratio. Using identical reference volume the estimate equals the ratio of volume fraction to surface density. For the mesangial matrix:
matrix-T = V_V(matrix/mes)/S_V(mesangial-urinary surface/mes)
is the arbitrary thickness of matrix, if spread in an even layer on the urinary surface of the mesangial regions. It increases with increasing mesangial volume (which implies decreasing S_V), and with increasing fraction of the matrix. It may be of interest in early stages, although a low precision should be taken into account.

Structural modifications associated with diabetic glomerulopathy

The parameters dealt with above are the main pillars of the characteristic glomerular changes. Along with these changes, several other structural modifications take place. Some of these are the decisive causes of functional abnormalities.

Area of glomerular interfaces: The structural variable relevant to GFR is the total area of filtration surface in the kidneys. Filtration surface has been used to denote the interface capillary-urinary space.

Estimates of filtration surface in kidney biopsies are expressed as surface area per mean size glomerulus, thereby taking into account the fraction of glomeruli that are totally occluded, i. e. with no surface left. Comparing data among individuals and among groups the assumption is that no systematic differences obtain in total glomerular number. The estimate is: Surface per nephron = S_V(PBM/glom), in open glomeruli · mean size of open glomeruli · fraction of open glomeruli.

The estimator surface density tends to vary considerably within groups. An analysis of variance showed that individual cases and levels within glomeruli contributed significantly to the total variance (Table 2). More than 80% of the variance lay within glomeruli, and the majority of this contribution was due to the counting, as shown by double counting.

The surface density estimates themselves are of only minor interest. They increase with increasing magnification [2]. They decrease as a necessary consequence of increase in mesangial volume fraction; but they also decrease with increasing glomerular volume, even in isomorphic enlargement [5, 23]. In enlarged glomeruli, with decreased surface density, the total surface area may well be increased.

Ratio of glomerular interfaces: Intercept counting provides direct estimates of the relationship between various interfaces. When orientation requirements are fulfilled for all surfaces the ratio of their areas equals the ratio of intercept countings. These very simple calculations have shown changes in the capillary and mesangial surfaces with developing glomerulopathy (Fig. 4).

Capillary diameter: Estimates of capillary diameter are of special interest with respect to capillary wall tension.

Three-dimensionally valid estimates of mean diameter are only obtainable by indirect measures. The ratio of volume to length, (which equals the volume fraction/length density, using identical reference space) gives average cross sectional area [24]. Or, the ratio of surface density of capillary wall and length density gives the average circumference [25]. To get from these measures to a diameter, the assumption of shape (circular!) enters. The ratio of surface to length has the advantage of being less sensitive to varying capillary collapse, but it is more biased if capillaries are not cylindrical. Permanent capillary concavities may be present in advanced glomerulopathy due to protruding mesangial-capillary interface. Thus diameter calculated from circumference is overestimated.

Epithelial cell configuration: Average foot process width can be obtained with two different methods. One uses the same basics as the estimation of membrane thickness: the distribution of distances between two neighbouring filtration slits [6]. It implies classification of a large number of apparent distances from which the mean and the distribution of foot process width are calculated. A bias enters due to curvature of the surfaces, in particular the mesangial surfaces. The alternative method is quick, but does not give distribution data. Mean width is calculated as the ratio of urinary surface of the tuft (i. e. the surface on which the feet are standing) and length of filtration slits, or the ratio of two densities, with identical reference volume. The rela-

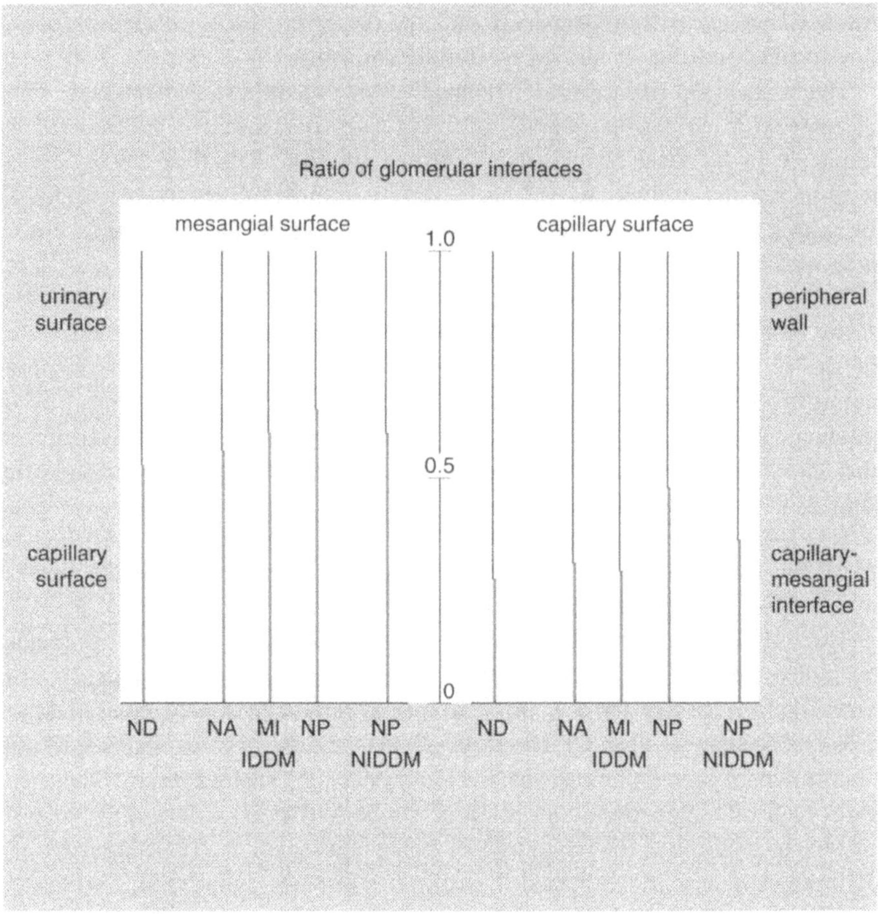

Fig. 4 The ratio of glomerular interfaces in patient groups: ND non-diabetic kidney donors; IDDM and NIDDM groups characterized by albumin excretion: NA: Normoalbuminuria, MI: microalbuminuria; NP: overt nephropathy with proteinuria. The two subsets of mesangial surface (shown to the left) are of equal size in normal glomeruli, but with increasing glomerulopathy the surface towards the capillary makes up a larger fraction. The two subsets of capillary surface (shown to the right) also show a shift in advanced stages, the peripheral part (filtration surface) constituting a smaller fraction of the total

tionship may be realized the other way round: total slit length factored by arithmetic mean width equals the entire surface.

The width of filtration slits, the interspaces between neighbouring foot processes, cannot be determined from random cuts with any orientation between slit axis and plane of sectioning, since the dimension of slits is in the order of section thickness. A method can be applied using classification of true width, determined by the appearance of triple layered cell membranes. High magnification is required (~ 120,000), and an elaborate protocol for the systematic random sampling (Bjørn, SF et al, unpublished).

Glomerular occlusion: The frequency of glomerular occlusion has been estimated from the count of open and occluded profiles, a process which underestimates of the fraction of occluded glomeruli, since they are smaller than open glomeruli. The bias can be corrected with estimates of the diameter of open and occluded glomeruli [26, 27]. An alternative procedure is the systematic sectioning of the biopsy and a count of the number of new appearing corpuscles, open and occluded [28]. This gives an unbiased estimate of the fraction, which may turn out to be very much different from that based on observed number of profiles in a limited number of sections. The still remaining problem is the small volume available in a biopsy, and the non-random distribution of occlusion within the kidney [29].

Glomerular volume

Estimation of glomerular volume is of interest in relationship to the hypertrophy early in the course of diabetes, and to the later compensatory enlargement. One major problem is the limited number of glomeruli available. A number of methods are available, with somewhat differing properties in terms of assumptions and workload.

Estimates from average profile area: The relationship between area and volume is: $\bar{V} = (\beta/K) \cdot \bar{A}^{3/2}$ [2, 19], where β depends on shape (1.38 for spheres). The factor K depends on the (unknown) size distribution characteristics. The requirement of spherical shape is sometimes reasonably fulfilled. For comparison among groups it is acceptable that the size distribution is unknown, so long as it is similar among the groups. This cannot be tested, and in different disease states it may well be different.

Average area is easily estimated by point counting, but the problem lies in sampling enough random profiles for the estimate. The necessary number depends on the variation in volume; but less than 30 profiles is not acceptable. The sampled profiles, on the other hand, need not belong to the same number of glomeruli, i. e. several levels may be sampled from one glomerulus.

Estimates using the disector: This method provides unbiased estimates, but it is time consuming. The simple derivation is: mean volume equals volume fraction (glom/cortex) divided by numerical density: number of glomeruli per cortex [30, 31]. The latter is estimated using the disector [12]: two parallel sections a known distance apart, with an unbiased sampling area within one section. New-appearing structures within the known sampling volume provides the numerical density. A major problem lies in sampling enough of these known volumes, since the numerical density of glomeruli varies considerably within different cortical areas.

Estimates using the Cavalieri principle: This estimate is unbiased, but time consuming. It requires exhaustive sectioning through a number of new-appearing glomeruli, i. e. sampled independently of size. A subset of equidistantly spaced sections is sampled from serial sections (systematic, random, as shown Fig. 3), and profile areas are measured (point counting). The average distance between levels must be estimated [32]. The number of glomeruli necessary for a reliable mean value depends on the variation in size. Measurement of ~ 10 glomeruli per biopsy showed an intra-biopsy CV of glomerular volume in the range 0.20–0.30.

Estimates from largest cross section: This is a perfect method so long as the glomeruli are perfect spheres. It requires some step-sectioning for the determination of the largest profile [30].

Volume-weighted mean glomerular volume: The point-sampled intercepts, as used for the matrix star volume, can be used also for estimation of a mean volume, the volume-weighted mean [33]. This procedure can be performed on random sections, i. e. it does not require the more elaborate sampling of level-sections or of known volumes. The method is particularly sensitive for detecting volume changes that imply a subpopulation of much enlarged glomeruli. Since the result is not the mean of the number-distribution it cannot be used for the calculation of total quantities, such as total filtration surface.

Number of glomeruli and cells

The total number of glomeruli in the kidney can be estimated as the product of numerical density and kidney volume. Such estimates are hardly reasonable within the space of a kidney biopsy. The method is useful in autopsy kidneys. For the whole kidney, an alternative method, the fractionator, may be used: Glomerular number is counted in a known, strictly random, fraction of the organ. The final counting within the chosen fraction includes exhaustive sectioning of a number of blocks. This method has been used in a series of cases, including IDDM and NIDDM patients and controls. The average number per kidney was in the order of ~ 600,000 with a CV of ~ 0.30 [34]. No differences were shown between the three groups.

The number of cell nuclei can be obtained with disector methods. In this case, the short-cut of using an optical disector, i. e. focusing into the depth rather than cutting, may be useful. It should be noted that unbiased estimates of numerical density have only been obtained with the fairly recently developed methods, and that older data may be neglected.

Cortical interstitium

The expansion of the interstitial tissue may be estimated by volume fraction, so the problems are those of sufficient and unbiased sampling (unbiased estimates are not obtained if 'abnormal fields' or 'normal fields' are considered) [35]. Advanced stages of fibrosis usually show a patchy distribution, therefore a renal biopsy may not be representative of the whole organ. The choice of reference space may be more efficient by using the part of the cortex outside glomeruli and the larger vessels, i. e. excluding the areas where interstitial tissue is never found, which furthermore may occupy a large fraction of a given section.

Extra-glomerular blood vessels

The diabetic arteriolar lesion is characterized by an increase in the proportion of matrix in the vessel wall and by a patchy occurrence [27]. Some arteriolar profiles often show marked changes, while other segments appear normal, so the main problem again is sufficient sampling. In semiquantitative studies, the number of profiles with a certain degree of abnormality have been counted. This estimate is difficult to interpret, since its meaning varies considerably with the size of individual profiles. Quantitative studies are not available, but unpublished data show an increase in matrix volume fraction, and in matrix-T for afferent and efferent arterioles in IDDM patients with only moderate glomerulopathy.

Interrelation of changes in various compartments

The development of individual structural changes over time has been considered by determining correlations between measures of the various components. Such correlations suffer from differences in the validity of estimates. Increase in BM thickness is detectable before mesangial expansion, which may or may not be due to the failure to measure the earliest mesangial changes, which requires extensive sampling. In advanced stages, the correlation has been reported to be poor. On this end of the spectrum, differences may obtain regarding interglomerular variation: Variation in BM thickness increases with developing glomerulopathy; whereas that of mesangial expansion perhaps decreases. The inclusion of endstage kidneys is particularly problematic: in the very few glomeruli, still-open, with only a few capillaries left, BM thickness is hardly a meaningful measure any more. Presently available data on the early stages of glomerulopathy are compatible with a concurrent development of changes in the PBM and in the mesangial matrix [36].

Whereas the individual structures must be considered separately for quantitation, it is the sum of changes in all compartments that is relevant to functional consequences.

To sum up glomerular changes an index of the glomerulopathy may be constructed and has been used for structure-function relationships. How the individual elements of the index should be balanced cannot be calculated in a rational manner. A glomerulopathy index (BM thickness/10 + V_V(matrix/glom) · 100) showed a correlation with an index summing up functional abnormalities in a series of IDDM patients with a broad range of functional involvement [25], and in a range of normal to slightly-impaired function [36]. The combination of glomerular and extra-glomerular changes is just as important, but this has not yet been approached.

Interrelation of structural changes and clinical variables

The questions raised concerning structure-function correlations differ somewhat in nature, depending on whether a very broad or narrow range of the two variables is considered. Looking at the full range of variables from almost normal to the end-stage situation, most correlations will be highly significant but do not provide detailed information. Several problems appear in taking more narrow ranges: it is sometimes unknown which is the relevant structural change, or rather the relevant combination of changes, to associate with a given clinical parameter, for instance albuminuria. The positive correlation with mesangial volume fraction found when end-stage kidneys are included is not helpful. Another problem may be the lack of sufficiently sensitive measurements of either structure or function, e. g. relationships between GFR and filtration surface if the range does not include the extremes. Furthermore, in this latter example, the structural dimension is but one of several determinants of the GFR. In structure-function relationships the interaction between different compartments should not be forgotten, and the nature of the questions should be made clear.

The rationale for quantitative structural studies of kidney biopsies

The intra-group variations in structural parameters overlap within groups, and the variation around regression lines raises questions regarding the rationale for kidney biopsies. Distinctions should be made between questions related to the *individual* patient, i. e. concerning diagnosis and prognosis, and research questions involving groups of patients. None of the measures described herein are 'specific' to diabetes, and so are not useful for diagnostic purposes.

Concerning prognosis, a very good agreement has been found in one NIDDM study between structural parameters and the ensuing course of renal function [28]. This finding, however, pertains to a group, and covers a rather broad range. Nothing is known about the variation in the pattern of development for individual patients over time, whether diabetic glomerulopathy usually progresses at a constant rate, or whether periods of deceleration may occur. Data to answer these questions require follow-up studies.

As for research questions, some very important questions exist, concerning possible intervention in the development of renal lesions.

It is suggested that the main task in future morphological studies is to evaluate intervention trials in relatively small, well-defined groups of patients. The best chances for intervention are likely to be in the early stages of micro-albuminuria or perhaps in patients with normal AER. Without clinical markers for the latter group, a structural analysis might be useful. Proof of this has not yet been presented. Whether the early increase in BM thickness is acceptable as the sign of 'incipient glomerulopathy' is decisive concerning the stage of micro-albuminuria. If only mesangial expansion is accepted as an endpoint, then the study is perhaps only feasible, when it is in fact too late: when mesangial expansion is detectable, with a practicable extent of the analysis, the progression may not be amenable to intervention. The level of measurement precision necessary for useful information is an important consideration regarding the questions dealt with. Improving precision in the analysis obviously makes the study more time-consuming. However, the invaluable gain of deriving useful data from small biopsy series, in order to address precise questions, should not be overlooked.

References

[1] Gundersen HJ. Stereology and sampling of biological surfaces. In: Echlin P, ed. The Analysis of Organic and Biological Surfaces. New York: J. Wiley & Sons, 1985; 477–506.

[2] Weibel ER. Stereological Methods. Practical Methods for Biological Morphometry, Vol. 1. New York: Academic Press, 1980.

[3] Gundersen HJ, Bendtsen TF, Korbo L et al. Some new, simple and efficient stereological methods and their use in pathological research and diagnosis. APMIS 1988; 96: 379–394.
[4] Jensen EB, Gundersen HJ, Østerby R. Determination of membrane thickness distribution from orthogonal intercepts. J Microsc 1979; 115: 19–33.
[5] Marcussen N, Ottosen PD, Christensen S. Ultrastructural quantitation of atubular and hypertrophic glomeruli in rats with lithium-induced chronic nephropathy. Virchows Arch A Pathol Anat Histopathol 1990; 417: 513–522.
[6] Gundersen HJ, Seefeldt T, Østerby R. Glomerular epithelial foot processes in normal man and rats. Distribution of true width and its intra- and inter-individual variation. Cell Tissue Res 1980; 205: 147–155.
[7] Gundersen HJ. Stereogogy – Or how figures for spatial shape and content are obtained by observation of structure in sections. Microsc Acta 1983; 83: 409–426.
[8] Østerby R, Nyberg G, Andersson C et al. Glomerular structural quantities in baseline biopsies from cadaveric donor kidney pairs. APMIS Suppl 1988; 4: 134–140.
[9] Gundersen HJ, Østerby R. Optimizing sampling efficiency of stereological studies in biology: or 'do more less well!' J Microsc 1981; 121: 65–73.
[10] Mayhew TM, Reith A. Introducing basic principles and methods of stereology and morphometry. In: Reith A, Mayhew TM, eds. Stereology and Morphometry in Electron Microscopy: Problems and Solutions. New York: Hemisphere Publishing Corporation, 1988; 1–12.
[11] Østerby R. A stereological study in practice. In: Reith A, Mayhew TM, eds. Stereology and Morphometry in Electron Microscopy, Problems and Solutions. New York: Hemisphere Publishing Corporation, 1988; 195–205.
[12] Sterio DC. The unbiased estimation of number and sizes of arbitrary particles using the disector. J Microsc 1984; 134: 127–136.
[13] Østerby R, Gundersen HJ. Sampling problems in the kidney. In: Miles RE, Serra J, eds. Lecture Notes in Biomathematics, Vol. 23. Heidelberg: Springer-Verlag, 1978; 185–191.
[14] Østerby R, Gundersen HJ. Stereology in experimental biology: Sampling universe, practical sampling procedures, and the biological interpretation of structural quantities. Mikroskopie 1980; 37: 161–164.
[15] Walker JD, Close CF, Jones SL et al. Glomerular structure in type-1 (insulin-dependent) diabetic patients with normo- and microalbuminuria. Kidney Int 1992; 41: 741–748.
[16] Bangstad HJ, Østerby R, Dahl-Jorgensen K et al. Early glomerulopathy is present in young, Type 1 (insulin-dependent) diabetic patients with microalbuminuria. Diabetologia 1993; 36: 523–529.
[17] Østerby R. Early phases in the development of diabetic glomerulopathy. Acta Med Scand Suppl 1974; 574: 3–82.
[18] Østerby R. Quantitative electron microscopy of the glomerular basement membrane. A methodologic study. Lab Invest 1971; 25: 15–24.
[19] Hirose K, Østerby R, Nozawa M et al. Development of glomerular lesions in experimental long-term diabetes in the rat. Kidney Int 1982; 21: 889–895.
[20] Steffes MW, Barbosa J, Basgen JM et al. Quantitative glomerular morphology of the normal human kidney. Lab Invest 1983; 49: 82–86.
[21] Chavers BM, Bilous RW, Ellis EN et al. Glomerular lesions and urinary albumin excretion in type I diabetes without overt proteinuria. N Engl J Med 1989; 320: 966–970.
[22] Østerby R, Nyberg G, Hedman L et al. Kidney transplantation in type 1 (insulin-dependent) diabetic patients. Early glomerulopathy. Diabetologia 1991; 34: 668–674.
[23] Østerby R, Gundersen HJ. Fast accumulation of basement membrane material and the rate of morphological changes in acute experimental diabetic glomerular hypertrophy. Diabetologia 1980; 18: 493–500.
[24] Ellis EN, Mauer SM, Sutherland DE et al. Glomerular capillary morphology in normal humans. Lab Invest 1989; 60: 231–236.
[25] Østerby R, Parving HH, Hommel E et al. Glomerular structure and function in diabetic nephropathy. Early to advanced stanges. Diabetes 1990; 39: 1057–1063.

[26] Østerby R, Parving HH, Nyberg G et al. A strong correlation between glomerular filtration rate and filtration surface in diabetic nephropathy. Diabetologia 1988; 31: 265–270.
[27] Harris RD, Steffes MW, Bilous RW et al. Global glomerular sclerosis and glomerular arteriolar hyalinosis in insulin dependent diabetes. Kidney Int 1991; 40: 107–114.
[28] Østerby R, Gall M-A, Schmitz A et al. Glomerular structure and function in proteinuric Type 2 (non-insulin-dependent) diabetic patients. Diabetologia 1993; 36: 1064–1070.
[29] Hørlyck A, Gundersen HJ, Østerby R. The cortical distribution pattern of diabetic glomerulopathy. Diabetologia 1986; 29: 146–150.
[30] Lane PH, Steffes MW, Mauer SM. Estimation of glomerular volume: a comparison of four methods. Kidney Int 1992; 41: 1085–1089.
[31] Schmitz A, Nyengaard JR, Bendtsen TF. Glomerular volume in Type 2 (non-insulin-dependent) diabetes estimated by a direct and unbiased stereologic method. Lab Invest 1990; 62: 108–113.
[32] Marcussen N, Ottosen PD, Christensen S et al. Atubular glomeruli in lithium-induced chronic nephropathy in rats. Lab Invest 1989; 61: 295–302.
[33] Sørensen FB. Quantitative analysis of nuclear size for objective malignancy grading: A review with emphasis on new, unbiased stereologic methods. Lab Invest 1992; 66: 4–23.
[34] Bendtsen TF, Nyengaard JR. The number of glomeruli in type 1 (insulin-dependent) and type 2 (non-insulin-dependent) diabetic patients. Diabetologia 1992; 35: 844–850.
[35] Lane PH, Steffes MW, Fioretto P et al. Renal interstitial expansion in insulin-dependent diabetes mellitus. Kidney Int 1993; 43: 661–667.
[36] Østerby R. Glomerular structural changes in type 1 (insulin-dependent) diabetes mellitus: causes, consequences, and prevention. Diabetologia 1992; 35: 803–812.

Measurement of pressure, flow and other parameters of the peripheral macro- and microcirculation in diabetes

J. E. Tooke, A. Bollinger

Introduction

Disease of the cardiovascular system accounts for the excess mortality and morbidity of patients with diabetes and involvement of the peripheral vasculature (which conventionally refers to leg vessels) is an important component. Indeed the age adjusted rate of lower limb amputations in people with diabetes is fifteen times that for people without the disease [1]; furthermore the prevalence of peripheral vascular disease (reduced ankle blood pressure one minute after exercise) may be as high as 30% in middle aged diabetics compared to matched controls (prevalence 10%) [2]. Although the debate continues as to the importance of involvement of the microvessels in peripheral ischaemia and foot ulceration there is no doubt that functional disturbances of the peripheral microvasculature may be found in diabetes [3].

Given the accessibility of this particular vascular bed it is no surprise that a variety of techniques have been applied to the extremeties to try and further our understanding of the pathogenesis of diabetic microangiopathy. The peripheral vasculature has the advantage of exhibiting many characteristics common to other regional circulations: Extrinsic and intrinsic control systems exist; functional and reactive hyperaemia can be demonstrated; autoregulation occurs; phasic fluctuations in flow (vasomotion) have been described. The disturbance of these various characteristics by the diabetic process may therefore be defined. However, it is important to emphasize that no one vascular bed is typical and conclusions regarding one particular regional circulation may not be applicable to another. Nonetheless, there is considerable conformity of the microvascular haemodynamic abnormalities observed in various organs which have been summarized as a haemodynamic hypothesis [4] (Table 1).

It is important to appreciate that study of the peripheral circulation presents a number of interpretative difficulties. Firstly, a large proportion of foot

Table 1 The haemodynamic hypothesis of diabetic microangiopathy

Early increased microvascular pressure and flow
↓
Microvascular sclerosis (injury response)
↓
Limited flow reserve
±
Loss of autoregulation

blood flow at room temperature occurs through thermoregulatory arteriovenous shunts which are under strong sympathetic nervous control. Estimates of total limb blood flow are therefore not a measure of nutritional flow as total flow will include this thermoregulatory element. Similarly some methods for estimating skin microvascular perfusion are incapable of distinguishing between shunted and nutritional flow. A further interpretative problem arises from the common concurrence of large vessel disease (atherosclerosis), neuropathy, and microangiopathy, all of which will have an impact on microvascular behaviour. Unless the degree of neuropathy and arterial stenosis is defined changes in microvascular function may be wrongly ascribed, although interestingly all three features tend to result in the same pattern of abnormalities, namely relative overperfusion at rest particularly on dependency, loss of capillary pressure regulation and limited flow reserve [5].

This chapter describes the various methods in contemporary use for examining the peripheral vasculature and their applicability to human diabetes.

Methods of measuring total limb flow

Venous occlusion plethysmography

Venous occlusion plethysmography is the classical method for non-invasive measurement of segmental blood flow in limbs. The principle consists of creating a sudden pressure of 40–60 mmHg within a venous occlusion cuff proximal to a volume sensor. The first steep volume increase after venous occlusion is proportional to the arterial inflow. Later as the capacitance vessels become completely filled by blood the rate of increase in limb volume lessens.

Different volume sensors are used, most often mercury-in-Silastic strain-gauges and air-filled cuffs. Water plethysmographs are more difficult to use because of sealing problems.

Segmental limb flow is expressed in ml/100 ml of tissue/min. The normal values at rest vary at the calf between 1 and 5 ml/100 ml/min and at the lower arm between 2 and 6 ml/100 ml/min [6, 7, 8]. Since values at rest do not reflect the situation distal to an arterial occlusion provocation tests such as reactive hyperaemia after 3–5 min of arterial occlusion are used to characterize impaired functional reserve in patients with ischaemic disease. Peak reactive hyperaemia flow at the calf reaches 20–40 ml/100 ml/min in normal subjects and is reduced and delayed in peripheral arterial occlusive disease [6, 7, 8]. In addition to peak flow, time to peak flow is a parameter that is often used for describing the pathological hyperaemia reaction.

Photocells may be attached to various skin regions and especially to digits. They allow one to record pulse volume tracings suitable for diagnostic purposes, but not for quantitative evaluation of skin blood flow.

For diagnosis of deep vein thrombosis venous volume at 40–60 mmHG cuff filling pressure (ml/100 ml) and maximal venous return after releasing the cuff (ml/100 ml/min) are valuable and frequently used parameters. In acute proximal above knee thrombosis venous volume and maximal venous outflow are decreased.

Doppler and Duplex sonography

According to the Doppler principle the flow velocity within a blood vessel is proportional to the difference of frequency between incident and back-scattered ultrasound beams (Doppler shift). Conventional Doppler probes are based on continuous emission of ultrasound waves; pulsed devices employ intermittent emission which opens the possibility to evaluate flow velocity within a determined intravascular sample volume. The combination of the latter technique with B-mode imaging is called Duplex sonography. Volume flow in single arteries may be computed by determination of vessel diameter and flow velocity in an area covering the whole diameter. If ten or more sample volumes are placed within a given vessel, flow velocity profiles may be determined. At bifurcations the flow profiles become asymmetrical, whereas in arterial aneurysms backflow may be documented in distinct sections. The most recent development consists of colour coding of different flow directions and speeds. Colour coding facilitates localisation of vessels and permits easy identification of arteries and veins.

Continuous wave ultrasound is used for segmental blood pressure and flow velocity measurements at different levels of the limb arterial tree [7, 9, 10]. The technique is simple, reliable with adequate experience and inexpensive. Since measurements of systolic ankle blood pressure depend upon the compressibility of the arteries underlying the sphygmomanometer cuff and medial calcification is more common at the ankle than at the toes, measurements at the latter location may be more informative [9, 11]. This is a particularly important consideration in the diabetic population where incompressibility of ankle vessels is frequently encountered and can be falsely reassuring unless its significance is understood.

More sophisticated information is gained by Duplex scanners [13, 14, 15]. The configuration and haemodynamic significance of arterial stenoses may be assessed with a high degree of accuracy. An occlusion is diagnosed when no flow can be detected within a vessel visualized by B-mode ultrasound. Even lesions that narrow the lumen by less than 50% may be detected. Turbulence provoked by wall changes or stenosis are evaluated by instantaneous spectral analysis. The arteries most often explored are extracranial, intestinal, renal and peripheral vessels. Figure 1 gives a typical example for evaluation of stenosis by colour coded Duplex. For planning therapy (peripheral transluminal angioplasty or direct vascular surgery) it may be essential to know the length of the occluded arterial segment. In some patients catheter therapy may be indicated without previous arteriography on the basis of the Duplex findings alone.

The configuration of the volume flow curve depends on the peripheral resistance in the vascular bed supplied by the artery explored. With high resistance as found in the leg at rest a postsystolic negative component and a positive flat diastolic wave is typical; with low resistance as found in the internal carotid and the renal artery diastolic flow is always positive. During hyperaemic conditions (physical exercise, distal to arterial obstructions) peak systolic flow increases less than diastolic flow which becomes positive even

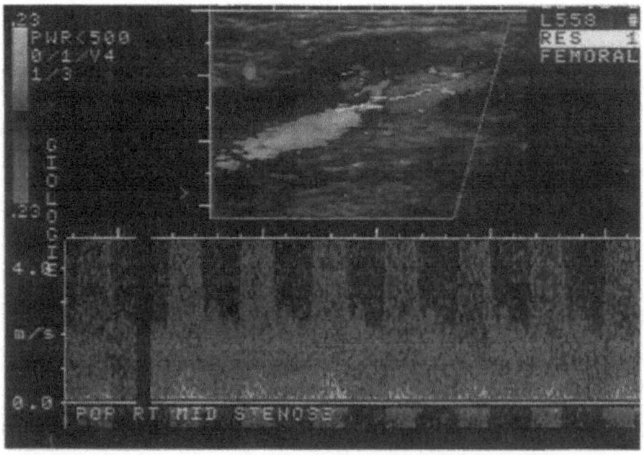

Fig. 1 Black and white representation of a clolour coded Duplex scan of a subtotal stenosis of the popliteal artery. Above: the segments either side of the stenosis are represented in different scales of grey (coded in red and blue on the original). Below: the Doppler signals are derived from a sample volume located in the stenotic area (high systolic and diastolic velocities, a lot of turbulence)

in high resistance circuits. Measurements may be rendered difficult in diabetics with medial calcification since calcium deposits in the walls tend to block the penetration of ultrasound beams. Pulsatile arterial flow in defined arteries may be measured by Duplex sonography not only under resting conditions, but also during reactive hyperaemia after arterial occlusion and other provocation tests [13, 14, 15].

Methods for examining arteriovenous shunt flow

The peripheral circulation in diabetes is characterized by high arteriovenous shunt flow which is secondary to release of sympathetic tone due to either the high metabolic rate which is a feature of poorly controlled diabetes, or sympathetic neuropathy, a common feature in long standing diabetes. A number of techniques have been employed to characterize this phenomenon, building on the clinical observation that foot veins tend to be full at heart level when shunt flow is high [16].

Foot venous oxygen tension and pressure

As the majority of peripheral blood flow bypasses the capillary bed during high shunt flow less oxygen is extracted by the tissues and the oxygen tension of blood sampled from a vein on the dorsum of the foot remains relatively high [17]. Recently raised pressure has been demonstrated in these veins using a conventional pressure transducer system, reflecting the reduction in arteriolar and shunt resistance [18].

Doppler signatures

As discussed above, the shape of the volume flow curve obtained using Doppler depends upon the peripheral resistance in the vascular bed supplied by the artery. The Doppler waveform in leg arteries of patients with diabetic neuropathy and high shunt flow exhibits changes characteristic of reduced peripheral vascular resistance, namely high forward flow with reduced reverse flow [19].

Deductive assumptions from measurements of total arterial inflow and nutritive capillary flow

If total arterial inflow is estimated by plethysmography and nutritive capillary flow by a specific technique such as videomicroscopy, an idea of the arteriovenous shunt flow can be obtained by comparing the relative flow values [20].

Microsphere partitioning

The definitive way to determine arteriovenous shunt flow is to inject micropheres (macroaggregates of radio labelled albumin) that in view of their size are incapable of passing through the nutritive capillary bed. A high count in the venous effluent reflects open thermoregulatory shunt vessels [21]. The radioactivity involved limits the usefulness of this specific technique.

Techniques for assessing microvascular perfusion

Microvascular flow velocity

In recent years techniques have developed for estimating microvascular perfusion close to the tissue surface.

Modern videomicroscopy systems are composed of an intravital microscope with incident illumination (mercury vapour lamp), a sensitive television camera, video timer and scale marker, a tape recorder and devices for optimizing video images [22]. At the nailfold of fingers and toes flow of corpuscular elements may be visualized and stored on tape. Final magnification on the television screen of approximately 250 times are required for capillary flow velocity measurements which may be performed on both the arterial and venous limbs of the capillary loops.

Three examining procedures are available for studying flow velocity in capillary loops:

1. The frame-by-frame technique is very accurate, but time consuming [23]. During the playback of a videotape one single frame after another is displayed and the displacement of a plasma gap between the flowing cells measured on the television monitor; the number of frames determines the time for a given displacement.
2. The flying spot method consists of projecting a spot on the television recording and manually moving the spot along the capillary under examination. Its speed is adjusted to coincide with the velocity of the flowing blood cells [24].
3. The combination of a dual window densitometer and the cross-correlation technique for processing of the signals allows continuous readings of flow velocity [25, 26]. Also the computerized measurements are based on dual-window densitometers (CapiFlow® [27]), but are easier to use. Prerequisites are good fixation of fingers or toes by a specially manufactured bracket, acceptable transparency of the skin and the presence of enough

plasma gaps between the flowing blood cells. Even this technique requires training and skill.

Flow velocity may be continuous or intermittent (flow motion). At rest mean velocity varies within a wide physiological range (0.01–2.2 mm/s). More valuable for characterizing the capillary flow conditions is again the determination of reactive hyperaemia after circulatory arrest. After one minute of arterial occlusion by a finger cuff inflated suddenly to suprasystolic pressure the normal time to peak velocity is very constant (7.8 ± 2.4 s [22]). It is prolonged distal to arterial obstructions, and also in diabetes [28]. The constrictor behaviour of precapillary arterioles is best tested by standardized cold provocation [29]. Decceleration of corpuscular speed occurs also in normal subjects after 1 min of blowing cold air or decompressed CO_2 on the nailfold. In most patients with primary or secondary Raynaud's phenomenon the blood cells stop completely.

Fluorescence videomicroscopy

Identical videomicroscopy systems equipped with tape recorders are suited for visualizing fluorescent tracers if adequate filters are inserted [12, 22]. *Na-fluorescein* binds only partially to plasma proteins and diffuses in detectable amounts through the capillary wall into a pericapillary area forming a halo around the capillary loop. In contrast to Na-fluorescein *indocyanine green* which couples almost completely to plasma proteins, fluoresces in the near infrared portion of the spectrum and requires sensitive infrared video cameras and special filters for its detection [22, 30]. Normal cameras are adequate for visualization of Na-fluorescein (fluorescence in the visible part of the spectrum).

The tracers are injected as a bolus into an antecubital vein. Both the time from the end of injection to the first appearance of the dye in the area under observation and the time elapsing between dye arrival in the first and last capillaries of a given field of observation are noted. The latter time describes microvascular flow distribution. At the nailfold, all capillaries are stained within 12 s, at the dorsum of the foot after 40–50 s [22]. Longer time intervals demonstrate inhomogeneous microvascular flow distribution occurring in vasospastic conditions and in severe skin ischaemia.

Laser Doppler fluxmetry

Laser Doppler instruments are used for recording blood cell flux in a sample volume of about 1 mm^3 [31]. Flux is the product of mean blood cell speed and number of blood cells within the sample volume. It is expressed in volts or better in arbitrary units. If arterial circulation is completely blocked by a cuff inflated to suprasystolic pressure the instrument still has a basic output called biological zero [32], which may relate to vasomotion of occluded vessels or Brownian motion within the tissue.

The instrument samples information from capillaries, arterioles, venules and arteriovenous shunts if present in the area [33]. It yields the most valuable information if provocation manoeuvres are performed. The most important ones are reactive hyperaemia after circulatory arrest, vasoconstriction induced by proximal venous occlusion, by standardized cold provocation or by orthostatis [31, 34, 35]. Moreover, it provides a unique opportunity to study spontaneous fluctuations of skin flux [36]. The latter include pulsatile

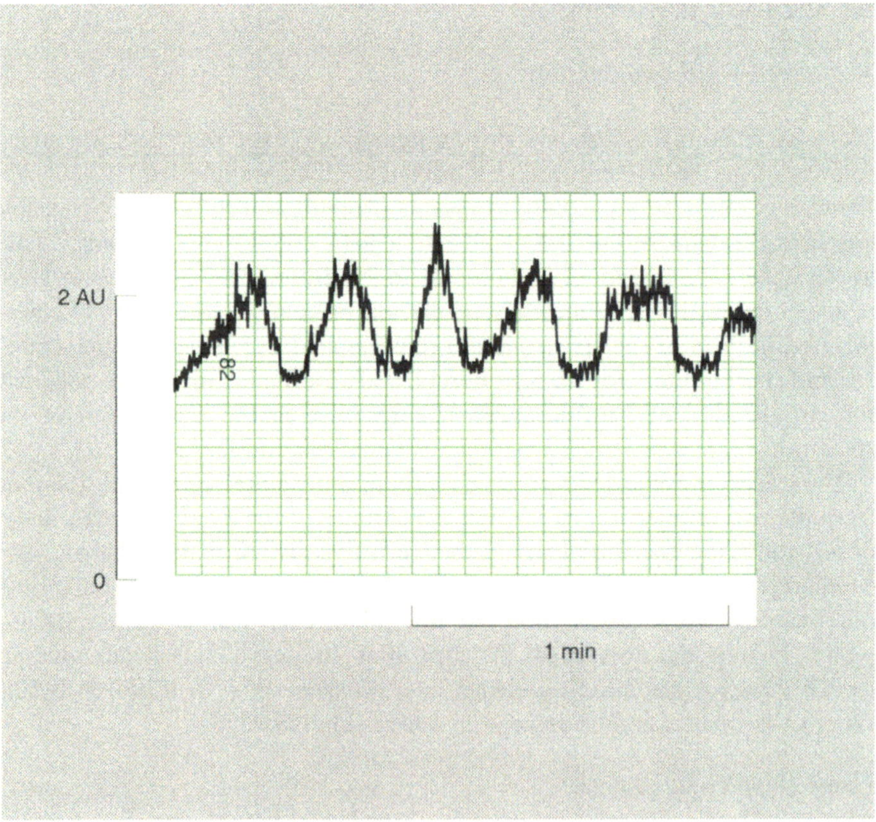

Fig. 2 Spontaneous rhythmic changes of laser Doppler flux at the foot dorsum in a patient with intermittent claudication. The waves correspond to arteriolar vasomotion

and respiratory flux waves and low frequency vasomotion caused by more or less rhythmic contractions of the arterioles (Fig. 2).

Skin flux at rest like arterial inflow is an insensitive parameter for characterizing the prevailing vascular condition at a given site of measurement. However, it may be used to assess hyperaemic states. Marked increases of skin flux have been observed in inflammation and chronic venous insufficiency [37, 38]. Vasomotion is abolished in severe skin ischaemia and reactive hyperaemia very low. Peak flux and time to peak flux are well suited to quantify the degree of ischaemia [35]. It must be emphasized that mild ischaemia distal to arterial occlusions or stenosis may be associated with almost normal skin microcirculation (still normal or only slightly impaired reactive hyperaemia).

In diabetic patients reactive hyperaemia and postural vasoconstriction may be reduced even in the absence of macroangiopathy [34, 39]. In these cases reactivity of skin vessels is decreased because of stiffened resistance vessels and/or loss of sympathetic nerve fibres involved in reflex vasoconstriction. Laser Doppler fluximetry opens a way to evaluate objectively one major component of functional diabetic microangiopathy.

Methods for measuring microvascular pressure

Although indirect techniques have been described for measuring peripheral capillary pressure comparison with direct methods discounts their worth [40]. Direct measurement of capillary pressure involves cannulation of nailfold capillaries with glass micropipettes with the aid of a micromanipulator and microscopy system (Fig. 3). Pressure may then be measured using a simple water manometry system [41] (which provides an estimate of mean pressure) or a complex electronic servonulling system [42] (which is capable of registering a dynamic pressure pulse waveform). In the manometry system manometer pressure is raised to balance the influx of red blood cells into the tip of the micropipette, mean pressure being taken as the point at which there is no net movement of red cells in or out of the pipette tip. In the servonulling system the electrical impedance across the pipette tip is measured. Influx of blood results in an increase in impedance and a pump drive is activated to restore the impedance to the starting position (i. e. the change is servonulled). The response time of the system is a few milliseconds and fluctuations in pressure resulting from the cardiac cycle can be recorded with a conventional pressure transducer attached to the pump drive. In practised hands pressure can be measured with an accuracy of 1 – 2 mmHg. Using such a technique the first demonstration of a control-related increase in peripheral capillary

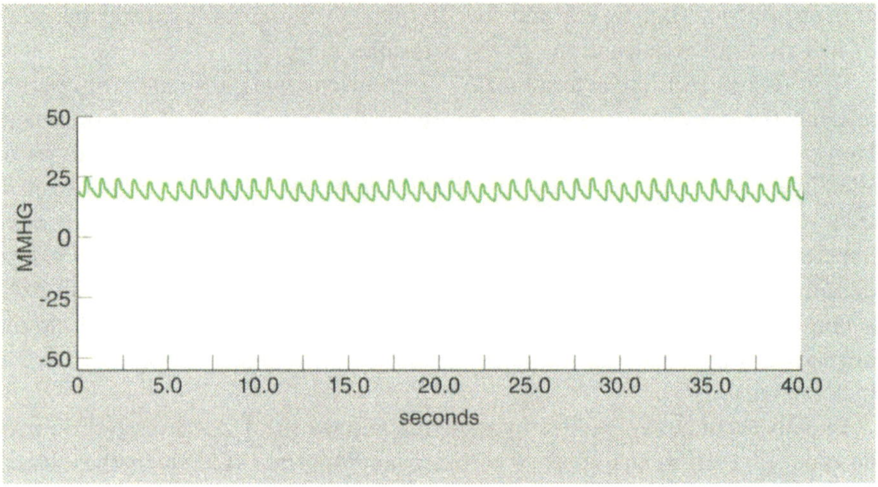

Fig. 3 Trace of human nailfold capillary pressure obtained using the Landis microinjection technique and servonulling pressure measurement; cardiac pulsatility is clearly visible

pressure in diabetes has recently been reported [43]. The technique has also been employed to measure peripheral lymphatic pressure, [44] although not in patients with diabetes.

Methods for measuring permeability

Plethysmography

As described above if venous outflow to a limb is obstructed with a cuff the initial increase in limb volume represents the filling of capacitance vessels. Once the capacitance vessels are full any further increment in limb volume provides an estimate of water flux across the capillary bed into the tissues. In practice the estimate of water flux is obtained by measuring the swelling rate of a limb in response to an increment in venous pressure using either mercury in silastic strain gauges or air or water displacement after several minutes have been allowed to elapse after onset of occlusion to prime the veins. It is assumed that the increase in venous pressure results in a similar step change in capillary pressure. It is therefore possible to estimate the capillary filtration coefficient (CFC) as millilitres of fluid accumulating per 100 g tissue per mmHg rise in pressure per minute [45]. As the capillary surface area available for exchange is unknown a true estimate of capillary wall hydraulic conductivity (the permeability term for water) cannot be derived.

A further compounding difficulty results from the fact that the increase in venous pressure resulting from venous occlusion invokes the venoarteriolar reflex, which causes precapillary vasoconstriction thereby limiting the rise in capillary pressure. This response is deficient in diabetes and hence it is likely that the increase in peripheral capillary pressure will be greater in patients with diabetes for a given increment in venous pressure. An observed apparent increase in CFC may thus reflect changes in peripheral haemodynamics rather than vessel wall permeability to water. More recently a computerized plethysmographic system has been developed which uses very small increments in venous pressure which are not thought to invoke the venoarteriolar reflex. Estimates of CFC using this system are thus likely to provide a more accurate estimate of capillary permeability is diabetes [46].

Tracer clearance techniques

An estimate of microvascular permeability of limb vessels may be obtained using tracer clearance techniques. Two approaches have been employed: The first measures the rate of disappearance of an injected depot [47] or superficial gaseous collection of radio active solute; the second is an indicator diffusion technique [48] which examines the clearance from the blood of radioactive tracers that are injected intra-arterially, tracer concentration being determined in venous blood draining the limb.

Not withstanding the problems associated with radioactive isotopes difficulties exist in relationship to the interpretation of the results obtained. In tracer clearance techniques the volume of distribution of the tracer is not accurately known nor is differential partitioning between different tissues. In the case of freely diffusible solutes clearance may be flow limited and thus it is usual to maximize flow and record this parameter using another tracer. Neither method is able to correct for the surface area for exchange and thus the capillary diffusion coefficients obtained are regarded at best as a measure of permeability surface area product.

The passage of ^{24}Na, ^{131}I, ^{51}Cr-EDTA have been examined in diabetes. From such studies it appears that the passage of small hydrophilic solutes is increased in longterm diabetes.

Fluorescence videomicroscopy

The same equipment as already described may be used for evaluation of transcapillary diffusion of the small solute Na-fluorescein (NaF) which binds only partially to plasma proteins and leaves the intravascular compartment even under physiological conditions. The passage of the intravital dye through the capillary wall and through the outer border of the pericapillary space (halo) is visualized by capillaroscopy after NaF bolus injection [12, 22]. The tape recordings are processed by videodensitometry. Fluorescent light intensities may be determined on an axis crossing one given capillary loop or in window-shaped areas encompassing a certain number of capillaries [22]. They are expressed in arbitrary units or as a percentage of the individual maximal intensity.

In Type I diabetes of more than 10 years duration transcapillary diffusion of NaF is enhanced. The videomicroscopy image becomes blurred by increased diffusion of the dye into the pericapillary and more remote interstitial space (Fig. 4). Fluorescence light intensity around nailfold capillaries and in skin areas of the forefoot are significantly higher in patients than in controls [12, 22].

Indocyanine green (ICG) which couples almost completely to plasma proteins is potentially suited to depict and quantify macromolecular permeability

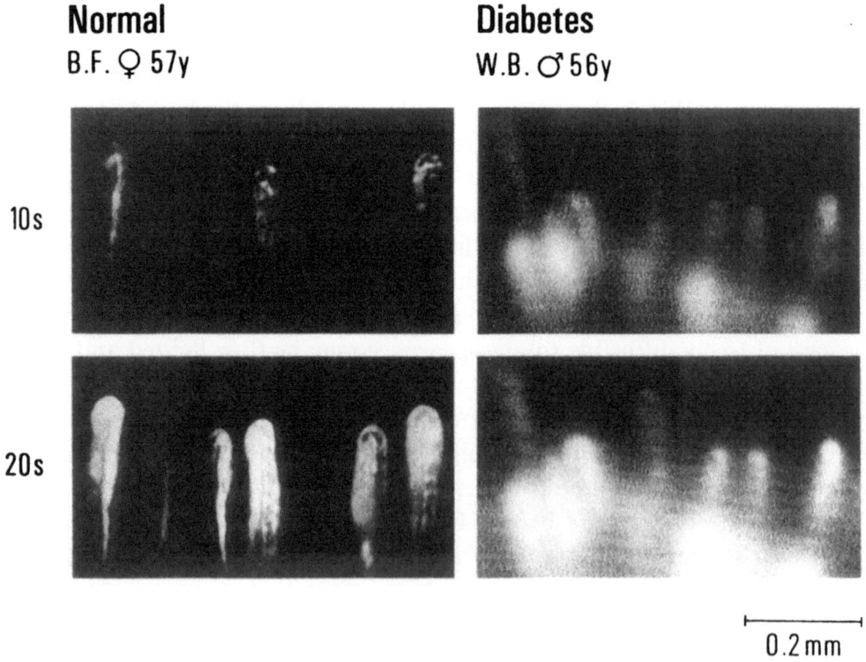

Fig. 4 Fluorescence videomicroscopy of nailfold capillaries after intravenous injection of 1 ml of Na-fluorescein. In the healthy controls the dye diffuses through the capillary wall and stains a pericapillary compartment called halo which acts as a second diffusion barrier. In the diabetic patient the fluorescent tracer promptly inundates the whole interstitial space causing "milky blurring" of the image

at the level of single capillary loops. Up to now the optical resolution due to the relatively low emission of fluorescent light in the near infrared portion of the spectrum is not high enough to reach this goal. However, the technique visualizes skin capillary aneurysms filled by plasma alone. Increased prevalence of capillary aneurysms has been documented in progressive systemic sclerosis and related disorders [30] and in Type 1 diabetes after 10 years of disease duration (unpublished own results).

Methods for measuring exchange function: transcutaneous oxygen tension ($tcPO_2$)

The diffusion of oxygen through the skin from superficial microvessels is dependent upon many factors including local blood flow, blood oxygen tension and the avidity with which oxygen binds to haemoglobin, as well as the diffusion distance. For this reason transcutaneous oxygen tension measurement provides a useful global measure of one aspect of exchange function. $TcPO_2$ is measured by modified Clark-type polarographic electrodes containing a platinum cathodes and silver–silver chloride anodes. Oxygen is reduced at the platinum cathode to produce a current proportional to the partial pressure of oxygen at the electrode surface. The electrode is attached to the skin by means of an adhesive ring after the application of a drop of distilled water as the contact agent. A heating element built into the anode produces an adjustable skin temperature. At 43–45 °C, the arterioles in the area studied are maximally dilated. Under these circumstances, $tcPO_2$ approximates PO_2 of arterial blood provided there are normal circulatory conditions [49]. At 37 °C, the amount of oxygen diffusing through the skin depends essentially on blood flow in the skin vessels and on the saturation of haemoglobin. Reactive hyperaemia after arterial occlusion or acute effects of vasoactive drugs are best monitored at this relatively low temperature.

At the dorsum of the foot, the normal values at 43–45 °C are scattered between 40 and 80 mmHg. When the temperature is reduced to 37 °C, $tcPO_2$ oscillates between 0 and 10 mmHg [16].

In peripheral vascular disease, determinations of $tcPO_2$ are mainly used to characterize skin ischaemia. Patients suffering from intermittent claudication exhibit values at the dorsum of the foot in the lower normal range or below 40 mmHg. Diabetic patients with peripheral arterial disease and ulceration have higher mean $tcPO_2$ values than non diabetic patients with ulcers. A significant number of diabetics develop ulcers despite adequate delivery of oxygen to the cutaneous tissue. Possible causes for this fact are neuropathy, impaired local metabolism, reduced resistance to infection and increased transcapillary diffusion of small solutes with a tendency to oedema formation [22]. The reactive increase in $tcPO_2$ after circulatory arrest is reduced in diabetic patients even in the absence of macroangiopathy [39].

Low or very low $tcPO_2$ values are not only observed in peripheral arterial disease. In severe chronic venous incompetence, especially in areas with spots of white atrophy, $tcPO_2$ may be zero, indicating danger of ulceration [50]. A direct correlation of capillary number and $tcPO_2$ becomes possible using probes with a transparent window for capillaroscopy.

Methods for measuring interstitial fluid parameters: tissue hydrostatic and colloid osmotic pressure

As the interstitium is predominantly in gel form under normal conditions of hydration, estimation of tissue pressure with needles attached to some form of manometer system is problematic: The introduction of even small amounts of fluid implies that the measurement is one of the compliance of the interstitial tissues. This potential criticism may be avoided by the introduction of a saline impregnated wick, a thin inert fibre which can be drawn through the subcutaneous tissue on the end of a needle and left in situ for several hours to equilibrate [51]. The wick is then connected to a pressure transducer and pressure recorded.

A criticism of this approach is the inevitable trauma that accompanies the introduction of the wick with associated inflammatory reaction and tissue swelling. The same criticism may be levelled at the use of this method to obtain samples of tissue fluid, the assumption being that tissue fluid protein will equilibrate with wick fluid over the period in situ. Clearly the fluid may be contaminated with blood proteins and it is customary to discard wicks that are discoloured by haemoglobin. Despite these reservations convincing changes in tissue oncotic pressure have been described in diabetes that are consistent with a rise in peripheral capillary pressure and net fluid filtration [52].

References

[1] Bild DE, Selby JV, Sinnock P et al. Lower-extremity amputation in people with diabetes: epidemiology and prevention. Diabetes Care 1989; 12: 24–31.

[2] Laing S, Ellis M, Greenhalgh RM. Who should be investigated for occult atherosclerotic disease? In: Salmasi and Nicolaides, eds. Occult Atherosclerotic Disease. Dordrecht, Boston, London: Kluwer, 1991.

[3] Flynn MD, Tooke JE. The aetiology of diabetic foot ulceration: A role for the microcirculation? Diabetic Medicine 1992; 8: 320–329.

[4] Tooke JE. Microvascular haemodynamics in diabetes mellitus. Clin Sci 1986; 70: 119–125.

[5] Jaap A, Tooke JE. The Diabetic Foot (2nd edn.) Chicester: John Wiley and Sons, 1993; (in press).
[6] Bollinger A. Durchblutungsmessungen in der klinischen Angiologie. Bern: Hans Huber, 1969.
[7] Fronek A. Noninvasive diagnosis in vascular disease. New York: McGraw-Hill Book Company, 1989.
[8] Sumner DS. Volume plethysmography in vascular disease: an overview. In: Bernstein EF, ed. Noninvasive diagnostic techniques in vascular diseases. St. Louis: The C. V. Mosby Company, 1985.
[9] Bernstein EF, ed. Noninvasive diagnostic techniques in vascular diseases. St. Louis: The C. V. Mosby Company, 1985.
[10] Carter SA. Role of pressure measurements in vascular disease. In: Bernstein EF, ed. Noninvasive diagnostic techniques in vascular diseases. St. Louis: The C. V. Mosby Company, 1985.
[11] Beinder E, Hoffmann U, Franzeck UK et al. Laser Doppler technique for the measurement of digital and segmental systolic blood pressure. Vasa 1992; 21: 15–21.
[12] Bollinger A, Frey J, Jäger K et al. Patterns of diffusion through skin capillaries in patients with long-term diabetes. N Engl J Med 1982; 307: 1305–1310.
[13] Labs KH, Jäger KA, Fitzgerald DE et al, eds. Diagnostic vascular ultrasound. London: Edward Arnold, 1992.
[14] Strandness DE. Duplex scanning in vascular disorders. New York: Raven Press, 1990.
[15] Bollinger A, Jäger K, Jünger M et al. The vascular laboratory: advances in noninvasive techniques. World J Surg 1988; 12: 724–731.
[16] Ward JD, Boulton AJM, Simms JM et al. Venous distension in the diabetic neuropathic foot (physical sign of arteriovenous shunting). J R Soc Med 1983; 76: 1011–1014.
[17] Boulton AJM, Scarpello JHB, Ward JD. Venous oxygenation in the diabetic neuropathic foot: evidence of arteriovenous shunting. Diabetologie 1982; 22: 6–8.
[18] Edmonds BMA '93
[19] Edmonds ME, Roberts VC, Watkins PJ. Blood flow in the diabetic neuropathic foot. Diabetologia 1982; 22: 9–15.
[20] Tymms DJ, Tooke JE. The effect of continuous subcutaneous insulin infusion (CSII) on microvascular blood flow in diabetes mellitus. Int J Microcirc Clin Exp 1988; 7: 347–356.
[21] Partsch H. Neuropathien vom ulzero-mutilierenden. Vasa 1977; 6 (Suppl.): 1–48.
[22] Bollinger A, Fagrell B. Clinical capillaroscopy: A guide to its use in clinical research and practice. Toronto, Lewiston NY, Bern, Göttingen, Stuttgart: Hogrefe and Huber, 1990.
[23] Bollinger A, Butti P, Barras JP et al. Red blood cell velocity in nailfold capillaries of man measured by a television microscopy technique. Microvasc Res 1974; 7: 61–72.
[24] Tyml K, Ellis CG. Evaluation of the flying spot technique as a television method for measuring red cell velocity in microvessels. Int J Microcirc: Clin Exp 1982; 1: 145–155.
[25] Fagrell B, Fronek A, Intaglietta M. A microscope television system for studying flow velocity in human skin capillaries. Am J Physiol 1977; 233: H318–H321.
[26] Intaglietta M, Silverman NR, Tompkins WR. Capillary flow velocity measurements in vivo and in situ by television methods. Microvasc Res 1975; 10: 165–179.
[27] Fagrell B, Eriksson SE, Malmström S et al. Computerized data analysis of capillary blood cell velocity. Int J Microcirc: Clin Exp 1988; 7: 276.
[28] Oestergren J, Fagrell B, Karlander SG. Skin capillary blood flow dynamics in patients with diabetes mellitus. Int J Microcirc: Clin Exp 1982; 1 (3): 300.
[29] Mahler F, Saner H, Boss Ch et al. Local cold exposure test for capillaroscopic examination of patients with Raynaud's syndrome. Microvasc Res 1987; 33: 422–427.
[30] Bollinger A, Saesseli B, Hoffmann U et al. Intravital detection of skin capillary aneurysms by videomicroscopy with indocyanine green in patients with progressive systemic sclerosis and related disorders. Circulation 1991; 83: 546–551.
[31] Belcaro G, Hoffmann U, Bollinger A et al, eds. Laser Doppler. London, Los Angeles, Nicosia: Med Orion, 1993.

[32] Caspary L, Creutzig A, Alexander K. Biological zero in laser Doppler fluxmetry. Int J Microcirc 1988; 7: 367.
[33] Tooke JE, Oestergren J, Fagrell B. Synchronous assessment of human skin microcirculation by laser Doppler flowmetry and dynamic capillaroscopy. Int J Microcirc: Clin Exp 1983; 2: 277–284.
[34] Rayman G, Hassan A, Tooke JE. Blood flow in the skin of the foot related to posture in diabetes mellitus. Brit Med J 1986; 292: 87–90.
[35] Seifert H, Jäger K, Bollinger A. Analysis of flow motion by the laser Doppler technique in patients with peripheral arterial occlusive disease. Int J Microcirc: Clin Exp 1988; 7: 223–236.
[36] Hoffmann U, Schneider E, Bollinger A. Flow motion waves with high and low frequency in severe ischaemia before and after percutaneous transluminal angioplasty. Cardiovasc Res 1990; 24: 711–718.
[37] Belcaro G, Christopoulos D, Nicolaides AN. Skin flow and swelling in post-phlebitic limbs. Vasa 1989; 18: 136–143.
[38] Leu AJ, Yanar A, Pfister G et al. Mikroangiopathie bei chronischer venöser Insuffizienz. Dtsch Med Wschr 1991; 116: 447–453.
[39] Franzeck UK, Stengele B, Panradl U et al. Cutaneous reactive hyperaemia in short-term and long-term type 1 diabetes. Continuous monitoring by a combined laser-Doppler and transcutaneous oxygen probe. Vasa 1990; 19: 8.
[40] Eichna LW, Bordley J III. Capillary blood pressure in man. Comparison of direct and indirect methods of measurement. J Clin Invest 1939; 18: 695–704.
[41] Tooke JE. A capillary pressure disturbance in young diabetics. Diabetes 1980; 29: 815–819.
[42] Williams SA, Wassermann S, Rawlinson DW et al. Dynamic measurement of human capillary blood pressure. Clin Sci 1988; 74: 507–512.
[43] Sandeman DD, Shore AC, Tooke JE. Relation of skin capillary pressure in patients with insulin-dependent diabetes mellitus to complications and metabolic control. New England Journal of Medicine 1992; 327; 760–764.
[44] Spiegel M, Vesti B, Shore AC et al. Pressure of initial lymphatics in human skin. Am J Physiol 1992; 262: H1208–H1210.
[45] Michel CC, Moyses C. in: Smaje LH, Tooke JE, eds. Clinical Investigation of the microcirculation. Kluwer-Nighoff, 1986.
[46] Jaap AJ, Shore AC, Gartside IB et al. Increased microvascular permeability to water in young Type I (insulin-dependent) diabetic patients. Diabetologia 1993; (in press).
[47] Trap-Jensen J, Lassen NA. Capillary diffusion capacity for small ions in skeletal muscle in long-term diabetics. Scand J Clin Lab Invest 1968; 21: 116–122.
[48] Trap-Jensen J. Increased capillary permeability to 131-I and 51Cr-EDTA in the exercising forearm of the long-term diabetic. 1970; 39: 39–49.
[49] Franzeck UK. Transkutaner Sauerstoffpartialdruck in der klinischen Mikrozirkulation. Bern: Huber, 1991.
[50] Franzeck UK, Bollinger A, Huch R et al. Transcutaneous oxygen tension and capillary morphologic characteristics and density in patients with chronic venous incompetence. Circulation 1984; 70: 806–811.
[51] Noddeland H, Hargens AR, Reed RK et al. Interstitial colloid osmotic and hydrostatic pressures in subcutaneous tissue of human thorax. Microvasc Res 1982; 24: 104–113.
[52] Fauchald P, Norseth J, Jervell J. Transcapillary colloid osmotic gradient, plasma volume and interstitial fluid volume in long-term type 1 (insulin-dependent) diabetes. Diabetologie 1985; 28: 269–273.

Conducting clinical trials in diabetic renal disease, including power analysis

M. Marre, G. Chatellier

Introduction

Several aspects of diabetic nephropathy and its companion vascular diseases make it a big challenge: first, from a social viewpoint, this complication is responsible for most of the reduced life expectancy and quality of life in diabetic subjects [1]; second, for medical scientists, observations made in diabetes may highlight some pathogenetic mechanisms of renal and vascular diseases in non-diabetic subjects; and third, it may also provide a model for people interested in comparing various cost-effectiveness strategies [2]. Advances in these three aspects are based primarily on data derived from clinical trials conducted with appropriate methodologies.

Background

In Tables 1 and 2, we present a sample of clinical trials conducted in diabetic nephropathy. They were organized according to type of intervention and the stage of diabetic nephropathy (Table 1). End-points are also mentioned (Table 2). Interestingly, the trials with the best design were those on the use of anti-hypertensive agents, of which angiotensin I converting enzyme inhibitors (ACEIs) are prominent. A recent meta-analysis of the effectiveness of anti-hypertensive agents in reducing UAE and protecting glomerular filtration rates in diabetic patients showed that ACEIs were more effective than other anti-hypertensive agents [25]. This positive result may have several explanations. First, ACEIs may truly be more effective than other agents in this indication. Second, there may be a difference in the quality of trials testing these agents, compared to those testing effectiveness of other anti-hypertensive agents, or other treatment strategies. Pirart's study, for instance, is the only one supporting the proposition that good glycemic control prevents diabetic nephropathy [17]. However, it was an observational cohort study, and not a randomized-controlled trial testing the effectiveness of an interven-

Table 1 Sample of clinical trials in diabetic nephropathy

Studies	Intervention Type (*)	Comparison Type	Design (+)	Number of subjects	Study Duration
A) Antihypertensive treatment					
Mogensen (1976) [3]	III	before/after treatment	O, self-controlled	8	47 days
Christensen (1985) [4]	II	before/after metoprolol	O, self-controlled	6	2.6 ± 1.0 years
Parving (1987) [5]	III	before/after treatment	O, self-controlled	11	72 months
Marre (1988) [6]	II	enalapril vs placebo	DB, P, R, MP	20	one year
Mimram (1988) [7]	II	captopril vs nifedipine vs placebo	DB, P, R	22	6 weeks
Romanelli (1990) [8]	I, II	captopril vs nifedipine vs placebo	DB, CO, R	65	acute
Rudberg (1990) [9]	II	before/after, normo/hypertensive	O	12	6 months
Melbourne (1990) [10]	II	perindopril vs nifedipine	O, P, R	50	one year
Mathiesen (1991) [11]	II	captopril ± lasix vs nil	O, P, R, MP	44	4 years
Bjork (1992) [12]	III	enalapril vs metoprolol	O, P, R	40	2.2 years
Weigman (1992) [13]	I, II	captopril vs placebo	DB, CO, R	18	3 months
Hallab (1993) [14]	II	enalapril vs hydrochlorothiazide	DB, P, R	25	1 year
Lewis (1993) [15]	II	captopril vs placebo	DB, P, R	409	3 years
Viberti (1994) [16]	II	captopril vs placebo	DB, P, R	92	2 years
B) Glycemic control					
Pirart (1977) [17]	I	good vs poor control	O, P	4398	25 years
Viberti (1983) [18]	III	CSII vs conventional	O, P, R	12	2 years
Feldt-Rasmussen (1986) [19]	II	CSII vs conventional	O, P, R, MP	36	2 years
Dahl-Jorgensen (1988) [20]	I, II	CSII vs intensified vs conventional	O, P, R	45	4 years
Reichard (1993) [21]	I, II, III	intensified vs standard	O, P, R	102	7.5 years
DCCT Research Group (1993) [22]	I, II	intensified vs conventional	O, P, R	1441	6.5 years
C) Low protein diet					
Cohen (1987) [23]	II	low vs normal protein diet	O, CO, R	8	3 weeks
Walker (1989) [24]	III	low vs normal protein diet	O, self-controlled	19	12–49 months

(*): I = primary, i.e., initial normoalbuminuria; II = secondary, i.e., initial microalbuminuria; III = tertiary, i.e., initial macroalbuminuria
(+): O = open; DB = double blind; P = parallel; CO = cross-over; R = randomized; MP = matched pairs

tion as compared to another. This was the rationale for setting-up the DCCT trial in 1985, which was specifically designed to demonstrate the effectiveness of intensified glycemic control for the primary or the secondary prevention of diabetic complications, including nephropathy. The results of this trial and of another one are available to date [21, 22].

As regards the low protein diet trials, most of them present one or more methodological problems, e. g. small sample size, insufficient study duration, flawed design, and confounding factors (i. e. concomitant anti-hypertensive treatment).

What would be the ideal clinical trial in diabetic renal disease? Certainly a prospective, randomized-controlled trial comparing the effectiveness of an experimental treatment to a reference one, or to placebo, using unquestionable end-points such as death or end-stage renal failure. However, such a study would last several decades for primary prevention studies (i. e., intervention before any prognostically useful sign of renal disease) and 5 to 10 years in secondary prevention studies. It would not be realistic to devote our entire efforts to such trials for both scientific and ethical reasons. Setting up such a trial with the present treatment strategies would mean that its results would not be available for several years. Meanwhile, a large number of diabetic subjects would not benefit from potentially effective intervention, raising ethical problems. Moreover, it is unrealistic to anticipate long-term adherence by both physicians and patients to a reference treatment strategy, due both to increased knowledge of the disease, and pressure from patients' groups and pharmaceutical industrials. Conversely, it is ethically questionable to give drugs without appropriate estimation of their benefit/risk ratio. Thus, valid surrogate end-points are urgently needed in this field.

Selection of end-points

Several end-points can be proposed. We shall focus on 3 critical variables: GFR, UAE and blood pressure. For each of them, the careful analysis of variability is a crucial issue. The two main sources of variability are intra- and inter-patient variabilities expressed by their coefficients of variation (CV). Intra-patient variability comprises spontaneous biological variability and measurement variability. To improve the strength of a trial, one should maximize the ratio of inter- over intra-patient variability by minimizing both biological variability and measurement error.

Glomerular filtration rate (GFR)

Methods for GFR measurement: The details of the different techniques are explored in another chapter of this book. A comprehensive analysis of the

Table 2 Sample of clinical trials in diabetic nephropathy

Types of diabetes	End-point	Confounding variables(*)			Final result on (**)		
		blood pressure	glycemic control	protein diet	UAE	GFR	renal failure/ death
I	Blood pressure, UAE	pre > post	pre = post	?	post > pre	pre > post	–
I	UAE reduction	pre > post	pre = post	?	post > pre	post = pre	–
I	GFR preservation	pre > post	controlled	unchanged	post > pre	post > pre	1 death
I, II	diabetic nephropathy onset	enalapril < placebo	controlled	controlled	enalapril > placebo	enalapril > placebo	–
I	UAE	captopril = nifedipine < placebo	controlled	?	captopril > nif > placebo	capto = nif = placebo	–
I, II	UAE	nifedipine < captopril = placebo	controlled	?	captopril > nif > placebo	?	–
I	UAE	pre = post	pre = post	controlled	post > pre	pre = post	–
I, II	UAE	perindopril = nifedipine	perind. = nif.	?	perind. = mif.	perind. = nif.	1 death
I	diabetic nephropathy onset	capto ± lasix = nil	capto = nil	capto = nil	capto > nil	capto > nil	–
I	GFR decline	enalapril = metoprolol	ena. = meto.	?	ena. > meto.	ena. > meto.	renal failure: E = 3 M = 3

Table 2 *Continued*

Types of dia-betes	End-point	Confounding variables(*)			Final result on (**)		
		blood pressure	glycemic control	protein diet	UAE	GFR	renal failure/ death
I	UAE, GFR	captopril < placebo	captopril = placebo	?	captopril < placebo	captopril < placebo	–
I	UAE	enalapril = hydrochlor.	controlled	controlled	ena. > HTZ	ena. = HTZ	–
I	doubling serum creatinine	captopril < placebo	controlled	controlled	captopril > placebo	captopril = placebo	–
I	diabetic nephropathy onset	captopril < placebo	controlled	controlled	–	captopril > placebo	23/42
I, II	diabetic nephropathy onset	?	good < poor	?	good < poor	unclear	?
I	GFR preservation	controlled	CSII < conv.	?	CSII = conv.	CSII = conv.	?
I	diabetic nephropathy onset	conv. > CSII	conv. > CSII	conv. = CSII	conv. > CSII	CSII > conv.	–
I	UAE	CSII = intens. = conv.	conv. < intens. < CSII	?	CSII < intens. < conv.	?	–
I	diabetic nephropathy	intensified = standard	stand < intens.	stand = in-tens.	intens. < stand.	intens. = stand.	–
I	UAE	conv. > intensified	conv. < intensified	?	intens. < conv.	intens. = conv.	–
I	UAE	low = normal	low = normal	low < normal	low < normal	low < normal	–
I	GFR decline	low < normal	low = normal	low < normal	low < normal	low > normal	?

(*): =: equality; >: higher; ?: unknown values between treatment strategies
(**): =: equality; >: superiority between treatment strategies

impact of various error sources on GFR measurement has been published by Levey et al [26]. The "gold standard" method remains a primed constant infusion technique with serial urinary clearance measurements of exogenous substances. A steady-state can be obtained through a progressive water load to be maintained during the test. Errors in plasma inulin measurements are numerous in diabetic subjects [26], so that radioactive tracers are preferred. If a constant infusion technique is used, intra-measure inter-period CV is mainly due to urine volume variability, because bladder neuropathy is frequent in diabetic patients, and bladder catheterization is harmful in them. Using 125 I-iodothalamate constant infusion, we found that mean intra-subject, intra-measure inter-period CV was 9%, inter-measure intra-patient CV was 7% [14]; inter-patients (selected for persistent micro-albuminuria) CV was 19% [27]. In using this technique, such values must be accounted for in calculating sample size for trials involving acute (intra-test) intervention, short-term (e. g., cross over), or long-term studies based on GFR changes.

The plasma disappearance technique of exogenous single shot substances (e. g., 51 Cr.EDTA) are largely used in routine practice. They are acceptable for long-term studies in spite of numerous sources of variation, i. e. absence of a steady-state, extra-renal elimination of the tracer, uncontrolled food intake and physical activity [26].

Regarding creatinine clearance, sources of errors are so numerous that the use of this method is not recommended [26]. However, plasma creatinine may be a sensitive indicator of small intra-subject GFR changes if GFR is already reduced [26].

The compatibility of GFR measurement methods is a crucial point when comparing different studies, or when pooling data from various studies, i. e. for meta-analysis purposes. Most frequently, 2 measurement methods are compared by regression analysis. This method is not appropriate. A statistically significant correlation coefficient is always expected, since the 2 methods are designed to estimate the same thing. This apparent good relationship is frequently associated with large differences at the individual level. Bland and Altman proposed replacing the correlation analysis with another graphical representation as illustrated in Fig. 1 [28]. We derived it from previously published data [29] on the correlation between 51 Cr.EDTA plasma disappearance technique, and 125 I-iodothalamate constant infusion technique. The correlation coefficient is relatively high (0.74) and highly statistically significant. However, three problems are obvious regarding the appropriate representation: first, the I 125 method gave higher GFR values than the 51 Cr.EDTA method; second, in some patients, differences of up to 70 ml/min/1.73 m^2 can be observed; third, the difference between the 2 methods decreases with the GFR level, meaning it is not possible to derive the GFR obtained with one method from the GFR measured by the other simply by subtracting or adding the mean difference between the 2 methods.

Choice of GFR measurement method: The choice of GFR measurement method depends on the type of trial and on the stage of nephropathy. In trials testing acute interventions (i. e., anticipated to change GFR within a few minutes, or hours), self-controlled infusion techniques with a steady-state are mandatory. Hommel et al published that acute blood pressure reduction reduced UAE acutely [30]. However, they measured blood pressure and UAE sequentially for the hours following I.V. clonidine, but they did not do so for GFR. Therefore, UAE reduction could have been due to acute GFR reduction, which could have recovered within 1–2 hours, thanks to intact renal auto-regulation. As a general rule, the shorter the study duration, the more precise the technique required. Regarding subjects with hyperfiltration, a constant infusion technique may be more sensitive than other techniques (see Fig. 1). Plasma disappearance techniques are easy to handle and well-suited for long-term studies. Plasma creatinine can be used only in studies dealing with renal insufficiency.

Choice of an endpoint for GFR assessment: For short-term studies, the endpoint for GFR is the intra- or inter-group differences between the experimental and the reference strategies. Hence, estimating sample size, or obtaining a statistical difference is a function of GFR measurement variability (see above), of the difference anticipated by clinicians and of the chosen statistical risks (alpha and beta).

For long term studies, the same general rule applies, but the effect of time must be taken into account when designing the study. First, when a regression to the mean phenomenon is anticipated (particularly in subjects having hyperfiltration), a control group must be present [6]. Moreover, a run-in period before assignment to treatment groups can be useful for reducing the phenomenon and avoiding a reduction of the power. Second, a given intervention may be deleterious for GFR in the short-term, and beneficial in the long-term [3, 5]. This is especially true in subjects with established or advanced diabetic nephropathy in whom renal auto-regulation is no longer effective causing GFR to decrease proportionally to blood pressure reduction. For both of these reasons, cross-over studies are not appropriate and parallel studies are preferred. GFR decreases with advancing age [26]. It can be useful to stratify the randomization by age to avoid any imbalance between groups in parallel trials or to allow for pre-planned subgroup analyses.

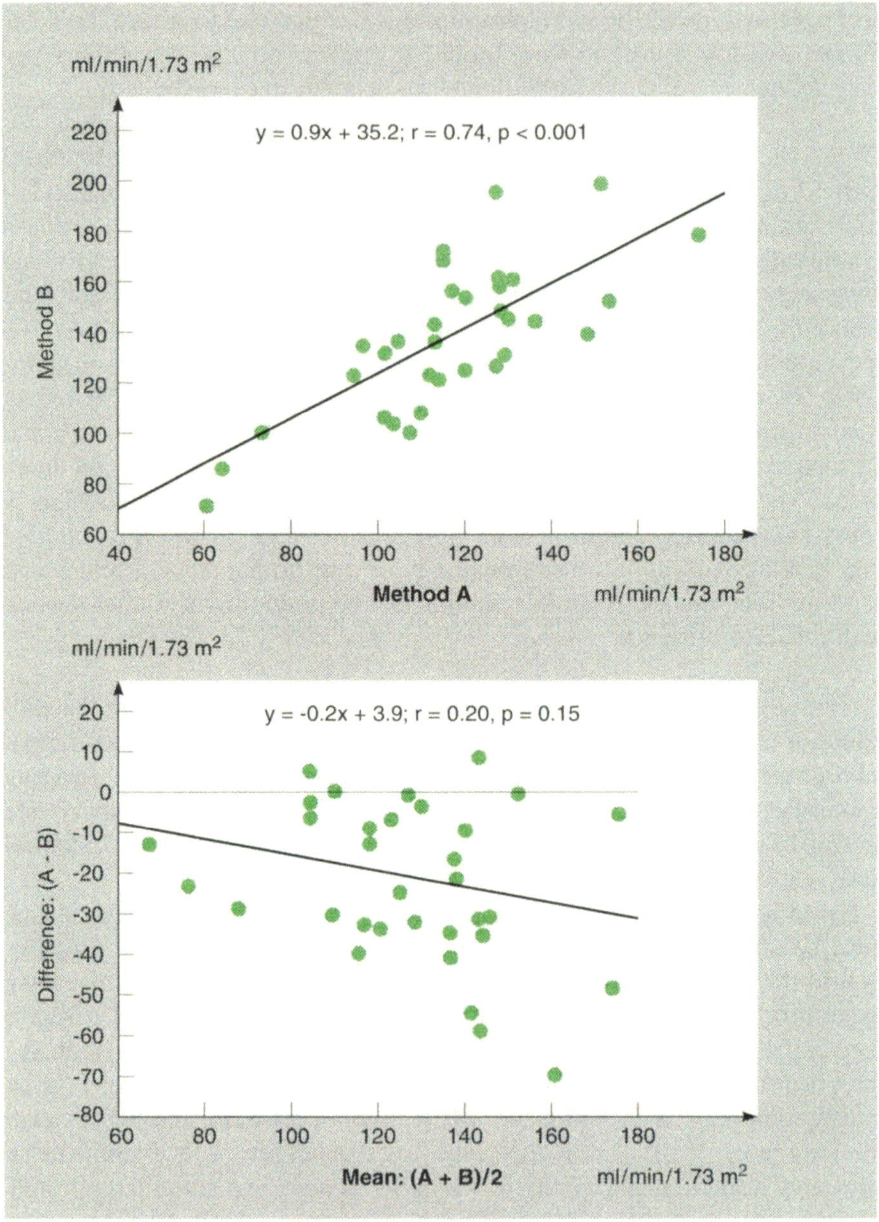

Fig. 1 Comparison of 2 ways of analyzing concordance between 2 methods of measurement:
- *Upper panel: Usual correlation method giving a highly statistically significant correlation coefficient*
- *Lower panel: Method of Bland and Altman [28], plotting the mean of the 2 measurements (x axis) over the difference between the 2 measurements (y axis)*

When repeated measurements of GFR are available, it is possible to use the slope of GFR decline as a surrogate end-point. It is frequently assumed that GFR decreases linearly with time. However, in long-term studies, such as Parving et al [5], the slope of the GFR decline varies with time. Therefore, it is important to maximize the power of the comparison by choosing the model best-fit to GFR decline. If standard statistical analysis such as repeated factor ANOVA are used, the model of the GFR decline should also be described. Describing the progression of reciprocal serum creatinine may be useful in patients with renal insufficiency. In earlier stages of diabetic renal disease (normo- or micro-albuminuria), progression assessment from one stage to another can be used (i. e., from hyper- to normo-, to hypo-filtration) and compared to the GFR values of age-matched controls.

Urinary albumin excretion (UAE)

Methods for UAE measurements: There are two aspects to UAE measurement. The first deals with the method used to measure albumin in urine, and the second with the type of urine collection. Regarding choice of measurement method, the assay sensitivity required to measure normal UAE is within 1 mg/l order, i. e. $10^{-7}-10^{-8}$ M. This can be achieved with many methods, including nephelometry, turbidimetry, and radial immuno-diffusion. RIA or ELISA may be useful, especially if urines are highly diluted. In such a case, the main problem is the avoidance of urinary albumin adsorption on reservoir, rather than assay sensitivity per se. A good inter-method correlation was reported on several occasions [31, 32].

There is no agreement to date regarding urine collection. It is presently recommended to quantify UAE on 24-hour or overnight basis, according to practical feasibility, but to maintain the same procedure for individual follow-up [33]. Whatever the urine collection technique used, intra-subject, inter-measure CV remains high (30–60%). The magnitude of this CV is independent of the urine collection technique and of the baseline UAE level [32]. The UAE inter-subject variability is also high: more than 50% of normal subjects excrete < 5 mg/24 h [32]. This high intra- and inter-subject variability is probably linked to glomerular permeation properties. Finally, the distribution of UAE values is skewed, whatever the sample group studied (diabetic or non-diabetic) or the study methodology used (cross-sectional or longitudinal). Consequently, statistical analysis must be based upon non-parametric tests, or be performed after log-transformation, if parametric analysis is chosen.

Choice of UAE measurement method: Although UAE variability is high, there is a good intra-subject concordance when UAE is graded as normal, micro or macro-albuminuria. Thus, random urine samples can be used for screening purposes to predict UAE stage [34]. For follow-up purposes, timed collections are preferable (see above).

Choice of an endpoint for UAE: Due to high UAE variability, the precision of a study will be proportional to UAE measurement frequency. Analysis of changes in UAE is the easiest assessment method. Due to skewed distribution, mean and standard deviation are inappropriate to summarize results. Geometric mean, or median and range are preferred. For the same reason, the expression of UAE changes should be based on relative changes rather than absolute differences. Since log-transformation is frequently used, be reminded that the difference between 2 log-transformed values is not equal to the log-transformed difference of the 2 raw values. If UAE is measured serially, it is essential to assess both the time effect and the intervention effect. For instance, glomerular permeability can be affected by an intervention within a very short time, but long-term interventions may, in addition, alter glomerular properties. Two different methods can be used to assess the effect of intervention while taking time into account. First, the slope of the regression line can be calculated for each individual after testing the linearity of the model [19], and the mean of these slopes will be compared between the two groups. Second, a two-way ANOVA can be used where intervention effect, time effect and time intervention interaction will be analyzed [6]. From a clinical viewpoint, progression from one stage of UAE to another (normo-, micro-, macro-albuminuria) may be more relevant and prognostically useful, however, this last method is less accurate than the previous ones.

Blood pressure

Methods for measurement: Blood pressure is normally distributed in the general population, and the risk associated with it is exponential. This situation contrasts with that of UAE or blood glucose and their attached risks. The hypertension definition is arbitrary and depends on associated risk factors. Consequently, the hypertension definition differs in diabetic and non-diabetic subjects [35]. It has varied according to evolving knowledge of the disease and/or the results of therapeutic trials. Thus, the last JNC V [35] recommendations included systolic blood pressure in the definition and the stages of hypertension for the first time. These variations in definition should be taken into account when analyzing different studies.

The definition of hypertension is based on blood pressure taken in the clinic and measured with a mercury sphygmomanometer. Nowadays, home blood pressure, automatic blood pressure measurement in the clinic, and ambulatory blood pressure monitoring are also available and technically validated. However, there is still no evidence that these alternative methods predict the cardio-vascular risk better than clinic blood pressure.

Improvement in precision can be achieved by the standardization of the circumstances and repetition of measurements. Standardization concerns many factors such as patient position, clock time, hour, physical activity, salt diet, etc. In addition, for clinic blood pressure, the presence of a physician is a major variability factor. Measurement repetition improves precision: usually, in therapeutic trials the mean of 3 clinic measurements is taken as the blood pressure value. Nevertheless, the "white-coat effect" is a major limitation on blood pressure measurement in the clinic. Home blood pressure and automatic blood pressure monitoring (either ambulatory or not) are devoid of such an effect, and allow multiple measurements. but there are two limitations in their use. First, automatic devices (portable or not) actually measure mean arterial pressure, and calculate systolic and diastolic pressures, while the reverse is done with clinic blood pressure. This explains some of the discrepancies in blood pressure values recorded automatically, as compared to clinic blood pressure. Second, blood pressure is usually lower with home or ambulatory than with clinic blood pressure, and there is no epidemiological description of risks attached to blood pressure values measured with the new methods. Recently, ambulatory devices were used to record blood pressure in type I, insulin-dependent diabetic subjects. A reduced nocturnal blood pressure decline was observed in patients with abnormal UAE [36]. This method may therefore be especially sensitive in detecting blood pressure burdens in diabetic subjects prone to nephropathy, especially during clinical trials.

Choice of method for blood pressure: In short-term trials, the highest precision is achieved by automatic measurement in the absence of the physician. For long-term trials an additional issue is the risk associated with blood pressure. For the reasons detailed above, casual blood pressure measurement is mandatory, but can be associated to ambulatory blood pressure measurements, particularly if circadian analysis is included.

Choice of endpoint for blood pressure: It is presently recommended to treat diastolic blood pressure > 90 mmHg in diabetics aged less than 40 years. The goal blood pressure is a blood pressure lower than 130/85 mmHg [35]. These statements must be considered when setting-up a clinical trial in diabetics. In clinical trials with hypotensive drugs, a pre-determined blood pressure reduction (e. g. a 5 mmHg reduction) can be used as an alternative.

Setting-up a clinical trial

Choice of primary outcome

Study duration, study design, and sample size calculation all depend on the choice of primary end-points.

Clinical end-points or biological surrogate end-points? Unquestionable clinical end-points are scarce: death, appropriately defined end-stage renal failure, or cardio-vascular events. As shown in Table 1, few studies reported these end-points as outcomes. Surrogate end-points are events occurring earlier in course of the disease, and predictive of the unquestionable clinical end-points. Candidate surrogate end-points have been listed above for GFR, UAE, and blood pressure. However, even a statistically significant change in any of these biological variables may not be prognostically significant. The prognostically useful endpoint based on one of these parameters could be the progression from one stage to another, e. g., progression from normal to reduced GFR, or from micro- to macro-albuminuria, or from normal blood pressure to hypertension. Nonetheless, the progression from one stage to another may ambiguous, e. g., what is the significance of progression from hyperfiltration to normal GFR?

Other surrogate end-points may be obtained by analyzing the raw values of GFR, UAE, or blood pressure (after appropriate mathematical transformation, if necessary), or the progression time of one variable to a portion of its baseline value (e. g., doubling serum creatinine, or halving UAE).

Practical example – the case for micro-albuminuria: Four independent studies reported that micro-albuminuria identification was prognostically useful in type I, insulin-dependent diabetics [37–40]. Three studies indicated that reducing micro-albuminuria with ACEIs may prevent, or postpone diabetic nephropathy onset [6, 11, 16]. To date, a number of issues are still uncertain. Does micro-albuminuria reduction protect against GFR reduction? If yes, what kind of effect can be anticipated? This is illustrated in Fig. 2. Do ACE inhibitors 1. postpone diabetic nephropathy onset, 2. prevent diabetic nephropathy onset but not cardiovascular disease, 3. prevent diabetic nephropathy onset and cardiovascular disease, 4. improve both glomerular function and prognosis, 5. deserve consideration for primary prevention of renal and cardiovascular disease?

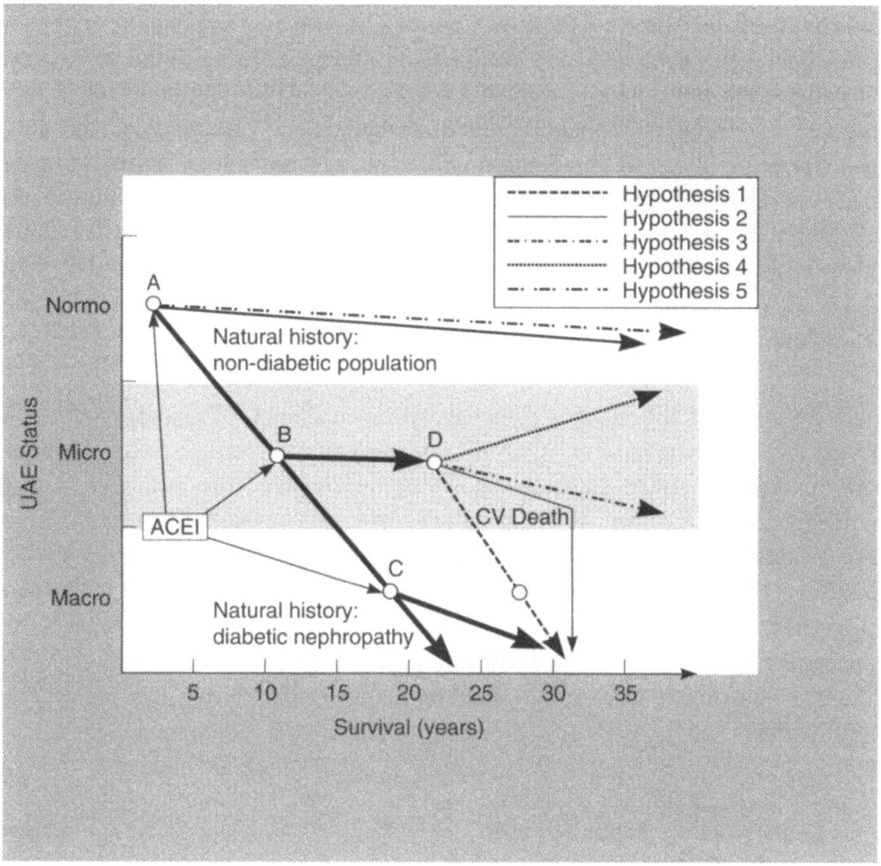

Fig. 2 Speculation on the potential effects of ACE inhibitors on the natural history of diabetic nephropathy

Plain lines indicate observed evolution.
Dotted lines indicate the various hypothesis.

Hypothesis 1: ACE inhibitors prevent macro-albuminuria but not renal failure
Hypothesis 2: ACE inhibitors prevent renal failure but not cardiovascular (CV) death
Hypothesis 3: ACE inhibitors prevent renal failure and cardiovascular death
Hypothesis 4: ACE inhibitors improve both kidney function and cardiovascular disease
Hypothesis 5: ACE inhibitors make prognosis of diabetics comparable to that of non diabetics

Study design

Cross-over trials are acceptable only in acute, or short-term (i. e., several-day) studies. Otherwise, parallel trials are mandatory due to the effect of time on GFR, UAE, and blood pressure. Double-blind, placebo-controlled studies are recommended. Single-center studies allow better precision but are rarely possible when a large number of subjects is required. Multi-center studies allow inclusion of large number of patients, but assessment of certain outcomes is less precise. Study design also differs according to the study goal. Organization, blinding and duration for example will be different when testing some pathophysiological aspect of diabetic renal disease (e. g., assessing the respective roles of the renin-angiotensin system and of systemic blood pressure in the constitution of micro-albuminuria [14]), or evaluating the effectiveness of various therapeutic attitudes (e. g., anti-hypertensive treatment with or without ACE inhibitors to prevent GFR degradation [12, 15]).

Duration of follow-up

The duration of follow-up varies according to choice of primary outcome. Once this outcome is chosen, study duration may be either fixed, or maximized. A fixed study duration allows comparison of the numbers of outcomes between groups. It requires previous follow-up studies to estimate the incidence of outcome. Alternatively, time-to-outcome may be chosen for analysis, thus allowing both time-to-event comparison between groups, or a stop-trial if a significant difference in the number of events is observable during one of the pre-planned interim analyses. In any case, a trial on GFR changes as primary outcome in diabetic nephropathy should last for 2 years minimally.

Sample size calculation

This crucial step is feasible with mathematical formula available in several statistical handbooks [41, 42]. Three parameters must be taken into account in every case:

- the expected incidence of chosen primary outcome
- the anticipated effectiveness of the experimental treatment compared to the reference treatment
- alpha and beta statistical risks.

If the outcome variable is qualitative (e.g., end-stage failure incidence), calculation can vary according to the type of design: fixed, or maximized period, presence or absence of interim analyses. If the outcome variable is quantitative, calculation will take into account its intra- and inter-subjects variability. The number of subjects will be dramatically influenced by the total variance of this variable. A pilot study can be useful to determine the best way of decreasing the variance: as seen above, the solution is a mixture of standardization and repetition of measurements.

Economic considerations

Due to increased health care costs, the number of economic analyses have increased rapidly in the literature. The 3 main types of analysis are cost-effectiveness, cost-benefit and cost-utility analysis. All involve the comparison of two or more strategies. In cost-effectiveness analysis, the strategies compared are based on the same outcome. For example one can compare the life expectancy or the number of patients with ESRF in patients treated or not with ACE inhibitors. In cost-benefit analysis, the outcome is valued in dollars. This unit allows comparison of strategies with various outcomes occurring with various frequencies. For example, the cost of premature death, hemodialysis, and cardiovascular events can be calculated and compared between the two strategies described above. In cost-utility analysis, natural units such as life expectancy are weighted by an index of utility. The quality of life is one measure of utility. Economists generally find this method of evaluating the effects of health care preferable to that of evaluating them in money terms. The QALY (Quality Adjusted Life Year) is the most frequently used unit allowing the comparison of several alternative therapeutic strategies.

All 3 types of analysis require a precise, unbiased estimate of the benefit of the interventions tested. In the absence of such estimates, the conclusion of different analyses may differ largely according to the studies on which the estimation of benefit is based. In the absence of a long-term trial comparing ACE inhibitors to other treatment strategies, published analyses should only be considered preliminary.

Bearing in mind this limitation, two recent studies have addressed the problem in the field of diabetic nephropathy. In the model used by Borch-Johnsen et al [2], the costs of screening and intervention for micro-albuminuria would balance the savings due to complications prevention in their worst hypothesis. In their best hypothesis, considerable economic savings could be expected. In an American study [43], the cost-effectiveness ratio of screening and intervention for micro-albuminuria with ACE inhibitors was estimated between 7,900 $ and 16,500 $ per year of life saved, according to the various hypothesis on the effectiveness of intervention. Interestingly, these figures were obtained in spite of relatively small improvements in life expectancy ranging from 0.5 to 1.2 years. These figures are comparable to those obtained for the treatment of mild hypertension (44). However, none of these 2 authors took into account some important aspects such as side-effects of treatments or poor compliance with long-term treatment which both decrease the cost-effectiveness of the programs.

From these analyses, it can be concluded that an aggressive screening and treatment program targeted at diabetics with micro-albuminuria is not unrealistic from a financial point of view. This is even more true if we consider the human value of the prevented complications (blindness, ESRF).

Acknowledgments

We thank Mrs. Line Godiveau for her secretarial assistance.

References

[1] Sepe SJ, Teutsch SM. Epidemiology of renal involvement in diabetes mellitus – Chap. 3. In: Mogensen CE, ed. The Kidney and Hypertension in diabetes mellitus. Den Haag: Martinus Nijhoff publishing, 1988; 17–23.
[2] Borch-Johnsen K, Wenzel H, Viberti GC et al. Is screening and intervention for microalbuminuria worthwhile in patients with insulin-dependent diabetes? B M J 1993; 306: 1722–1725.
[3] Mogensen CE. Progression of nephropathy in long-term diabetics with proteinuria and effect of initial anti-hypertensive treatment. Scand J Clin Lab Invest 1976; 36: 383–388.
[4] Christensen CK, Mogensen CE. Effect of antihypertensive treatment on progression of incipient diabetic nephropathy. Hypertension 1985; 7 (Suppl. II): 109–113.
[5] Parving HH, Andersen AR, Smidt UM et al. Effect of antihypertensive treatment on kidney function in diabetic nephropathy. B M J 1987; 294: 1443–1447.
[6] Marre M, Chatellier G, Leblanc H et al. Prevention of diabetic nephropathy with enalapril in normotensive diabetics with microalbuminuria. B M J 1988; 297: 1092–1095.
[7] Mimram A, Insua A, Ribstein J et al. Comparative effects of captopril and nifedipine in normotensive patients with incipient diabetic nephropathy. Diabetes Care 1988; 11: 850–853.
[8] Romanelli G, Giustina A, Bossoni S et al. Short-term administration of captopril and nifedipine and exercise-induced albuminuria in normotensive diabetic patients with early-stage nephropathy. Diabetes 1990; 39: 1333–1338.
[9] Rudberg S, Aperia A, Freyschuss U et al. Enalapril reduces microalbuminuria in young normotensive type 1 (insulin-dependent) diabetic patients irrespective of its hypotensive effect. Diabetologia 1990; 33: 470–476.
[10] Melbourne Diabetic Nephropathy Study Group. Comparison between perindopril and nifedipine in hypertensive and normotensive diabetic patients with microalbuminuria. B M J 1991; 302: 210–216.

[11] Mathiesen ER, Hommel E, Giese J et al. Efficacy of captopril in postponing nephropathy in normotensive insulin dependent diabetic patients with microalbuminuria. B M J 1991; 303: 81–87.
[12] Björk S, Mulec H, Johnsen SA et al. Renal protective effect of enalapril in diabetic nephropathy. B M J 1992; 304: 339–343.
[13] Wiegmann TB, Gish Herron K, Chonko AM et al. Effect of angiotensin-converting enzyme inhibition on renal function and albuminuria in normotensive type 1 diabetic patients. Diabetes 1992; 41: 62–67.
[14] Hallab M, Gallois Y, Chatellier G et al. Comparison of reduction in microalbuminuria by enalapril and hydrochlorothiazide in normotensive patients with insulin dependent diabetes. B M J 1993; 306: 175–182.
[15] Lewis EJ, Hunsiker LG, Bain RP et al. The effect of angiotensin-converting-enzyme inhibition on diabetic nephropathy. N Engl J Med 1993; 329: 1456–1462.
[16] Viberti GC, Mogensen CE, Groop LC et al. Effect of Captopril on progression to clinical proteinuria in patients with insulindependent diabetes mellitus and microalbuminuria. JAMA, 1994; 271: 275–279.
[17] Pirart J. Diabète et complications dégénératives. Présentation d'une étude prospective portant sur 4400 cas observés entre 1947 et 1973. Diabète Métab 1977; 3: 97–107, 173–182, 245–256.
[18] Viberti GC, Bilous RW, Makintosh D et al. Long term correction of hyperglycæmia and progression of renal failure in insulin-dependent diabetes. B M J 1983; 286: 598–602.
[19] Feldt-Rasmussen B, Mathiesen ER, Deckert T. Effect of two years of strict metabolic control on progression of incipient nephropathy in insulin-dependent diabetes. Lancet 1986; II: 1300–1304.
[20] Dahl-Jorgensen K, Hanssen KF, Kierfulf P et al. Reduction of urinary albumin excretion after 4 years of continuous subcutaneous insulin infusion in insulin-dependent diabetes mellitus; the Oslo study. Acta Endocrinol 1988; 117: 19–25.
[21] Reichard P, Nilsson BY, Rosenqvist U. The effect of long-term intensified insulin treatment on the development of microvascular complications of diabetes mellitus. N Engl J Med 1993; 329: 304–309.
[22] The Diabetes Control and Complications Trial Research Group: The effect of intensive treatment of diabetes on the development and progression of long-term complications in insulin-dependent diabetes mellitus. N Engl J Med 1993; 329: 977–986.
[23] Cohen D, Dodds R, Viberti GC. Effect of protein restriction in insulin-dependent diabetics at risk of nephropathy. B M J 1987; 294: 795–798.
[24] Walker JD, Bending JJ, Dodds RA et al. Restriction of dictary protein and progression of renal failure in diabetic nephropathy. Lancet 1989; II: 1411–1415.
[25] Kasiske BL, Kalil RS, Ma JZ et al. Effect of antihypertensive therapy on the kidney in patients with diabetes: a metaregression analysis. Ann Int Med 1993; 118: 129–138.
[26] Levey AS, Madaio MP, Perrone RD. Laboratory assessment of renal disease: clearance, urinalysis, and renal biopsy. Chap. 22. In: Brenner BM, Rector FC, eds. The Kidney. New York: W. B. Saunders Company, 1991; 919–968.
[27] Marre M, Leblanc H, Suarez L et al. Converting enzyme inhibition and kidney function in normotensive diabetic patients with persistent microalbuminuria. B M J 1987; 294: 1448–1452.
[28] Bland JM, Altman DG. Statistical methods for assessing agreement between two methods of clinical measurement. Lancet 1986; I: 307–310.
[29] Marre M, Hallab M, Roy J et al. Glomerular hyperfiltration in type I, type II, and secondary diabetes. J Diab Complic 1991; 6: 19–24.
[30] Hommel E, Mathiesen ER, Edsberg B et al. Acute reduction of arterial blood pressure reduces urinary albumin excretion in type I (insulin-dependent) diabetic patients with incipient nephropathy. Diabetologia 1986; 29: 211–215.

[31] Feldt-Rasmussen B, Dinesen B, Deckert M. Enzyme immunoassay: an improved determination of urinary albumin in diabetics with incipient nephropathy. Scand J Clin Lab Invest 1985; 45: 539–544.
[32] Marre M, Claudel JP, Ciret P et al. Laser immunonephelometry for routine quantification of urinary albumin excretion. Clin Chem 1987; 33: 209–213.
[33] Mogensen CE, Chachati A, Christensen CK et al. Microalbuminuria: an early marker of renal involvement in diabetes. Uremia Investigation 1985–1986; 9: 85–95.
[34] Bouhanick B, Berrut G, Chameau AM et al. Predictive value of testing random urine sample to detect microalbuminuria in diabetic subjects during outpatient visits. Diabète Métab 1992; 18: 54–58.
[35] Joint National Committee on Detection, Evaluation, and Treatment of High Blood Pressure: the fifth report of the Joint National Committee on Detection, Evaluation, and Treatment of high Blood Pressure (JNCV). Arch Intern Med 1993; 153: 154–183.
[36] Hansen KW, Mau Pedersen M, Marshall SM et al. Circadian variation of blood pressure in patients with diabetic nephropathy. Diabetologia 1992; 35: 1074–1079.
[37] Viberti RC, Hill RD, Jarret RJ et al. Microalbuminuria as a predictor of clinical nephropathy in insulin dependent diabetes mellitus. Lancet 1982; I: 1430–1432.
[38] Parving HH, Oxenboll B, Svendsen PAA et al. Early detection of patients at risk of developing diabetic nephropathy. A longitudinal study of urinary albumin excretion. Act Endocrinologia 1982; 100: 550–555.
[39] Mathiesen ER, Oxenboll B, Johansen K et al. Incipient nephropathy in type 1 (insulin-dependent) diabetes. Diabetologia 1984; 26: 406–410.
[40] Mogensen CE, Christensen CK. Prediciting diabetic nephropathy in insulin-dependent patients. N Engl J Med 1984; 311: 89–93.
[41] Schwartz D, Flamant R, Lellouch J. Nombre de sujets nécessaire Chap. X, XI, XII, XIII, XIV. In: L'essai thérapeutique chez l'homme. Paris: Flammarion Médecine – Science, eds, 1990; 93–128.
[42] Pocock SJ. Clinical Trials: A practical Approach. New York: John Wiley & sons, eds, 1987.
[43] Siegel JE, Krolewski AS, Warram JH et al. Cost-effectiveness of screening and early treatment of nephropathy in patients with insulin-dependent diabetes mellitus. J Am Soc Nephrol 1992; 3: S111–119.
[44] Kawachi I, Malcolm LA. The cost-effectiveness of treating mild-to-moderate hypertension: a reappraisal. J Hypertension 1991; 9: 199–208.

Methods for estimating the kinetics of lipid fuels in vivo

J. M. Miles, R. L. Judd, M. Persson, S. W. Coppack

Introduction

The discovery of the relationship between the pancreas and diabetes the late nineteenth century [1] heralded an interest in intermediary metabolism that continues to the present. Over the years, most investigators have focused attention on the derangements in glucose metabolism in diabetes rather than abnormalities in protein or lipid metabolism which are known to be present in this condition [2, 3]. Part of the reason that glucose metabolism has received the most attention is because of a bias, sometimes unspoken, that abnormalities in non-glucose metabolism are of secondary importance. This bias may relate to the serendipity of scientific discovery, however, as pointed out by McGarry [4]. Over the past decade, a number of studies have been published which indicate that abnormal lipid metabolism may have a more central role in the pathogenesis of diabetes (at least the type II variety) than has been previously appreciated [5–7]. The demonstration that the glucose-fatty acid cycle of Randle [8] is operative in the *in vivo* situation [6] suggests that competition by fatty acids for mitochondrial oxygen could contribute to insulin resistance, leading to chronic hypersecretion of insulin and eventually an insulin secretory defect in genetically susceptible individuals [9]. Such competition with glucose does not derive solely from circulating free fatty acids (FFA); metabolically active triglyceride (TG) depots are present in muscle [10], liver [11] and myocardium [12], and are likely the proximal source of fatty acids for oxidation in these tissues [13]. Preliminary evidence from muscle biopsies in individuals with type II diabetes suggests that intramuscular TG stores may be significantly increased in this condition [7]. Thus, the metabolism of lipid metabolites and its relationship to the pathogenesis of diabetes has recently received increased attention.

A second reason for the relative paucity of studies of lipid fuel metabolism is that the laboratory analyses of these substances are tedious and technically demanding, especially when compared with the relative ease of glucose measurements. In this chapter, we shall address a variety of methodological issues relating to the *in vivo* study of the lipid fuels: FFA, TG (i.e., the TG present in TG-rich lipoproteins) and ketone bodies (KB).

The use of tracers in lipid fuel research

The rationale for the use of tracers in the field of metabolism can be traced to early work demonstrating that circulating substances turn over in a dynamic steady state [14]. Although FFA kinetic rates have often been inferred from plasma concentrations, this approach can yield misleading information. First of all, it should be recognized that the kinetics of most (if not all) metabolizable substrates are non-linear; this is true for both FFA [15] and KB [16], and is likely the case for TG as well [17]. Secondly, the clearance rate of a substance may not only change inversely with turnover rate [15, 16, 18], but may also vary under different metabolic conditions. Thus, FFA clearance may be altered during exercise [19], in obesity [20], and in diabetes [21]. Both FFA and KB concentrations may remain unchanged during exercise in spite of an increase in the turnover rate of these substances [19, 22]; this is due to an increase in clearance rate for both FFA and KB, and in the absence of kinetic measurements could lead to an underestimation of the importance of lipid fuels in submaximal exercise.

Most tracer studies of FFA and KB metabolism have used the constant infusion technique, which is less mathematically formidable and which lends itself more easily to the study of nonsteady-state conditions. In the case of FFA, it is necessary to choose a single fatty acid as a paradigm for all long chain fatty acids. While this approach is generally valid [23], it should be remembered that there are subtle but potentially important differences in the metabolism of the different FFA [24]. For this reason, a tracer of one of the three major FFA in plasma – palmitate, oleate, or linoleate – should be used except in special circumstances. We have found that palmitate labelled with ^{3}H gives essentially identical results when compared to ^{14}C-labelled palmitate [25]. ^{3}H-labelled FFA are therefore preferable because of lower cost and lower radiation exposure. Although direct data concerning the comparability of FFA labelled with stable isotopes of hydrogen and carbon are to our knowledge not available, they are likely interchangeable based on experience with radiolabelled tracers. Whereas carbon labelled FFA have been used by us [26] and others [27, 28] to estimate FFA oxidation, this practice should be discouraged. Because of the presence of unlabelled intracellular TG, the specific activity (or enrichment) of the precursor pool for oxidation is unknown, and estimates of oxidation rates will be in error [13].

Because of the nature of the required laboratory analyses, FFA kinetics are more difficult to measure than glucose kinetics. However, the FFA method is actually easier in one respect. Because of the short half life and high fractional turnover of FFA, the difficulties encountered with estimates of nonsteady-state glucose turnover [29] are generally not a problem. The equations of Steele [30] adopted for nonsteady-state conditions perform quite well when applied to the study of FFA metabolism [31]. Moreover, the tracer recycling which can create errors in the estimation of glucose [32] and leucine [33] kinetics is not a problem in FFA studies [15]. Finally, there is no significant interconversion among the FFA [12], unlike branched-chain amino acids [34] and KB [35].

The interconversion which occurs between the KB anions β-hydroxybutyrate and acetoacetate creates a special challenge for the investigator who wishes to measure KB kinetics. Regardless of the choice of tracer, isotope disequilibrium, or inequality in specific activity between the two KB, has consistently been found [35, 36]. This phenomenon creates difficulty in the calculation of KB turnover [35, 36]. Several investigators have attempted to minimize the potential errors associated with the use of a single tracer by simultaneously infusing two KB isotopes [36, 37]. Although more accurate measurements of KB turnover can be obtained with two isotopes, this approach is technically difficult and requires steady-state conditions [38]. A single tracer method generates estimates of KB carbon flux which are usually sufficiently accurate to be useful [38]. For this reason, *in vivo* studies of the regulation of KB metabolism may best be accomplished with a single isotope. This would not be the case in specialized studies which examine regional KB metabolism with the powerful combination of arteriovenous sampling and tracer infusion; in this instance, two simultaneous KB tracers are needed [39].

TG metabolism is more difficult to study than FFA or KB metabolism. This is due in part to the much longer half life of TG-rich lipoproteins and in part to the unavailability of an ideal TG tracer. In earlier studies, VLDL was isolated from plasma, labelled with ^{131}I and reinjected into the subject [40]. Other investigators have used an indirect method in which the TG pool of interest is labelled by administering a labelled precursor [41, 42]. If one is interested in the fate of the lipoprotein particle, one can label apolipoproteins with an amino acid tracer and measure the fractional decay of the particle [43]. On the other hand, if the chief interest is the fate of the lipoprotein TG, it can be labelled with a bolus injection of an FFA or glycerol tracer [41, 42] in the case of very low density lipoproteins (VLDL), or with a meal containing labelled TG-fatty acids in the case of chylomicrons [44]. A glycerol tracer is preferable to an FFA tracer because the FFA tracer traverses an intrahepatic TG pool [11], delaying and prolonging its entry into VLDL. This can result in ongoing entry of FFA tracer into VLDL-TG during measurement of plasma VLDL kinetics, and can potentially underestimate the fractional disappearance of VLDL-TG. In contrast, glycerol disappears from plasma (and presumably from liver) extremely rapidly, resulting in near-instantaneous labelling of intrahepatic VLDL-TG.

Another approach to measuring VLDL kinetics is to infuse a radiolabelled VLDL precursor (labelled glycerol or FFA), isolate the newly labelled VLDL from plasma, and then use it as a tracer in another animal [45]. Wolfe et al used an ingenious method to label both the glyceride and fatty acid moieties of VLDL-TG in dogs [46]. They administered ^{3}H-labelled glycerol and ^{14}C-labelled palmitate via the portal vein and isolated VLDL-TG from arterial blood. This "biosynthetic" VLDL tracer was then administered in subsequent experiments to determine the actual turnover rate (rather than fractional disappearance) as well as the separate fates of the glyceride and fatty acid moieties [46]. The tracer produced by this method is ideal for determining VLDL-TG kinetics, but practical application of this approach in humans is obviously limited by the relative inaccessibility of the hepatic vein, the near-absolute inaccessibility of the portal vein and limitations on tracer dose imposed by dosimetry considerations. The use of labelled TG to study chylomicron metabolism has not received much attention, but has considerable potential. It is easy to generate measurable specific activities in chylomicron-TG fatty acids with relatively modest doses of radiolabelled TG (Coppack et al, unpublished results). The tracer can be administered as part of a synthetic liquid meal [44] or a mixed meal (Coppack et al, unpublished results). As this is an indirect method, it provides only a measurement of fractional disappearance. It is possible to estimate actual turnover rates from chylomicron-TG pool size, derived in turn from estimates of the concentration and volume of distribution of chylomicron-TG, provided that the amount and specific activity of the TG in the mixed meal is known and a sufficient number of blood samples are taken.

Analytical methods for the study of lipid fuel metabolism

Over the past 10−15 years, high performance liquid chromatography (HPLC) and gas chromatography/mass spectrometry (GC/MS) have achieved widespread use in research laboratories. These technologies have been improved, simplified and made less expensive so that they are now within the reach of most investigators. We shall review the impact of these developments on lipid fuel research below.

Free fatty acids

As stated above, FFA measurements have been historically difficult. The earliest studies of FFA kinetics were reported in the 1950s [47]. In an informal review of the literature, we found over 20 papers describing the administration of an FFA tracer to human subjects published between 1950 and 1975 (unpublished data). Interestingly, no more than 3 to 4, and usually fewer, of these articles were by the same authors. It is tempting to speculate that investigators working in this field found the analytical techniques available for measuring FFA specific activity sufficiently unsatisfactory or demanding (or both) that they lost interest in measuring FFA kinetics. The older methods typically involved infusion of a radiolabelled tracer and determination of radioactivity on an extract of plasma either with [47] or without [48] an attempt to separate FFA from esterified fatty acids. It is important to separate plasma FFA from TG when an FFA tracer is used, since significant labelling of plasma TG occurs within 15 min of tracer administration in such studies in humans [47]. An alternative approach for isolation of plasma FFA radioactivity involves thin layer chromatography [10, 12, 20], which is a more specific method but rather tedious. In either case, it is necessary to separately measure either individual [49] or total [47] FFA concentration in order to calculate specific activity.

The advent of GC/MS has made it possible to use stable isotopic tracers for *in vivo* kinetic measurements [50]. Stable isotopes have the obvious advantage of avoiding radiation exposure, desirable for studies in adults and mandatory for studies in children or pregnant women. In addition, the measurement of stable isotopic enrichment wich mass spectrometry avoids the imprecision which is inherent when tracer and tracee concentrations are determined separately, as was the case with the early studies of FFA metabolism. Since stable isotopic enrichment is essentially a tracer : tracee ratio determined simultaneously in a single analytical procedure, the recovery of tracer and tracee is linked and thus does not affect the results. The use of stable isotopes does have a significant disadvantage when applied to FFA studies, however, because FFA tracers are insoluble in water and thus must be infused after binding to albumin. An experiment lasting several hours in an adult subject may require infusion of several hundred milliliters of 4% albumin, potentially affecting such parameters as plasma volume and, indirectly, the metabolic processes which one is attempting to measure. Measurement of FFA enrichment with GC/MS is tedious in its own right, as it requires a thin layer chromatography (TLC) step prior to derivatization [51]. For these reasons, the use of radioactive tracers has an advantage over stable isotopes that is unique to studies of FFA metabolism.

Nearly 10 years ago, we attempted to develop a method for measuring FFA concentration and specific activity which would take advantage of the specificity and precision of HPLC. This procedure was initially applied to validate the measurement of palmitate kinetics [15] and has since undergone modification. The method involves a simple Folch-type extraction from plasma and the preparation of a phenacyl derivative of the FFA [15], without need for a TLC step because there is no hydrolysis of esterified fatty acids during the derivatization (unpublished data). The measurement of individual

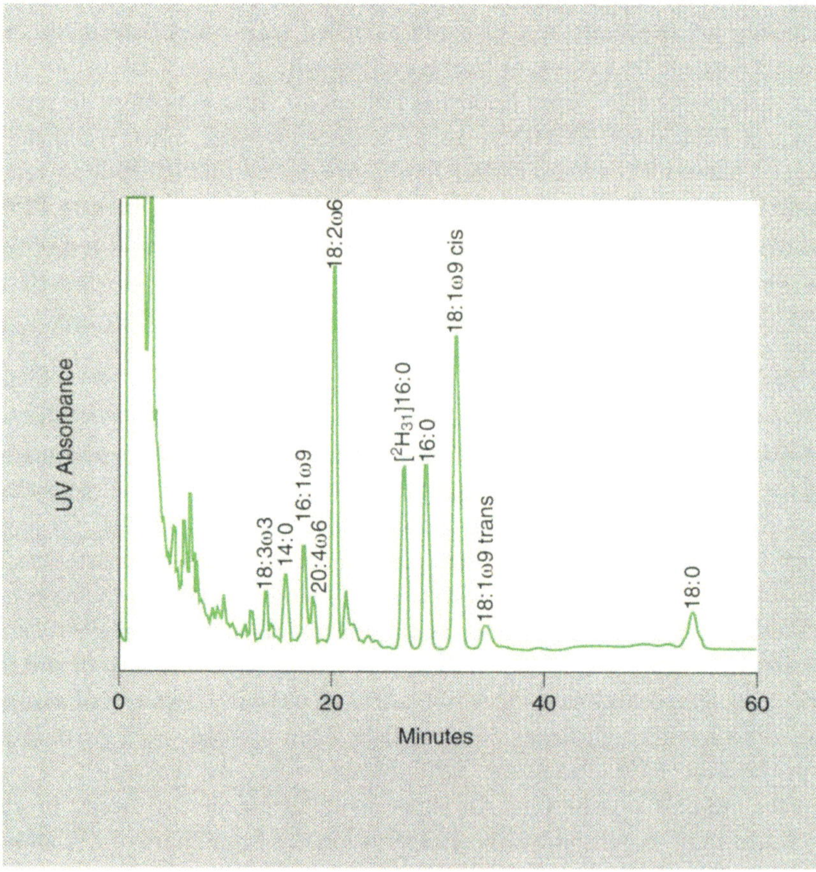

Fig. 1 An HPLC chromatogram of plasma free fatty acids. 18:3ω3 = α-linolenate, 14:0 = myristate, 16:1ω9 = palmitoleate, 20:4ω6 = arachidonate, 18:2ω6 = linoleate, [$^2H_{31}$] 16:0 = perdeuterated palmitate (internal standard), 16:0 = palmitate, 18:1ω9cis = oleate, 18:1ω9trans = elaidate, and 18:0 = stearate

FFA concentrations was facilitated by the use of [$^{2}H_{31}$] palmitate as an internal standard [25]. Chromatographic conditions can be adjusted in order to quantify 8–10 separate long chain fatty acids (Fig. 1). Although detection is typically performed at 214 or 254 nm (to accommodate fixed wavelength detectors and to reduce sensitivity for the analysis of relatively large aliquots of plasma from human studies), sensitivity can be increased as needed for small plasma aliquots by lowering the detection wavelength to ~ 240 nm. With this approach, individual FFA concentrations and specific activities can be determined on 10–20 μl specimens, making the procedure ideal for studies in rodents. The coefficient of variation for this method is < 2% for both concentration and specific activity. Thus, the precision of FFA specific activity analysis by HPLC is equal to that of isotopic enrichment measurements using gas chromatography-mass spectrometry.

Triglycerides

Several methods have been used historically to analyze TG labelled for kinetic studies. The simplest approach is to extract whole plasma with an organic solvent and either count the radioactivity directly [41] or isolate the TG using TLC. In either case a meaningful specific activity cannot be obtained from the analysis; in the first instance, the fatty acids are derived from total plasma lipids, not TG, and in the second instance the extracted TG derives from a variety of lipoproteins, including VLDL, low density lipoproteins (LDL), high density lipoproteins (HDL) and, when present, chylomicrons. For this reason, it is best to isolate the lipoprotein of interest as a first step. Some investigators have determined specific radioactivity in a lipid extract of plasma after removing FFA with dilute base [41] with or without removal of phospholipids; here, contamination of the sample with fatty acids from cholesterol esters will create analytical errors that may be greater than those encountered with TLC isolation of whole plasma TG.

Isolation of VLDL and chylomicrons is traditionally accomplished by ultracentrifugation [52]. This procedure is well established but is limited by the number of samples that can be processed from a typical experiment in a human volunteer. The principles of gel filtration chromatography have been adapted to more efficient and powerful HPLC systems to allow separation of lipoprotein classes based on molecular size [53]. We have developed a method for isolating chylomicrons and VLDL using automated HPLC in which 1.2 ml aliquots of fresh plasma are loaded onto a refrigerated autosampler (Waters WISP) and 1.0 ml is injected onto three BioRad SEC-50XL columns connected in series. The columns are eluted with a 2 μM

Na_2PO_4 buffer containing 0.2% sodium azide at 0.5 ml/min. Fractions are collected by a fully automated, computer-driven fraction collector (ISCO Retriever IV, Omaha, NB USA). Arterialized venous blood samples were taken from a volunteer subject 3 hours after ingestion of a mixed meal labelled with 100 μCi [1-^{14}C] triolein and after labelling VLDL TG with a 200 μCi injection of [2-^{3}H] glycerol. An HPLC chromatogram of ^{14}C and ^{3}H radioactivity is shown in Figure 2. As can be seen, the major chylomicron peak, labelled with ^{14}C, is easily separated from ^{3}H VLDL and a second peak of ^{3}H which coelutes with $^{3}H_2O$. This method can be used to rapidly separate chylomicrons from VLDL in plasma samples obtained from an acute experi-

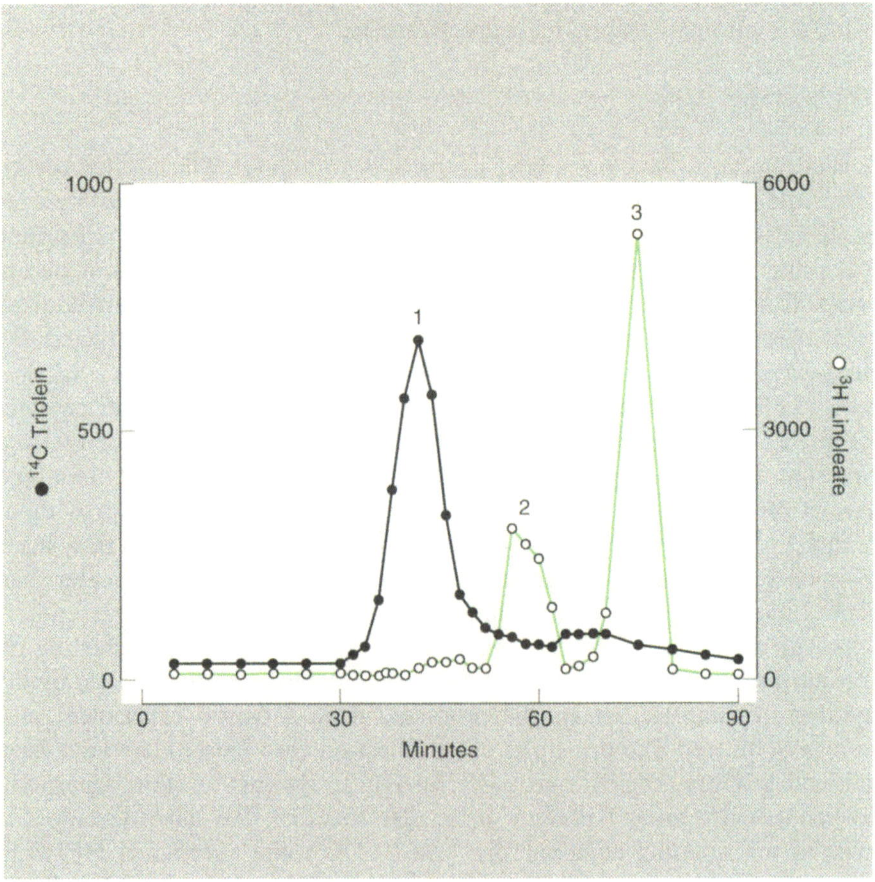

Fig. 2 An HPLC radiochromatogram of labelled lipoproteins from a human volunteer. 1 = ^{14}C-labelled chylomicrons; 2 = ^{3}H-labelled very low density lipoproteins; and 3 = $^{3}H_2O$ (a metabolite of ^{3}H linoleate). Units are dpm

ment; a sample can be injected as often as every 60 min without interfering with the preceding run. If more rapid throughput is desired, two automated HPLC systems can be set up in parallel to accomplish the analysis. Just as is the case with sequential floatation ultracentrifugation, smaller chylomicron remnants can potentially coelute with VLDL, so that the VLDL fraction will not be as pure as the chylomicron fraction.

Once the lipoprotein of interest has been isolated, a second HPLC step can be used to separate TG from cholesterol esters, FFA and phospholipids. We have modified the method of Christie [54] for more rapid throughput, allowing isolation of TG from 30–35 samples during an overnight run, using automated sampling and fraction collecting. This TG fraction is then saponified and the FFA extracted and derivatized as described for the plasma FFA analysis [15]. Thus, the specific activity of chylomicron or VLDL TG fatty acids can be determined with high sensitivity, precision and accuracy by taking advantage of the versatility and power of HPLC.

Glycerol

Glycerol is an important product of adipose tissue lipolysis. Glycerol kinetics have been measured for over 20 years as a measure of lipolytic rate, and have been touted as superior to FFA kinetics because of concern that local adipose tissue reesterification of FFA [55] might result in falsely low estimates of lipolysis. Recent *in vitro* work [56], together with studies combining highly accurate stable isotope methods for measuring glycerol and FFA turnover [57, 58], indicate that adipose tissue FFA reesterification is minimal under most circumstances. Nonetheless, glycerol tracers remain a useful tool for assessing lipolytic rates, and when a carbon-labelled tracer is used have the additional feature of providing an estimate of gluconeogenesis [59].

Glycerol is in some respects quite different from FFA; it is water soluble and does not bind to plasma proteins. However, like FFA it presents an analytical challenge to the investigator. It is therefore not surprising that highly divergent and sometimes implausible results have been obtained in studies where glycerol kinetics were measured with a radioactive tracer, with FFA : glycerol turnover ratios ranging from 1.4: to 5.2 : 1 [60, 61]. Glycerol is hydrophilic, does not absorb UV light well, and the small amounts found in a plasma sample can be volatile when isolated and subjected to vacuum during a drying procedure. It is possible to isolate plasma glycerol radioactivity using borate columns [62], but this procedure is tedious and still depends upon a separate measurement of glycerol concentration, introducing potential errors. The advent of GC/MS procedures for determining glycerol kinet-

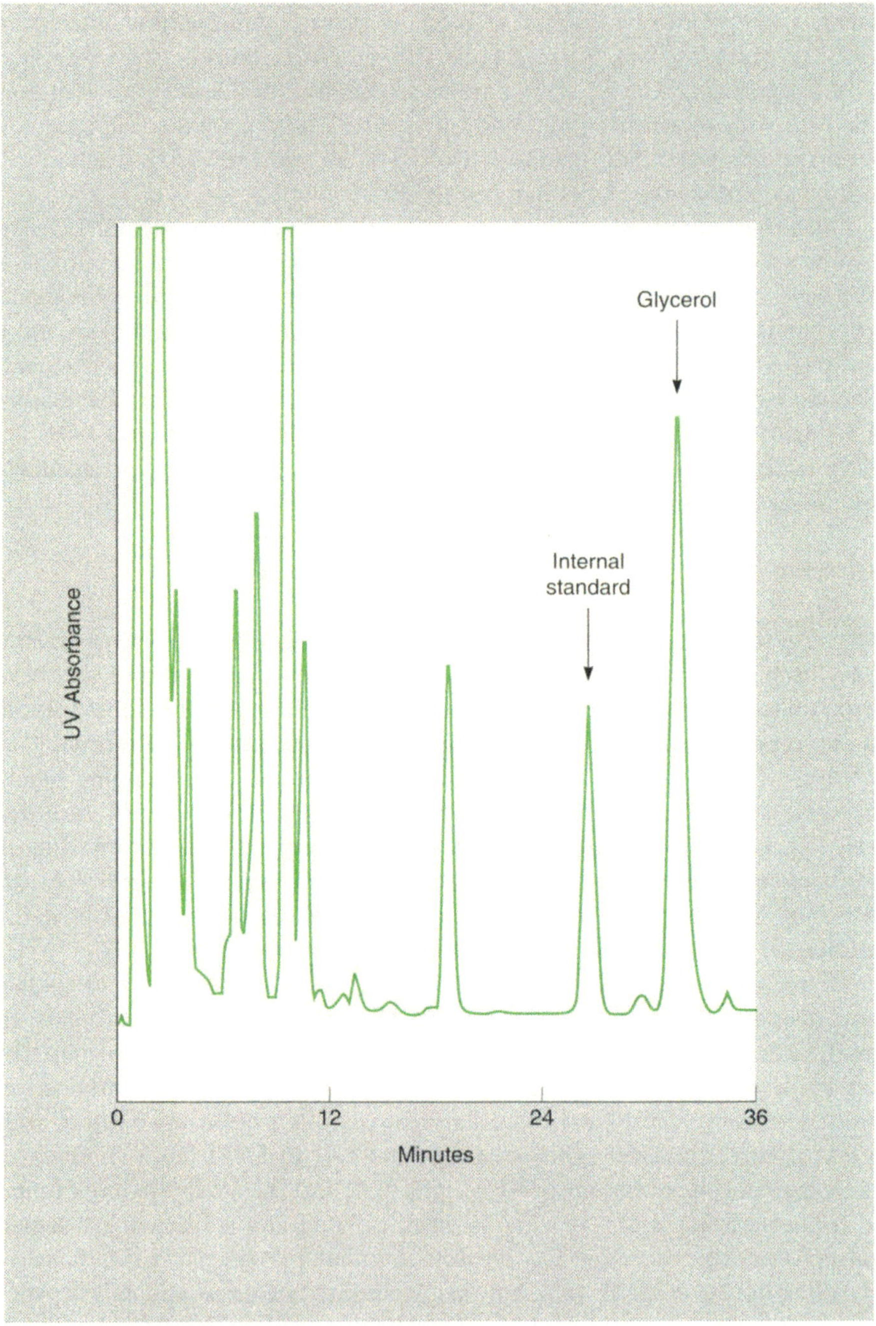

Fig. 3 An HPLC chromatogram of glycerol in human plasma. The internal standard is pentanediol

ics [63] represents a real advance in the study of this important substrate. We have developed a new HPLC method for measuring glycerol concentration and specific activity which is specific, precise and highly sensitive [64]. The key to the method is preparation of a benzoyl derivative. This technique is able to detect glycerol concentrations < 10 mol/L, and has a coefficient of variation < 3%. A chromatogram of plasma glycerol is shown in Figure 3.

Ketone bodies

The measurement of KB kinetics presents special modelling problems which have been addressed in a recent review [38]. Numerous methods are available for the laboratory measurement of KB specific activity; initially, most investigators isolated KB radioactivity using a precipitation method [65] or the method of Mayes and Felts [66]. Both of these procedures are time consuming, neither is ideally suited to batch analysis, and both require a separate measurement of KB concentration. We initially developed a streamlined method based on the binding of B-hydroxybutyrate to an anion exchange resin and the heat lability of acetoacetate [67]. This approach accomplished the goal of more rapid analysis with reasonable accuracy, but remained nonspecific and somewhat imprecise because of the need for a separate concentration measurement. We then developed a method which isolates radioactivity in the two KB anions by ion suppression reversed phase HPLC [68]. This method can be automated and is quite specific; imprecision can be minimized by measuring KB concentration directly on the HPLC fraction. However, it does not accomplish the goal of measuring specific activity in a single step. More recently, we reported an HPLC method which is capable of determining β-hydroxybutyrate specific activity [69]. This procedure, which involves preparation of a phenacyl ester, cannot measure acetoacetate. It is useful, however, for measuring the kinetics of acetate [70] and could be applied to the study of other short chain fatty acids.

The use of stable isotopes was a significant advance in the study of ketone body metabolism. A highly precise and sensitive method was developed which involves preparation of tert-butyl dimethylsilyl derivatives, utilizing capillary GC/MS and utilizes [$^{13}C_4$]-labelled ketone bodies as internal standards [71]. This method can detect KB concentrations < 10 mol/L and isotopic enrichments as low as 0.6%. Other investigators have reported similar success with slightly different derivatives [72]. Because these techniques involve stable isotopes, they are not suitable for determination of kinetics using bolus injections of tracer, but are quite useful for constant infusion experiments.

Summary

Major advances have occurred in the laboratory analysis of the lipid fuels FFA, TG, KB and glycerol. Older methods have been replaced by new procedures which utilize GC/MS and HPLC. These procedures are accurate, sensitive and precise. Together with the growing appreciation of the potential major role of lipid fuels in the pathogenesis of insulin resistance and type II diabetes, they will facilitate major advances in our understanding of lipid metabolism in the years to come.

Acknowledgements

JMM acknowledges Dr. Harold Jeskey for inspiring generations of students about the wonders of organic chemistry. Supported in part by grants from the U. S. Public Health Service (DK38092) and from St. Luke's Hospital Foundation for Education and Research.

References

[1] Houssay B. The discovery of pancreatic diabetes: The role of Oscar Minkowski. Diabetes 1952; 1: 112–116.
[2] Jensen MD, Caruso M, Heiling VJ et al. Insulin regulation of lipolysis in nondiabetic and IDDM subjects. Diabetes 1989; 38: 1595–1601.
[3] Nair KS, Garrow JS, Ford C et al. Effect of poor diabetic control and obesity on whole body protein metabolism in man. Diabetologia 1983; 25: 400–403.
[4] McGarry JD. What if minkowski had been ageusic? An alternative angle on diabetes. Science 1992; 258: 766–770.
[5] Felber JP, Ferrannini E, Golay A et al. Role of lipid oxidation in pathogenesis of insulin resistance of obesity and type II diabetes. Diabetes 1987; 36: 1341–1350.
[6] Ferrannini E, Barrett EJ, Bevilacqua S et al. Effect of fatty acids on glucose production and utilization in man. J Clin Invest 1983; 72: 1737–1747.
[7] Falholt K, Jensen I, Lindkaer Jensen S. et al. Carbohydrate and lipid metabolism of skeletal muscle in type 2 diabetic patients. Diabetic Med 1988; 5: 27–31.
[8] Randle PJ, Garland PB, Hales CN et al. The glucose fatty-acid cycle. Its role in insulin sensitivity and the metabolic disturbances of diabetes mellitus. Lancet I, 1963; 785–789.
[9] Ward WK, Beard JC, Halter JB et al. Pathophysiology of insulin secretion in non-insulin dependent diabetes mellitus. Diabetes Care 1984; 7: 491–502.
[10] Dagenais GR, Tancredi RG, Zierler KL. Free fatty acid oxidation by forearm muscle at rest, and evidence for an intramuscular lipid pool in the human forearm. J Clin Invest 1976; 58: 421–431.
[11] Woodside WF, Heimberg M. Hepatic metabolism of free fatty acids in experimental diabetes. Israel J Med Sci 1972; 8: 309–319.
[12] Wisneski JA, Gertz EW, Neese RA et al. Myocardial metabolism of free fatty acids. Studies with ^{14}C-labelled substrates inhumans. J Clin Invest 1987; 79: 359–366.

[13] Heiling VJ, Miles JM, Jensen MD. How valid are isotopic measurements of fatty acid oxidation? Am J Physiol 1991; 261: E572–E577.
[14] Shoenheimer R. The Dynamic State of Body Constituents. Cambridge: Harvard University Press, 1942.
[15] Miles JM, Ellman MG, McClean KL et al. Validation of a new method for determination of free fatty acid turnover. Am J Physiol 1987; 252: E431–E438.
[16] Fery F, Balasse EO. Ketone body production and disposal in diabetic ketosis. Diabetes 1985; 34: 326–332.
[17] Brunzell JD, Hazzard WR, Porte D et al. Evidence for a common, saturable, triglyceride removal mechanism for Chylomicrons and very low density lipoproteins in man. J Clin Invest 1973; 52: 1578–1585.
[18] Verdonk CA, Rizza RA, Gerich JE. Effects of plasma glucose concentration on glucose utilization and glucose clearance in man. J Clin Invest 1981; 65: 682–689.
[19] Havel RJ, Naimark A, Borchgrevink CF. Turnover rate and oxidation of free fatty acids of blood plasma in man during exercise: studies during continuous infusion of palmitate-1-C^{14}. J Clin Invest 1963; 42: 1054–1063.
[20] Nestel PJ, Ishikawa T, Goldrick RB. Diminished plasma free fatty acid clearance in obese subjects. Metabolism 1978; 27: 589–597.
[21] Taskinen MR, Bogardus C, Kennedy A et al. Multiple disturbance of free fatty acid metabolism in noninsulin-dependent diabetes. J Clin Invest 1985; 76: 637–644.
[22] Fery F, Balasse EO. Ketone body turnover during and after exercise in overnight-fasted and starved humans. Am J Physiol 1983; 245: E318–E325.
[23] Miles JM, Jensen MD. Determination of plasma-free fatty acid kinetics with tracers: methodological considerations. J Parenter Enteral Nutr 1991; 15 (suppl.): 90S–92S.
[24] Hagenfeldt L, Wahren J, Pernow B et al. Uptake of individual free fatty acids by skeletal muscle and liver in man. J Clin Invest 1972; 51: 2324–2330.
[25] Jensen MD, Rogers PJ, Ellman MG et al. Choice of infusion-sampling mode for tracer studies of free fatty acid metabolism. Am J Physiol 1988; 254: E562–E565.
[26] Bowyer BA, Fleming CR, Haymond MW et al. L-carnitine: effect of intravenous administration of fuel homeostasis in normal subjects and home parenteral nutrition patients with low plasma carnitine concentrations. Am J Clin Nutr 1988; 49: 618–623.
[27] Groop LC, Bonadonna RC, Shank M et al. Role of free fatty acids and insulin in determining free fatty acid and lipid oxidation in man. J Clin Invest 1991; 87: 83–89.
[28] Bonadonna RC, Groop LC, Zyck K et al. Dose-dependent effect of insulin on plasma free fatty acid turnover and oxidation in humans. Am J Physiol 1990; 259: E736–E750.
[29] Finegood DT, Bergman RN, Vranic M. Estimation of endogenous glucose production during hyperinsulinaemic euglycaemic glucose clamps: comparison of unlabelled and labelled exogenous glucose infusates. Diabetes 1987; 36: 914–924.
[30] Steele R, Wall JS, DeBodo RC et al. Measurement of size and turnover rate of body glucose pool by the isotope dilution method. Am J Physiol 1956; 18: 15–24.
[31] Jensen MD, Heiling VJ, Miles JM. Measurement of non-steady-state free fatty acid turnover. Am J Physiol 1990; 258: E103–E108.
[32] Bell PM, Firth RG, Rizza RA. Effects of hyperglycemia on glucose production and utilization in humans. Measurement with [2-3H]-, [3-3H]-, and [6-14C]glucose. Diabetes 1986; 35: 642–648.
[33] Rodriguez N, Schwenk WF, Beaufrère B et al. Trioctanoin infusion increases in vivo leucine oxidation: a lesson in isotope modeling. Am J Physiol 1986; 251: E343–E348.
[34] Schwenk WF, Beaufrère B, Haymond MW. Use of reciprocal pool specific activities to model leucine metabolism in humans. Am J Physiol 1985; 249: E646–E650.
[35] Miles JM, Schwenk WF, McClean KL et al. A dual-isotope technique for determination of in vivo ketone body kinetics. Am J Physiol 1986; 251: E185–E191.
[36] Bailey JW, Haymond MW, Miles JM. Validation of two-pool model for in vivo ketone body kinetics. Am J Physiol 1990; 258: E850–E855.

[37] Bougneres P-F, Ferre P. Study of ketone body kinetics in children by a combined perfusion of Carbon-13 and 2H(sub3) tracers. Am J Physiol 1987; 253: E496–E502.
[38] Miles JM. Techniques for the measurement of ketone body and lactate kinetics in vivo. Diabetes Rev 1994; in press.
[39] Bailey JW, Haymond MW, Miles JM. Metabolism of ketone bodies by skeletal muscle in starvation and uncontrolled diabetes. Metabolism 1990; 39: 1039–1043.
[40] Kissebah AH, Alfarsi S, Adams PW et al. Role of insulin resistance in adipose tissue and liver in the pathogenesis of endogenous hypertriglyceridaemia. Diabetologia 1976; 12: 563–571.
[41] Ryan WG, Schwartz TB. Dynamics of plasma triglyceride turnover in man. Metabolism 1965; 14: 1243–1254.
[42] Howard BV, Reitman J, Vasquez B et al. Very-low-density lipoprotein triglyceride metabolism in non-insulin-dependent diabetes-mellitus. Diabetes 1983; 32: 271–276.
[43] Eaton RP, Crespin S, Kipnis M. Incorporation of 75Se-selenomethionine into human apoproteins. III. Kinetic behavior of isotopically labelled plasma apoprotein in man. Diabetes 1976; 25: 679–690.
[44] Roust LR, Jensen D. Postprandial free fatty acid kinetics are abnormal in upper body obesity. Diabetes 1993; 42: 1567–1573.
[45] Steiner G, Haynes FJ, Yoshino G et al. Hyperinsulinemia and in vivo very-low-density-lipoprotein-triglyceride kinetics. Am J Physiol 1984; 246: E187–E192.
[46] Wolfe RR, Shaw JHF, Durkot MJ. Effects of sepsis on VLDL kinetics: responses in basal state and during glucose infusion. Am J Physiol 1985; 248: E732–E740.
[47] Fredrickson DS, Gordon RS. The metabolism of albumin-bound C^{14}-labelled unesterified fatty acids in normal human subjects. J Clin Invest 1958; 37: 1504–1515.
[48] Birkhahn RH, Cardwell RJ, Birkhahn GC et al. Palmitic acid kinetics in fasting, traumatized patients. J Trauma 1992; 32: 427–432.
[49] Hagenfeldt L. Turnover of individual free fatty acids in man. Federation Proc 1975; 34: 2246–2249.
[50] Wolfe RR. Tracers in metabolic research: radioisotope and stabel isotope/mass spectrometry methods. New York: Alan R. Liss, Inc., 1987.
[51] Wolfe RR, Evans JE, Mullany CF et al. Measurement of plasma free fatty acid turnover and oxidation using [1-^{13}C]palmitic acid. Biomed Mass Spectrom 1980; 7: 168–171.
[52] Havel RJ, Eder HA, Bragdon JH. The distribution and chemical composition of ultracentrifugally-separated lipoproteins in human serum. J Clin Invest 1955; 34: 1345–1353.
[53] Hara I, Okazaki M. High-performance liquid chromatography of serum lipoproteins. In: Segrest JP, Albers JJ, eds. Methods in enzymology. Vol 128. Plasma lipoproteins. Part A. Preparation, structure and molecular biology. Orlando: Academic Press Inc., 1986; 57–78.
[54] Christie WW. Rapid separation and quantification of lipid classes by high performance liquid chromatography and mass (light-scattering) detection. J Lipid Res 1985; 26: 507–512.
[55] Vaughan M. The production and release of glycerol by adipose tissue incubated in vitro. J Biol Chem 1962; 237: 3354–3358.
[56] Edens NK, Leibel RL, Hirsch J. Mechanism of free fatty acid re-esterification in human adipocytes in vitro. J Lipid Res 1990; 31: 1423–1431.
[57] Shaw JHF, Wolfe RR. The integrated effect of adrenergic blockade on glucose, fatty acid, and glycerol kinetics: responses in the basal state and during hormonal control with somatostatin-hormonal infusion. J Surg Res 1987; 42: 257–272.
[58] Wolfe RR, Peters EJ, Klein S et al. Effect of short-term fasting on lipolytic responsiveness in normal and obese human subjects. Am J Physiol 1987; 252: E189–E196.
[59] Nurjhan N, Consoli A, Gerich JE. Increased lipolysis and its consequences on gluconeogenesis in non-insulin-dependent diabetes mellitus. J Clin Invest 1992; 89: 169–175.
[60] Winkler B, Steele R, Altszuler N. Effects of growth hormone administration on free fatty acid and glycerol turnover in the normal dog. Endocrinology 1969; 85: 25–30.
[61] Bjorntorp P, Bergman H, Varnauskas E et al. Lipid mobilization in relation to body composition in man. Metabolism 1969; 18: 840–851.

[62] Nurjhan N, Campbell PJ, Kennedy FP et al. Insulin dose-response characteristics for suppression of glycerol release and conversion to glucose in humans. Diabetes 1986; 35: 1326–1331.
[63] Klein S, Young VR, Blackburn GL et al. Palmitate and glycerol kinetics during brief starvation in normal weight young adult and elderly subjects. J Clin Invest 1986; 78: 928–933.
[64] Judd R, Klein S, Morse D. et al. A new HPLC method for the determination of plasma glycerol kinetics. FASEB J 1993; 7: A170.
[65] Peters JP, Van Slyke DP. Quantitative Clinical Chemistry. London: Bailliere, Tindall and Cox, 1932; 626 pp.
[66] Mayes PA, Felts JM. Determination of Carbon14-labelled ketone bodies by liquid-scintillation counting. Biochem J 1967; 102: 230–235.
[67] Miles J, Haymond M, Rizza R et al. Determination of 14C radioactivity in ketone bodies: a new, simplified method and its validation. J Lipid Res 1980; 21: 646–650.
[68] Miles JM, Haymond MW, Nissen S et al. Effects of free fatty acid availability, glucagon excess and insulin deficiency on ketone body production in postabsorptive man. J Clin Invest 1983; 71: 1554–1561.
[69] Persson M, Bleiberg B, Kiss D et al. Measurement of plasma acetate kinetics using high-performance liquid chromatography. Anal Biochem 1991; 198: 149–153.
[70] Bleiberg B, Beers TR, Persson M et al. Systemic and regional acetate kinetics in dogs. Am J Physiol 1992; 262: E197–E202.
[71] Miles JM, Schwenk WF, McClean KL et al. Determination of ketone body turnover in vivo with stable isotopes, utilizing gas chromatography/mass spectrometry. Anal Biochem 1984; 141: 110–115.
[72] Bougneres PF, Balasse EO, Ferre P et al. Determination of ketone body kinetics using a D-(-)-3-hydroxy[4,4,4-$^{2}H_{3}$]butyrate tracer. J Lipid Res 1986; 27: 215–220.

Methods in protein metabolism in diabetes

T. P. Almdal, H. Vilstrup

Introduction

Two thousand years ago, Areatus the Cappodocian, a Greek medical scientist of the first century, described diabetes as being: "the melting down of the body and the limbs in the urine" [1]. It has thus long been known that diabetes, if untreated, is a catabolic disease.

Atchley et al demonstrated in 1932 that a withdrawal of insulin leads to negative N-balance, and that this can only partly be normalized by insulin treatment [2]. Although this study only comprised two patients, it is generally referred to as the standard study demonstrating that diabetes is a catabolic disease. This suggests that the literature on most aspects of protein metabolism in patients with diabetes is rather limited, which is in fact the case.

This chapter focuses on human diabetes, but as the literature is so scarce, a few basic results from animal studies are reviewed as an introduction. These studies are based on the fact that in comparison with other substances in the body protein and amino acids are unique in that they possess one or more nitrogen atoms, which means that the amount of nitrogen in a tissue precisely reflects its protein content. The importance of diabetes for tissue protein content was examined experimentally in diabetic rats treated with 4 different insulin and glucagon regimens: one with uncontrolled diabetes, one with poorly controlled diabetes, one optimally controlled with insulin, and one group optimally controlled, but also given glucagon, selectively re-establishing the hyperglucagonaemia of uncontrolled diabetes [3–5]. From the results shown in Figure 1, two main conclusions can be drawn with potential relevance to human diabetes. In uncontrolled diabetes, nitrogen is lost from muscles and the heart but not from other organs, and this can only be fully corrected by optimum insulin treatment. The other finding, which may relate to the pathogenesis of nitrogen loss in diabetes, is that the total nitrogen loss in the animals also given glucagon amounts to ⅓ of that in uncontrolled diabetes. In uncontrolled diabetes, both lack of insulin and increased glucagon levels are present, and the results suggest that about ⅔ of the total nitrogen loss is due to lack of insulin, whereas the last third is due to the hyperglucagonaemia, which is shown to accelerate hepatic elimination of amino acids and lead to an increased flux of amino acids from organs to the liver.

These findings support the conclusions of the classical studies, that diabetes leads to loss of tissue proteins.

This chapter will focus on methods for assessing protein content and metabolism in human diabetes. Table 1 gives an overview of the various methods which will be addressed.

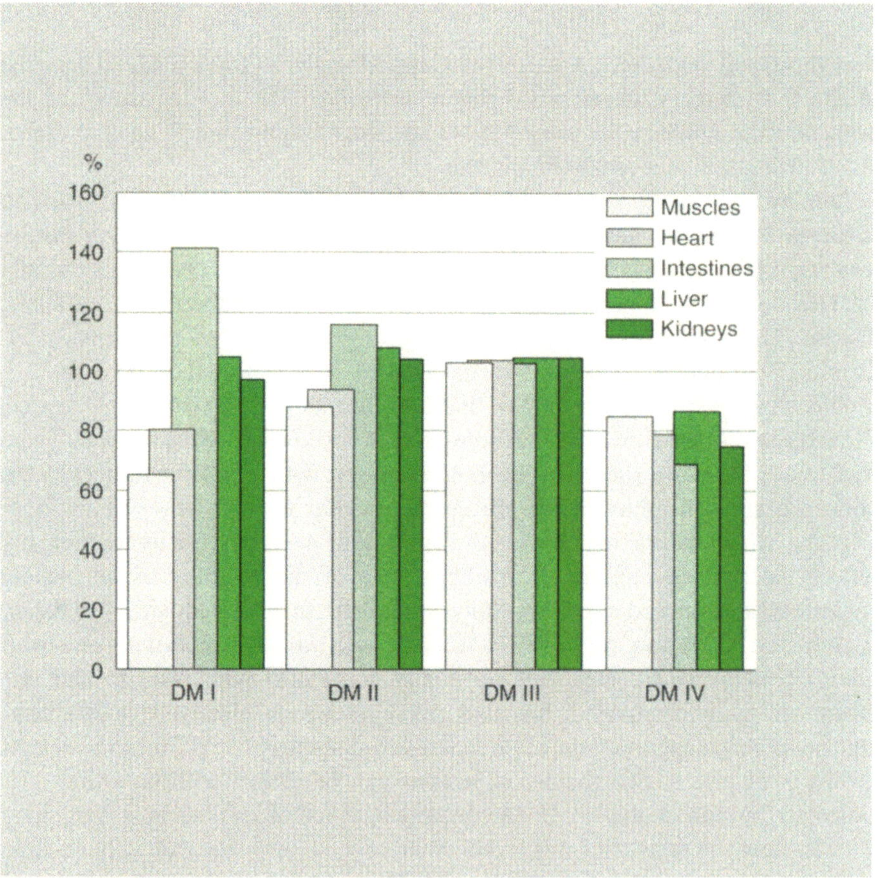

Fig. 1 The protein content of various organ systems given as % of control values in 4 groups of rats with experimental diabetes:

DM I: diabetic rats uncontrolled with insulin
DM II: diabetic rats poorly controlled with insulin
DM III: diabetic rats well controlled with insulin
DM IV: diabetic rats well controlled with insulin, but with hyperglucagonaemia as in DM I

Table 1 Areas of investigation and techniques in which they can be applied. The methods and their pro's and con's are discussed in the text

Body protein content (body composition)
Neutron activation analysis
Four compartment of body composition including:
Total body water by isotope techniques
Body density by water submersion
DEXA-scanning
DEXA-scanning
K^{40} in total body
24 h creatinine excretion
Body electrical impedance
Skinfold thickness
Protein and amino acid requirement
N-balance techniques
(Amino acid oxidation by isotope techniques)
Protein synthesis and breakdown
Isotope techniques
(A-V difference methods)
Amino acid and urea metabolism of the liver
A-V difference techniques
Kinetics of urea synthesis

Body composition

Methods

It is not possible to determine the nitrogen or protein content of individual organs *in vivo.* In principle however, the body consists of four basic components or compartments: water, fat, minerals and proteins, and, with various techniques, it is possible to determine and quantitate these compartments. In the present context, special focus is put on how to determine the body protein content.

In vivo total body N-contents can be determined with neutron activation analysis, and figures for this are available for the average healthy male [6]. There are, however, few facilities in the world for this complicated and expensive technique.

In practice, the methods available are more or less complicated ways of determining the fat-free or lean body mass, of which body protein constitutes the major component. The reference method is based on the so-called four compartment model, which segregates body into water, fat, minerals and protein [7, 8]. It uses a combination of the following techniques: isotope dilution technique, using labelled water for determination of total body water, underwater weighing for determination of body density and volume, and dual energy X-ray absorptionmetry (DEXA-scanning) for determination of bone mineral mass. By combining these techniques, and given knowledge of the density of fat and protein, it is possible to calculate the size (in kg) of the four compartments. This method is laborious and requires simultaneous access to all the techniques as well as experienced staff.

Most potassium is contained within non-fat cells, i. e. cells of the lean body mass. The potassium contents of the body can be determined by whole body scintillation counting, as there is a naturally and constantly occurring potassium isotope, K^{40}, and as the amount of K^{40} per kg lean body mass is known from cadaver analysis [9]. Compared to the four compartment model, the potassium method at mean is accurate, but gives large individual variations [8]. Moreover, it requires access to a whole body scintillation counter which is expensive and technically demanding to use.

In recent years DEXA-scanning (Dual Energy X-ray Absorptiometry) has been used not only for determination of bone mineral content, but also for determination of fat-mass and lean body mass [10]. Compared to the reference method, it is precise and the individual variation is quite small [8]. In practice, the method is technically easy to perform and the examination of a patient only takes 1 – 1½ hours. The equipment is moderately expensive, but is now available in many hospitals, as it is also used for bone research.

Fat is essentially water-free, and fat-free or lean body mass can be calculated by determination of total body water, if assuming a constant hydration fraction of the lean body mass [11]. The method is as precise as DEXA scanning [8], but the assumption of a constant hydration fraction cannot be taken as a given in diabetes. Another problem is that use of tritiated water implies a large dose of radiation, possibly raising ethical problems. Alternatively, deuterium can be used, but this requires access to mass spectrometry facilities for the determination of deuterium. Creatinine is released at a constant rate from muscles, and a precise correlation between 24 h creatinine and lean body mass, as assessed by the K^{40}-method, has been shown [12]. This method has, however, not been compared with the four compartment method, so its precision is not known. Its advantage is that it requires only standard biochemical analyses; the disadvantage is that, due to large day-to-day variations, three 24 h urinary collections are needed in order to obtain a good estimate, so that the method relies heavily on patient compliance [12].

Finally, there are various bedside techniques such as whole body impedance [13] and determination of skinfold thickness [14] at various sites, from which lean body mass can be approximated by use of various equations and nomograms. These methods seem to be fairly precise, but with some variation. In each study they probably require inclusion of a local control population for reference.

Diabetes

The literature on body composition in diabetes is very scarce. There is one study, using neutron activation analysis in 6 patients with newly diagnosed diabetes. Neither normal values nor adequate details concerning metabolic control are given. Nonetheless, the study suggests that the body nitrogen contents increases by about 20% during the first half year of insulin treatment [15]. The K^{40}-method has been used in some studies, but in only one study were matched controls included, and this study reports essentially normal values of total K^{40} with no trend towards reduced values in patients with poor metabolic control [16]. In a longitudinal study based on 24 h urinary creatinine excretion values, a large group of patients was followed the initial 7 years after the diagnosis of diabetes. During this period, the patients maintained lean body mass at normal levels, including those in poor metabolic control [17].

In conclusion, a number of methods exist for determination of lean body mass in humans, but very few studies have actually been undertaken in diabetes, and primarily in insulin-dependent diabetes. For future studies, DEXA scanning at present seems to be the most promising method currently available, as it is technically easy to use and is becoming more readily available. However, this method has not yet been validated in patients with diabetes.

Protein and amino acid requirements

Methods

The assessment of protein requirements in man has for many years relied on the N(itrogen)-balance technique, and this is still the standard method. The N-content of the food eaten and of all the excretes, urine and feces, are determined by the Kjeldahl technique. The figure for output is then subtracted from input. The balance obtained is positive if the person is retaining nitrogen and negative if nitrogen is lost from the body. The minimum protein requirements can be determined by feeding persons with increasing amounts of proteins, until a zero balance is reached. Most studies of this type were carried out in healthy students in the US more than 50 years ago, and therefore, the degree to which these figures can be used in various groups of patients has come into question [18]. However, figures for protein requirements published by the Food and Drug Administration (FDA) still relies on these early studies, and the most current version of the Recommended Dietary Allowances (RDA) still recommends a protein intake of 0.75 g/kg per day for healthy adults [19].

The requirements of essential amino acids, i. e. amino acids which can not be synthesized by the body, can also be determined by the N-balance technique. The amino acid in question is removed from the food and the person reverts into negative N-balance irrespective of the total amount of protein in the food. Then, an increasing amount of the amino acid is added to the food until neutral N-balance is reached. The requirement for this amino acid is then the amounts which leads to a return to neutral N-balance.

In recent years, it has been suggested that if amino acid requirements are equal to the rate of oxidation of a given amino acid, this could be assessed by tracer techniques (for details see [20]).

Diabetes

Neither the total protein requirement, nor the requirement of individual amino acids has ever been established in diabetes. One reason is probably that large amounts of dietary proteins have always been recommended for diabetic patients, and still are [21, 22]. This recommendation is given in order to reduce the amount of carbohydrate in the food, and is not based on knowledge of high protein requirements in diabetes.

During recent years, some studies have suggested that a restriction of dietary protein intake may delay the progression of diabetic renal failure [23, 24], and it has also been suggested that vegetarian proteins, as compared to meat proteins, are less damaging to the failing kidneys [25]. In these studies, not much emphasis has been put on whether a protein restriction, or a change to vegetarian proteins, causes a loss of body proteins, i. e. negative N-balance.

Only one short-term study has examined the relationship between metabolic control and protein requirements in diabetic patients, and it suggests that protein requirements increase during poorer metabolic control [26].

In conclusion, the method of choice for assessing of protein and/or amino acid requirements still is the N-balance technique. At present, the actual requirements for diabetics and their possible relation to metabolic control and/or diabetic complications (kidney disease) remain unknown.

Dynamics of protein metabolism

With body composition techniques and nitrogen balance studies it is possible to describe the actual size of and net changes in the whole body protein mass, i. e. whether or not the body protein contents are normal, and whether or not a net protein loss takes place. These methods, however, do not provide any information about the dynamics of the metabolic processes that regulate body protein metabolism. In an adult man of 70 kg, the total body protein mass amounts to about 10,000 g. All body proteins undergo constant turnover; they are broken down and new ones are synthesized. The rate of these processes probably varies substantially from organ to organ and from situation to situation, but it has been estimated that the total body protein turnover amounts to 250–300 g/24 hrs., i. e. 2,5–3% of the total amount/24 hrs. When proteins are broken down to amino acids, they are released into the blood-free-amino-acid pool which amounts to about 100 g in an adult man. The size of the free-amino-acid pool is thus determined, among other factors, by organ protein breakdown, which tends to increase it, and by organ protein synthesis, which tends to decrease it. However, a number of experimental studies also suggest that the size of the pool regulates the protein synthesis rate, i. e. a high amino acid concentration tends to increase protein synthesis rates. The size and composition of the free-amino-acid pool is also regulated by the liver. Following a meal, the liver regulates the proportion of amino acids released into systemic circulation, and thus made available to protein synthesis. The liver can deplete the pool of amino acids by converting them into glucose and urea, and hence abnormalities in the control of these processes affect the free-amino-acid pool and thereby organ protein turnover. Therefore, in order to study the dynamics of protein metabolism, it is necessary to have methods which assess protein turnover (synthesis and breakdown), the blood-free-amino-acid pool, and hepatic amino acid metabolism.

Determination of whole body protein turnover

In order to enable determination of whole body protein metabolism/turnover a simplified model of the body is assumed.

The body is divided into two pools, one homogenous pool of all free amino acids, and one pool in which all proteins are located. It is assumed that all amino acids, whether derived from food or endogenous, enter the amino-acid pool and are evenly distributed in it. Body proteins are synthesized from the pool of amino acids, and amino acids can also be lost from the pool by oxidation and urea formation. During a steady-state concentration of all amino acids within the pool, the whole body turnover or flux (Q) of an amino acid is equal to the sum of the processes supplying the amino acid, i. e. exogenously as dietary intake (Ra_{ex}), plus endogenously as released from proteins (Ra_{end}). This is equal to the sum of all processes removing the amino acid, i. e. oxidation (Rd_{ox}) plus non-oxidative disposal ($Rd_{non\text{-}ox}$) [27, 28]:

$$Q = (Ra_{ex}) + (Ra_{end}) = (Rd_{ox}) + (Rd_{non\text{-}ox})$$

When protein turnover is studied under postabsorptive conditions, dietary intake is zero and the equation reduces to:

$$Q = (Ra_{end}) = (Rd_{ox}) + (Rd_{non\text{-}ox})$$

It is necessary to keep track of the amino acids by use of an amino acids tracer, labelled either in radioactive (C^{14}) or stable (C^{13}) carbon atoms, or in the nitrogen by the stable isotope (N^{15}) (there is no radioactive nitrogen isotope). If radioactive isotopes are used, a scintillation counter is the only necessary analytical equipment in principle, whereas if stable isotopes are used, a mass spectrometer is needed. Due to radiation problems most studies are now carried out with stable isotopes despite the higher cost of isotopes and equipment.

Most studies have used the indispensable branched-chain amino acid leucine. Leucine transverses all membranes and moves rapidly within the cells. Reversibly, it transaminates to its keto acid, alpha-ketoisocaproate (KIC). KIC may undergo irreversible decarboxylation of its 1. carbon, thereby releasing CO_2, and if leucine is labelled in this atom, the label can be measured in the expiratorial gases [29]. Whole protein turnover can be measured during infusion of a leucine tracer in the fasting state and up to the steady-state. It has been shown that the plasma enrichment of KIC reflects the intracellular leucine enrichment [29]. Leucine flux is calculated as:

$$Q = i(E_i/E_p - 1)$$

where i is the rate of leucine infusion (μmol/min), E_i is the enrichment of the tracer, and E_p is the enrichment of plasma (of KIC). When the patient is fasting, Q equals breakdown (Ra_{end}). Oxidation of leucine (O_L) is calculated as

$$O_L = (VCO_2 \times E_{CO2})/(E_p \times 0.81)$$

where VCO_2 corresponds to the volume of expired CO_2, E_{CO2} the specific activity of CO_2, E_p the enrichment of plasma KIC, and 0.81 a correction for fixation of CO_2 in body tissues [29, 30]. The synthesis can then be calculated as the difference between flux and oxidation.

It should be emphasized that different amino acid tracers do not supply identical results, suggesting that the model is not entirely correct. Most studies, however, have been carried out with leucine.

Determination of organ protein turnover

The whole body protein flux is the mean of what is occurring in all the various organs and types of proteins, and will not reflect abnormalities in specific organs. Therefore, it is desirable to study single organs. In principle, this has been attempted in two ways, either by studying the A−V balance of one or more amino acids across the organ, or by direct determination of the incorporation of a tracer into the organ. In order to measure net A−V differences, reliable and precise measurement of perfusion of the organ is required. Colour, thermo, or radio-isotope dilution techniques are available and have been reliably validated. It has to be realized, however, that with regard to extremities, which are often taken to represent skeletal muscle tissue for the most part, the flow measured stems, not only from muscles, but also from skin, adipose and bone tissues. A−V differences can be measured over the splanchnic area and include both intestines and liver. By multiplying perfusion flow with A−V concentration differences, it is possible to determine the net uptake or release of one or more amino acids. Such measurements do not, however, give any information on actual rates of synthesis or breakdown.

By combining the A−V difference technique with isotope incorporation in tissues, synthesis can be measured directly, but until now this has only been done in muscles. In practice, during leucine infusion, one biopsy is taken once isotope steady-state has been reached and another is taken later. The synthesis rate is then calculated as the increase in leucine enrichment divided by the product of plasma leucine enrichment (or KIC) and time between the biopsies. If the A−V difference of leucine enrichment is also determined, breakdown can be calculated from the synthesis rate.

Protein metabolism in diabetes

The majority of studies on protein metabolism in diabetes have been carried out in patients with insulin-dependent diabetes mellitus (IDDM), and have mainly focused on whole body protein metabolism, using leucine as tracer.

Following insulin withdrawal in IDDM patients, the leucine flux or protein breakdown increases, typically to values of about 140% of those found in the control group [31–37]. After insulin is resumed, most studies report that the leucine flux falls to values within the normal range. One study, however, reports that leucine flux is still higher than that found in control persons at identical concentrations of insulin [33]. During the period when insulin is lacking, the leucine oxidation determined from labelled KIC is increased, but returns to normal values upon resumption of insulin [33, 35, 37]. Protein synthesis, which, as mentioned earlier, is a calculated value and not measured directly, is slightly increased during lack of insulin, but normal during insulin treatment [31, 34, 35, 37]. The whole body protein turnover in non-insulin-dependent diabetes mellitus has only been examined on few occasions, and they do not suggest abnormalities in protein metabolism [38, 39]. There are only a few studies on the protein turnover of separate organs of patients with insulin-dependent diabetes, all dealing with muscles. When muscle protein syntheses before and after insulin replacement were compared, no abnormalities were identified [40, 41]. In one study, measurements were performed before and after raising plasma amino acid concentrations by infusions, and it was found that this did not increase the muscle protein synthesis in IDDM patients, which it did in the controls [42].

In conclusion, lack of insulin leads to increased whole body protein breakdown as well as muscle protein breakdown, as well as to an increased rate of whole body protein oxidation. These abnormalities can be fully corrected by insulin replacement. Whole-body protein synthesis increases slightly when insulin is lacking, and it normalizes during insulin treatment. In muscles, lack of insulin does not affect the rate of protein synthesis. However, it appears that muscle protein synthesis is not stimulated by amino acids to same extent as it is in normal subjects.

The free-amino-acid pool in diabetes

The free-amino-acid pool is, as stated earlier, equal to total blood amino acid content. If, assuming that the plasma volume is unchanged in diabetes, the free-amino-acid pool can be assessed by determination of plasma amino acid concentration. Apart from access to an amino acid analyser, this does not represent a technical problem.

In both insulin-dependent diabetes [43, 45] and in non-insulin-dependent diabetes [43], it has been found that the gluconeogenic amino acids are slightly reduced or not different from control, whereas the branched chain amino acids tend to be increased during poor control, and normal during good metabolic control.

Amino acid metabolism in the diabetic liver

Methods

Amino acids metabolism in the liver plays a dominant role in whole body amino acid homeostasis.

The amino acid metabolism of the liver can be assessed in various ways. The net uptake or release of amino acids over the splanchnic bed, i. e. intestines and liver, can be studied by using the liver vein catherization technique.

Urea is synthesized from the alpha-amino-N-atoms of all amino acids within the liver. It is an irreversible process, whereby the nitrogen incorporated into urea cannot be reused. Quantitatively, urea synthesis is by far the most important metabolic process removing nitrogen from the body. Urea synthesis can be measured simply as the urinary output of urea, corrected for accumulation in its distribution space, for total body water, and for gut hydrolysis that seems to be fairly constant [44]. In humans, there is a linear relationship between amino acid concentration and the rate of urea synthesis, so that the kinetics of urea synthesis can be studied as the slope of this relation [45].

Diabetes

Using the liver vein catherization technique, it has been shown in fasting and insulin-deprived IDDM patients that the splanchnic uptake of amino acids is substantially increased [45]; whether this is also the case during insulin replacement has not been examined. Splanchnic amino acid exchange has also been examined in insulin-withdrawn IDDM patients following protein ingestion, and no difference between patients and controls could be demonstrated [46].

The kinetics of urea synthesis have been studied in insulin-withdrawn IDDM patients, and a marked increase in urea synthesis was found [47]. Whether this is also the case during insulin therapy has not been examined to date. In diet-controlled, fasting NIDDM patients, urea synthesis is also increased, but not as markedly as in IDDM patients [48].

In conclusion, in fasting and insulin-withdrawn diabetic patients, the liver takes up more amino acids and converts them into glucose and urea, but no abnormalities in amino acid metabolism in response to protein ingestion have been demonstrated.

Conclusion

The protein and amino acid metabolism of human diabetes has thus far been the object of few studies.

Whether the body protein contents of patients with diabetes is normal or reduced is still an open question. At the moment, the most promising technique for examining this question on a large scale appears to be DEXA-scanning. Likewise, the exact protein requirements of patients with diabetes have not been studied; this question merits attention, especially as protein restriction may well become part of the treatment of patients with diabetic nephropathy. The problem can be addressed with nitrogen balance techniques, possibly combined with repeated DEXA-scans. The processes regulating protein turnover have been studied to some extent, but due to methodological limitations only measurements of whole-body and, to some degree muscle (leg), turnover have been conducted. It is not clear what the measured whole-body protein metabolism actually represents. In order to obtain better estimates of protein turnover, improved techniques are needed. In contrast, good techniques are available for estimating liver amino acid metabolism, (i. e. liver vein catherization techniques) and for quantitating urea synthesis and its kinetics and regulation.

Finally, whether the abnormalities in protein metabolism of patients with diabetes carry any prognostic significance is completely unknown. In insulin-dependent diabetes, poor prognosis is very strongly associated with diabetic kidney disease. Although it is not known for certain, these patients may well have a reduced lean-body mass, which could be of prognostic importance. In non-insulin-dependent diabetes there is an increased mortality for the whole group of patients. In this disease, there also exists a strong association between kidney disease and mortality, but, as in insulin-dependent diabetes, the presence and possible importance of decreased lean body mass is unknown.

There are many open questions regarding protein and amino acid metabolism in patients with diabetes that may well be of both scientific and clinical significance. In general, the technologies to address the questions are available. Thus far, however, the problems have received very little attention because of the prevailing focus on other aspects of the disease.

References

[1] Reed JA. Aretaeus, the Cappadocian. Diabetes 1954; 3: 419–421.

[2] Atchley DW, Loeb RF, Richards DW et al. On diabetic acidosis. J Clin Invest 1933; 12: 297–326.

[3] Almdal TP, Vilstrup H. Effects of streptozotocin-induced diabetes and diet on nitrogen loss from organs and the capacity of urea synthesis in rats. Diabetologia 1987; 30: 952–956.

[4] Almdal TP, Vilstrup H. Strict insulin treatment normalizes the organ nitrogen contents and the capacity of urea nitrogen synthesis in experimental diabetes in rats. Diabetologia 1988; 31: 114–118.

[5] Almdal TP, Vilstrup H. Exogenous hyperglucagonaemia in insulin controlled diabetic rats increases urea excretion and nitrogen loss from organs. Diabetologia 1988; 31: 836–841.
[6] Cohn SH, Vartshy D, Yasumura S et al. Compartmental body composition based on total-body nitrogen, potassium, and calcium. Am J Phys 1980; 239: E524–E530.
[7] Heymsfield SB, Lichtman S, Baumgartner RN et al. Body composition of humans: comparison of two improved fourcompartment models that differ in expense, technical complexity, and radiation exposure. Am J Clin Nutr 1990; 52: 52–58.
[8] Fuller NJ, Jebb SA, Laskey MA et al. Four-compartment model for the assessment of body composition in humans: comparison with alternative methods, and evaluation of the density and hydration of fat-free mass. Clinical science 1992; 82: 687–693.
[9] Forbes GB, Gallup J, Hursh JB. Estimation of total body fat from potassium-40 content. Science 1961; 133: 101–102.
[10] Sartois DJ, Resnick D. Dual-energy radiographic absorptiometry: current status and perspective. Am J Roentgenol 1989; 152: 214–246.
[11] Brodie DA. Techniques of measurement of body composition. Part I. Sports Medicine 1988; 5: 11–40.
[12] Forbes GB, Bruining GJ. Urinary creatinine excretion and lean body mass. Am J Clin Nutr 1976; 29: 1359–1366.
[13] Fuller NJ, Elia M. Potential use of bioelectrical impedance of the whole body and of body segments for assessment of body composition: comparison with densitiometry and antropometry. Eur J Clin Nutr 1989; 43: 779–791.
[14] Durnin JVGA, Womersley J. Body fat assessed from total body density and its estimation from skinfold thickness: measurements on 481 men and women aged 16–72 years. Br J Nutr 1974; 32: 77–97.
[15] Walsh CN, Soler NG, James H et al. Studies in the whole body potassium and whole body nitrogen in newly diagnosed diabetics. Q J Med 1976; 178: 295–301.
[16] Goodship THJ, Butler PC, Clayton B et al. Total-body potassium in insulin dependent diabetes mellitus. Clinical Science 1990; 78: 377–381.
[17] Rosenfack AM, Snorgaard O, Almdal T et al. Creatinine height index and lean body mass in adult patients with insulin dependent diabetes mellitus followed for 7 years from onset. J Parenteral Enteral Nutr, accepted 1993.
[18] Hegsted DM. Assessment of nitrogen requirements. Am J Clin Nutr 1978; 31: 1669–1677.
[19] Recommended dietary allowances. 10th ed. Washington DC: National Academy Press, 1989.
[20] Young VR, Bier DM, Pellett PL. Atheoretical basis for increasing current estimates of the amino acid requirements in adult man with experimental support. Am J Clin Nutr 1989; 50: 80–92.
[21] American Diabetes Association. Nutritional recommandations and principles for individuals with diabetes mellitus. Diabetes Care 1986; 10: 126–132.
[22] Diabetes and Nutrition Study Group of the European Association for the Study of Diabetes. Nutritional recommandations for individuals with diabetes mellitus. Diab Nutr Metab 1988; 1: 145–149.
[23] Walker JD, Bending JJ, Dodds RA et al. Restriction of diatary protein and progression of renal failure in diabetic nephropathy. Lancet 1989; II: 1411–1415.
[24] Zeller K, Whittaker E, Sullivan L et al. Effect of restricting dietary protein on the progression of renal failure in patients with insulin-dependent diabetes mellitus. N Eng J Med 1991; 324: 78–84.
[25] Wiseman MJ, Hunt R, Goodwin A et al. Dietary composition and renal function in healthy subjects. Nephron 1987; 46: 37–42.
[26] Lariviere F, Kupranycz DB, Chiasson JL et al. Plasma leucine kinetics and urinary nitrogen excretion in intensively treated diabetes mellitus. Am J Physiol 1992; 263: E173–E179.
[27] Protein Turnover in Mammalian Tissues and in Whole Body. Waterlow JC, Garlick PJ, Millard DJ, eds. Amsterdam: North Holland, 1978.
[28] Matthews DE, Motil KJ, Rihrbaugh DK et al. Measurement of leucine metabolism in man from primed, continuous infusion of L (1-^{13}C)leucine. Am J Physiol 1980; 238: E473–E479.

[29] Matthews DE, Schwartz HP, Yang RD et al. Relationship of plasma leucine and alfa-ketoisocaproate during L (1-^{13}C)leucine infusion in man: a method for measuring human intracellular leucine tracer enrichment. Metabolism 1982; 31: 1105–1112.

[30] Bier DM. Intrinsically difficult problems: The kinetics of body proteins and amino acids in man. Diabetes Metab Rev 1989; 5: 111–132.

[31] Nair KS, Garrow JS, Ford C et al. Effect of poor diabetic control and obesity on whole body protein metabolism in man. Diabetologia 1983; 25: 400–403.

[32] Robert JJ, Beaufrere B, Koxiet J et al. Whole body de novo amino acid synthesis in type I (Insulin dependent) diabetes studied with stable isotope-labelled leucine, alanine and glycine. Diabetes 1985; 34: 67–73.

[33] Tessari P. Nosadini R, Trevisan R et al. Defective suppression of leucine-carbon appearance and oxidation in type 1, insulin dependent diabetes mellitus. J Clin Invest 1986; 77: 1797–1804.

[34] Umpleby AM, Boroujerdi MA, Brown PM et al. The effect of metabolic control on leucine metabolism in type 1 (insulin-dependent) diabetic patients. Diabetologia 1986; 29: 131–141.

[35] Nair KS, Ford CG, Halliday D. Effects of intravenous insulin treatment on in vivo whole body leucine kinetics and oxygen consumption in insulin-deprived type I diabetic patients. Metabolism 1987; 491–495.

[36] Tessari P, Pehling G, Nissen SL et al. Regulation of whole-body leucine metabolism with insulin during mixed-meal absorption in normal and diabetic humans. Diabetes 1988; 37: 512–519.

[37] Luzzi L, Castellino P. Simonson DG et al. Leucine metabolism in diabetes. Diabetes 1990; 39: 38–48.

[38] Staten MA, Matthews DE, Bier DM. Leucine Metabolism in type 2 diabetes mellitus. Diabetes 1986; 35: 1249–1253.

[39] Biolo G, Tessaari P, Inchiostro S et al. Fasting and postmeal phenylalanine metabolism in type 2 diabetes. Am J Phys 1992; 263: E877–E883.

[40] Pacy PJ, Nair KS, Ford C et al. Failure of insulin infusion to stimulate fractional muscle protein synthesis in type 1 diabetic patients: anabolic effect of insulin and decreased proteolysis. Diabetes 1989; 38: 618–624.

[41] Bennet WM, Connacher AA, Smith K et al. Inability to stimulate whole body protein synthesis in type 1 (insulin-dependent) diabetic patients by insulin-plus-glucose during amino acid infusion: studies of incorporation and turnover of tracer L (1-^{13}C)leucine. Diabetologia 1990; 33: 43–51.

[42] Bennett WM, Connacher A, Jung RT et al. Effect of insulin and amino acids on leg proteinturnover in IDDM patients. Diabetes 1991; 40: 499–508.

[43] Vannini P, Marchesini G, Forlani G et al. Branched-Chain amino acids and alanine as indices of metabolic control in type I (insulin-dependent) and type 2 (Non-Insulin-Dependent) diabetic patients. Diabetologia 1982; 22: 217–219.

[44] Vilstrup H. Synthesis of urea after stimulation with amino acids: relation to liver function. Gut 1980; 21: 990–995.

[45] Wahren J, Felig P, Cerasi E et al. Splanchnicand peripheral glucose and amino acid metabolism in diabetes mellitus. J Clin Invest 1972; 51: 1870–1878.

[46] Wahren J, Felig P, Hagenfeldt L. Effect of protein ingestion on splanchnic and leg metabolism in patients with diabetes mellitus. J Clin Invest 1976; 57: 987–999.

[47] Almdal TP, Jensen T, Vilstrup H. Increased hepatic efficacy of urea synthesis from alanine in insulin dependent diabetes mellitus. Eur J Clin Invest 1990; 20: 29–34.

[48] Almdal TP, Jensen T, Vilstrup H. Control of non insulin dependent diabetes mellitus partly normalizes the increased hepatic efficacy for urea synthesis. Metabolism, 1994; 43: 328–332.

Research methodologies in the evaluation of pancreas and islet cell transplantation

R. G. Bretzel, B. J. Hering, K. F. Federlin

Introduction

Replacement of the patient's islets of Langerhans either by pancreas transplantation or by isolated islet transplantation is the only treatment of type 1 diabetes mellitus to achieve an insulin-independent, constant normoglycemic state [1,2] The expense for this benefit is the need for immunosuppressive treatment of the recipient with all its potential risks. Thus, indications for pancreas or islet transplantations at present exist almost exclusively in patients with end-stage renal disease waiting on dialysis for a kidney graft or in diabetics with already established kidney graft being and going to be obligated to immunosuppression for this reason, respectively. Pancreas transplants alone are primarily performed in only highly selected non-uremic patients with extreme problems of the diabetes [3]. Recent studies demonstrated that pancreas transplantations finally delay the progression of diabetic secondary complications and probably prolong patients' life expectancy [4]. Furthermore, there is no doubt on the dramatic improvement of quality of life [5]. However, pancreas transplantation confers a certain risk and has its complications whereas islet transplantation is a rather minor procedure associated with only small risk, if any [4]. Islet transplantation offers the possibility to alter in vitro the islet immunogenicity and antigenicity, to induce an immunotolerant state or to encapsulate the islets so as to introduce only temporary immunosuppressive treatment of the recipient or to obviate the need for immunosuppression after islet allo- or xenotransplantation [4]. The effectiveness of this concept was demonstrated in animal experiments and may be successfully transferred into the clinical situation [6, 7, 8]. In that case the indications for islet transplantation may be extended to non-uremic type 1 diabetics including diabetic children. This group of patients is the ultimate target group for this treatment concept. But, up to now, islet transplantations have been performed only simultaneously to or after kidney transplantations and this method is still a clinical investigational procedure.

Nevertheless, the progress during the last three years period has provided evidence that islet transplantation may in principle establish insulin independence also in man albeit prolonged insulin independence has been achieved in only a small number of cases [9].

Experimental pancreas transplantation

The discovery that the pancreas is an organ essential for carbohydrate metabolism was made by von Mering and Minkowski when they demonstrated in 1889 that pancreatectomy produced diabetes mellitus in dogs [10]. In the years to follow this discovery, treatment of diabetes mellitus by transplantation of (non-vascularized) pancreatic tissue was suggested and attempted by several investigators in animal models and even in man [12, 13, 14]. These series of experimental pancreatic tissue grafting were initiated about 30 years before the discovery of insulin [15]. Finally, the first successful transplants of immediately vascularized pancreatic grafts were made in dogs in the late 1920's by Gayet and Guillaumie [16], Houssay [17], and Lexer [18].

A main obstacle to successful pancreas transplantation has been the anatomic peculiarity of the pancreas, which comprises about 1 million endocrine islets of Langerhans randomly distributed in an organ which consists mainly (more than 96%) of exocrine tissue. Technical problems of vascularized pancreatic transplantation mainly concern the exocrine part of the gland and the predisposition of the graft to vascular thrombosis. The surgical techniques meanwhile proven to be very effective in clinical transplantation were first elaborated in experimental models, mostly on dogs and pigs as auto- and allotransplantations. Another major obstacle to either pancreas or islet transplantation, graft rejection, and its prevention by immunosuppressive treatment, will be discussed in the chapters on clinical pancreatic and islet transplantation. In principle, the immunosuppressive regimens used to prevent rejection of pancreas allografts are similar to those used for other solid organ transplants [19].

Duct drainage procedures

A dog model for drainage of the exocrine pancreas by transplanting the duodenum along with the pancreas was described as early as 1929 and was further developed performing cutaneous duodenostomy or by jejunal anastomy [17, 20, 21]. Open duct drainage to the abdominal cavity was well tolerated in some experimental animals but was followed by subsequent ductal obstruction and acinar atrophy in long-term studies [22, 23]. Alternative duct drainage procedures were developed using ductal anasthomosis to the ureter or to the bladder [24, 25].

Duct occlusion procedures

Preservation of endocrine pancreatic function after occlusion of the pancreatic duct and subsequent atrophy of the exocrine parenchyma was demonstrated in early experimental studies [14, 15, 26]. Simple duct ligation proved as incomplete obstruction prone to cause pancreatitis and fistulae where as duct occlusion by injection of polymers like vinyl-plastic, acrylate glue, neoprene, prolamine, polyisoprene, and silicon rubber components was shown to give excellent results in large animals and was later successfully adopted in clinical pancreas transplantation [27–32].

Revascularization procedures

In the early experimental studies with pancreas organ transplantation a high incidence of vascular thrombosis had to be realized, probably due to the considerable low pancreatic blood flow [33]. Following this explanation various methods of vessel constructions were experimentally tested but the increased risk of vascular thrombosis is still a relevant problem in clinical pancreatic organ transplantation [34, 35].

Clinical pancreas transplantation

The first pancreas transplant in man was performed by Kelly, Lillehei and associates at the University of Minnesota on December 17, 1966 [36]. A cadaver donor segmental (body and tail) duct-ligated pancreas graft was transplanted to the iliac fossa of an uremic diabetic woman. A kidney was transplanted to the opposite iliac fossa. The patient became normoglycemic and insulin-independent, but died two months post transplant from a rejection and sepsis. The American College of Surgeons/National Institute of Health [37] maintained an Organ Transplant Registry until June 30, 1977, and up to that time received information on 57 pancreas transplants in 55 diabetic recipients [37]. The one-year patient survival rate and the one-year pancreas graft function rate in these pioneering cases was only 40% and 3%, respectively [38]. However, at that time, kidney transplantation was still in the early stages of development and clinical immunosuppressive protocols had just been formulated.

Pancreas procurement

Of all the organs procured for transplantation, the pancreas is considered the most difficult. The ultimate success of a functioning graft is often predicated upon expertise by which the organ is recovered. Presently, the majority of transplant centers perform combined liver-pancreas procurement. Experimental work was started in the early 1970's when the advantage of protein gel solutions compared to electrolyte solutions for pancreas flushing and preservation was first emphasized [39]. Other preservation solutions tested mainly in dog experiments were Collins solution [40], Euro-Collins solution [41], Silica-gel-filtered plasma [42], and Belzer-University of Wisconsin (UW) solution [43]. The preservation techniques using presently in most of the clinical cases either Euro-Collins or UW solution are aimed to protect against tissue and cell damage during hypothermic ischemia in order to preserve satisfactory endocrine graft function. In particular, ion exchange across the cell membrane may be limited, cell swelling may be prevented and energy substrates conserved.

Technical aspects

In the following years various surgical techniques emerged for solving the problems with pancreatic duct management. Today, the three most popular techniques are bladder drainage, polymer injection and enteric drainage [44]. Simultaneous pancreas/kidney (SPK) transplants comprise the vast majority of the cases with pancreas after kidney (PAK) and pancreas transplants alone (PTA) in non-uremic patients being much less frequent.

Immunosuppressive treatment of the recipient

The immunosuppressive regimens used to prevent rejection of pancreas allografts are similar to those used for other solid organ transplants [19]. Theoretically, new organs are as susceptible to the basal autoimmune process (insulitis) in type 1 diabetes mellitus as the one being replaced. But in practical terms the amount of immunosuppression required to prevent allograft rejection is nearly always sufficient to prevent autoimmune disease recurrence [45].

Success rates and effects on glucose metabolism

The development of pancreatic organ transplantation has been documented by the International Pancreas Transplant Registry, created in 1980 and since that time maintained at the University of Minnesota [44]. The data of the previous ACS/NIH Registry were incorporated. Since October 1, 1987, all US cases have also been reported to the United Network for Organ Sharing (UNOS) Registry and the cases have been depicted by Pre-UNOS and UNOS era, respectively (Figure 1). As of July 31, 1994, the International Pancreas Transplant Registry (IPTR) had received reports on 6,060 pancreas transplants (Figure 1). An analysis of all simultaneous pancreas – kidney transplants, regardless of duct management technique, reported to the Registry between October 1, 1987 and April 30, 1994, are shown in table 1. The one-year survival rate of the patients, kidney and pancreas was 91%, 84% and 74%, respectively. The five-year survival rate was 81% for the patients, 70% for the kidney and 62% for the pancreas. Approximately less than half

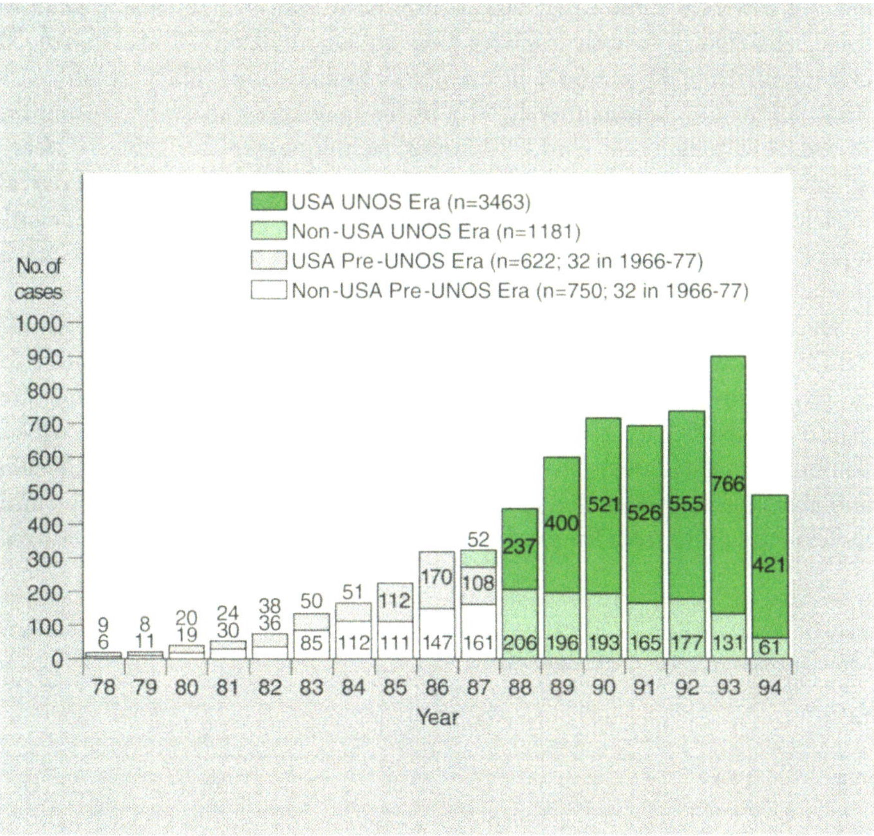

Fig. 1 World pancreas transplants (total of 6016 cases) by location and year. IPTR, Minneapolis, as of Aug 1, 1994; 54 cluster cases excluded

Table 1 World Simultaneous Pancreas-Kidney (SPK) transplant outcome. Cases reported to the IPTR in Minneapolis between Oct 1, 1987 and Apr 30, 1994

Category	n	1 yr survival (%)	5 yr survival (%)
Patient	3629	91	81
Kidney	3597	84	70
Pancreas	3623	74	62

of PAK and PTA recipients were insulin-independent at one year but, later on the survival rate significantly decreased (Table 2). Loss from acute rejection was much higher in the latter two categories, perhaps because of the inability to use the kidney as a marker for rejection. Patient survival rates did not differ in three categories, being more than 91% at one year in all three. However, previous analysis have shown that with 0–1 HLA-A, B, DR mismatches the same results can be obtained with solitary as with SPK transplants [46]. Approximately 90% of the pancreas transplants during this period were done by the bladder drainage technique (see also Table 3). Nearly all enteric drained or duct injected grafts were done in Europe. The overall technical failure rate of 18% for non-US cases (141 of 797) was significantly higher than the technical failure rate of 12% (234 of 1.948) for US cases ($p<0.001$)[46].

Several metabolic indices can be used to measure transplant effects. Successful pancreas transplantation has been shown to eliminate the need for exogenous insulin and to result in normal or much improved glucose metabolism as measured by glucose tolerance tests and glycosylated hemoglobin determinations [47–49]. However, in pancreas transplant recipients, insulin and glucagon responses to a glucose challenge, and certain other biochemical indices may differ from those of non-diabetic patients. The long-term clinical-

Table 2 Pancreas graft survival by category and by continent. Cases reported to the IPTR in Minneapolis between Oct 1, 1987 and Apr 30, 1994

Category		n	1 yr survival (%)	5 yr survival (%)
SPK	USA	2713	75	59
	Europe	889	72	66
PAK	(US only)	244	48	18
PTA	(US only)	178	48	21

Table 3 Pancreas graft survival by duct management. Cases reported to the IPTR in Minneapolis between Oct 1, 1987 and Apr 30, 1994

Category		n	1 yr survival (%)	5 yr survival (%)
BD	USA	2574	76	60
	Europe	576	78	73
ED	USA	89	57	48
	Europe	70	63	49
DI	(Europe only)	243	61	59

BD bladder drainage; ED enteric drainage; DI duct injection

significance of these disturbances is unclear. It should be further noted that a pancreas transplant closely approximates, but does not duplicate, the function of a normal pancreas. For example, in most cases, venous drainage of the transplant is into the systemic rather than the portal vein system, thus, secreted insulin initially bypasses the liver and produces an elevated peripheral-portal venous insulin ratio, the ultimate significance of which remains to be determined [50]. In addition, drugs used in immunosuppression regimens (e.g., glucocorticoides) may independently affect metabolism [51].

Effects on diabetic secondary complications

Most diabetic pancreas organ recipients were suffering from advanced secondary complications. Nevertheless, analysis of the data show that there is an impact of correcting the diabetic condition by pancreas organ transplantation on established complications. However, for several reasons, only preliminary and incomplete data exist with regard to the effect of pancreas transplantation on these complications. Secondary intervention studies are hampered by the difficulty in assessing the window of reversibility for each complication. The possibility that pancreas transplantation can arrest and, to a limited extent, reverse the progression of diabetic polyneuropathy has been suggested by some studies [52–54].

It has been demonstrated that pancreas transplantation prevents kidney graft diabetic nephropathy [55]. Another study of subjects who received pancreas transplants after having undergone renal transplantation found that they had significantly less severe histological changes in the glomerulus than a control group of diabetic renal transplant patients treated with conventional insulin therapy [56]. These data support the hypothesis that normoglycemia achieved by pancreas transplantation may prevent or retard the progression of diabetic renal disease.

Transplantation safety

The mortality risk of pancreas transplantation procedures either alone or combined with kidney transplants, is similar to that of kidney transplantation, that is small but not negligible. In combined kidney – pancreas transplants, the risk is small enough so that such surgery can be considered as an alternative to dialysis and continued insulin therapy in many uremic diabetic patients. However, uremic recipients of kidney - pancreas transplants have a higher renal rejection episode rate and longer hospitalization than recipients of kidney – only transplants [57]. Surgical complications of pancreas transplantation include bleeding, local infection, urinary leak, graft pancreatitis, bicarbonate loss, and urethritis [58]. Recipients of kidney allografts require life-long immunosuppression, the risk of which, also significant, generally is outweighed by the poor quality of life and mortality of end-stage renal disease. Combining a pancreas transplantat with a kidney transplant imposes little additional risk of drug toxicity beyond that which already exists from the immunosuppression needed by the renal graft. This is not true for pancreas – only transplants; such patients incure a substantial exposure to drug-induced nephropathy and other adverse effects from immunosuppression that they otherwise would not experience. Therefore, at present the risk-benefit ratio for pancreas – only transplants in non-uremic patients is more difficult to assess and, in principle, islet cell transplantation with its potential to obviate the need for life-long post transplant immunosuppression may be considered in non-uremic type 1 diabetics.

Experimental islet transplantation

Pancreatic islets were first described by Paul Langerhans in 1869, when his thesis on his research as a medical student in Virchow's laboratory was published [59]. After the successful autologous transplantation of pancreatic fragments in a dog by Minkowski in 1892 in order to prevent the development of diabetes mellitus, the idea of separating the islet tissue from the exocrine tissue of the pancreas before transplantation was suggested by Ssobolew [11, 14]. Only experimental studies on isolated adult islet tissue will be described; the various aspects of fetal islet transplantations will not be considered.

Islet isolation and purification

The message of Ssobolew was not well taken and it took a further sixty years until the first method was described to isolate islets by handdissection under the microscope [60]. But this method yielded only a small number of islets whereas the discovery of the action of collagenase on pancreatic fragments was a real breakthrough that led to high yields of isolated islets from murine pancreas [61, 62]. In the original method the pancreatic duct was distended with saline solution followed by handchopping to small pieces before incubation with collagenase. This method has been used by many groups, sometimes with minor variations, e.g. we preferred an arterial perfusion-distension protocol instead of the original pancreatic duct distension [63]. The advantage of the latter is that the islets are selectively stained by neutral red which eases the identification when doing handpicking under a dissecting microscope for further purification of the preparation. Meanwhile, the most widely used method involves pancreatic duct distension with collagenase before chopping as first investigated on mouse pancreatic tissue [64]. Very recently, we modified the established automated digestion-filtration method including air bubbling during the separation process in the stainless chamber for application on rodent pancreas [65, 66].

A critical step in the islet isolation process has been the purification procedure. Simple sedimentation is the easiest but also the most inefficient method. In rodent experiments centrifugation on Ficoll gradients proved as most effective compared to sucrose or albumin [67]. It was learned that the islet purification technique determines the mass and the viability of islets as well as the purity which may greatly affect the degree of islet implantation, islet immunogenicity, and safety for the islet recipient [68–70]. Standard methods for purification are currently performed using Ficoll-sodium diatrizoate, nicodenz or bovine serum albumin, and a COBE 2991 cell-separator for large-scale purification of islet preparations from higher mammalian and human pancreas [71–73].

Islet culture and cryopreservation

Preservation of islets has been performed by culture techniques. Rodent islets maintained in culture for days or weeks can synthesize and secrete insulin in response to appropriate stimuli [74–76]. It was further demonstrated that cultured isolated rodent islets may reverse diabetic metabolic state after transplantation into diabetic animals [74–76]. Long-term preservation of large amounts of isolated islets of Langerhans may be preferentially done with cryopreservation techniques. Isolated adult islets of Langerhans derived from rodent pancreas can be frozen and stored at -196°C for months or years without evident loss of viability [77–79]. Preserved endocrine function of frozen-thawed rat and human islets was demonstrated in vitro [80]. Meanwhile, numerous studies have shown that rodent islets can be successfully cryopreserved, as evidenced by preservation of beta-cell responsiveness in vitro and in vivo resulting in a reversal of diabetes after implantation into experimentally diabetic animals [81]. Cryopreservation methods have been recently extended to long-term preservation of higher mammalian and human isolated islet tissue [82, 83]. These data indicated that indefinite storage of islets is possible by cryopreservation and the methods have been used to successfully freeze islets from most species. Cryopreservation of islets is the only reliable way for long-term storage, which probably will facilitate the clinical use of islet transplantation.

Islet implantation sites

Various routes for implantation of isolated islets of Langerhans in rodent recipients have been tested with different outcome. The most advantageous sites are vascular access via the portal vein with final lodging of the islets in the liver, vascular injection into the spleen and the only successful extravascular implantation site, the peritoneal cavity and the renal subcapsular space [84]. Other routes, embolisation of islets to the lung via systemic vein, direct injection into the liver or into the spleen, subcutaneous tissue, and intramuscular, intratesticular, intrapancreatic, intraprostatic or an intrasalivary gland approach proved to be less effective [84]. Other sites such as the anterior chamber of the eye, the cheek pouches of hamsters, implantation into the brain or intraventricularly gave some success for the results in small animals but may not be applicable in human diabetics.

Metabolic outcome of islet transplantation in rodents and large animals

Rodent adult pancreatic islet transplantation has been performed in experimentally diabetic small animals or in naturally occurring diabetes in various species: mice, rats, hamsters, guinea pigs and rabbits. In general, if adequate numbers of syngeneic islets are transplanted via a reliable implantation site, the metabolic abnormalities in diabetic recipients are reversed. Weight gain is restored, polyuria, polydipsia and polyphagia are alleviated, plasma glucose levels return to normal as do glycosylated hemoglobin levels, and glycosuria is abolished. Glucose tolerance test curves are markedly improved or normalized, circulating insulin levels become nearly normal or elevated and other metabolic abnormalities, such as elevated pancreatic glucagon, plasma lipids, articular cartilage enzymes, liver enzymes and other markers of a diabetic state disappear. Perturbations in glucose tolerance and of blood glucose homeostasis during stress-situations may be attributed to the ectopic location of the islets, an at least initial lack of innervation although signs of re-innervation are observed. It may also be attributed to a disruption of the entero-insular axis or to less than normal islet mass [85].

Studies of large animal islet transplantation have been conducted with dogs, pigs, and primates. The greatest success has been observed in the dog. Studies as early as 1892 [11] showed evidence for functional autologous grafts of canine pancreas transplanted into a subcutaneous pouch. Subsequent reports of islet transplantation in this model have appeared since 1977. It could be demonstrated that if sufficient islet mass was present near-normal insulin response to intravenous glucose challenge was sustained [86]. Despite low circulating insulin levels, insulin sensitivity was preserved and glucose effectiveness was maintained after islet autotransplantation into the spleen following total pancreatectomy in dogs [87]. In the pig, when isolated islets were initially transplanted into the peritoneal cavity of totally pancreatectomized recipients, a minimal effect on diabetes was observed [88]. Recent studies appear more promising. Using more purified preparations of autologous islets transplanted into the spleen of apancreatic pigs, one group observed long-term normoglycemia, while another group has reported euglycemia in pigs that received intraportal infusions of purified allogeneic islets [89, 90]. In primate studies, serum insulin and K values were found to be improved after intraportal transplantation of isolated islets in Rhesus monkeys that were rendered diabetic by partial pancreatectomy and streptozotocin [91]. More recent studies have shown function of allografts of purified islets in streptozotocin-diabetic Cynomolgus monkeys [92].

Effect on diabetic secondary complications

The ultimate goal behind islet transplantation is to prevent or reverse diabetic secondary complications. One of the most exciting aspects of islet transplantation in rodents has been the demonstration that renal and other organ lesions associated with diabetes mellitus in animals can be prevented by early islet grafting. Even established, but early lesions may either regress or stabi-

Table 4 Effect of islet transplantation on diabetic late complications in the rat

• Prevention of cataracts	
• Prevention, delay, or reversal of:	• nephropathy
	• retinopathy
	• neuropathy
	• cardiopathy
	• skeletal disorders

lize following successful islet transplantation (Table 4). Transplantation of syngeneic islet or successful immunosuppressive treatment in case of islet allografting resulted in a beneficial effect on renal glomerular and tubular lesions [93, 94]. This effect at first observed by lightmicroscopic studies has been confirmed with immunohistological methods, electronmicroscopic studies and quantitative analysis [95, 96]. Furthermore, function-structural parameters as the turnover rate of type 4 collagen, phagocytic and clearance function of mesangial cells, renal collagen glucosyl transferase activity and tubular enzymuria normalized after successful islet transplantation [63, 97–99]. Although it has been clearly demonstrated that the mesangial matrix volume normalizes after islet transplantation, the basement membrane thickening observed by electronmicroscopic analysis remained unchanged and could not be reversed by islet transplantation [100]. Beneficial effects of successful adult islet transplantation on diabetic retinopathy, neuropathy, cardiopathy and skeletal disorders have been reported by various authors and our own group [6, 85, 102–106].

In contrast to studies of the metabolic function of islet grafts in large animals, there is comparatively little data on the effect of islet transplantation on chronic complications in large animal models. Renal morphology appeared to be preserved in dogs bearing functional intrasplenic islet autografts for 1–2 years [107]. No data is available on neural or retinal changes.

Restoration of pancreatic beta cells after experimental islet transplantation

We have found indications of a restoration of beta cells after successful metabolic normalization by islet transplantation in our earlier investigations on islet transplantation in experimental diabetes of rats [108]. Meanwhile, quantitative analysis revealed intrainsular beta cell regenerates, neoformation of beta cells evidently appearing in the duct epithelium of the exocrine pancreas and finally resulting in an about sixfold increase of the entire beta cell mass of the residual pancreas following successful intraportal islet transplantation in rats [109, 110]. It is not yet known which factors bring out this regeneration. However, this might provide an approach to clinical therapy by raising the critical beta cell mass during the early remission phase of type 1 diabetics.

Prevention of islet allograft rejection

Early studies with transplants of isolated adult islets have shown that islet allografts are highly susceptable to the recipient's immune mechanisms and will be destroyed within a few days after implantation. Some immunologically privileged properties have been ascribed to the portal venous bed or to the liver in mice and to the renal subcapsular space in rats. But, freshly isolated adult islet allografts are rejected rapidly if no measures are taken to prevent rejection. Most of the classical techniques found to be successful for other organ allografts in rodents, they have been in general proved much more difficult to suppress rejection of islet allografts. Furthermore, multiple factors such as heterogenous combinations of donor – recipient pairs used, variability of donor source, the site of implantation and the number of islets transplanted and the lack of uniformity in the definition of rejection make it difficult to interprete and compare the results of the islet allograft experiments reported by various investigators. In the following chapter, we discuss only those allograft experiments using a sufficient number of islets transplanted to an appropriate site that established normoglycemia before rejection occurred.

Induction of immunotolerance: First attempts with injection of donor antigens and antilymphocyte serum according to defined protocols resulted in a prolonged but not ultimate survival of islet allografts [111]. Difficulties appeared in using enhancement protocols with different sera [112]. Very recently, rat islet allografts have been transplanted into the thymus of recipients treated with a single injection of anti-lymphocyte serum [113]. These islet allografts survived indefinitely. Interestingly, a state of donor-specific unresponsiveness was achieved by this procedure which permitted survival of a second donor strain islet allograft transplanted to an extrathymic site. The authors speculate that maturation of precursors in a thymic microenvironment that is harbouring foreign alloantigen may induce the selective unresponsiveness [113]. Tolerance to islet allografts was also induced in mice and rats by donor-specific bone marrow (intrathymic) inoculation [114, 115]. But in general, many of the experiments with the objective to induce immunotolerance were performed under highly artificial conditions and the specific protocols are currently not much relevant to transplantation in humans. Therefore, another approach that has been demonstrated to prevent rejection in rodents is to manipulate the islet immunogenicity in vitro before transplantation.

Table 5 Methods known for in vitro immunoalteration of isolated adult pancreatic islets

- Culture 22 °C, 24 °C, 27 °C
- Hyperbaric/high oxygen culture
- Megaislets, pseudoislets
- UV-light
- Gamma-irradiation
- Cryopreservation
- Monoclonal antibodies against class-II antigen-bearing cells, dendritic cells or lymphocyte subpopulations
- Antineoplastic drugs
- Gangliosides

Immunoalteration: This concept starts with the hypothesis that antigen-presenting cells or passenger leukocytes within the graft are responsible for the induction of islet graft rejection exerted by the recipient's immunocompetent cells. The objective is to selectively eliminate or reduce donor immune cells or to suppress their antigen expression by various in vitro manipulations. It has been shown that prolonged in vitro culture at low (22–24°C) or 37°C temperature, in high oxygen concentrations, by cryopreservation, by ultraviolet or gamma-irradiation and by pretreatment of islets with antibodies or

Table 6 Success rates of intraportal islet allografts in diabetic rats in terms of normoglycemia of the recipient for more than 120 days. Islet pretreatment by different measures. (Data derived from Bretzel et al. 1986 [118])

Treatment	Success rate (%)
• Fresh islets	0
• Fresh islets + ALS	0
• Fresh islets + CYA	0
• Cultured islets	0
• Cultured islets + ALS	90
• Cultured islets + CYA	0
• Cryopreserved islets	44
• Cryopreserved islets + ALS	64
• Cryopreserved islets + CYA	80

ALS: Antilymphocyte serum; CYA: Cyclosporine A

substances directed to class-II antigens of the donor indeed significantly reduces islet allograft immunogenicity [116–126] (Table 5). These methods are very effective and induce, in many cases with only a temporary immunosuppressive treatment of the recipient, e.g. a single dose of ALS at the day of operation, an indefinite prolongation of islet allograft survival across major histocompatibility barriers. Moreover, in our hands a combined cryopreservation – culture protocol induced a tremendous decrease of class-II antigen expression in isolated adult rat pancreatic islets enabling long term islet allograft survival in 80% of the cases after transplantation across a major histocompatibility barrier without any immunosuppressive treatment of the recipient [118] (Table 6).

Immunoisolation (micro- and macroencapsulation): Immunoisolation of islets has been performed using an artificial membrane as a barrier to exclude cells or molecules able to mediate rejection while allowing flux of insulin and glucose. Millipore chambers and hollow fibers have been used with temporary but not ultimate islet allograft and even xenograft survival [127–133]. More recently, our group provided evidence for the protection of islets inside the hollow fiber membrane from interleukin-1 toxicity [134]. While the survival of isolated rat islets in hollow fibers lasts only a few weeks there is one observation of much longer-lasting function of insulinoma cells or adult rat islets even in vivo [135, 136]. More promising are the results using the technique of microencapsulation. In these cases, isolated islets are encapsulated in semipermeable hydrogels [137]. It has been clearly demonstrated that these microcapsules are permeable to glucose, arginine, theophylline, and insulin, but they are nevertheless able to efficiently protect pancreatic beta cells against cytotoxic anti-islet antibodies and immuno-competent cells [138, 139]. A prolonged (more than 100 days) islet endocrine function was observed in vitro as well as after allografting in spontaneously diabetic BB rats or in experimentally diabetic mice, also by our group [140–143]. But, the excellent in vitro function of encapsulated islets demonstrated by many groups has not been widely matched in transplantation experiments, with relatively few groups reporting long-term graft function. The major obstacle appears to be pericapsular fibrosis. Although recent advances in the purification of alginates provide a potential solution to this problem, much work is still required, particularly relating to the problems posed by spontaneously occurring long-term diabetic recipients. However, the ability to reduce greatly the size of the capsules and the advent of purified alginate preparations should allow considerable progress towards transplantation of encapsulated islets into type 1 diabetic patients.

Prevention of diabetes recurrence: Islet grafts are susceptible to another immune-mediated pathway of destruction exerted by autoimmune mechanisms inherent in type 1 diabetes mellitus or in experimental models of spontaneously occurring diabetes mellitus in small animals (NOD mice; BB rats). Both experimental models and probably also the model of the immune-mediated low-dose streptozotocin diabetes mellitus provide an effective approach to study the mechanisms of recurrence of diabetes mellitus as it has been observed in non-immunosuppressed human recipients of pancreatic segment grafts from non-diabetic identical twin donors and also in the BB rat model when MHC – compatible islets had been grafted [144–146]. Most of the studies show that the disease of the BB rats as well as diabetes recurrence after the islet transplantation is restricted to the major histocompatibility complex (MHC) although two studies revealed conflicting results [147–151]. Also in the natural model of autoimmune diabetes in non-obese diabetic mice (NOD) the pathogenic process seems to be MHC-restricted [152]. Furthermore, isolated islets are more vulnerable to recurrent diabetes than vascularized pancreas grafts [153]. The MHC-restriction of the disease would suggest that the problem of diabetes recurrence could be obviated by implanting an MHC-incompatible graft whose allograft immunogenicity had been controlled by pretreatment prior to allografting, since primed islet-autoreactive T cells would not recognize the islets. In fact, this has been recently evidenced by different measures in various studies in the NOD mice and in the BB rat model and in the NOD mice model including our own experiments (Table 7): culture pretreatment of the isolated adult or neonatal islets or pancreatic single islet cell preparations, UV light irradiation of the islet graft, immunosuppressive treatment of the recipient with various specific monoclonal antibodies or complete Freund's adjuvant (CFA), an immunomodulating agent, or with a lymphocyte transfer from normoglycemic rats to diabetic BB rats bearing syngeneic islet grafts (from the diabetes-resistant BB rat line) or treatment with antioxidative agents (desferrioxamine; nicotinamide) directed towards protection from inflammatory tissue damage [126, 154–164]. Considering recurrence of autoimmune diabetes, the survival of isolated islet grafts was highly dependent on the site of the islet implantation as it has been evidenced years before with respect to islet allograft rejection revealing the kidney subcapsular space superior to the liver, at least in rats [165]. Our group recently found that autoimmune damaging has been avoided in all cases by adult rat pancreatic islet implantation into the renal subcapsular space of BB rats where the islets survived indefinitely [166]. In principle, disease recurrence may be also prevented by any of the methods used for immunoisolation of islets by biomembrane constructs. But so far the results in spontaneous diabetes of small animals, in particular the NOD mouse, are not that much encouraging and an additional recipient treatment (e.g. with monoclonal anti-CD4$^+$ antibodies) may be required [167, 168]. The interesting finding that composite kidney-islet transplants in a model of spontaneously occurring diabetes function indefinitely suggests that the revascularizing endothelium of the islets may play a role in resistance or susceptibility to autoimmune beta cell destruction [169].

Table 7 Survival of Wistar-Furth (WF) and Lewis rat islets transplanted immediately after isolation or after 14 days in tissue culture (22°C) to BB rats. (Data derived from Woehrle et al. 1986 [126]; and Woehrle et al. 1987 [165] with permission of the author)

Donor strain	Islet treatment	Type of diabetes	Posttransplant normoglycemia (days)	Median survival time (days)
WF	None	Spontaneous	10, 10, 12, 25, 45	12.7 ± 0.35
WF	None	Streptozotocin	7, 14, 16, 17, >90	13.0 ± 0.37
WF	Culture	Spontaneous	9, 12, 12, 14, 17	13.4 ± 0.21
WF	Culture	Streptozotocin	14, 14, 20, 55, 69	20.0 ± 0.46
Lewis	None	Spontaneous	4, 4, 5, 7, 8	4.7 ± 0.19
Lewis	None	Streptozotocin	5, 5, 5, 9, 12	5.6 ± 0.24
Lewis	None	Spontaneous	12, 16, 16, 18, >20	14.6 ± 0.15
Lewis	Culture	Spontaneous	>35, >35, >35, >18	>25.1 ± 0.38
Lewis	Culture	Spontaneous	23, 39, >100 × 3, >150	>100
Lewis	Culture	Streptozotocin	>100 × 3, >125 × 2	>100

Clinical islet transplantation

Ultimately, islet transplantation will probably supersede pancreas transplantation as a method of endocrine replacement therapy [170]. Unfortunately, islet isolation is still not as efficient as desired, and prevention of rejection of islet allografts appears to be even more difficult than prevention of pancreas allograft rejection [171, 172]. However, insulin independence has been preserved with intraportal islet autotransplantation following total pancreatectomy for benign disease, and in this situation (no possibility of rejection), normoglycemia can be maintained with a relatively small number of intrahepatic islets [173–175].

R. G Bretzel, B. J Hering, K. F Federlin

Assessment of human islet preparations and guidelines for islet quality control

Clinical islet cell transplantation is still an investigational procedure and several centers are currently at the early beginning of clinical islet isolation and transplantation programs. Therefore, guidelines were set for human islet quality control in order to facilitate clinical islet transplant programs, to make results from various centers more comparable and finally, to facilitate future multicenter studies [176].

Several quality control measures (Table 8) need to be evaluated to ascertain whether an islet preparation merits transplantation into a patient. Before organ donation, (pre-donation) factors such as pancreas procurement and distension have to be considered, and parameters such as islet yield in terms of islet number and islet volume, islet purity, islet viability, and islet sterility must be assessed. The most crucial point will be the transplantability, or what in-vitro parameter best predicts the in-vivo endocrine effect after islet transplantation?

Table 8 Islet quality control testing

- Islet quantity
    - Counting by size
    - Islet equivalent count
    - Islet volume
- Islet purity
    - Determined by dithizone stain
- Islet viability and function
    - Counting living and dead islets
    - In-vitro
        - Perifusions
        - Insulin stimulation index
    - In-vivo
        - Rodent transplants
- Islet sterility
    - Samples
        - Donor pancreas
        - Reagents
        - Processing steps
        - Preserved islets
        - Culture media
    - Testing
        - Filtration culture
        - 24 °C + 37 °C
        - Bacteria + Fungus

Pre-organ donation factors, pancreas procurement and distension: The impact of pre-organ donation factors on the outcome of islet isolation has been addressed elsewhere and recently studied in a small number of organ donors [177, 178]. It appeared that young (< 21 yr) donor age, low body mass index (< 21), blood glucose levels above 10 mmol/L (it should be mentioned that hyperglycemia more often reflects insulin resistance and central dysregulation of the brain-death donor than does beta-cell failure), and prolonged intensive care management are associated with significantly reduced or lower islet yields, whereas increased serum amylase levels are not associated with low islet yields [178–180].

Critical issues of human pancreas procurement are the warm ischemia time, which should be as short as possible; an in-situ vascular perfusion with cold University of Wisconsin (UW) solution which appears superior to, e.g. Eurocollins; no overperfusion and no intrapancreatic venous hypertension; cold ischemia time of no more than 12 hr and, interestingly, no less than 2 hr; and a well-preserved pancreatic capsule that allows subsequent intraductal collagenase distension [177–184].

At present, most centers with own experience in human adult islet isolations prefer to start the pancreas dispersion procedure with intraductal administration of collagenase followed by an automated digestion-filtration using recirculating collagenase solution [185–188] (Figure 2). A critical factor in the successful isolation of islets is the collagenase reagent but will not be discussed in detail here. The persistent problems with and the lack of standardized formulations of collagenase preparations have been recently addressed [189].

Islet number and volume: Based on calculations from historical and more recent work the average human pancreas, weighing 70 g, contains between 305,000 and 1.5 million islets of 150 μm equivalent diameter (IEQ)(4), corresponding to between 0.5% and 4% of the total pancreatic volume [190–193]. In case of absence of any form of insulin resistance including diabetogenic immunosuppressive substances such as cortison and cyclosporine A, a minimum of 265,000 human adult islets (3,500/kg body weight of the recipient) may be enough to produce insulin independence with perfect metabolic control (fasting blood glucose, glycated hemoglobin, oral glucose test) after intraportal islet autotransplantation as demonstrated in patients after undergoing total pancreatectomy [194]. However, islets to be transplanted into type 1 diabetic patients more often will be confronted with an environment characterized by long-lasting glucose toxicity and microangiopathy (perhaps

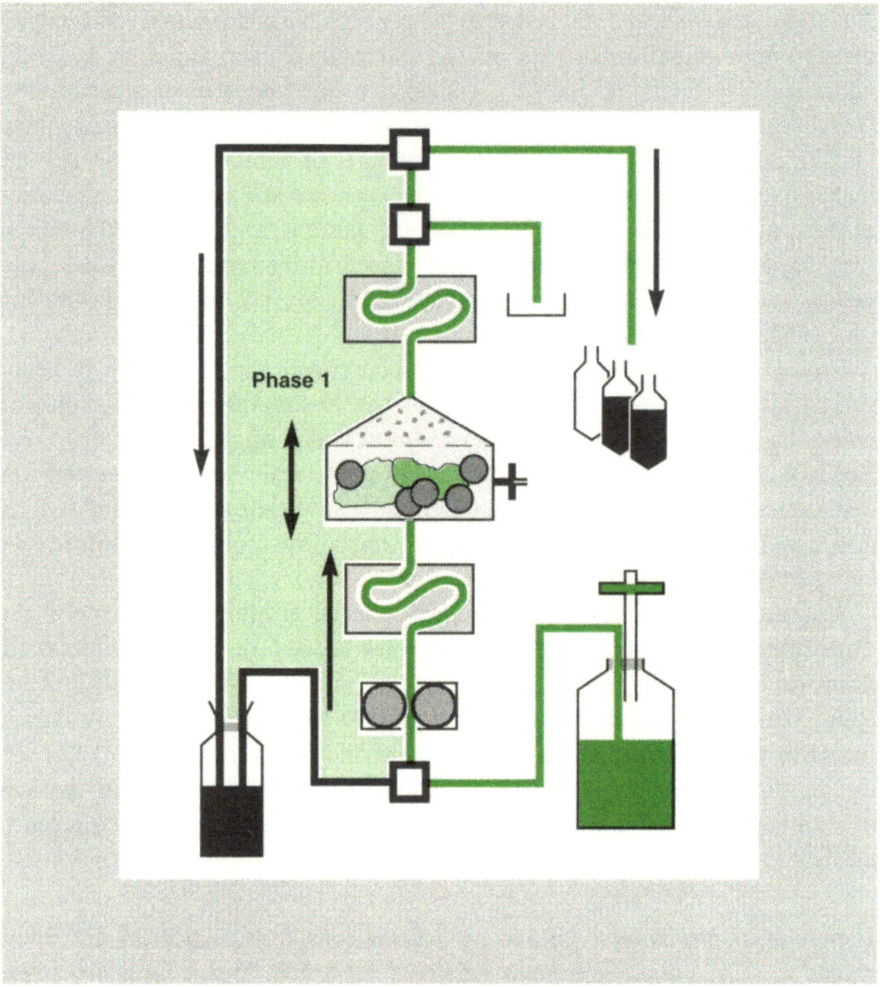

Fig. 2 Schematic drawing of pancreatic enzyme digestion and islet isolation. Pancreas within digestion chamber (middle) surrounded by glass beads and covered by a mash with 500 μm pore size
Phase 1: Recirculating enzyme solution passes digestion chamber until islets are liberated (above mash)
Phase 2: Dilution of proteolytic enzyme and collagenase with enzyme free buffer and collection of free islets and exocrine fragments of < 400 μm

also in the portal system) insulin-resistance, and autoimmune disease recurrence. It is therefore not surprising that the minimal number of islets required to render an adult type 1 diabetic patient insulin independent has been about 8,000 IEQ/kg [195].

Table 9 Determination of islet volume for each 50 μm-diameter range and conversion into islet equivalents (IEQ) with a diameter of 150 μm

Islet diameter range (μm)	Mean volume (μm3)	Conversion factor (counted islet number × conversion factor)
50–100	294,525	0.16
100–150	1.145,373	0.66
150–200	2.977,968	1.7
200–250	6.185,010	3.5
250–300	11.159,198	6.3
300–350	18.293,231	10.4
>350	27.979,808	15.8

The sampling technique represents a critical factor that could affect the results of an islet count as well as insulin content from any islet preparation. It is preferable to collect multiple samples, e.g., five aliquots of 100 μL after suspension of the islet preparation in a 200 mL flask. As a specific stain for islet tissue, dithizone (DTZ), which stains zinc in the insulin granules and results in a characteristic red stain, proved to be most appropriate. An easy and rapid way to stain islets is to add a few drops of freshly prepared and filtered (4–5 – 8 μ) solution. The solution is prepared as follows. Add 50 mg DTZ to 5 mL dimethylsulfoxide (DMSO) stock solution, and dilute 1 mL of this solution with 20 mL of Hank's with 2% fetal calf serum (FCS); add a few drops of the final solution to a sample contained in a petri dish. The addition of DMSO accelerates the staining process.

Stained islets are counted according to diameter classes using a calibrated grid in the eyepiece of the phase contrast microscope. Particles smaller than 50 μm are not considered and islets larger than 350 μm are no further subdivided. Table 9 gives the mean volume for each diameter class and the relevant conversion factor into islets of 150 μm diameter. The total islet volume of the final preparation also can be estimated and may be a further useful parameter to characterize an islet preparation. The potential use of automated methods using computerized imaging analyzers appears to be an attractive alternative to visual methods and may provide a more objective and standardized quantitative evaluation. Although this technology appears promising, it is expensive and too early in development to be proposed as a general standard.

Islet purity: Transplanting highly purified islet preparations holds potential advantages of increased safety, reduced immunogenicity of the graft and probably improved islet implantation, although these issues recently have been questioned in light of new results obtained in a few diabetic patients using unpurified islet preparations (196–199). However, reports of severe portal hypertension and in three deaths resulting from intraportal autotransplantation of unpurified islet tissue should be a warning to use only highly purified (i. e. > 80%) islet preparations for transplantation purposes [200–203].

Large-scale, continuous-gradient centrifugation established on a COBE 2991 cell processor using different or specifically designed gradient media is at present the preferred technique for rapid, effective, and reproducible human islet purification (204, 205). To run in parallel a test gradient for each individual pancreas may help to further increase islet recovery and islet viability.

Although many approaches for determination of islet purity have been proposed, including insulin/amylase ratio and algebraic equations, each approach has inherent problems that result in assessment variabilities that are not easily controlled. Again, it is possible that the automatic methods using either specific stains or highly specific monoclonal antibodies ultimately will be used. For now, however most investigators use the dithizone stain as an easy method to roughly estimate the approximate degree of purity of the islets in any preparation.

Islet viability and endocrine function: Islet viability is a critical factor that determines the outcome of transplantation. However, there is currently no entirely reliable method for standardizing viability assessment (Table 10). In-vitro methods include light and electron microscopic morphology, fluorometric membrane integrity tests, colorimetric tests of mitochondrial function, and glucose-stimulated insulin release determined in static incubation or in

Table 10 Islet viability and endocrine function tests. Stimuli and inhibitors commonly used

	Stimuli	Inhibitors
• Insulin secretion in vitro	D-Glucose	Mannoheptulose
	Fatty acids	
• Static uncubation	Amino acids	
• Dynamic incubation (perifusion)	Theophylline	
• Insulin biosynthesis in vitro (Preopro-, proinsulin)	D-Glucose	
Incorporation of (^{3}H)-Leucine or (^{3}H)-Phenylalanine		
• Insulin secretion and biosynthesis (Bioassy)		
Islet transplantation into nude mice or rats		

continuous perifusion systems [206–218]. Moreover, in studies of basic islet physiology and responses to pharmacological agents insulin and protein synthesis and glucose utilisation have also been used to assess vital islet functions [216, 218, 219].

For rapid assessment of islet viability before islet transplantation, a fluorometric assay using inclusion and exclusion dyes that allows discrimination between intact and damaged cells is now widely used and recommended (208, 209). The combination of the inclusion and exclusion dyes acridin orange (AO) and propidium iodide (PI) have minimal background fluorescence, and when used in optimal concentrations (AO – 0.67 μmol/L; PI – 75 μmol/L), they stain living cells green and dead cells red. Using this fluorometric method, viable and non-viable whole islets may be differentiated, as may viable and non-viable components within an islet. The stability, cytotoxicity, and reproducibility of the assay has been demonstrated on animal and human islets.

It is crucial that the isolated islets be shown not only to be viable but also able to respond appropriately to a glucose challenge. The standard in assessing in-vitro islet endocrine function is the perifusion of islets with glucose, which provides a dynamic profile of the characteristics of glucose-mediated insulin release from pre-stored and newly synthesized insulin and of the ability of the islet endocrine cells to downregulate insulin secretion after the glycemic challenge is interrupted (return to baseline)[215, 217]. Technical details have been described previously [171, 176](see also Figure 3). In brief, duplicate groups of 200–300 islets of comparable size are perifused with Krebs-Ringer bicarbonate solution, which is maintained at 37°C and gassed with 95% O_2 and 5% CO_2. The perfusate is pumped through the chambers for 3 consecutive hours, during which time the glucose concentration is 50, 300 (500) and 50 mg/dL, respectively. The effluent from the chamber is sampled every 10 min after subjecting the islets to perifusion for 40 minutes to eliminate an artificial increase in insulin due to mechanical stimulation from the transfer procedure. During the second hour, samples are removed at 1, 2.5, 5, 7.5, 10, 20, 30, 40, 50, and 60 min, and during the final hour every 10 minutes. The samples are collected at 4°C and stored at – 20°C until assay for insulin is initiated using a double-antibody radioimmunoassay technique [220].

Standards for reporting results of perifusion studies are critical for the accurate comparison of data. The absolute levels of insulin secretion during the prechallenge baseline period, the high glucose challenge, and the last period of perifusion after return to low glucose concentration should be re-

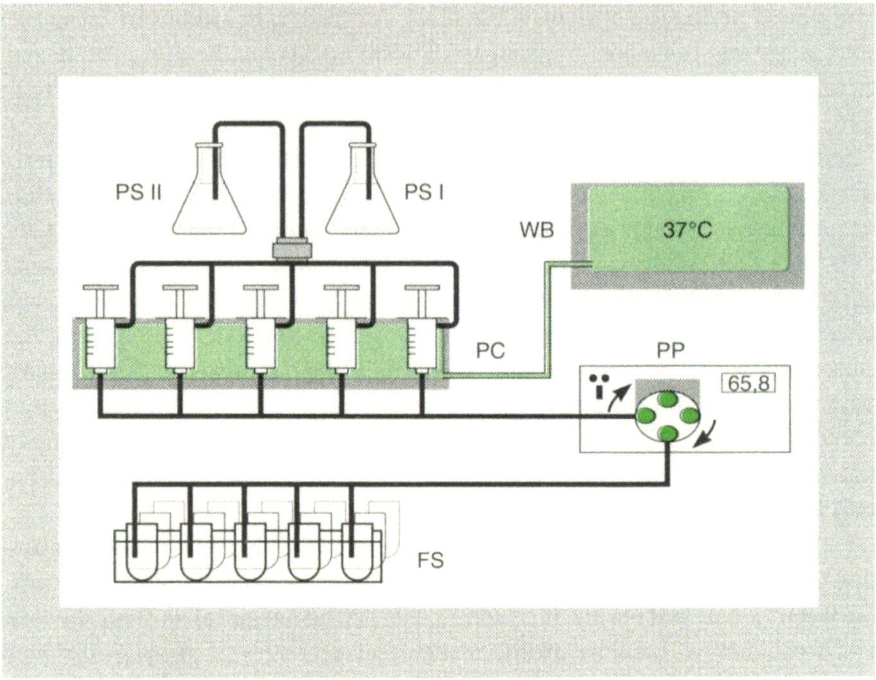

Fig. 3 Schematic drawing of a perifusion apparatus; PS Perifusion Solution, PP Peristaltic Pump, WB Water Bath, FS Fraction Sampler, PC Perifusion Chamber

ported (Figure 4). The profile of insulin release is best reported as a plot that shows the release during the three consecutive periods [221]. Stimulation index estimated by determining the ratio between basal (last 15 minutes before high glucose and last 15 minutes after return to basal conditions) and stimulated insulin release (first 15 minutes and last 15 minutes of stimulation) identifies the secretory capacity but lacks details on basal insulin release, the quality of the biphasic response and return to basal secretion [222]. However, in-vitro insulin release does not necessarily predict in-vivo transplant outcome, and the results of islet perifusion studies should therefore be interpreted with caution. Thus, cryopreserved rodent islets showed normal perifusion response but later failed to reverse diabetes, and vice versa, cryopreserved canine islets that failed to secrete insulin during perifusion induced normoglycemia after autotransplantation and it has been reported that a poor response from human islets during perifusion did not predict their in-vivo function after transplantation [223–225].

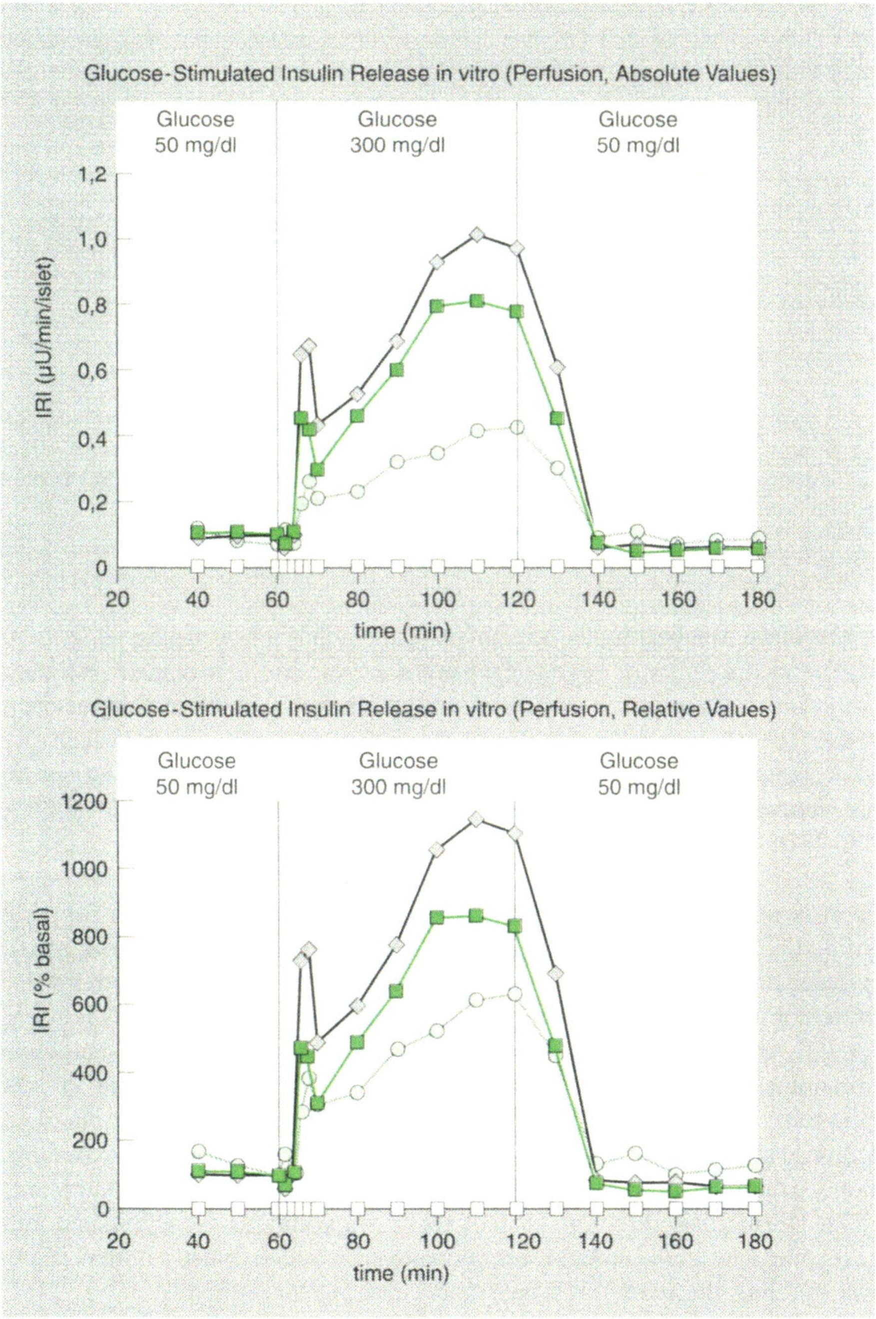

Fig. 4 Example of a perifusion test performed on isolated adult human pancreatic islets

Table 11 Interactions between islet graft and host environment

Islet cell structures	• Cell-mediated immunity
	• Humoral immunity
	  • Islet cell antibodies (ICA)
	  • Complement-fixing ICA (CF-ICA)
	  • Islet cell surface antibodies (ICSA)
	  • 64 KD and 37 KD islet cell antibodies
	  • GAD (glutamate decarboxylase) – antibodies
	  • Anti-ganglioside antibodies
	  • Virus activity

Islet cell insulin secretion	• Insulin autoantibodies (IAA)
	• Insulin resistance
	  • Abnormalities in hepatic glucose production
	  • Islet amyloid polypeptide (amylin)
	  • Insulin receptor and postreceptor defects
	  • Abnormal contrainsular hormone levels
	  • Abnormalities in lipid oxidation
	  • Down-regulation of glucose transporter-systems by chronic hyperglycemia (glucose toxicity)
	  • Unknown factors of heterotopic implantation

Therefore, the best index of viability is the ability of transplanted islets to withstand the rigors of engraftment in an ectopic site of a diabetic recipient until revascularisation is complete and to reverse diabetes in this recipient (Table 11). In-vivo endocrine function of human islets can be tested after transplantation (bioassay) of aliquots of the final islet preparation beneath the renal capsule of diabetic immunodeficient and athymic mouse or rat [223, 226, 227].

Islet sterility: Testing should start as usual with donor screening for viral antibodies (hepatitis A, B, and C; human immunodeficiency viruses 1 and 2; cytomegalo-virus). The demonstration that islets to be transplanted are free from bioburden risk is an important quality control test. This issue should be carefully considered because a period of tissue culture may amplify microbial contamination and the induction of an immunosuppressed state in islet transplant recipients may render them susceptible to infections. It has been demonstrated that 42% of human donor pancreas had low level contaminants, usually of gram positive bacteria, and 15% had fungal contaminants (229). During islet isolation, 97% of these contaminants are eliminated and only some new environmental contaminants are added, mostly fungal. However, holding the islets for 7 days and culturing the samples both at 24 °C and at 37 °C has been prevented contaminated islet preparations from being transplanted into immunosuppressed recipients [229]. By contrast, other cen-

Table 12 Minimal requirements to be met by islet preparations intended for clinical islet transplantations

• Islet mass	>8.000 IEQ/kg body wt in type 1 diabetic recipient >3.500 IEQ/kg body wt in patients to be autotransplanted after pancreatectomy
• Islet purity	>80% (percentage of the islet volume in the total cell volume)
• Islet viability	>80% (assessed by a microfluorometric membrane integrity test)
• Islet in-vitro function	Documented biphasic response to a glucose challenge and return to baseline phenomenon
• Islet culture	Exclusion of microbial contamination

ters transplanting freshly isolated islets have reported septicemia in two cases whereas another center observed no clinical apparent infection despite retrospectively demonstrable microbial contamination of the islet preparations [230, 231].

The various issues of the quality control program suggested should serve as guidelines for investigators going to initiate clinical islet transplantation programs. The main message should be that only an islet preparation with well-documented quantity, purity, viability, function, and sterility (Table 12) before transplantation fulfills the criteria of transplantability and merits transplantation into a patient to mimic the complexicity of the (carbohydrate) metabolism in normal subjects (Table 13).

Table 13 Characteristics of the carbohydrate metabolism in normal subjects

• Hepatic glucose production (mg/kg × min)	
• Newborn	4.2 – 5.4
• Adult	2.3 ± 0.1
• Suppression by an OGTT	55 ± 5%
• Basal peripheral glucose utilization	2.0 mg/kg × min
• Hepatic glucose extraction	10 – 25%
• Insulin production rate	
• Basal	0.7–1.0 U/h
• Prandial	1.35 U/12 g glucose
• Ratio basal/prandial (24 h)	about 1.0
• Periodicity of pulses 12 min	
• Hepatic insulin extraction	about 50%
• Modulators of the insulin effects by increasing hepatic glucose production and peripheral insulin resistance: catecholamines, cortisol, growth hormone and glucagon	

OGTT: oral glucose tolerance test

Success rates and effects on glucose metabolism

Islet transplantation in man can be subdivided into three categories: a) islet autotransplantation; b) islet allotransplantation in pancreatectomized patients; c) islet allotransplantation in type 1 diabetic recipients.

Islet autotransplantation: Chronic pancreatitis may lead to severe continuously or recurring pains which may increase to nearly untractable situations. One choice of treatment with definite pain relief is pancreatectomy which, however, has the consequence of diabetes. The isolation of islets from the completely removed gland and transplantation as a free graft may help to avoid diabetes as well as diabetic complications in the future of those patients. In Europe, the first patient received his own islets as pancreatic fragments transplanted into the portal vein in 1978 [232]. Although the transplantation resulted in significant C-peptide secretion, the patient did not become insulin independent with nowadays, 15 years later, still low insulin requirement of 10–12 units per day. In the following years 105 autotransplants have been reported from 13 centers, and 50 patients (48%) were insulin independent post-operatively. The Minneapolis group quite recently published remarkable data [173–175]. They performed islet autografts in 26 patients and five patients are still insulin independent with a maximum of now 9.5 years after the implantation. Along with insulin independence normal glycosylated hemoglobin A_{1c} levels were achieved.

Islet allotransplantation in pancreatectomized patients: The first report of insulin independence in this category of patients came from Altman et al. in 1988 and concerned a patient with hemochromatosis who was serum C-peptide negative prior to combined liver and islet transplantation [233]. The islets were placed into an epiploic flap and the patient remained insulin independent for 49 months post transplantation. The second group to report insulin independence after islet allotransplantation in non-type 1 diabetic patients was Pittsburgh with their cluster/islet transplants after upper abdominal exenteration for abdominal malignancies [234]. These ten patients received pancreatic islet grafts obtained from the pancreas of the liver allograft donor only in five cases, a third party donor in one case and a combination of the two in four cases. Seven of these patients developed periods of insulin independence post-operatively, one of whom is still insulin independent after more than four years. More recently, ongoing insulin independence was reported of a patient after combined liver – islet transplantation after pancreatectomy and hepatectomy for carcinoma at the center in Milan [235]. In all cases, islet allotransplantation was followed by a better metabolic control in terms of glycosylated hemoglobin A_{1c} levels.

Islet allotransplantation in type 1 diabetic recipients: A few years after the first successful attempts to treat experimental diabetic animals by transplantation of isolated islets, the Minneapolis group initiated clinical islet allotransplantations in diabetic patients. At this time, there was much hope that human islet isolation could be simply achieved and that clinical islet transplantation would supersede pancreatic organ transplantation. However, already the first preliminary report of Najarian, Sutherland and their colleagues in 1977 demonstrated that this was not the case [236]. The authors described their first attempts of intraperitoneal and intraportal transplantation of dispersed human pancreas from adult or infant donors in seven patients with long-lasting insulin-dependent diabetes. The mass of islet tissue transplanted varied from 0.4% to 14.5% of that present in a normal adult pancreas [236, 237]. Although no patient became insulin independent, there were intervals of reduced insulin requirement in four patients with transplantation of islets into the liver and in three patients who received intraperitoneal transplantation. The main message from this pioneer work was, however, that in principle also human islets start insulin secretion in a heterotopic environment, liver, peritoneal cavity, that the transplantation procedure itself is safe and that there will be no increase of rejection episodes of a previously transplanted kidney. From another rough calculation one could estimate that the number of islet transplanted in this first series range between 15–150 thousands. So, at this time it could be argued that the number or the islet mass was too low to reach insulin independence in those patients apart from other reasons as insufficient immunosuppression or contamination with exocrine tissue. Human islet allotransplants following these pioneer cases were reported to the International Pancreas and Islet Transplant Registry at the University of Minnesota until 1989, when responsibility for data collection and analysis was transferred to our Department of Internal Medicine, Justus-Liebig-University, Giessen, Germany. Previous reports of the Islet Transplant Registry have been made [238, 239]. The following refers to the last report of the International Islet Transplant Registry (ITR) at Giessen University [240].

Between December 12, 1893, and December 31, 1993, 215 adult islet allografts and one adult islet xenograft have been performed at 30 different institutions, including 130 at 12 institutions in North America, 83 at 18 institutions in Europe, and one elsewhere (Table 14). One type 1 diabetic recipient

Table 14 Summary of adult islet allografts (and one xenograft) according to institution and year through December 31, 1993; ITR 1994 [240]*

Institution	Year of tx	No. of cases
• Bristol*	1893	1
• Newcastle-upon-Tyne	1916	2
• Padova	1927	2
• New York	1935	1
• Leiden	1944	1
• Petah Tikva	1968	1
• Minneapolis	1974–1993	38
• Zurich	1977–1988	8
• Genoa	1978–1979	13
• Hannover	1978	2
• Detroit	1980–1985	7
• Giessen	1980–1993	8
• Berlin (East)	1982–1987	8
• St. Louis	1985–1993	25
• Miami	1985–1993	13
• Paris	1988–1991	7
• Perugia	1989–1991	5
• Berlin (West)	1989	1
• Edmonton	1989–1993	5
• Milan	1989–1993	15
• St. Louis/London, Ontario	1990–1992	4
• Pittsburgh	1990–1993	30
• Leicester	1991–1992	3
• Oxford	1991–1993	3
• Charlestown	1991	2
• Los Angeles I	1992–1993	4
• Madrid	1992–1993	3
• Los Angeles II	1993	1
• Verona	1993	1
• Homburg/Saar	1993	1
Total no. of cases:		215
Total no. of institutions:		30

of an islet-after-kidney (IAK) allograft in Milan and one type 1 diabetic recipient of a simultaneous islet-kidney (SIK) allograft in Edmonton have been insulin independent for 2.6 and for 2.3 years, respectively. Thus, the principle feasibility of clinical islet transplantation has clearly been proven. However, only six type 1 diabetic recipients of adult islet allografts are currently insulin independent (Table 15). Since the number of transplants remains low – during the last four years approximately 30 transplants have been performed per year at 18 institutions – it is evident that the impact of different approaches can only be substantiated through a careful analysis of all data available.

Table 15 Insulin independence after adult islet transplantation into type I diabetic patients. Summary of cases through October 15, 1994; ITR 1994 [240]

Institution	Year of Tx	No. of sonors		IEQ*/kg	Islet purity	Site of Tx	Type of Tx	# of Shared HLA-Ag		Induction immunosuppression	Period of insulin independence Days post Tx	Glucose control †
		Fresh	Cryo					AB	DR			
St. Louis	1989	2	–	12,661	p. v.$^{\Delta}$	IAK*	1/3 2/1	ALG (+P)		10	−25 i. v. Insulin	
St. Louis	1990	1	+2	14,733	98%	p. v.$^{\Delta}$	IAK*	1/2/2	1/1/0	ALG (+P)	33 – 341	i. v. Insulin
St. Louis	1993	1	+7	22,197	90%	p. v.$^{\Delta}$	SIK*	2 (fresh)	1 (fresh)	OKT3 (+P−C−A)	92 –> 425$^{\#}$	i. v. Insulin
St. Louis	1993	3	+2	27,370	87%	p. v.$^{\Delta}$	SIk	NA	NA	ALG (+P−C−A)	274 –> 309$^{\#}$	i. v. Insulin
Edmonton	1990	1	+4	9,698	70%	p. v.$^{\Delta}$	SIK*	3 (fresh) 1/0/2/0	0 (fresh) 0 (cryo)	ALG (+P−C at day 10−A)	69 – 821	i. v. Insulin
Edmonton	1992	1	+5	9,867	55%	p. v.$^{\Delta}$	SIK*	3 1/0/0/1/0	1 (fresh) 1/1/0/0/1 (cryo)	ALG (+P−C at day 8−A)	155 – 166 +837 –> 909$^{\#}$	i. v. Insulin
Milano	1990	1	–	10,767	95%	p. v.$_{\Delta}$	IAK*	1	0	ALG (+P−C−A)	120 – 330	i. v. Insulin
Milano	1990	2	–	8,607	75%	p. v.$^{\Delta}$	IAK*	1/2	1/0	ALG (+P−C−A)	60 – 1,178	i. v. Insulin
Milano	1991	1	+2	15,241	80%	p. v.$^{\Delta}$	SIK*	NA	NA	ALG (+P−C−A)	210 – 360 +480 – 635	i. v. Insulin
Milano	1992	2	–	11,566	80%	p. v.$^{\Delta}$	IAK*	NA	NA	ALG (+P−C−A)	150 –> 760$^{\#}$	i. v. Insulin
Milano	1994	1	+2	15,945	50%	p. v.$^{\Delta}$	IAK*	NA	NA	ALG (+P−C−A)	43 – 90	i. v. Insulin
Miami	1990	3	–	18,700	55%	p. v.$^{\Delta}$	IAK*	0/2/0	1/1/0	OKT3 (+P−C−A)	42 – 78	i. v. Insulin
Miami	1990	3	–	18,891	50%	p. v.$^{\Delta}$	IAK*	0/0/0	0/1/0	OKT3 (+P−C−A)	87 – 125	i. v. Insulin
Mnpls	1992	1	–	7,882	1%	p. v.$^{\Delta}$	SIK*	1	1	ALG (+P−C−D)	326 –> 968$^{\#}$	i. v. Insulin
Mnpls	1992	1	–	13,319	1%	p. v.$^{\Delta}$	SIK*	2	0	ALG (+P−C−A)	123 – 348	i. v. Insulin
Giessen	1992	1	–	6,158	92%	p. v.$^{\Delta}$	IAK*	2	1	ATG (+P−C)	400 –> 688$^{\#}$	i. v. Insulin

* IEQ: Islet Equivalents (150 μm islets)
IAK: Islet After Kidney
SIK: Simultaneous Islet and Kidney

P: Prednisone
C: Cyclosporine A
A: Azathioprine

Δ portal vein
† in the early posttransplant period
\# as of Oct. 15, 1994

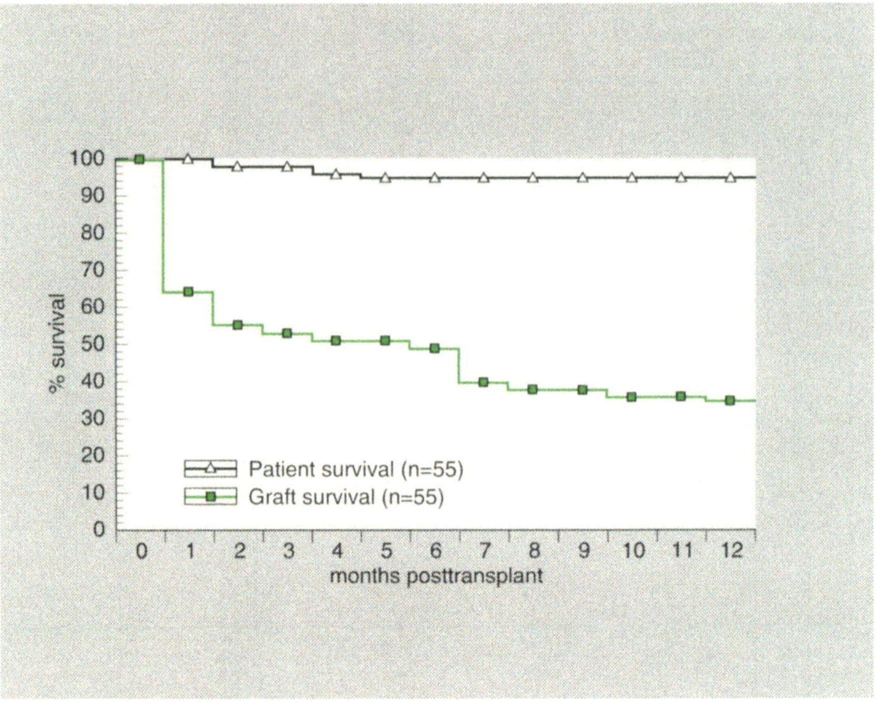

Fig. 5 One-year patient and islet allograft survival (basal C-peptide ≥ 1 ng/ml) in 55 pretransplant C-peptide negative IDDM recipients (1990–1992); ITR 1994 [240]

From a detailed analysis of 55 well-documented adult islet allografts into pretransplant C-peptide negative type 1 diabetic recipients performed from 1990 to 1992 the following lessons emerged: results have improved compared to previous reports; one-year patient survival rate was 95%; one-year islet allograft survival rate assessed by basal C-peptide ≥ 1 ng/ml was 33% (Figure 5). Eleven percent of the recipients were insulin independent at one year follow-up. Insulin independence after single donor islet allotransplantation was demonstrated and unequivocal examples of insulin independence were only obtained in association with other organ allografts. Patients who became insulin independent had pretransplant insulin requirements and HbA1c levels varying from 0.6 to 1.2 units per kg per day and from 6.5 to 11.5%, respectively. Values were available in only 32 of 55 cases pre- and one year post transplant. The one-year post transplant HbA1c levels ranged from 5% to about 8.5%. Thirty-six percent of all recipient lost their graft function within the first month post transplant.

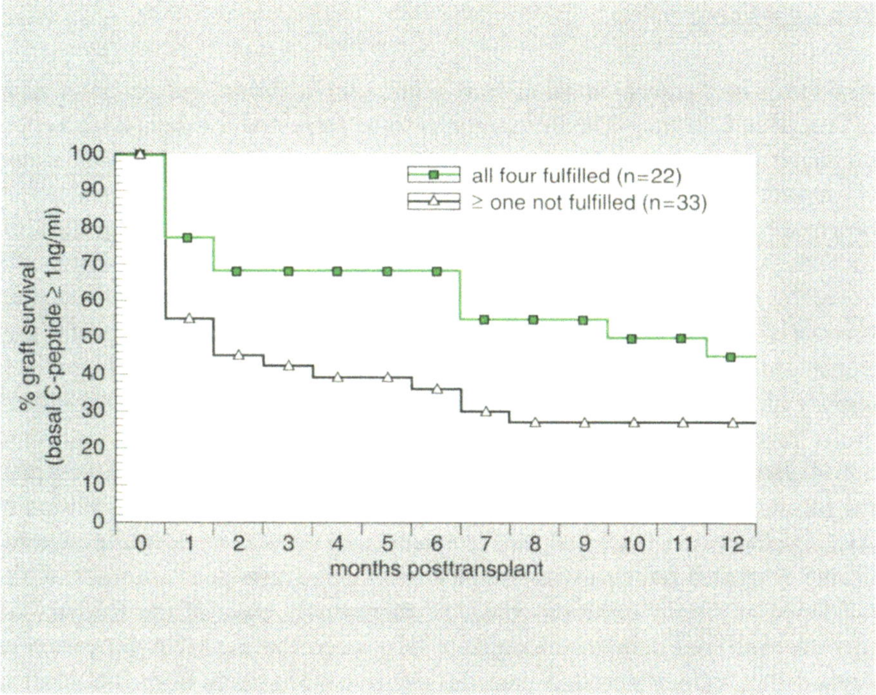

Fig. 6 One-year islet allograft survival in 55 pre-transplant C-peptide negative IDDM recipients (1990–92 cases) according to common characteristics; ITR 1994 [240]

All pretransplant C-peptide negative type 1 diabetic patients who ever became insulin independent following islet transplantation shared four common characteristics: mean pancreatic preservation time was less than 8 hours, islet mass was at least 6.000 IEQ per kg bodyweight; the liver served as implantation site; and ALG/ATG/ALS or OKT3 was given for induction immunosuppression. When all four criteria were met, 47% of all recipients were insulin independent at one-year follow-up (Figure 6).

Effects on diabetic secondary complications

At present, there is no data available and the follow-up studies are too short a post transplant period to draw any conclusions concerning effects on diabetic secondary complications. But, significant plasma C-peptide concentrations achieved in 33 percent of the cases at one year posttransplant may prevent progression of early lesions as recently demonstrated in a prospective manner by C-peptide injections [242].

Transplantation safety

Reporting islet transplantation – related complications represents an issue of crucial importance. The Edmonton is to be respected for their frank report on bacterimia in two of their patients due to transplantation of contaminated cryopreserved pancreatic islets [242]. Portal hypertension represents an actual potentially life-threatening risk if unpurified pancreatic digest is grafted intraportally. The recent analysis of the Registry revealed that islet purity did not affect islet allograft survival. However, there is increasing agreement that, for safety reasons, islet purification should be performed if intraportal islet transplantation is intended. The Pittsburgh group reported on a higher frequency of kidney rejection episodes in recipients of simultaneous islet-kidney grafts receiving FK506 and steroids compared with diabetic patients and non-diabetic patients who had a kidney transplant alone [243]. In contrast, the Minneapolis group presented data suggesting that islet transplantation in ALG/cyclosporine – treated SIK recipients and in ALG/cyclosporine azathioprine – treated patients with established kidney grafts does not increase the incidence of kidney rejection episodes. Regrettably, data of the Registry on this relevant issue remains incomplete. However, the available data seem to suggest that kidney rejection episodes are not more likely if an islet graft is added to the kidney graft.

The Giessen Center experience

In the meantime, we have achieved insulin independence by islet transplantation in one autografted patient following pancreatectomy due to chronic pancreatitis, and in one liver-islet allografted patient following pancreatectomy and hepatectomy due to abdominal malignancy.

A clinical islet transplantation program in type 1 diabetic recipients was started at our institution in 1992. On November 26, 1992, a 37-year old female diabetic patient received 6.140 IEQ per kg bodyweight from a single donor into the liver by percutaneous transhepatic catheterization of the portal vein in local anesthesia. The donor was 26 years old, AB0 identical, HLA-haploidentical, CMV negative, and the serum crossmatch test was negative. The patient had been kidney grafted due to end-stage renal diabetic disease five years earlier by donation of a kidney of her mother. This patient, first of a series, became insulin independent at day 400 post transplant and remains so at the present time, more than 650 days post transplant [244] (Figure 7). Her metabolic control is nearly optimal (postprandial blood glucose

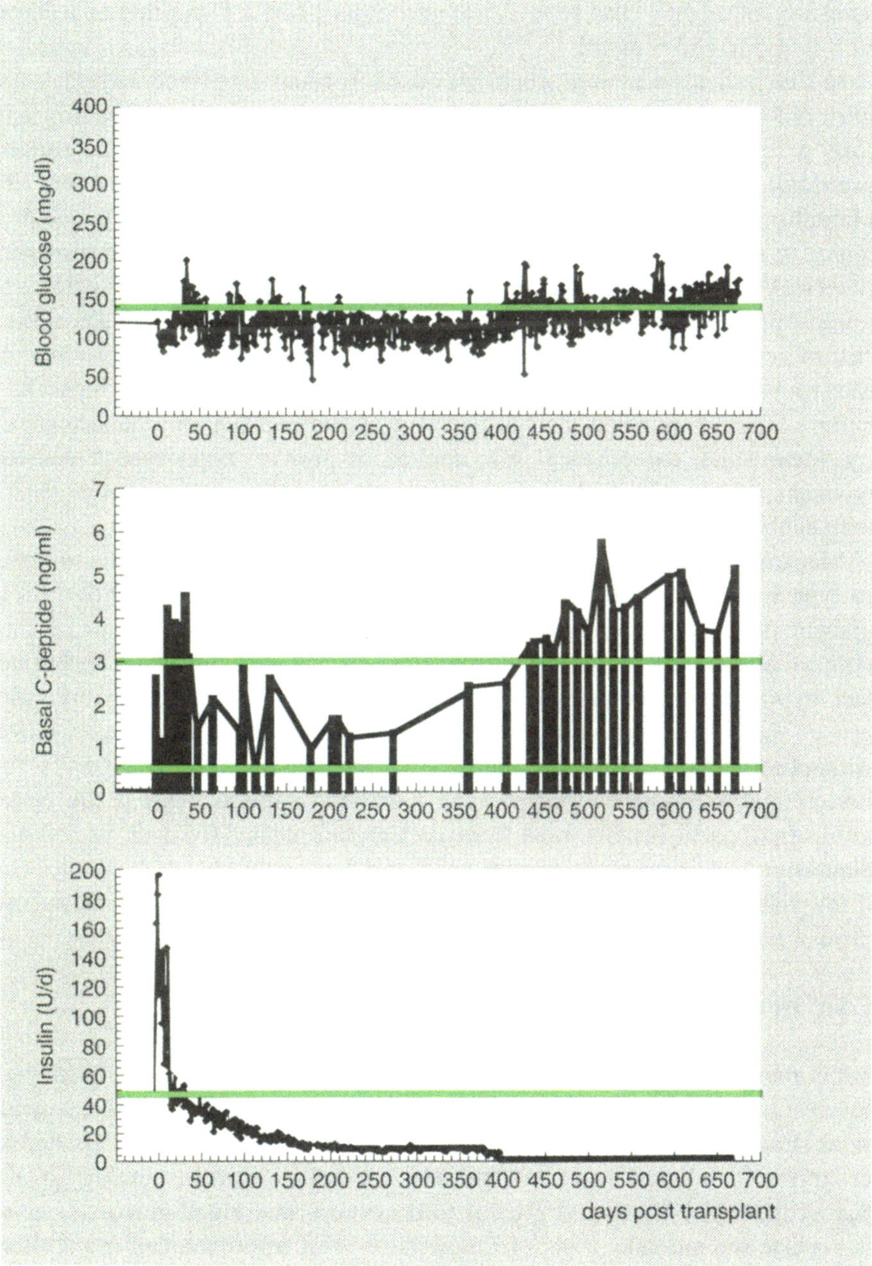

Fig. 7 Major metabolic parameters in a patient following islet transplantation in November 1992 at Justus-Liebig-University Giessen. Temporary increase in insulin dosage due to peritransplant treatment with steroids and to parenteral nutrition

levels < 150 mg/dl; HbA1c < 7.5%) and basal plasma C-peptide concentration is about 4 to 5 ng/ml.

In this patient, a new protocol was used in order to overcome early allograft failure as: 1. Technically related: islets of proven viability; Biostator and total parenteral nutrition to ensure normoglycemia and to avoid potentially islet-toxic substrate concentration in the portal circulation during islet implantation; intensified insulin therapy from day +12 to day +90; nicotinamide to stimulate islet cell replication. 2. Immunologically related: prospective HLA-matching to make islet rejection episodes less likely; induction immunosuppression beginning at day -3 using T-cell antibodies and steroids to ensure peripheral T-cell depletion and macrophage inhibition at the time of islet transplantation; pentoxyfilline to inhibit TNF release; low temperature culture of highly purified islets to reduce graft antigenicity and immunogenicity. Meanwhile, the protocol was applied to another eight type 1 diabetic recipient with established kidney grafts and in one type 1 diabetic patient with simultaneous kidney graft.

Islet transplantation at our center will be extended in the months to come to type 1 diabetic patients with overt cardiac autonomic neuropathy, overt diabetic nephropathy but still ≥ 50 ml/min glomerular filtration rate, and to type 1 diabetic patients suffering from hypoglycemia unawareness and/or defect hypoglycemia counter regulation. Because it has been unequivocally proven that islet transplantation can be performed successfully in association with other organ transplants, more attention should be now given to the non-uremic, non-kidney grafted type 1 diabetic patients. This is the target group that could benefit most from islet replacement. However, islet transplantation in this recipient category will only have an undisputable indication if low-risk but effective methods other than lifelong immunosuppression to protect the islet graft from rejection can be developed.

Conclusion

Experimental pancreas and islet transplantation in animals has been very successful in different models of type 1 diabetes mellitus. The valuable conclusions drawn from these studies have been meanwhile successfully applied in programs for clinical pancreas and islet transplantation in humans. It appeared that the only way at present to restore normal blood glucose levels is to replace the patient's islets of Langerhans. This approach can more effectively normalize glucose metabolism than any current form of exogenous insulin treatment [245, 246]. Indeed, intraportal islet autografts in totally pancreatectomized patients are characterized by an entirely normal pulsatile insulin secretion pattern [247]. Replacement of the patient's islets can be achieved by the transplantation of either an intact vascularized pancreas or isolated islets. Although transplantation of single beta cells is a theoretical alternative, its feasibility has only been demonstrated in the rat [248].

According to a recent position statement of the American Diabetes Association (ADA) [4] successful pancreas transplantation has been demonstrated to improve significantly the quality of life of people with diabetes primarily by eliminating the need for exogenous insulin, frequent daily blood glucose measurements, and many of the dietary restrictions imposed by the disorder. Transplantation also can eliminate the acute complications commonly experienced by patients with insulin-dependent diabetes (e.g. hypoglycemia). However, there is no strong evidence from prospective controlled studies that pancreas transplantation can prevent or retard the development and/or progression of the long-term complications of diabetes. Nor is there evidence that pancreas transplantation can prolong the life of patients with diabetes mellitus. The reason for this observation which was so disappointing for transplant surgeons, diabetologists and patients alike are based on the fact that pancreas transplantation is in almost every case performed simultaneously with a kidney transplant in uremic recipients, that is to say at a time at which the neurovascular complications of the disease are too far advanced for a beneficial influence to the exerted (beyond the point of no return).

Although many issues in the field of pancreas transplantation are contentious there is general agreement that pancreas transplantation is unlikely to be useful for young adults or children who have recently developed diabetes, because it is impossible to predict whether the surgical and immunosuppressive risks of the procedure will be greater than the risks posed by the disease itself [249]. This is particularly important when one considers that roughly half of diabetic patients will not develop any serious long-term complications. These principle limitations imposed by the concept of pancreatic organ transplantation may explain why pancreas transplantation has failed to achieve widespread acceptance among diabetologists and patients despite 25 years of surgical experience with the method.

Islet transplantation, however, is a minor procedure and because it is a cellular transplant that can be maintained in culture and/or cryopreserved, it offers the potential advantages of pre-transplant reduction of immunogenicity (islet immunomodulatioin) and prospective donor/recipient matching. These procedures could obviate the need for recipient immunosuppression and thus theoretically, islet transplantation could become available to patients prior to the onset of devastating complications and thereby prevent them. With these considerations in mind, the American Diabetes Association (ADA) concluded that pancreatic islet cell transplants hold significant potential advantages over whole-gland transplants [4]. However, at this time, islet transplantation is a clinical investigational procedure.

Obviously, a number of fundamental steps will have to be taken before this appealing concept can attain clinical importance in the treatment of diabetic patients. Nevertheless, the feasibility studies demonstrated that following total pancreatectomy and islet autotransplantation ongoing insulin independence has been achieved for more than 9.5 years, for more than 4 years following simultaneous islet – liver allotransplantation, and for a maximum of 3.2 years following simultaneous islet – kidney allotransplantation in type 1 diabetic patients (status by 1994). With these remarkable achievements in mind it is our task to make islet transplantation available to more patients and to make long-term islet graft function more likely. It is only through a joint effort on the part of diabetologists, nephrologists, surgeons, immunologists, transplant coordinators and organ exchange organisations, through a thorough analysis of the successes and failures and through continued investigation that islet transplantation can one day assume clinical importance for the treatment of type 1 diabetes mellitus.

Acknowledgements

The authors wish to express their thanks to colleagues of the Third Medical Department and Policlinic, University of Giessen, Germany, Dr. C. Bollen, Dr. H. Brandhorst, Dr. D. Brandhorst, C. Geier, R. Grossmann, F. Helf, R. Mahler, C. Meyer, Dr. G. Raptis, A. Schultz and R. Schulz-Gabel, and to Prof.Dr. W.S. Rau, Department of Radiology, University of Giessen; Dr. S. Friemann and Dr. W. Ernst, Second Medical Department, University of Giessen; PD Dr. E.H. Scheuermann and Prof.Dr. W. Schoeppe, Department of Nephrology, University of Frankfurt/Main and Prof.Dr. H.D. Becker, Dr. J. Mellert and Prof.Dr. U.T. Hopt, Department of Surgery and Policlinic, University of Tübingen, for their excellent cooperation. The author's work was substantially supported by Deutsche Forschungsgemeinschaft, Bonn, Bundesministerium für Forschung und Technologie, Bonn; EUROTRANSPLANT and Bioimplant Services, Leiden/The Netherlands; Deutsche Stiftung Organtransplantation, Neu-Isenburg, and numerous cooperating transplant centers, in particular Berlin, Erlangen-Nürnberg, Essen, Frankfurt/Main, Halle, Rostock, Tübingen and Würzburg. We are grateful to our technicians.

References

[1] Sutherland DER. Pancreatic transplantation. An update. Diab Rev 1993; 1: 152–165.

[2] Bretzel RG, Browatzki CC, Schultz A et al. Klinische Inseltransplantation bei Diabetes mellitus. Diab Stoffw 1993; 2: 378–390.

[3] Sutherland DER, Kendall DM, Moudry KC et al.. Pancreas transplantation in nonuremic, type I diabetic recipients. Surgery 1988; 104: 453–463.

[4] American Diabetes Association (ADA). Pancreas transplantation for patients with diabetes mellitus. Diab Care 1992; 15: 1668–1672.

[5] Zehrer CL, Gross CR. Quality of life of pancreas transplant recipients. Diabetologia 1991; 34 suppl 1: S145–149.

[6] Federlin KF, Bretzel RG. The effect of islet transplantation on complications in experimental diabetes of the rat. World J Surg 1984; 8: 169–178.

[7] Lacy PE. Status of islet cell transplantation. Diab Rev 1993; 1: 76–92.

[8] Hering BJ, Browatzki CC, Schultz A et al. Clinical islet transplantation – Registry report, accomplishments in the past and future research needs. Cell Transplant 1993; 2: 269–282.

[9] Federlin KF, Bretzel RG, Hering BJ. Islet transplantation: state-of-the-art. Diab News 1994; 15: 6–8.

[10] Mering J von, Minkowski O. Diabetes mellitus nach Pankreasexstirpation. Arch Exp Pathol Pharmacol 1889; 26: 371–379.

[11] Minkowski O. Weitere Mittheilungen über den Diabetes mellitus nach Exstirpation des Pankreas. Berl Klin Wochenschr 1892; 29: 90–93.

[12] Hedon ME. Greffe sous-cutance du pancreas. Arch Physiol Norm Path 1892; 5: 617–628.

[13] Williams PW. Notes on diabetes treated with extract and by grafts of sheep's pancreas. Br Med J 1894; 2: 1303–1304.

[14] Ssobolew LW. Zur normalen und pathologischen Morphologie der inneren Secretion der Bauchspeicheldrüse. Virch Arch Pathol Anat 1902; 168: 91–128.

[15] Banting FG, Best CH. The internal secretion of the pancreas. J Lab Clin Med 1922; 7: 251–266.

[16] Gayet R, Guillaumie M. La regulation de la secretion interne pancreatique par un processus normalisateur demontrée par des transplantations de pancreas. Cr Soc Biol 1877; 97: 1613–1627.

[17] Houssay BA. Technique de la greffe pancreaticoduodenale an cou. Cr Soc Biol (Paris) 1929; 100: 138–140.

[18] Lexer E. Die freien Transplantationen. Ferdinand Emke, Stuttgart 1929.

[19] Sutherland DER. Immunosuppression for pancreas transplantation. Clin Transplant 1991; 5: 549–583.

[20] De Jode LR, Howard JH. Studies in pancreaticoduodenal homotransplantation. Surg Gyn Obstet 1962; 114: 553–558.

[21] Largiader F, Lyons GW, Hidalgo F et al. Orthotopic allotransplantation of the pancreas. Am J Surg 1967; 113: 70–76.

[22] Kyriakides GK, Nuttall FQ, Miller J. Segmental pancreatic transplantation in pigs. Surgery 1979; 85: 154–158.

[23] Cutfield RG, Polonsky K, Olson L et al. Long-term follow-up of canine segmental pancreatic autografts. Diabetes 1985; 34: 174–178.

[24] Gliedman ML, Gold M, Whittaker J et al. Pancreatic duct to ureter anastomosis for exocrine drainage in pancreatic transplantation. Am J Surg 1973; 125: 245-252.

[25] Cook K, Sollinger HW, Warner T et al. Pancreaticocystostomy: an alternative method for exocrine drainage of segmental pancreatic allografts. Transplantation 1983; 35: 634–636.

[26] Thiroloix J. Note sur la physiologie du pancreas. Arch Physiol Norm Pathol 1892; 4: 716–720.

[27] Anlyan WG, Isley JK, Fetter BF et al. A study of some pathophysiologic disturbances resulting from diffuse pancreatic duct obstruction. Surgery 1957; 42: 29–38.

[28] Little JM, Lauer C, Hogg J. Pancreatic duct obstruction with an acrylate glue: a new method for producing pancreatic exocrine atrophy. Surgery 1977; 81: 243-249.
[29] Dubernard JM, Traeger J, Neyra P. Suppression of the exocrine function as an aid to segmental pancreatic transplantation in dogs. Biomedicine 1977; 27: 172-174.
[30] Gebhardt Ch, Stolte M. Pankreasgang-Okklusion durch Injektion einer schnellhärtenden Aminosäurenlösung. Langenbecks Arch Chir 1978; 346: 149-166.
[31] McMaster P, Gibby O, Calne RY et al. Human pancreatic transplantation – preliminary studies of carbohydrate control. Transplant Proc 1981; 13: 371–373.
[32] White DC, Sutherland DER, Zweber B et al. Pancreatic endocrine function following exocrine ablation with silicone polymers. Trans Am Soc Artif Intern Organs 1981; 27: 254–258.
[33] Rausis C, Choudhury A, Ogota Y. Influence of pancreatic duct anastomosis on function of autotransplanted canine pancreatic segments. J Surg Res 1970; 10: 551–557.
[34] Vanek I, Bartos V, Kocandrle V. Prognosis of experimental pancreatic transplantation in relation to vascular reconstructive procedure. Transplant Proc 1984; 16: 716–720.
[35] Calne RY, McMaster P, Rolles K et al. Technical observations in segmental pancreas allografting: observations on pancreatic blood flow. Transplant Proc 1980; 12 suppl 2: 51–57.
[36] Kelly WD, Lillehei RC, Merkel FK et al. Allotransplantation of the pancreas and duodenum along with the kidney in diabetic nephropathy. Surgery 1967; 61: 827–837.
[37] American College of Surgeons/National Institute of Health (ACS/NIH). Organ Transplant Registry: first scientific report. JAMA 1971; 217: 1520–1529.
[38] Sutherland DER. International Human Pancreas and Islet Transplant Registry. Transplant Proc 1980; 12 suppl 2: 229–236.
[39] Serrou B, Solassol C, Michel H et al. Transplantation 1973; 16: 398–402.
[40] Baumgartner D, Sutherland DER, Heil J et al. J Surg Res 1980; 29: 249–257.
[41] Schilfgaarde R van, Gooszen HG, Bosman FT et al. Transplant Proc 1984; 16: 809–810.
[42] Florack G, Sutherland DER, Heil J et al. Surgery 1982; 92: 260–269.
[43] Belzer FO, Southard JH. Principles of short-term preservation by cold storage. Transplantation 1988; 45: 673–676.
[44] Sutherland DER, Moudry KC. Pancreas Transplant Registry: history and analysis of cases 1966 to October 1986. Pancreas 1987; 2: 473–488.
[45] Sanchez-Urdazpal L, Czaja AJ, van Hoek B et al. Prognostic features and role of liver transplantation in severe corticosteroid-treated autoimmune chronic active hepatitis. Hepatology 1992; 15: 215–221.
[46] Sutherland DER, Gruessner A, Moudry-Munns K. International Pancreas Transplant Registry Report. Transplant Proc 1994; 26: 407–411.
[47] Pozza G, Bosi E, Secchi A et al. Metabolic control of type I (insulin dependent) diabetes after pancreas transplantation. Br Med J 1985; 291: 510–513.
[48] Morel P, Goetz FC, Moudry-Munns K et al. Long-term glucose control in patients with pancreatic transplants. Ann Intern Med 1991; 115: 694–699.
[49] Katz H, Homan M, Velosa J et al. Effects of pancreas transplantation on postprandial glucose metabolism. N Engl J Med 1991; 325: 1278–1283.
[50] Diem P, Abid H, Redmon JB et al. Systemic drainage of pancreas allografts as independent cause of hyperinsulinemia in type I diabetic patients. Diabetes 1990; 39: 534–540.
[51] Smith JL, Hunsicker L, Yuh WTC. Appearance of type II diabetes mellitus in type I diabetic recipients of pancreas allografts. Transplantation 1989; 47: 304-311.
[52] Kennedy WR, Navarro X, Goetz FC et al. Effects of pancreatic transplantation on diabetic neuropathy. N Engl J Med 1990; 322: 1031–1037.
[53] Bently FR, Jung S, Garrison RN. Neuropathy and psychosocial adjustment after pancreas transplant in diabetics. Transplant Proc 1990; 22: 691–695.
[54] Solders G, Gunnarsson R, Persson A et al. Effects of combined pancreatic and renal transplantation on diabetic neuropathy: a two-year follow-up study. Lancet 1987; 2: 1232–1235.
[55] Bohmann SO, Tyden G, Wilczek Het al. Prevention of kidney graft diabetic nephropathy by pancreas transplantation in man. Diabetes 1985; 34: 306–308.

[56] Bilous RW, Mauer SM, Sutherland DERet al. Effects of pancreas transplantation on the glomerular structure of renal allografts in patients with insulin-dependent diabetes. N Engl J Med 1989; 321: 80–85.
[57] Sutherland DER, Dunn DL, Goetz FCet al. A ten year experience with 290 pancreas transplants at a single institution. Ann Surg 1989; 210: 274–288.
[58] Sasaki T, Pirsch JD, Ploeg RJ et al. Effects of DR mismatch on long-term graft survival in simultaneous kidney-pancreas transplantation. Transplant Proc 1993; 25: 237–238.
[59] Langerhans P. Beiträge zur mikroskopischen Anatomie der Bauchspeicheldrüse. Inauguraldissertation, Medizinische Fakultät, Friedrich-Wilhelm-Universität Berlin, Lange, Berlin, 1869.
[60] Hellerström C. A method for the microdissection of intact pancreatic islets of mammals. Acta Endocrinol 1964; 45: 122.
[61] Moskalewski S. Isolation and culture of the islets of Langerhans of the guinea pig. Gen Comp Endocrinol 1965; 5: 342.
[62] Lacy PE, Kostianovsky M. Method for the isolation of intact islets of Langerhans from the rat pancreas. Diabetes 1967; 16: 35.
[63] Bretzel RG. Inseltransplantation und Diabetes mellitus. Experimentelle Grundlagen und klinische Versuche. München: R. Pflaum, 1984.
[64] Gotoh M, Maki T, Kiyoizumi T et al. An improved method for isolation of mouse pancreatic islets. Transplantation 1985; 40: 437–438.
[65] Ricordi C, Lacy PE, Finke EH et al. Automated method for the isolation of human pancreatic islets. Diabetes 1988; 37: 413–420.
[66] Hering BJ, Milde K, Busam J et al. Oxygen bubbling enhanced collagenase digestion: A new approach to islet isolation. Proc Int Congress on Pancreatic and Islet Transplantation, Lyon, June 6–8, 1991.
[67] Scharp DW, Kemp CB, Knight MJ et al. The use of Ficoll in the preparation of viable islets of Langerhans from the rat pancreas. Transplantation 1973; 16: 686
[68] Mittal VK, Toledo-Pereyra LH, Sharma M et al. Acute portal hypertension and disseminated intravascular coagulation following pancreatic islet autotransplantation after subtotal pancreatectomy. Transplantation 1981; 31: 302.
[69] Gray DW, Sutton R, McShane P et al. Exocrine contamination impairs implantation of pancreatic islets transplanted beneath the kidney capsule. J Surg Res 1988; 45: 432–442.
[70] Gotoh M, Maki T, Satomi S et al. Immunological characteristics of purified pancreatic islet grafts. Transplantation 1986; 42: 387–390.
[71] Hering BJ, Muench KP, Schelz J et al. The evaluation of neutral density separation utilizing Ficoll-sodium diatrizoate and Nycodenz and centrifugal elutriation in the purification of bovine and canine islet preparations. Horm Metabol Res 1990; Suppl Ser 25: 57–63.
[72] Lake SP, Anderson J, Chamberlain J et al. Bovine serum albumine density gradient isolation of rat pancreatic islets. Transplantation 1987; 43: 805–808.
[73] Lake SP, Bassett PD, Larkins A et al. Large-scale purification of human islets utilizing discontinuous albumin gradient on IBM 2991 cell separator. Diabetes 1989; 38 suppl 1: 143–145.
[74] Andersson A, Buschard F. Culture of isolated pancreatic islets: Its application for transplantation purposes. Trans Am Soc Artif Intern Organs 1977; 23: 342.
[75] Nakagawara G, Yamasaki G, Kimura S et al. Insulin-releasing activity and successful transplantation of pancreatic islets preserved by tissue culture. Surgery 1978; 83: 188.
[76] Bretzel RG, Beule B, Federlin K. Function and morphology of adult rat islets after culture and transplantation. In: Federlin K, Bretzel RG, eds. Islet Isolation, Culture and Cryopreservation. Stuttgart: G Thieme, 1981: 96.
[77] Rajotte RV, Steward HL, Voss WAG et al. Viability studies on frozen-thawed rat islets of Langerhans. Cryobiology 1977; 14: 116.
[78] Bank HL, Davis RF, Emerson D. Cryogenic preservation of isolated rat islets of Langerhans: Effect of cooling and warming rates. Diabetologia 1979; 16: 195.

[79] Bretzel RG, Beule B, Schaefer S et al. Cryopreservation and tissue culture of pancreatic islets for transplantation in experimental diabetes mellitus. Diabetes 1979; 25: 377.
[80] Bretzel RG, Schneider J, Dobroschke J et al. Islet transplantation in experimental diabetes of the rat. VII. Cryopreservation of rat and human islets. Preliminary report. Horm Metabol Res 1980; 12: 274.
[81] Bretzel RG, Flesch B, Brendel M et al. Cryopreservation of islets of Langerhans. In: Albarran AJ, Martin AA, Melero VMA, Gomez SA, eds. Islet Transplantation. Madrid: Editorial Medica Panamericana, 1992: 97.
[82] Rajotte RV, Warnock GL, Bruch LC et al. Transplantation of cryopreserved and fresh rat islets and canine pancreatic fragments: comparison of cryopreservation protocols. Cryobiology 1983; 20: 169–184.
[83] Warnock GL, Gray DWR, McShane Pet al. Survival of cryopreserved isolated adult human pancreatic islets of Langerhans. Transplantation 1987; 44: 75–82.
[84] Bretzel RG, Hering BJ, Stroedter D, Zekorn T, Federlin KF. Experimental islet transplantation in small animals. In: Pancreatic Islet Cell Transplantation. C. Ricordi (ed.), R.G. Landes Company, Austin, 1992, pp 249–260.
[85] Bretzel RG, Hering BJ, Linn T et al. Islet transplantation in rodents. In: Bretzel RG, ed. Diabetes mellitus. Immunological and Dynamic Aspects of Insulin Substitution. Berlin: Springer, 1990: 229.
[86] Warnock GL, Ao Z, Cattral MS et al. Experimental islet transplantation in large animals. In: Ricordi C (ed.) Pancreatic Islet Cell Transplantation, R.G. Landes Company, Austin, 1992, pp 261–278.
[87] Finegood DT, Warnock GL, Kneteman NM et al. Insulin sensitivity and glucose effectiveness in long-term islet autotransplanted dogs. Diabetes 1989; 38 (suppl 1): 189–191.
[88] Sutherland DER, Steffes MW, Mauer SM et al. Isolation of human and porcine islets of Langerhans and islet transplantation in pigs. J Surg Res 1974; 16: 102–111.
[89] Hesse UJ, Weyer J, Meyer Get al. Long-term results after porcine islet transplantation. Transplant Proc 1989; 21: 2763–2764.
[90] Mellert J, Hering BJ, Brandhorst H et al. Experience with islet allografts in immunosuppressed pigs. Horm Metabol Res 1990; 25 (suppl 1): 187–189.
[91] Scharp DW, Murphy JJ, Newton WT et al. Transplantation of islets of Langerhans in diabetic Rhesus monkeys. Surgery 1975; 77: 100–105.
[92] Stegall MD, Chabot J, Weber C et al. Pancreatic islet transplantation in Cynomolgus monkeys. Transplantation 1989; 48: 944–950.
[93] Bretzel RG, Federlin K. Rückbildung diabetischer Nierenläsionen durch Inseltransplantation bei der Ratte. Quantitative Morphologie. Verh Dtsch Ges Inn Med. 1977; 83: 1373.
[94] Mauer SM, Sutherland DER, Steffes MW et al. Pancreatic islet transplantation: Effects on the glomerular lesions of experimental diabetes in the rat. Diabetes 1974; 23: 748.
[95] Steffes MW, Brown DM, Basgen JM et al. Amelioration of mesangial volume and surface alteration following islet transplantation in rats. Diabetes 1980; 29: 509.
[96] Bretzel RG, Breidenbach DH, Hofmann J et al. Islet transplantation in experimental diabetes of the rat. VI. Rate of regression in diabetic kidney lesions after isogeneic islet transplantation. Quantitative measurements. Horm Metabol Res 1979; 11: 200.
[97] Bretzel RG, Menden A, Richardt M et al. Renal collagenglucosyltransferase activity following islet transplantation in streptozotocin-diabetic rats. Diabetologia 1981; 21: 428.
[98] Bretzel RG, Schneider J, Zimmermann I et al. Urinary excretion of alanine aminopeptidase and total proteinuria in experimental diabetes mellitus before and after islet transplantation. Contr Nephrol 1981; 24: 153.
[99] Koesters W, Seelig HP, Stauch M. Reversibility of function and morphologic glomerular lesions by islet transplantation in long-term diabetic rats. Diabetologia 1977; 13: 409.
[100] Steffes MW, Brown DM, Basgen JM et al. Glomerular basement membrane thickness following islet transplantation in the diabetic rat. Lab Invest 1979; 41: 116.

[101] Schmidt RE, Plurad SB, Olack BJ et al. The effect of pancreatic islet transplantation and insulin therapy on experimental diabetic autonomic neuropathy. Diabetes 1983; 32: 532–540.

[102] Gray BN, Watkins E. Prevention of vascular complications of diabetes by pancreatic islet transplantation. Arch Surg 1976; 111: 254.

[103] Krupin T, Waltman SR, Scharp DW et al. Ocular fluorophotometry in streptozotocin diabetes mellitus in the rat: Effect of pancreatic islet isografts. Invest Ophthalmol Visual Sci 1979; 18: 1185.

[104] Stroedter D, Schuster KR, Bretzel RG et al. Der Effekt von Diabetes mellitus und Inselzelltransplantation auf Funktion und Stoffwechsel des isoliert arbeitenden Rattenherzens. Klin Wochenschr 1987; 65 Suppl. 9: 207.

[105] Britland ST, Zimmermann O von, Sharma AK et al. The effect of pancreatic islet transplantation on experimental diabetic neuropathy. J Neurol Sci 1991; 105: 168–174.

[106] Silberberg R, Hirshberg G, Lesker P. Enzyme studies in the articular cartilage of diabetic rats and of rats bearing transplanted pancreatic islets. Diabetes 1977; 26: 732.

[107] Warnock GL, Rajotte RV, Kneteman NM et al. Oral glucose tolerance and response to mixed meals in dogs bearing long-term transplanted islets of Langerhans. Transplant Proc 1987; 19: 969–973.

[108] Bretzel RG, Federlin K. Islet transplantation in experimental diabetes mellitus of the rat. Biochemical and morphological findings. In: Bibergeil H, Zühlke H, Poser U, eds. Early Diabetes. Pathogenesis, Diagnosis, Prevention. Karlsburg: Central Institute for Diabetes, 1980: 290.

[109] Richardt M, Menden A, Bretzel RG et al. Islet transplantation in experimental diabetes of the rat. VIII. B-cell restoration following islet transplantation. Preliminary results. Horm Metabol Res 1984; 16: 551–552.

[110] Bretzel RG, Federlin K. Perspectives from experimental islet transplantation: The restorative effect on the diabetic pancreas. Pediat Adolesc Endocrinol 1986; 15: 398.

[111] Vialettes B, Sutherland DER, Payne WA et al. Synergystic effect of donor specific soluable membrane antigen injection and antilymphocyte globulin administration on the survival of islet allografts in rats. Transplantation 1978; 25: 336.

[112] Sutherland DER. Pancreas and islet transplantation. I. Experimental studies. Diabetologia 1981; 20: 161.

[113] Posselt AM, Barker CF, Tomaszewski JEet al. Induction of donor-specific unresponsiveness by intrathymic islet transplantation. Science 1990; 249: 1293-1295.

[114] Markees TG, De Fazio SR, Gozzo JJ. Prolongation of impure murine islet allografts with antilymphocyte serum and donor-specific bone marrow. Transplantation 1992; 53: 521–527.

[115] Posselt AM, Odorico JS, Barker CF et al. Promotion of pancreatic islet allograft survival by intrathymic transplantation of bone marrow. Diabetes 1992; 41: 771–775.

[116] Lacy PE, Davie JM, Finke EH. Prolongation of islet allograft survival following in vitro culture (24 C) and a single injection of ALS. Science 1979; 204: 312.

[117] Forsen JW, Blum BE, Bretzel RG et al. Islet transplantation in experimental diabetes of the rat. IX. In vitro culture reduces Ia-bearing cells in rat islets. Horm Metabol Res 1984; 16: 671–672.

[118] Bretzel RG, Blum BE, Höll E et al. Rat islet allograft survival following different immunomodulative and immunosuppressive treatment. Exc Med ICS 1986; 717: 181.

[119] Flesch BK, Bretzel RG, Otto DA et al. Pretreatment of rat pancreatic islets with MHC I-A monoclonal antibody: in vitro and in vivo effects on islet antigenicity. Horm Metabol Res 1991; 23: 357–361.

[120] Flesch BK, Entenmann H, Milde Ket al. Islet transplantation in experimental diabetes of the rat. XIII. Cryopreservation reduces MHC class II but not class I antigens of rat pancreatic islets. Horm Metabol Res 1991; 23: 1–6.

[121] Bretzel RG, Flesch BK, Willig J, et al. Effects of ganglioside (Cronassial) treatment on MHC Ia antigen expression and allograft survival of pancreatic islets in diabetic rats. Diabetologia 1990; 22: 112–114.

[122] Bowen KM, Andrus L, Lafferty K. Successful allotransplantation of mouse pancreatic islets to nonimmunosuppressed recipients. Diabetes 1980; 29: 98.

[123] Lau H, Reemtsma K, Hardy MA. Pancreatic islet allograft prolongation by donor-specific blood transfusions with ultraviolet irradiation. Science 1983; 221: 754–756.

[124] Kanai T, Porter J, Gotoh M et al. Effect of gamma-irradiation on mouse pancreatic islet allograft survival. Diabetes 1989; 38 suppl 1: 154–156.

[125] Faustman DL, Hauptfeld V, Lacy PE et al. Prolongation of murine islet allograft survival by pretreatment of islets with antibody directed to Ia determinants. Proc Natl Acad Sci USA 1981; 78: 5156.

[126] Woehrle M, Markmann JF, Silvers WK et al. Transplantation of cultured pancreatic islets to BB rats. Surgery 1986; 100: 334–341.

[127] Strautz RL. Studies of hereditary-obese mice (ob/ob) after implantation of pancreatic islets in Millipore filter capsules. Diabetologia 1970; 6: 306.

[128] Maratos E, Taub RN, Bramis J. Amelioration of streptozotocin-induced diabetes in mice by the implantation of pancreatic islets in diffusion chambers. Mt Sinai J Med 1976; 43: 415.

[129] Weber C, Weil R, McIntosh R et al. Xenotransplantation of piscine islets into hyperglycaemic rats. Surgery 1975; 77: 208.

[130] Archer J, Kaye R, Mutter G. Control of streptozotocin diabetes in Chinese hamsters by cultured mouse islet cells without immunosuppression: A preliminary report. J Surg Res 1980; 28: 77.

[131] Chick WL, Perris JJ, Lauris V et al. Artificial pancreas using living beta cells: Effect on glucose homeostasis in diabetic rats. Science 1977; 197: 780.

[132] Tze WJ, Wong FC, Chen LM et al. Implantable artificial endocrine pancreas unit used to restore normoglycemia in the diabetic rat. Nature 1976; 264: 466.

[133] Altman JJ, Houlbert D, Chollier A et al. Encapsulated human islet transplants in diabetic rats. Trans Am Soc Artif Intern Organs 1984; 30: 382–386.

[134] Zekorn T, Siebers U, Bretzel RG et al. Protection of islets of Langerhans from interleukin-1 toxicity by artificial membranes. Transplantation 1990; 50: 391-394.

[135] Zekorn T, Bretzel RG, Siebers U et al. Protein coat causes improved insulin diffusion through membranes for immunoisolated islet transplantation: improved islet survival by pretreatment of membranes and islets. Transplant Proc 1990; 22: 867–869.

[136] Altman JJ, Houlbert D, Callard P et al. Long-term plasma glucose normalization in experimental diabetic rats with macroencapsulated implants of benign human insulinomas. Diabetes 1986; 35: 625–633.

[137] Lim F, Sun AN. Microencapsulated islets as bioartificial endocrine pancreas. Science 1980; 210: 908.

[138] Darquy S, Reach G. Immunoisolation of pancreatic B cells by microencapsulation. An in vitro study . Diabetologia 1985; 28: 776–780.

[139] Taunton-Rigby A. Transplantation of encapsulated islets. Transplant Proc 1986; 18: 1841.

[140] Iwata H, Amemiya H, Matsuda Tet al. Evaluation of microencapsulated islets in agarose gel as bioartificial pancreas by studies of hormone secretion in culture and by xenotransplantation. Diabetes 1989; 38 suppl 1: 224–225.

[141] Fan MY, Lum ZP, Fu XW et al. Reversal of diabetes in BB rats by transplantation of encapsulated pancreatic islets. Diabetes 1990; 39: 519–522.

[142] Siebers U, Zekorn T, Horcher A et al. In vitro testing of rat and porcine islets microencapsulated in barium alginate beads. Transplant Proc 1992; 24: 950-951.

[143] Zekorn T, Siebers U, Horcher A et al. Barium-alginate beads for immunoisolated transplantation of islet of Langerhans. Transplant Proc 1992; 24: 937–939.

[144] Sibley RK, Sutherland DER, Goetz F et al. Recurrent diabetes mellitus in the pancreas iso- and allograft: A light and electron microscopic immunohistological analysis of four cases. Lab Invest 1985; 53: 132–144.

[145] Naji A, Silvers WK, Dafoe D et al. Successful islet transplantation in spontaneous diabetes. Surgery 1979; 86: 218.
[146] Naji A, Silvers WK, Bartlett ST et al. Immunologic factors in pathogenesis and treatment of human and animal diabetes. World J Surg 1984; 8: 214–220.
[147] Colle E, Guttmann RD, Seemayer R. Spontaneous diabetes mellitus in the rat. I. Association with the major histocompatibility complex. J Exp Med 1981; 154: 1237.
[148] Prud'homme GJ, Colle E, Fuks A et al. Major histocompatibility complex restriction of T-lymphocyte response to islet cell antigens in IDDM rats. Diabetes 1987; 36: 237–239.
[149] Naji A, Silvers WK, Kimura H et al. Influences of islet and bone marrow transplantation on the diabetes and immunodeficiency of BB rats. Metabolism 1983; 32: 62–68.
[150] Prowse SJ, Bellgrau D, Lafferty KJ. Islet allografts are destroyed by disease occurrence in the spontaneous diabetic BB rat. Diabetes 1986; 35: 110–114.
[151] Weringer EJ, Like AA. Immune attack on pancreatic islet transplants in the spontaneous diabetic BioBreeding/Worcester (BB/W) rat is not MHC restricted. J Immunol 1985; 134: 2383–2386.
[152] Terada M, Salzler M, Lennartz K et al. The effect of H-2 compatibility on pancreatic beta cell survival in the nonobese diabetic mouse. Transplantation 1988; 45: 622–627.
[153] Roza A, Markmann JF, Brayman KL et al. Isolated islet cells are more vulnerable to recurrent diabetes than vascularized pancreas grafts. Surg Forum 1987; 38: 373.
[154] Hegre OD, Serie JR, Weinhaus AJet al. Cultured neonatal islet transplants in Alloxan-treated and spontaneously diabetic rats. In: Federlin K, Bretzel RG, Hering BJ, eds. Methods in Islet Transplantation Research. Horm Metabol Res 1990; Suppl Ser 25: 108–116.
[155] Pipeleers D, Pipeleers-Marichal M, Markholst H et al. Transplantation of purified islet cells in diabetic BB rats. Diabetologia 1991; 34: 390–396.
[156] Chabot JA, Lau H, Reemtsma K et al. Successful islet transplantation in BB rats without chronic immunosuppression. Transplant Proc 1987; 19: 974–975.
[157] Jacobson JD, Markmann JF, Brayman KL et al. Prevention of recurrent autoimmune diabetes in BB rats by anti-asialo-GM 1 antibody. Diabetes 1988; 37: 838–841.
[158] Markmann JF, Jacobson JD, Brayman KLet al. Prevention of recurrent diabetes in BB rats after islet transplantation by monoclonal antibody therapy. Diabetes 1989; 38 suppl 1: 165–167.
[159] Markmann JF, Woehrle M, Roza A et al. Islet transplantation to study autoimmune pathogenesis of diabetes in BB rat. In: Federlin K, Bretzel RG, Hering BJ, eds. Methods in Islet Transplantation Research. Horm Metabol Res 1990; Suppl Ser 25: 116–119.
[160] Matsuo S, Mullen Y, Wicker LS et al. Prolongation of islet isograft survival in diabetic NOD mice by anti-L3T4 and anti-LYT2 monoclonal antibodies. Transplant Proc 1990; 22: 880–881.
[161] Wang T, Singh B, Warnock GL et al. Prevention of recurrence of IDDM in islet-transplanted diabetic NOD mice by adjuvant immunotherapy. Diabetes 1992; 41: 114–117.
[162] Hahn HJ, Kuttler B, Lucke S et al. Effect of temporary IL-2 receptor mab therapy on islet allografts in autoimmune diabetes. Transplant Proc 1989; 21: 2711–2713.
[163] Kuttler B, Dunger A, Volk HD et al. Prevention and suppression of autoimmune pancreatic beta-cell destruction in BB rats by syngeneic lymphocytes obtained from long-term normoglycaemic donors. Diabetologia 1991; 34: 74–77.
[164] Nomikos IN, Prowse SJ, Carotenuto P, Lafferty KJ. Combined treatment with nicotinamide and desferrioxamine prevents islet allograft destruction in NOD mice. Diabetes 1986; 35: 1302–1304.
[165] Woehrle MF, Markmann JF, Armstrong J et al. Effect of transplant site on islet allograft survival in BB rats. Transplant Proc 1987; 19: 925–927.
[166] Woehrle M, Pullmann J, Bretzel RG et al. Prevention of recurrent autoimmune diabetes in the BB rat by islet transplantation under the renal capsule. Transplantation 1992; 53: 1099–1102.
[167] Darquy S, Chicheportiche D, Capron F et al. Comparative study of microencapsulated rat islets implanted in different diabetic models in mice. In: Federlin K, Bretzel RG, Hering

BJ, eds. Methods in Islet Transplantation Research. Horm Metabol Res 1990; Suppl Ser 25: 209–213.
[168] Weber CJ, Zabinski S, Koschitzky TS et al. Microencapsulated dog and rat islet xenografts into streptozotocin-diabetic and NOD mice. In: Federlin K, Bretzel RG, Hering BJ, eds. Methods in Islet Transplantation Research. Horm Metabol Res 1990; Suppl Ser 25: 219–226.
[169] Bartlett ST, Hadley GA, Dirden B et al. Composite kidney-islet transplantation prevents recurrent autoimmune beta-cell destruction. Surgery 1993; 114: 211-217.
[170] Warnock GL, Rajotte RV. Human pancreatic islet transplantation. Transplant Rev 1992; 6: 195–208.
[171] Ricordi C, Hering BJ, London NJM et al. Islet isolation assessment. In: Pancreatic Islet Cell Transplantation. Ricordi C (ed.), R.G. Landes Company, Austin, 1992, pp 132–142.
[172] Ricordi C, Tzakis AG, Carroll PB et al. Human islet isolation and allotransplantation in 22 consecutive cases. Transplantation 1992; 53: 407–414.
[173] Farney AC, Najarian JS, Nakhleh RE et al. Autotransplantation of dispersed pancreatic islet tissue combined with total or near-total pancreatectomy for treatment of chronic pancreatitis. Surgery 1991; 110: 427–439.
[174] Pyzdrowski KL, Kendall DM, Halter JB et al. Preserved insulin secretion and insulin independence in recipients of islet autografts. N Engl J Med 1992; 327: 220–226.
[175] Farney AC, Najarian JS, Nakhleh RE et al. Long-term function of islet autotransplants. Transplant Proc 24: 969–971.
[176] Bretzel RG, Alejandro R, Hering, BJ et al. Clinical islet transplantation: guidelines for islet quality control. Transplant Proc 1994; 26: 388–392
[177] Scharp DW. The elusive human islet: variables involved in its effective recovery. In: van Schilfgaarde R, Hardy MA (eds), Transplantation of the Endocrine Pancreas in Diabetes Mellitus, Amsterdam, Elsevier, 1988, 97.
[178] Klitscher D, Brandhorst H, Hering B et al. Can donor data predict human islet isolation outcome? Horm Metabol Res 1993; 25: 60.
[179] Zeng Y, Torre MA, Karrison T. The correlation between donor characteristics and human pancreatic islet yield and purity. Transplantation 1994; 57: 954-958.
[180] Yao QX, Yao Z, Heintz R et al. Effect of donor age and cold ischemia time (CIT) on yield, purity and function of human islets isolated from fifty-four (54) consecutive pancreas donors. Transplant Proc (in press).
[181] Brandhorst H, Klitscher D, Hering BJ et al. Influence of organ procurement on human islet isolation. Horm Metabol Res 1993; 25: 51.
[182] Kneteman NM, de Groot TJ, Warnock GL et al. The evaluation of solutions for pancreas preservation prior to islet isolation. In: Methods in Islet Transplantation Research. Federlin K, Bretzel RG, Hering BJ (eds.), Horm Metabol Res 1990; Suppl Ser 25: 4–9.
[183] Kneteman NM, Lakey JRT, Warnock GL et al. Human islet isolation after prolonged cold storage. Diab Nutr Metab 1992; 5 suppl 1: 33.
[184] Ricordi C, Mazzeferro V, Casavilla A et al. Pancreas procurement from multiorgan donors for islet transplantation. Diab Nutr Metab 1992; 5 suppl 1: 39.
[185] Gray DW, McShane P, Grant A et al. A method for isolation of islets of Langerhans from the human pancreas. Diabetes 1984; 33: 1055–1061.
[186] Horaguchi A, Merrell RC. Preparation of viable islet cells from dogs by a new method. Diabetes 1981; 30: 455.
[187] Ricordi C, Lacy PE, Finke EH et al. Automated method for isolation of human pancreatic islets. Diabetes 1988; 37: 413–420.
[188] Socci C, Davalli AM, Vignali A et al. A significant increase of islet yield by early injection of collagenase into the pancreatic duct of young donors. Transplantation 1993; 55: 661–663.
[189] Scharp DW. Commentary. Cell Transplant 1993; 2: 299.
[190] Ogilvie F. A quantitative estimation of the pancreatic islet tissue. Quart J Med 1937; 6: 287.
[191] Gepts W. Method for the quantitative determination of islands of Langerhans. Can Roy Soc Biol 1958; 152: 879.

[192] Hellman B. The frequency distribution of the number and volume of the islets of Langerhans in man. 1. Studies on non-diabetic adults. Acta Soc Med Upsal 1959, 64: 432.
[193] Saito K, Iwama N, Takahashi T. Morphometrical analysis on topographical difference in size distribution, number and volume of islets in the human pancreas. Tohoku J Exp Med 1978; 124: 177.
[194] Pyzdrowski KL, Kendall DM, Halter JB et al. Preserved insulin secretion and insulin independence in recipients of islet autografts. N Engl J Med 1992; 327: 271–273.
[195] Gores PF, Najarian JS, Stephanian E et al. Insulin independence in type I diabetes after transplantation of unpurified islets from single donor with 15-deoxyspergualin. Lancet 1993; 341: 19–21.
[196] Gray DW. The role of exocrine tissue in pancreatic islet transplantation. Transplant Int 1989; 2: 41–45.
[197] Gores PF, Sutherland DER. Commentary. Cell Transplant 1993; 2: 291.
[198] Ulrichs K, Mueller-Ruchholtz W. Mixed lymphocyte islet culture (MLIC) and its use in manipulation of human islet alloimmunogenicity. Horm Metabol Res 1990; Suppl Ser 25: 123–127.
[199] Zeevi A, Rilo HLR, Fontes PA et al. Effect of purity and culture on human islet immunogenicity in vitro. Transplant Proc (in press).
[200] Memsic L, Busuttil RW, Traverso LW. Bleeding esophageal varices and portal vein thrombosis after pancreatic mixed-cell autotransplantation. Surgery 1984; 95: 238–242.
[201] Cameron JL, Mehigan DG, Broe PJ et al. Distal pancreatectomy and islet autotransplantation for chronic pancreatitis. Ann Surg 1981; 193: 312.
[202] Toledo-Pereyra LH, Rowlett AL, Cain W et al. Hepatic infarction following intraportal islet cell autotransplantation after near total pancreatectomy. Transplantation 1984; 38: 88–89.
[203] Grodsinsky C, Malcolm S, Goldman J et al. Islet cell autotransplantation after pancreatectomy for chronic pancreatitis. Arch Surg 1981; 116: 511.
[204] Robertson GM, Chadwick DR, Contractor H et al. The optimization of large scale density gradient human islet isolation. Acta Diabetologica 1993; 30: 93-98.
[205] London NJM, Robertson GSM, Chadwick DR et al. Purification of human pancreatic islets by large scale continuous density gradient centrifugation. Horm Metabol Res 1993; 25: 61.
[206] Andersson A, Sandler S. Viability tests of cryopreserved endocrine pancreatic islet cells. Cryobiology 1983; 20: 161–168.
[207] Rajotte RV, Stewart HL, Voss WAC et al. Viability studies on frozen-thawed rat islets of Langerhans. Cryobiology 1977; 14: 116.
[208] Bank HL. Assessment of islet cell viability using fluorescence dyes. Diabetologia 1987; 30: 812–816.
[209] Bank HL. Rapid assessment of islet cell viability using fluorescent dyes. In Vitro Cell Dev Biol 1988; 24: 266–273.
[210] London NJM, Contractor H, Lake SP et al. A microfluorometric viability assay for isolated human and rat islets of Langerhans. Diab Res 1989; 12: 141–149.
[211] Gray DW, Morris PJ. The use of fluorescein diacetate and ethidium bromide as a viability stain for isolated islets of Langerhans. Stain Technol 1987; 62: 373-381.
[212] Gutte N, Kuhn F, Matthes G et al. The MTT-dye test for the in vitro vitality control of fresh as opposed to cryopreserved rat pancreatic islets for syngeneic intraportal islet transplantation. Z Éxp Chir Transplant Kuenstliche Organe 1989; 22: 323–329.
[213] McKay DB, Karow AM. Factors to consider in the assessment of viability of cryopreserved islets of Langerhans. Cryobiology 1983; 20: 151–160.
[214] Kuhn F, Abri O, Lohde E et al. In vitro rapid calorimetric assay for viability control of fresh isolated and deep-frozen huma pancreatic islets. Diabetes 1989; 38 suppl 1: 278.
[215] Lacy PE, Walker BS, Fink CJ. Perifusion of isolated rat islets in vitro: participation of the microtubular system in the biphasic release of insulin. Diabetes 1972; 21: 987.
[216] Ashcroft SJH, Bassett JM, Randle PJ. Isolation of human pancreatic islets capable of releasing insulin and metabolizing glucose in vitro. Lancet 1971; i: 888.

[217] Lacy PE, Finke EH, Conant S et al. Long-term perifusion of isolated rat islets in vitro. Diabetes 1976; 25: 484.
[218] Kneteman NM, Rajotte RV. Isolation and cryopreservation of human pancreatic islets. Transplant Proc 1986; 18: 182.
[219] Scharp DW, Lacy PE, Finke E et al. Low temperature culture of human islets isolated by the distension method and purified with Ficoll and Percoll gradients. Surgery 1987; 102: 869–879.
[220] Morgan CR, Lazarow A. Immunoassay of insulin: antibody system. Plasma insulin levels of normal, subdiabetic and diabetic rats. Diabetes 1963; 12: 115.
[221] Warnock GL, Ellis D, Rajotte RV et al. Studies of the isolation and viability of human islets of Langerhans. Transplantation 1988; 45: 957–963.
[222] Ricordi C, Scharp DW, Lacy PE. Reversal of diabetes in nude mice after transplantation of fresh and 7-day-cultured (24°C) human pancreatic islets. Transplantation 1988; 45: 994–996.
[223] Rajotte RV, Evans MG, Warnock GL et al. Islet cryopreservation. In: Methods in Islet Cell Transplantation. Federlin K, Bretzel RG, Hering BJ (eds.). Horm Metabol Res 1989; Suppl Ser 25: 72–81.
[224] Evans MG, Rajotte RV, Warnock GL et al. Viability studies on cryopreserved isolated canine islets of Langerhans. Transplant Proc 1989; 21: 3368–3370.
[225] Socci C, Davalli AM, Vignali A et al. Evidence of in vivo human islet graft function despite a weak response to in vitro function. Transplant Proc 1992, 24: 3056–3057.
[226] London NJ, Thirdborough SM, Swift SM et al. The diabetic "human reconstituted" severe combined immunodeficient (SCID-hn) mouse: a model for isogeneic, allogeneic, and xenogeneic human islet transplantation. Transplant Proc 1991; 23: 749.
[227] Lake SP, Chamberlain J, Bassett PD et al. Successful reversal of diabetes in nude rats by transplantation of isolated adult human islets of Langerhans. Diabetes 1989; 38: 244–248.
[228] Scharp DW, Lacy PE, McLear M et al. The bioburden of 590 consecutive human pancreata for islet transplant research. Transplant Proc 1992; 24: 974-975.
[229] Scharp DW. Islet quality control testing and the islet isolation laboratory. In: Ricordi C (ed), Pancreatic Islet Cell Transplantation, R.G. Landes Company, Austin, Georgetown, 1992, pp 82–88.
[230] Warnock GL, Lakey JRT, Taylor GD et al. Microbial studies of a tissue bank of cryopreserved human islet cells. Transplant Proc 1994; 26: 827.
[231] Lloveras JJ, Farney AC, Sutherland DER et al. Significance of contaminated islet preparation in clinical islet transplantation. Transplant Proc (in press).
[232] Dobroschke J, Schwemmle K, Langhoff G et al. Autotransplantation von Langerhansschen Inseln nach totaler Duodenopankreatektomie bei einem Patienten mit chronischer Pankreatitis. Dt Med Wschr 1978; 103: 1905–1910.
[233] Altman JJ, Cugnenc PH, Tessier C et al. Epiploic flap: a new site for islet implantation in man. Horm Metab Res 1990; suppl 25: 136–137.
[234] Ricordi C, Tzakis AG, Carroll PB et al. Human islet isolation and allotransplantation in 22 consecutive cases. Transplantation 1992; 53: 407–414.
[235] Socci C, Falqui L, Bertuzzi F et al. Islet transplant: a successful procedure for the replacement of pancreatic endocrine function. Diabetes 1993; 42 suppl 1: 53A.
[236] Najarian JS, Sutherland DER, Matas AJ et al. Human islet transplantation: A preliminary report. Transplant Proc 1977; 9: 233–236.
[237] Gores PE, Najarian JS, Sutherland DER. Clinical islet allotransplantation. In: Ricordi C (ed.). Pancreatic Islet Cell Transplantation. R.G. Landes, Austin, 1992, pp 423–433.
[238] Bretzel RG, Hering BJ, Federlin KF. Islet transplantation registry report 1991. Diab Nutr Metab 1992; suppl 1: 177–181.
[239] Federlin K, Bretzel RG, Hering BJ. Recent achievements in experimental and clinical islet transplantation. Diabetic Med 1991; 8: 5–12.
[240] Hering BJ, Geier C, Schultz AO, Bretzel RG, Federlin K. Islet Transplant Registry Newsletter No. 5, Vol 4, 1994.

[241] Fernqvist-Forbes E, Borg K, Johansson B-L et al. Effects of C-peptide on autonomic nerve dysfunction in patients with type 1 diabetes. Proceedings 15th IDF Congress, Kobe, 1994; 481 (Abstr).
[242] Taylor D, Kirkland T, Lakey J et al. Bacteremia due to transplantation of contaminated cryopreserved pancreatic islets. Cell Transplant 1994; 3: 103–106.
[243] Carroll PB, Ricordi C, Shapiro R et al. Frequency of kidney rejection in diabetic patients undergoing simultaneous kidney and pancreatic islet cell transplantation. Transplantation 1993; 55: 761–765.
[244] Bretzel RG, Hering BJ, Brandhorst D et al. Insulin independence in type 1 diabetes achieved by intraportal transplantation of purified pancreatic islets. Diabetologia 1994; 37 suppl 1: A38.
[245] Morel P, Goetz FC, Moudry-Munns K et al. Long-term glucose control in patients with pancreatic transplants. Ann Intern Med 1991; 115: 694–699.
[246] Katz H, Homan M, Velosa J et al. Effect of pancreas transplantation on postprandial glucose metabolism. N Engl J Med 1991; 325: 1278–1283.
[247] Sutherland DR, Goetz FC, Sibley RK. Recurrence of disease in pancreas transplants. Diabetes 1989; 38 suppl 1: 85–87.
[248] Pipeleers DG, Pipeleers-Marichal M, Hannaert JC et al. Transplantation of purified islet cells in diabetic rats. I. Standardization of islet cell grafts. Diabetes 1991; 40: 908–919.
[249] London NJM, Bell PRF. Pancreas and islet transplantation. Br J Surg 1992; 79: 6–7.

Survival studies related to diabetes mellitus

K. Borch-Johnsen

Introduction

Before the introduction of insulin in the treatment of diabetes, the median life expectancy of children with insulin-dependent diabetes mellitus (IDDM) was 1½ to 2 years [1], and the patients died from acute complications such as ketoacidosis or infections. The introduction of insulin in 1922 by Banting et al. [2] dramatically changed the prognosis and immediately increased the median survival by a factor 10 to 20. Since then, treatment has changed, the treatment of complications has become possible, and the syndrome has been subdivided into several different types of diabetes – but what has happened to prognosis and survival?

Survival-studies – why?

Survival data is of interest for the diabetic patient, for the clinician, for the provides of health care and for institutions such as life insurance companies and pension funds. For the *patient*, the prognosis, in terms of life expectancy and the risk of developing complications, represents a relevant measure of the severity of the disease. For the *clinician*, studies of survival serve as a parameter for the quality of the treatment. If major efforts are made to improve care and prevent development of late diabetic complications, an increase in life expectancy would be expected. Thus, analysis of survival serves as an indicator of the effectiveness of the treatment we are offering. For the *health care providers and health authorities*, survival studies and studies of the incidence of late diabetic complications are necessary in the planning and dimensioning of future need for services. For *insurance companies and pension funds*, studies of the prognosis are essential as the necessary additional premiums are calculated on the basis of these excess mortality rates.

The prognosis of IDDM-patients

In the pre-insulin era, patients with IDDM died from acute complications such as ketoacidosis and infections [1]. Since 1923, life-expectancy has increased (Fig. 1) and the development of late diabetic complications has become the primary cause of death [3]. Age-adjusted mortality rates, however, also decreased in the non-diabetic population (Fig. 2), and thus the question of whether the improved prognosis was specific for patients with IDDM remained unanswered. In 1984, Panzram was justified in concluding his review of the topic by stating "whether the prognosis of IDDM has improved within the last decades remains uncertain" [4]. As discussed later, subsequent studies, using statistical models that enable corrections for changes in the mortality for the general population, have demonstrated that the excess mortality of IDDM-patients decreased gradually from 1930 to 1980.

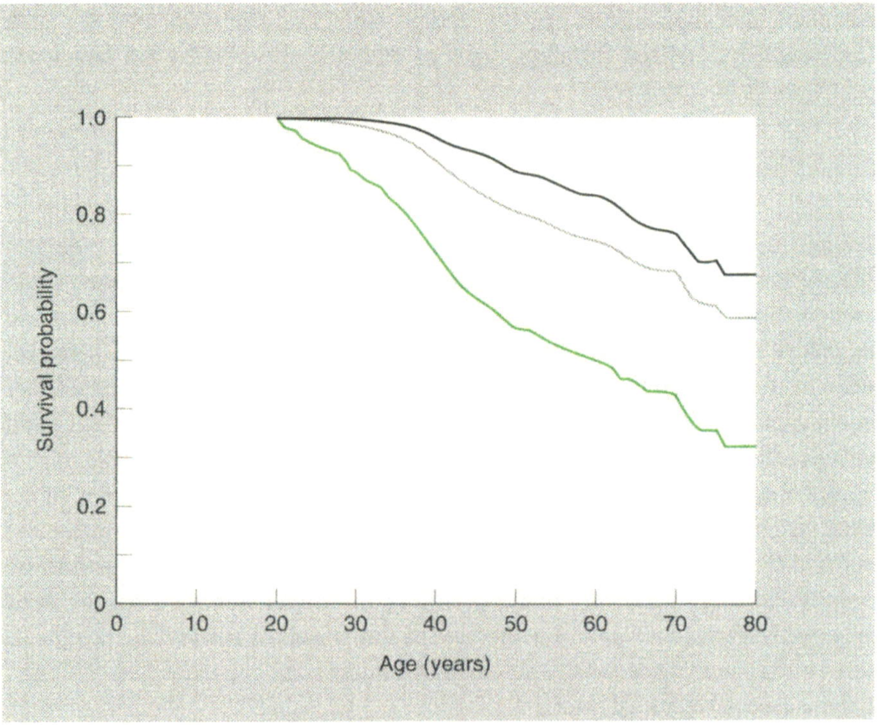

Fig. 1 Estimated survival probability of male, Danish IDDM patients diagnosed 1932 (–), 1952 (---) and 1972 (...) (Age at diagnosis: 20 years)

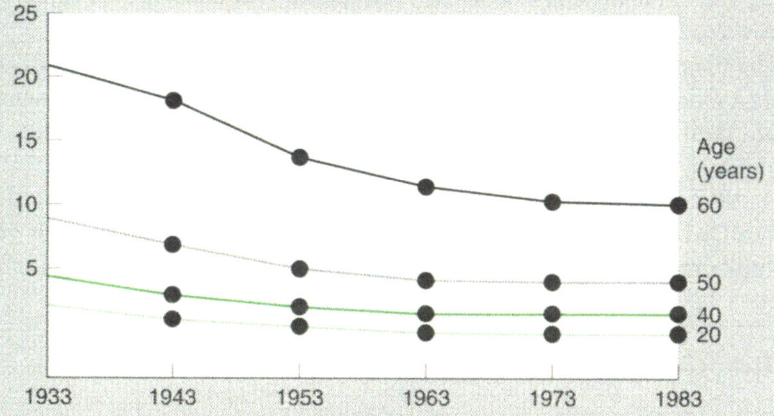

Fig. 2 Age-adjusted mortality rates (per thousand per year) for females in Denmark 1933 to 1983

The prognosis of NIDDM-patients

The prognosis of NIDDM-patients varies considerably between individuals, countries, and populations. Furthermore, the epidemiological pattern of NIDDM (e. g. age at diagnosis, incidence, prevalence, and degree of heritability) varies considerably between countries and between ethnic groups [5, 6]. In the European Caucasoid population, NIDDM is a disease of the elderly, very rare before the age of 40 years [6], and very strongly associated with the development of cardiovascular disease [7]. In other ethnic groups, like the Pima Indians and certain Pacific populations [6], the incidence of NIDDM is high even before the age of 40 years, showing a very strong familial inheritance pattern that is apparently different from what is seen in

Caucasoid populations [8], and less closely linked to cardiovascular disease. These differences in the epidemiological pattern are also reflected in studies of survival after the onset of disease, and thus NIDDM-patients cannot be looked upon as one homogeneous group world-wide.

Survival studies are, furthermore, difficult to perform in NIDDM-patients, as the onset of NIDDM may precede clinical diagnosis by many years [9]. In using the clinical diagnosis as entry to a survival analysis, we understand it as a surrogate variable for time of onset.

The diagnostic classification of patients as NIDDM and IDDM also represents a major problem in epidemiological studies, especially for patients diagnosed between the ages of 30 and 60 and for non-Caucasian populations. An analysis of data based on type of treatment will not solve the problem, but it is still better than what many studies do, namely present mortality data for IDDM and NIDDM-patients together, leaving the reader with virtually no information regarding the specific prognosis for NIDDM-patients [10, 11].

Current challenges in survival studies

For IDDM-patients, some of the major problems related to survival studies are:

1. creating population-based study samples for the study of prognosis. Most of the studies so far have been based on samples from highly specialized centers in the USA and Denmark [1, 3, 12, 13], and these studies may have been affected by selection bias;
2. creating a better understanding of the prognostic markers. It has been convincingly demonstrated that the development of late diabetic complications – especially development of microalbuminuria and diabetic nephropathy [14] – are important prognostic markers, but our understanding of the reasons for the considerable inter-individual variability in the susceptibility for developing these complications is far from complete. It is likely that yet-unidentified genetic factors are of major importance in determining the susceptibility of the individual patient [15], but at present we can only hypothesize regarding potential genetic candidates for the "prognostic genes".

For NIDDM-patients there are similar challenges and problems, and some of which are:

3. establishing population-based studies of survival and prognostic markers in NIDDM;

4. establishing study-cohorts based on truly incident cases and not only on clinically-diagnosed cases. This is necessary because of the strong association between cardiovascular disease (CVD), where NIDDM may lead to death from CVD before a diagnosis of NIDDM is ever made;
5. elucidating why the mortality from cardiovascular disease in Caucasoid NIDDM-patients is apparently independent of diabetes duration [7]. NIDDM may not be a traditional risk-factor for development of cardiovascular disease, and a common underlying (genetic) pathogenetic mechanism has been suggested [7]. One potential candidate would be insulin resistance [16, 17].

Methodological problems related to the design of mortality studies

The specific problems related to the design of a study involve: identification of the ideal sample with respect to a) type of diabetes, b) selection problems and c) sample size, and the choice of a proper and relevant reference group to ensure comparability with other national and international studies.

Sample or study group

Type of diabetes: IDDM is a disease with the highest incidence before the age of 25 years, a low, but still significant, mortality from acute complications and a high incidence of diabetic nephropathy and end-stage renal failure. In contrast to this, NIDDM is a disease of the elderly with virtually no mortality from acute complications and a low incidence of diabetic nephropathy, but a high incidence of and mortality from cardio-vascular disease. Despite these differences, several previous studies have analysed diabetes-related mortality without separating IDDM and NIDDM-patients [10, 11], a procedure that may lead to misleading results. Goodkin [18] studied the mortality and potential prognostic factors in 10,538 diabetic patients applying for life insurance. The patients were subdivided according to type of medication (insulin, oral drugs or diet), and the highest excess mortality was found among patients receiving insulin. This type of analysis ignores the fact that NIDDM-patients with complications and poor metabolic control are more likely to be treated with insulin than well-controlled, uncomplicated NIDDM-patients. Therefore, by comparing on the basis of type of treatment only, he compared patients with an a priori bad prognosis with those with a good prognosis.

Differentiation of patients into IDDM and NIDDM is possible on the basis of measurement of endogenous insulin production using C-peptide [19].

This is, however, expensive, time-consuming and not feasible in large-scale epidemiological studies. In the epidemiological setting, simpler characteristics must be used for the classification of patients as IDDM- or NIDDM-patients. These include:

6. Age at diagnosis
7. Type of treatment

A combination of age at diagnosis and type of treatment will classify most of the patients correctly with onset before the age of 40 years [20] and after the age of 60 years, while it will be difficult in the interval between.

These simple criteria for classification can, however, be used only in European, Caucasian low-incidence populations. In populations such as Pima Indians and Pacific Islanders [6, 8] where the age at onset is typically low (20 to 40 years) for NIDDM-patients, age at diagnosis and type of treatment does not in itself ensure a diagnosis of IDDM or NIDDM – it should be combined with information on ethnicity.

Therefore, in the practical classification of patients in relation to survival studies, patients should be classified according to age at diagnosis, mode of treatment and ethnicity; and data should be analysed and reported accordingly.

Selection of study sample: The fundamental requirement for the study population is that it is representative of the disease under study. Thus, the ideal study base is a population-based inception cohort of all incident cases of diabetes within a specified region and period of time.

IDDM: Previous studies of the prognosis of IDDM-patients have generally used hospital-based patient cohorts, and followed these patients for a period of up to 60 years [21]. The advantages of this design are that the patients can generally be followed for decades, that long-term changes in mortality and diabetes related morbidity can be analyzed, and that the basic data available are often of high quality and standardized. These factors are of vital importance to the interpretation and validity of the study. The major disadvantage is that the patients are referred to the hospital, and thus, that only selected patients are referred. The criteria for referral are difficult to identify and may vary over time. Due to this potential selection bias the main objection has been that these studies are not representative and that conclusions and interpretations can therefore not be generalized [22]. In one study, the results from a population-based group of IDDM-patients and a hospital-based group were compared with respect to excess mortality and factors affecting mortality, and in this particular study no difference was found between the results from the two populations [23]. This result is, however, valid only for this particular clinic-based population at that specific point of time, and cannot be used as a general validation for the use of clinic-based populations.

The growing number of registers, based on incident cases of IDDM and the internationally accepted procedures for ascertainment, have made register-based mortality studies possible [24]. The obvious advantage is that selection bias is excluded. In most countries, the registers are based on obligatory reporting of all newly diagnosed cases of IDDM from the departments of pediatrics to the register. The same procedure has not proven to be feasible for cases of IDDM developing in adolescence, early adulthood and later, as the number of departments and doctors treating these patients are much larger in number. Therefore population-based, register-based studies of the prognosis of IDDM has so far been confined to patients developing IDDM during childhood, and this represents the major disadvantage.

For future research, the establishment of registers including patients in the age interval 16 to 30 (or 40) years should be encouraged, as future mortality studies of IDDM-patients should be based on these registers. Several sources can be used for case identification, and insulin prescriptions have been successfully used as an alternative to registers [25].

NIDDM: Mortality studies of NIDDM-patients have been based on clinic-based cohorts [26], populations with life insurance [18], populations from general practice, and follow-up from newly-diagnosed cases in screening programs [28, 29].

Patients admitted to specialized care centres for treatment of their disease will represent highly selected and probably complicated cases of the disease, and will therefore not be representative of the entire population of NIDDM-patients.

Patients with life insurance have been used in USA for the study of the prognosis of NIDDM [18], but the population showed a heavy male predominance (94%) and furthermore, it consisted of white, middle-to-upper class individuals in permanent jobs. Thus it was not representative of the entire population of NIDDM-patients.

Follow-up studies based on patients treated in general practice might be regarded as more representative than a clinic-based population. This is not necessarily the case as: a) the most complicated cases may be missing due to selective referral to specialized centres, b) diabetic patients will seek general practitioners with a special interest for treating diabetes, leading to potential selection bias and c) prevalent, but still undiagnosed cases of NIDDM will still be missing from the study population.

Population based registries covering all patients with NIDDM would represent the ideal study population. These registers very seldom exist, and the second best alternative is follow-up studies of population based surveys for DM, using the oral glucose tolerance test. This type of data would represent unselected and unbiased samples for studies of the prognosis of NIDDM-patients.

Sample size: Calculation of sample sizes has become an accepted and necessary part of the planning of controlled clinical trials. In epidemiological studies, including survival studies, there has been a tendency to overlook this need. Conduction of an epidemiological study without calculation of sample sizes is, however, quite as unethical as it is in controlled clinical trials. In relation to mortality studies the prerequisites necessary for sample size calculations are a priori expectations regarding: Mortality rates, excess mortality and the relative risk associated with the risk factors under study. The literature describing the methods is rapidly expanding, and within the field of epidemiology a WHO-publication by Lemeshow et al. from 1990 represents a clear and easy-to-read presentation of the methods [29].

The reference group

The descriptive study of the mortality of diabetic patients does not need a reference group, but if the question is raised of whether the mortality of the diabetic patients is higher than expected, a reference group will also be needed.

The most widely used reference group as a parameter for standardization is the age- and gender-specific mortality of the general population. In principle, the reference should be the mortality of the general population, excluding the diabetic population, but due to the relatively low prevalence of diabetes in the population this adjustment is not necessary. In high-risk populations, adjustment of the reference mortality-rates to include only non-diabetic individuals may be necessary to obtain a correct estimate of the diabetes-related excess mortality.

Studying secular changes in (excess) mortality, the age- and gender-specific reference mortality rates may vary considerably, as shown in Fig. 2. Thus, careful adjustment of the reference mortality rates must be performed, as skewed estimates of the true excess mortality would otherwise be obtained.

International comparability of studies

Comparing crude mortality rates between countries is, at best, confusing and is more likely to be misleading. The living conditions vary between countries and continents, and this is reflected in the life expectancy. In Europe or Japan, the median life expectancy is between 70 and 80 years, while in some developing countries it is 30 to 40 years. This must be considered when comparing mortality rates, and standardization of mortality rates by regional or international standardized rates represents one such possibility which will be discussed in more detail later.

Furthermore, international comparison will rely on the comparability of the study samples. Here, ethnicity is only one of many features that must be reported upon to enable international comparison. Regional variations will also exist with respect to treatment (e. g. the use of insulin in NIDDM-patients). Thus, criteria for classification must be clearly specified in the methods of the study.

Methodological problems related to data analysis

Incomplete data

In clinical studies, or experimental studies, missing data reflects that a test went wrong, the test tube was lost, etc. This may also be the case in survival studies, where some of the variables measured at base-line or during follow-up might be missing in some patients. This type of missing data might create problems in the data analysis, but they can often be solved in the data analysis by technical procedures described in standard textbooks. More important in survival studies are the problems related to delayed entry into the study and loss to follow-up.

Delayed entry can be seen in all design types. In clinic-based studies, patients are referred to the hospital with a delay from disease onset to referral that will varies between patients. Thus, the patient has a certain survival as a diabetic at entry to the population. If these years of survival are included in the analysis the patient will be immortal during the first years of disease, as he was alive at entry! This must be accounted for in the analysis and graphical presentation. In a population-based study, based on screening for diabetes with OGTT, a similar problem exists with all individuals known to have diabetes at the time of the study. But even in the newly-diagnosed patients identified through the survey, the unknown time duration from diabetes onset to clinical diagnosis will represent a case of delayed entry. The first two situations can be solved by applying statistical techniques allowing for left censoring or delayed entry, while the latter problem represents a methodological problem where the duration of the delay can only be based on assumptions, and where the choice of solution must be made by the investigator and not be left to the statistician.

Incomplete follow-up is another frequently occurring problem in survival analyses. For a number of patients in a study we typically know that they survived for a period of time, but we do not know what happened thereafter. This type of incomplete observation is called right censoring. It is obvious that the individual contributes to the study with a significant amount of information, as we know that he was alive at entry, and we know that he was alive at the time where we lost him for follow-up. Thus, the information given by the case should also be included in the analysis. Again, statistical techniques are available that can use data with right censoring (as discussed below).

Bias and confounding

Bias may be defined as "any systematic error in an epidemiological study that results in an incorrect estimate of the association between the exposure and risk of disease (or death)" [30]. Bias occurs because epidemiology deals with free living human beings, where even the most rigorously designed investigation will have the potential for one or more types of bias. Some of the potential types of bias have been discussed already. One important type of bias is selection bias due to selective referral or non-population based study samples [31]. The second major source of bias is observation or information bias, where the likelihood of obtaining valid information on exposure is directly associated to the outcome of the disease. Potential sources for bias must be identified before the start of the study and – wherever possible – eliminated, as data analysis and interpretation of the results may be misleading if bias is introduced. The possibility of adjusting for selection bias or other types of bias in the data analysis is generally very limited, and therefore the design of the study should be adjusted according to the potential for bias.

Confounding factors are a consequence of the complex interrelationship between several potential risk factors for the disease (or death). Only in very rare cases will disease or death be the consequence of one single event. For most diseases several risk factors exist. If two different factors (e. g. gender and diabetic nephropathy) are associated with the mortality, and at the same time associated to each other (incidence of nephropathy differs between genders), then gender would act as a confounding factor in the analysis of diabetic nephropathy as a risk factor for mortality. Ignoring this in the analysis will lead to false estimates of the association between a risk factor (nephropathy) and event (death). Potential confounding variables should, however, not be controlled in the design. They are to be included in the analysis, as inclusion of all potential confounding factors is the only way to obtain a true understanding of the complex interrelationship between different factors leading to disease and death.

Statistical models in survival studies

Survival studies may either look at crude mortality rates among diabetic patients, or compare mortality rates of diabetic patients with those of selected control groups (excess mortality, relative mortality of standardized mortality rates). Furthermore, survival studies will be interested in factors affecting the risk of death for the individual patient (risk factors or markers). It is not the intention here to review all methods available and to discuss advantages, disadvantages and problems to any degree of detail. The interested reader is referred to relevant textbooks [32]. The following will discuss in only brief terms some selected methods for data analysis.

Crude survival data

The simple survival function S(t) expresses the probability of being alive at time t, and the figure can be drawn directly from observational data (incomplete data, due to loss to follow up and other reasons for "right censoring", can be relatively easily accounted for by making a Kaplan-Meier plot). The information obtained from these very simplified models is, however, limited, and generally we are interested in comparing survival of several groups of patients in an attempt to identify factors affecting the survival probability. This can be done by comparing survival functions for male and female diabetic patients, for example, using a log-rank test or Gehan's test. If we do, however, want to include more parameters in the analysis, and if we want to analyse potential interactions between several factors, other multivariate models or logistic models must be used for analysis, as discussed later.

Relative or excess mortality

The interesting question in survival analysis is not whether diabetic patients die; as the immortal state is not a part of life – even for the non-diabetic individual. The interesting question is, whether the mortality of diabetic patients is higher than that of the general population or the non-diabetic population. It will be therefore relevant to compare the observed number of deaths in the diabetic population with the number of deaths that would have been expected if the diabetic population had the same mortality rate as the general population. Methods for this type of calculation, using direct or indirect standardization, are described in epidemiology [30] and statistics [32] textbooks. The estimate obtained may be expressed as a standardized mortality ratio or relative mortality. Both of these represent the mortality of the diabetic population as a percentage of the mortality of the general population. It may also be expressed as an excess mortality, representing the percentile excess in mortality of the diabetic population.

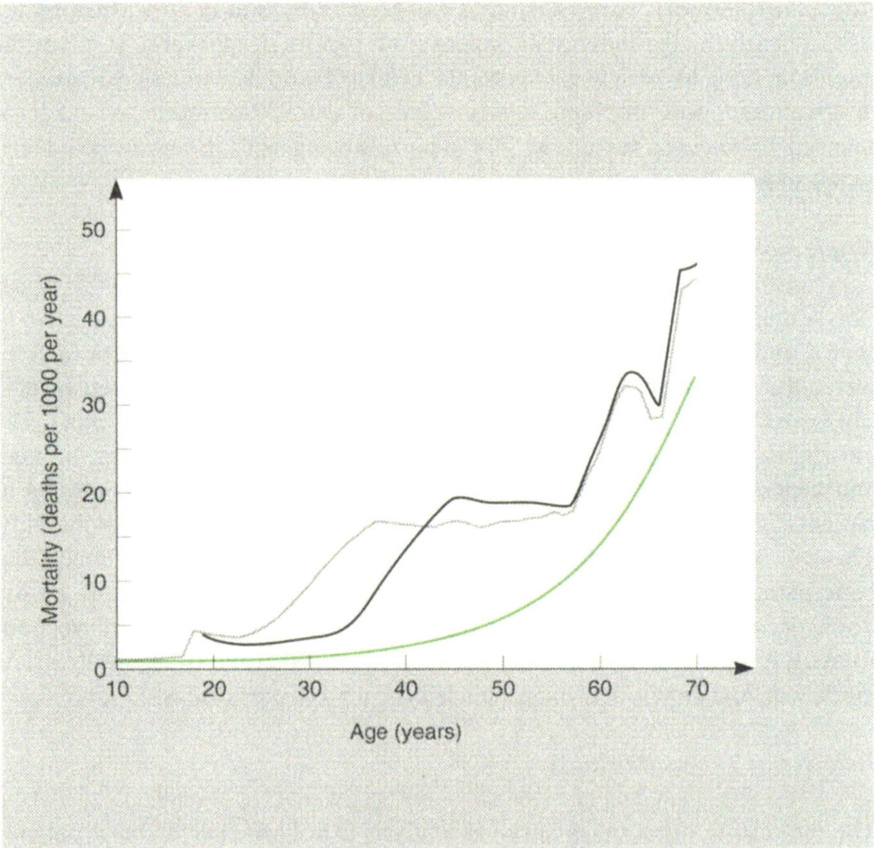

Fig. 3 Estimated mortality rates for Danish male IDDM-patients diagnosed 1965, age at diagnosis 10 years (–) and 20 years (---), and the mortality rates of the general male population (...)

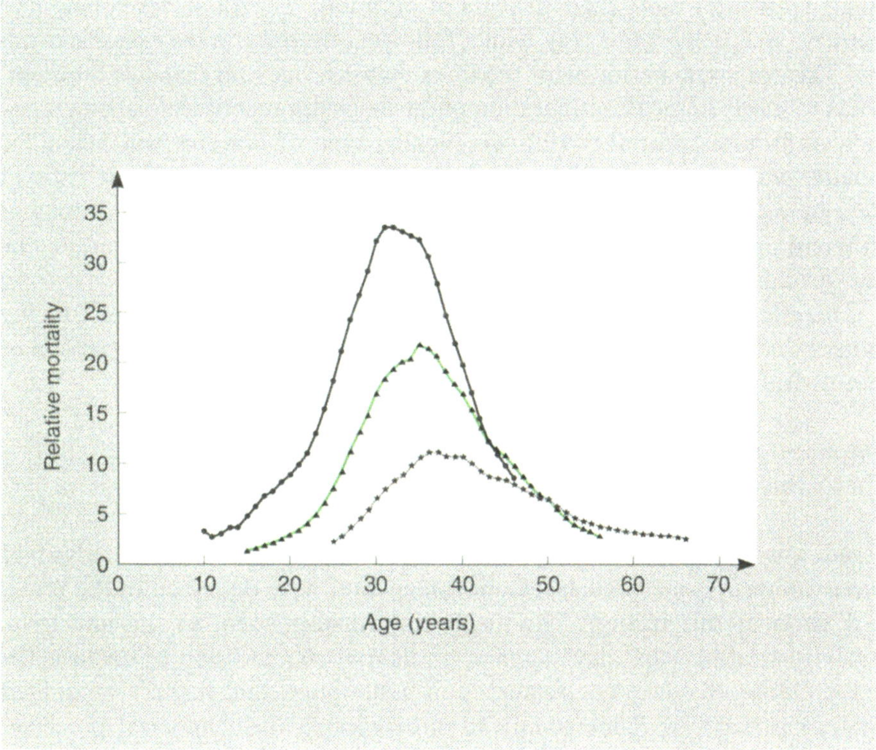

Fig. 4 Excess mortality of Danish male IDDM-patients in relation to age at diagnosis (Age at diagnosis: ● = 5 years, ▲ = 15 years and ★ = 25 years)

Measures of relative mortality are, however, not necessarily comparable. In diabetes, three factors are important: the age group, the diabetes duration and the type of diabetes of the population under study. The expected number of deaths in a population increases with increasing age. If the additional effect due to diabetes is additive and not multiplicative, the excess mortality will decrease by age. This phenomenon is well described in IDDM, where IDDM-patients have an increasing mortality with increasing age (Fig. 3), but the increasing mortality in the general population leads to a bell-shaped relationship between relative mortality and age (Fig. 4).

Diabetes duration influences the risk of developing (or having) potentially lethal complications. In IDDM-patients this risk is low during the first 10–15 years of duration [3, 21]. Thus these patients will have a relatively low mortality in this range of diabetes duration. From 15 to 35 years of duration the prevalence of complications is high, and therefore the mortality is also high, while after more than 40 years of duration, the risk of developing diabetic nephropathy is low [14], with a following decrease in the excess mortality. This (in combination with the links between age and diabetes duration) leads to a bell-shaped configuration of the association between diabetes duration and excess mortality (Fig. 4). Finally, type of diabetes will affect the relative mortality as IDDM- and NIDDM-patients have different risks of developing potentially lethal complications, they develop complications at different ages and different diabetes durations, and the age structure of the two groups is different, as discussed previously.

Therefore, interpretation of relative mortality data for diabetes (or any other disease) should be done with great care, as an uncritical comparison of results from different studies may be invalid and even misleading.

Advanced models (regression analysis, graphical models and frailty models)

Regression models: Four simple and univariate models for the analysis of crude mortality rates and excess mortality rates were described in the previous parts of this section. The theoretical correspondent to the univariate analysis would be that development of disease, complication or death is the consequence of one single factor – an assumption that has a very limited biological basis. To understand the more complicated biological processes leading to disease and death, and to understand the interrelation between different risk factors, some kind of multivariate analysis must be applied. The two most often used models are the Cox regression model and the logistic regression model. Both models can be used for analysis of crude mortality as well as for excess mortality [14, 33]. The Cox regression model [34] has several advantages, the most important being that problems related to censored data are relatively easy to solve within this model. For the non-statistician, the fact that the effect of each risk factor is expressed as a regression coefficient can create problems in the interpretation, as the regression coefficients cannot be directly converted to a relative risk. Regarding this difficulty, the logistic regression analysis has an advantage, in that the analysis is based on odds ratios (i. e. the odds of dying within the next interval of time for a person with a given risk factor compared to one without this risk factor). The interpretation of the data may therefore be easier for the non-statistician. It should, however, be noticed that both the Cox regression model and logistic regression models are based on various sets of assumptions regarding the structure of the data-set. Therefore, in survival studies, multivariate models should only be used by the non-statistician in close collaboration with statisticians or experienced users of the models. A review of the medical literature would probably disclose a large number of misinterpretations based on incorrect application of these models, and the inclusion of these models in routine statistical packages would increase this risk.

Graphical models: In the traditional studies of risk factors for death, we generally use a base-line observation, and the cohort is then followed up from the base-line. In many cases, however, we do have additional information about the individual from subsequent follow-up studies, hospital records, etc. The traditional models for survival analysis do not allow inclusion of this type of information. Recent developments within the framework of graphical models [34, 35] have tried to solve these problems. These graphical models [35] (partly built on the Rasch item analysis [36]) can disclose the latent structures describing how different risk factors affect each other over time; but at present they cannot define the magnitude of the effect of each parameter. These models may, however, play an important role in the future analyses of survival studies with repetitive observations.

Frailty models: The diabetic individual's risk of dying is only in part determined by the fact that the individual has developed diabetes. Other factors are also involved, some of them probably related to genetic factors and family environment. Thus, some diabetic patients will be more susceptible to the development of nephropathy, atherosclerosis or hypertension than others. Studies of inter-individual variability in susceptibility may look at some families as being more frail than others, indicating that genetic factors, family environment, or both combined affect the mortality of the diabetic individual. This highly relevant hypothesis can be analysed by extending the studies to include non-diabetic family members in the data analysis. Taking advantage of the recently developed frailty models for survival studies [32, 37] would probably be helpful in the analysis of the relative importance of genes and environment in the prognosis of diabetic patients.

Concluding remarks

The rapidly changing methods and strategies for prevention of diabetes and its complications raise the need for follow-up with survival studies, as this is the only way to make sure that changes in treatment are also followed by improvements in prognosis. Population-based registries of IDDM-patients are being established world-wide, and these registries will serve as a natural base for survival studies. At the same time, they will enable international comparison of results. It is, however, crucial that international guidelines for data analysis are developed and followed (as suggested by the WHO-DIAMOND group). Every effort should be made to ensure the representativeness of the study base and to make clear separations between true insulin-dependent patients and NIDDM-patients. Finally, advantage should be taken of the rapidly developing theories and models within the field of biostatistics – and this cannot be done without academic collaboration between diabetologists, epidemiologists and statisticians.

References

[1] Marks HH. Longevity and mortality of diabetics. Am J Publ Health 1965; 55: 416–423.
[2] Banting FJ, Best CH, Collip JB et al. Pancreatic extracts in the treatment of diabetes mellitus. Can Med Assoc J 1922; 2: 141–146.
[3] Borch-Johnsen K. The prognosis of insulin-dependent diabetes mellitus. Dan Med Bull 1989; 36: 336–348.
[4] Panzram G. Epidemiological data on excess mortality and life expectancy in insulin-dependent diabetes mellitus – critical review. Exp Clin Endocrinol 1984; 83: 93–100.
[5] WHO Study Group on the prevention of diabetes mellitus. WHO, Geneva: Technical Report Series, 1993; (in print).
[6] Bennett P, Bogardus C, Tuomilehto J et al. The epidemiology of non-insulin dependent diabetes – Non-obese and obese. In: Alberti KGM, DeFrozo RA, Keen H et al, eds. International Textbook of Diabetes. New York: John Wiley & Sons, 1992.
[7] Jarrett RJ. The epidemiology of coronary heart disease and related factors in the context of diabetes mellitus and impaired glucose tolerance. In: Jarrett J, ed. Diabetes and heart disease. Amsterdam: Elsevier Science Publishers, 1984; 1–23.
[8] Zimmet P. Challenges in diabetes epidemiology – from West to the rest. Diabetes Care 1992; 15: 232–252.
[9] Harris MI, Klein R, Welborn TA et al. Onset of NIDDM occurs at least 4–7 years before clinical diagnosis. Diabetes Care 1992; 15: 815–819.
[10] Kessler II. Mortality experience of diabetic patients. Am J Med 1971; 51: 715–724.
[11] Kaplan MH, Feinstein AR. A critique of methods in reported studies of long-term vascular complications in patients with diabetes mellitus. Diabetes 1973; 22: 160–174.
[12] Borch-Johnsen K, Kreiner S, Deckert T. Mortality of Type 1 (insulin-dependent) diabetes mellitus in Denmark. Diabetologia 1986; 29: 767–772.
[13] Krolewski AS, Warram JH, Christlieb AR. Onset, course, complications and prognosis of diabetes mellitus. In: Marble A, Krall LP, Bradley RF et al, eds. Joslin's Diabetes Mellitus. 12th edn. Philadelphia: Lea & Fibiger, 1985.
[14] Borch-Johnsen K, Andersen PK, Deckert T. The effect of proteinuria on relative mortality in Type 1 (insulin-dependent) diabetes mellitus. Diabetologia 1985; 28: 590–596.
[15] Borch-Johnsen K, Nørgaard K, Hommel E et al. Is diabetic nephropathy an inherited complication? Kidney Int 1992; 41: 719–724.
[16] Reaven GM. Role of insulin resistance in human disease. Diabetes 1988; 37: 1595–1607.
[17] Flier JS. Syndromes of insulin resistance: from patient to gene and back again. Diabetes 1992; 41: 1207–1219.
[18] Goodkin G. Mortality factors in Diabetes. J Occup Med 1975; 17: 716–721.
[19] Hother-Nielsen O et al. Classification of newly diagnosed diabetic patients as insulin-requiring or non-insulin requiring based on clinical and biochemical variables. Diabetes Care 1988; 11: 521–537.

[20] Agner T, Damm P, Binder C. Remission in IDDM: Prospective study of basal C-peptide and Insulin Dose in 268 Consecutive Patients. Diabetes Care 1987; 10: 164–169.
[21] Kroleswki AS, Warram JH, Christlieb AR et al. The changing natural history of nephropathy in Type 1 diabetes. Am J Med 1985; 78: 785–794.
[22] Green A. On relative survival as a measure in prognosis evaluation. Dan Med Bull 1981; 28: 260–263.
[23] Green A, Borch-Johnsen K, Andersen PK et al. Relative mortality of Type 1 (insulin-dependent) diabetes in Denmark: 1933–1981. Diabetologia 1985; 28: 339–342.
[24] Diabetes Epidemiology Research International (DERI) Group. Secular trends in incidence of childhood IDDM in 10 countries. Diabetes 1990; 39: 858–864.
[25] Green A, Hauge M, Holm NN et al. Epidemiological studies of diabetes mellitus in Denmark, II. A prevalence study based on insulin prescriptions. Diabetologia 1981; 20: 468–470.
[26] Pirart J. Diabetes mellitus and its degenerative complications: A prospective study of 4,400 patients observed between 1947 and 1973. Diabetes Care 1978; 1: 168–188.
[27] Garcia MJ, McNamara PM, Gordon T et al. Morbidity and mortality in diabetics in the Framingham population. Diabetes 1974; 23: 105–111.
[28] Jarrett RJ, McCartney P, Keen H. The Bedford survey: ten-year mortality rates in newly diagnosed diabetics, borderline diabetics and normoglycaemic controls and risk indices for coronary heart disease in borderline diabetics. Diabetologia 1982; 22: 79–84.
[29] Lemeshow S, Hosmer DW, Klar J et al. Adequacy of sample size in health studies. Chichester: John Wiley & Sons, 1990.
[30] Hennekens CH, Buring JE. Epidemiology in Medicine. Boston: Little, Brown and Company, 1987.
[31] Melton LJ, Ochi JW, Palumbu PJ et al. Referral bias in diabetes research. Diabetes Care 1984; 7: 12–18.
[32] Andersen PK, Borgan Ø, Gill RD et al. Statistical models based on counting processes. New York: Springer Verlag, 1992.
[33] Cox DR. Regression models and life tables (with discussion). J Royal Stat Soc 1972; Series B 34: 187–220.
[34] Whittaker J. Graphical models in applied multivariate analysis. New York: Wiley, 1990.
[35] Kreiner S. Validation of index scales for analysis of survey data: The symptom Index. In: Dean K, ed. Population health Research: Linking theory and Methods. London: Sage Pub, 1994; (in print).
[36] Rasch G. An Item analysis which takes individual differences into account. Brit J Mathemat and Statist Psychol, 1966; 19: 49–57.
[37] Nielsen GG, Gill RD, Andersen PK et al. A counting process approach to maximum likelihood estimation in frailty models. Scand J Statist 1992; 19: 25–43.

Pitfalls in patient selection and statistical procedures in diabetes research

J. M. Stephenson, P. M. McKeigue

Introduction

This chapter discusses problems of design and analysis of clinical studies of outcome, and examines their relevance to the timing, size and purpose of trials in diabetes research. The strengths and limitations of randomized trials are discussed, together with alternative study designs for evaluating outcomes in diabetes. Pitfalls in patient selection and statistical procedures are illustrated by reference to some of the main recent clinical trials in diabetes. Methods for the design and analysis of clinical trials have advanced considerably since the University Group Diabetes Program [1] (UGDP), one of the first multicentre randomized trials conducted in the 1960s. Techniques to reduce bias, such as randomization and blinding, have generally been applied effectively in diabetes trials. Other principles of trial design have sometimes been neglected in diabetes research; innovations in other fields such as cardiovascular research and tropical public health have not been applied to their full potential in diabetes research. It may be possible to resolve some current controversies in diabetes management by large, simple trials which keep costs down by collecting a minimum of information and relying on easily-determined end-points such as mortality. For further reading about the conduct of clinical trials [2, 3] and observational studies [4, 5] we recommend books by Pocock [2], Meinert [3], Rothman [4] and Schlesselman [5].

Patient selection: when and in whom to conduct a randomized trial

The randomized controlled trial is the definitive study design for evaluating a new treatment or intervention [6]. In non-randomized trials the patient or investigator can influence the type of intervention received, and this is likely to produce bias in the selection of patients for the treatments being compared. Randomization is the only sure way to eliminate this bias.

Uncontrolled studies have been used to study the efficacy of antihypertensive treatment in slowing the progression of diabetic nephropathy [7, 8] but the comparison of rate of progression before treatment with that during treatment is likely to be biased by regression to the mean. If the outcome measure, such as rate of decline of renal function, has some random variation within individuals, any intervention when the outcome measure is especially poor will tend to be followed by relative improvement. Thus patients selected because their renal function is declining rapidly will tend to have a slower rate of decline when re-examined. For other outcomes, which are even less predictable than the progression of nephropathy, a controlled evaluation is essential.

The selection of patients who can be invited to participate in a randomized trial depends on a combination of ethical and statistical considerations. This chapter is not concerned with the more general ethical issues such as informed consent and the balance between individual and collective interests, but with how to define patient selection criteria that will make the trial ethically acceptable. For this the timing of a trial is important. Initially, there may be insufficient preliminary evidence of potential benefit and lack of harm to justify a trial on ethical grounds. But if the intervention becomes widespread before its effects have been adequately evaluated, the need for a definitive trial may no longer be accepted. Most treatments in current clinical practice have not been subject to rigorous scientific evaluation, but have become widespread on the basis of a general belief that they are beneficial. In this situation, even though definitive evidence of benefit may be lacking, a randomized trial designed to measure the benefits and risks of the treatment will often encounter opposition.

There was, for example, considerable controversy [9] about the Diabetes Control and Complications Trial (DCCT), a randomized trial of the effect of strict versus conventional glycaemic control on diabetic complications [10]. Observational studies [11–15] had consistently shown that poor glycaemic control was a strong risk factor for diabetic complications, but small short-term randomized trials [16–21] of improved glycaemic control had yielded equivocal results. The most consistent finding was that improved control caused transient worsening of retinopathy [19–21]. Nonetheless, in the ensuing controversy, some researchers claimed that the "benefits of the best possible metabolic control for Type 1 diabetic patients are well documented and proven" [22]. Interim analysis of the DCCT showed that strict control caused a three- to four-fold increase in severe hypoglycaemia, to an absolute rate of 0.5 episodes per patient-year [23]. Since the trial has now shown that strict control confers benefit also, by reducing the incidence of long term complications, informed patients can weigh the measured benefits against the risks of strict control in a meaningful way [24]. This illustrates the importance of quantifying the negative as well as the positive effects of an intervention.

The problems with timing of a trial are illustrated by trials of antihypertensive drugs in insulin dependent patients with diabetic nephropathy. Two uncontrolled studies of antihypertensive therapy in 6 [7] and 11 [8] patients with nephropathy found that glomerular filtration rate (GFR) fell less rapidly after treatment than before the start of therapy. The conclusion of these limited studies that antihypertensive therapy postpones renal failure was generally accepted. It is now not possible to conduct a randomized trial to get a reliable estimate of the effectiveness of such intervention in reducing the risk of renal failure. Retrospective studies [25, 26] suggest that antihypertensive therapy has improved survival in diabetic nephropathy, but these studies suffer from the inherent biases of nonrandomized comparison, compounded in one study [25] by the use of historic control groups.

The ethics of randomization depend also on the type of control intervention and the risk status of the patients. It may be necessary to modify the treatment protocols so that the trial becomes a study of a new intervention, or more intensive intervention versus whatever is considered as usual intervention. Thus when a new or unevaluated treatment is being compared against standard treatment of known effectiveness, all patients in the trial will receive either the best available treatment, or one which is potentially superior. In a placebo-controlled trial, a proportion of patients will be randomized to no active treatment. This is not a problem for trials in low risk, asymptomatic patients, where the most important consideration is lack of evidence of harm associated with the active intervention. For patients with more advanced disease, randomization into a placebo-controlled trial is ethically justifiable only if there is no available treatment or if those above an agreed level of risk are excluded from the trial.

One way to modify the design to make a trial ethically acceptable is to define the patient selection criteria to include an intermediate group between those at high risk (whom it is considered unethical to randomize) and those at low risk (whom it is considered unreasonable to treat) (Fig. 1). For instance, in a trial of antihypertensive treatment in diabetes, it would no longer be considered ethical to randomize patients with definite hypertension or established nephropathy, and it would not be reasonable to treat patients with normal renal function whose blood pressures were in the lower part of the normal range. Somewhere between these high-risk and low-risk groups lies an intermediate category, perhaps those with microalbuminuria or blood pressures in the upper part of the normal range, in whom it is neither unethi-

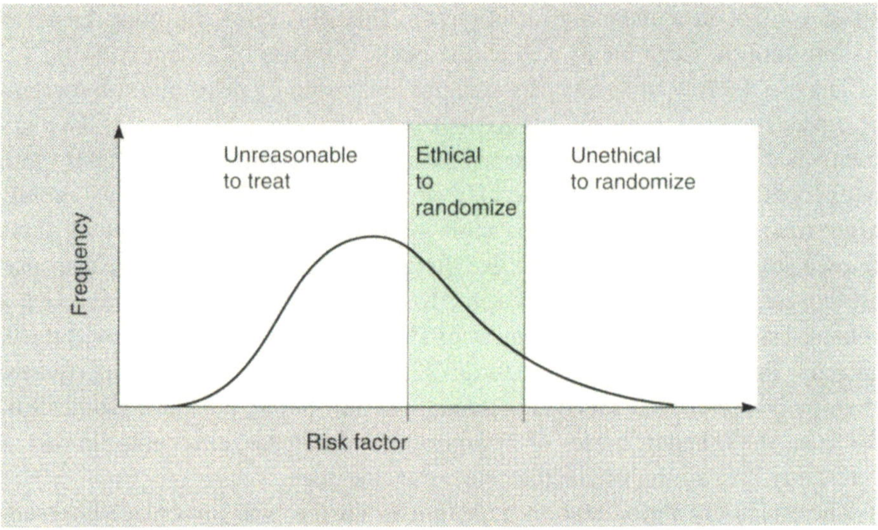

Fig. 1 Defining a borderline risk category where it is ethical to randomize patients

cal to withold treatment nor unreasonable to consider treatment. For any proposed trial such a borderline category can be defined, although the cut-off points that define it are often controversial.

Explanatory versus pragmatic trials

The nature of the trial influences the criteria for patient selection. Clinical trials fall broadly into two categories: explanatory and pragmatic. An explanatory trial seeks to establish a cause-effect relationship between intervention and outcome. Questions about large scale, practical application of the intervention, as administered in the trial, are secondary. Entry criteria to an explanatory trial are usually designed to define a homogeneous group of patients best suited to testing a causal hypothesis. In contrast, a pragmatic trial seeks to evaluate a realistic clinical or public health option. In such a trial it is usually desirable to minimize exclusion criteria, so that the results will be applicable to all patients at risk. Most trials have both explanatory and pragmatic elements, but the balance between these may vary.

The DCCT is a good example of a mainly explanatory trial, in which highly-motivated patients prepared to pursue either strict or conventional control were carefully recruited. The trial was designed to determine whether an intensive treatment regimen, maintaining blood glucose as close to normal as possible, affects the appearance or progression of early vascular complications in patients with insulin dependent diabetes [27]. The unequivocal answer to this question has advanced understanding of the aetiology of complications as well as defining the efficacy of intervention. However, the intervention depends on extensive support provided by a team of diabetes specialists to maintain patients' motivation. Though this support is crucial to the aims of the trial, it does not reflect typical diabetes care. One of the remaining key issues is the extent to which the findings can be applied to the wider population of insulin-dependent patients.

Statistical procedures in the design and analysis of clinical trials

A crucial question that arises during the planning of a clinical trial is how many patients to select. The size of a trial should be determined by the scientific objectives of the trial as well as by financial and practical constraints. One of the most important advances in trial design in the last ten years has come from the realization that valid results can be obtained from large, but simple randomized trials in which outcome is assessed by some easily measured end-point such as mortality [28]. The tendency in diabetes research has been to conduct a series of small trials of the same question in preference to one or two large trials. For instance, only 3 [29–31] of 19 trials [29–47] of angiotensin converting enzyme (ACE) inhibitors in insulin-dependent patients, studied more than 20 patients for at least one year. Although it is clear from these small trials that ACE inhibition lowers the rate of albumin excretion, estimates of the magnitude of albuminuria lowering are very imprecise and the long term effects of such intervention are not clear [48, 49]. In other fields, particularly cardiovascular research, the effects of intervention have been more precisely determined by meta-analysis, or systematic overviews [50] in which the results of a number of similar trials are pooled. This approach is most useful where trials have used easily-defined clinical end-points such as mortality, myocardial infarction or end-stage renal failure. Since few trials in diabetes research have used such "hard" end-points, the potential benefit of meta-analysis is limited.

The key steps in assembling the information required to estimate the required number of patients in a trial are as follows:

1. define the primary outcome measure,
2. estimate the rate of adverse outcomes in the control group,
3. decide how small a treatment effect it is important to detect, and
4. decide what chance of failing to detect this effect is acceptable.

From this information, the number of patients required in the trial can be estimated; details of the statistical methods for these power calculations can be found elsewhere [3, 51].

It is desirable to use morbid events, such as end stage renal failure or blindness as the primary outcome measure in a trial. Since major clinical events are rare and trials using such outcome measures have to be very large, it is common to use surrogate end-points. These surrogate end-points are intermediate events or measurements which are likely to predict the clinical outcome, such as heavy proteinuria, glycated haemoglobin. The predictive value of the surrogate end-point is therefore crucial, particularly when the natural history of the disease is prolonged, as in diabetic nephropathy.

When considering the expected rate of adverse outcomes in the control group, it is important to realize that the rate in the control group will be lower than expected on the basis of observational studies. This results from the usual tendency to favourable outcome among trial participants compared with non-participants, and may also occur because the control group has adopted some of the changes intended for the intervention group. It is also important to start with realistic estimates of the likely size of effect: few interventions will produce a 50% reduction in mortality or incidence of serious complications. The smaller the expected treatment effect, the larger the trial required to detect a genuine effect. It is not usually necessary to include complex measurements of covariates at baseline or repeated measurements of intervening variables other than the main end-point under study. For instance in a trial with cardiovascular disease as the end-point it is not necessary to include repeated measurements of cardiovascular risk factors throughout the progress of the trial.

It is important to decide at the outset what size of effect the trial should not fail to detect, and what should be the criteria for stopping the trial, either because there is evidence of poorer outcome in one of the groups, or because enough outcome data have accumulated to make it unlikely that the treatment has an effect large enough to be worth detecting. The smallest treatment effect that warrants detection is an important concept. It is necessary to strike a balance between the costs of seeking to detect small, but clinically meaningful effects which would require very large numbers of patients in the trial, and the implications for patient care of failing to detect such an effect. Where the sample size has to be large, it is sometimes possible to simplify the trial protocol so as to reduce the cost per participant.

This problem is illustrated by The United Kingdom Prospective Diabetes Study (UKPDS), a large randomized trial of management of patients with non-insulin-dependent diabetes. The objective was to determine whether improved blood glucose control would prevent complications and reduce the associated morbidity and mortality. The target size of effect to be detected was not clearly stated at the outset of the study, though subsequently a reduction of 20% in the incidence of complications in the intervention compared with the control group was defined as the minimum detectable effect [52]. The trial has not yet been able to demonstrate such an effect [52]. If intervention has a small beneficial effect, the clinical and public health consequences of not detecting a treatment effect of less than 20% need to be considered against the additional expense that detection of a modest effect would require. In other words, can we afford to detect a modest treatment effect, or can we afford to miss one?

The UKPDS was initiated in 1977, before the usefulness of large simple trials had been promoted by Collins and Peto [28]. The design of the UKPDS was extremely complex, with opportunities for randomization at three different stages. The original design specified that the outcome measure was to be the incidence of major clinical events: cardiovascular disease, amputations, blindness and renal failure. Follow-up, however, was not limited to recording these events but included annual biochemical measurements and triennial retinal photography, tests of autonomic function, biothesiometry, chest X-ray and ECG. This must have considerably increased the cost of the study. With hindsight, it would have been preferable to simplify the protocol into a straightforward comparison of three treatment strategies, and to reduce the measurements of baseline characteristics and follow-up to a minimum. Statistical power, rather than design complexity, could thereby have been increased.

By contrast, the design of the DCCT was much simpler. There were only two hypotheses (related to primary and secondary prevention) to be tested, one main end-point (retinopathy), and two treatments to compare (intensive versus conventional treatment). A 33% reduction was chosen during the design stage as the effect to be detected or excluded by the trial. Large resources were made available. Table 1 summarizes comparison of the UKPDS and DCCT.

In one area of diabetes research an alternative solution to the large simple trial has been exploited usefully. In randomized trials of the efficacy of photocoagulation (laser) therapy in preventing blindness from diabetic retinopathy [53–56], eyes, rather than patients, at high risk of visual loss, were randomized to receive the intervention. These trials were highly successful in demonstrating the effects of laser therapy on retinopathy and visual loss, allowing reliable estimation of the efficacy (around 73%) of laser therapy in preventing blindness from diabetic retinopathy [57]. Randomizing eyes also meant that all trial patients could be offered treatment.

Table 1 Comparison of the Design of the Diabetes Control and Complications Trial and the UK Prospective Diabetes Study

	DCCT	UK PDS
Primary Outcome Measure	Onset or progession of retinopathy	Major clinical events, including cardiovascular disease, renal failure, amputations, and blindness
Effect to be detected	33% reduction in incidence	20% reduction in event rate (Not made explicit at outset)
Planned follow-up:	Mean 7 years	9 years for glucose study 7 years for hypertension study
Sample size	700 primary prevention, 700 secondary prevention	4072 in glucose study
Intervention	Intensive versus conventional insulin therapy	Diet alone versus diet plus insulin or sulphonylurea; tight versus less tight therapy for hypertension study
Resources	Well funded	More limited funding

For the results of a randomized trial to be free from bias it is essential to analyze the results by intention-to-treat, so that patients are included in the treatment groups to which they were originally randomized whatever their subsequent adherence to treatment. If assessment of outcome is based on clinical examination at follow-up, as with a study of retinopathy, there will inevitably be some losses to follow-up. Otherwise all patients randomized should be included in the analysis, whether or not they complied with the treatment protocol. The size of the bias that can be introduced by ignoring defaulters is illustrated by data from the Coronary Drug Project: in the placebo group, five-year mortality was 15% in those who adhered to treatment and 28% in those who failed to adhere to treatment with placebo [58]. It is possible that similar biases would apply to trials of drug therapy in diabetes where patients who did not comply with the intervention were dropped from the analysis [59].

Subgroup analyses and interactions of treatment efficacy with baseline characteristics

It is common in analysing large trials to look for evidence of effects which are significant in one subgroup but not in another: for instance, to show that treatment was of benefit in the subgroup with abnormal ECGs at baseline, but not in those with normal ECGs. This is part of the rationale for including detailed measurements of baseline characteristics in the design of large trials. Clinicians emphasize that they want to know which patients will benefit from treatment, and are reluctant to apply the results of trials showing modest benefit in low-risk patients. We suggest that this emphasis on identifying subgroups in which treatment is beneficial may be misguided. Most treatments which are of value do not confer benefit only in one subgroup of patients, and the statistical requirements for detecting such associations are not widely appreciated. Subgroup analyses of the effects of treatment are usually of doubtful validity, unless they are based on testing hypotheses defined in advance and unless the test for statistical significance is a test for interaction. Interaction between two variables (treatments or baseline characteristics) means that the relative risk associated with one variable depends on the level of the other variable. Thus an effect of treatment in one subgroup but not in another is an interaction. It is generally the case that to detect interactions, a sample size four times larger than that to detect main effects is required [60].

Patient selection in observational studies

It is important to recognize circumstances in which randomized trials are not ethically or financially justifiable and to appreciate alternative study designs which can be used to investigate factors determining the outcome of diabetes. Observational designs include clinical follow-up studies, studies using historical controls, and case-control studies.

In general there have been relatively few large observational studies of outcome in diabetes. Our understanding of the incidence of complications such as blindness or amputation, and the factors associated with incidence is therefore limited, particularly in non-insulin-dependent diabetes. Almost all follow-up studies of the outcome of diabetes are clinic-based. Only two large-population-based cohorts of subjects with IDDM [61, 62] have received much attention, and there are only two detailed follow-up studies of NIDDM in Caucasians [63, 64]. Unless follow-up is based on all cases in a defined population, the sample of cases included in a follow-up study is likely to be biased towards those with complications. For instance, patients may be referred to a clinic because they are already developing complications such as peripheral vascular disease. Although this makes it difficult to rely on clinic-based studies for estimates of the prevalence and incidence of complications, it is less likely that selection bias will affect the associations of risk factors with complications. For instance, patients seen at a clinic may be worse (or better) controlled and have higher (or lower) prevalence of retinopathy than those not attending the clinic, but this will not necessarily affect the association of retinopathy with elevated levels of glycated haemoglobin, as long as the selective forces for poor glycaemic control are independent of those for retinopathy. With longer follow-up the effects of selection bias on outcome tend to wear off.

Observational studies can be particularly useful in situations where witholding treatment would be ethically unacceptable [65]. For example, although the efficacy of laser therapy in preventing blindness from diabetic retinopathy is now established, evidence that *screening* for diabetic retinopathy has reduced the incidence of blindness in the diabetic population is lacking. It would be unethical to conduct a randomized trial of screening for diabetic retinopathy in which some patients were not offered examination of their eyes, yet it is clearly important to know whether screening is effective. An alternative approach to this problem is to use the case-control design. (Comparing rates of blindness before and after introduction of laser therapy is difficult because few countries routinely collect the necessary data). The case-control technique was originally developed by epidemiologists investigating the aetiology of rare diseases such as cancer to estimate the relative risk of disease associated with an exposure. A more recent extension of the technique has been to study adverse outcomes some of which might have been prevented by early diagnosis and treatment. For instance, to test the efficacy of screening for diabetic retinopathy in preventing blindness, we could study new cases of blindness caused by diabetes, together with a control group from the general population. The "exposure" under study would be a screening examination for diabetic retinopathy and the efficacy of screening could then be calculated from the relative risk of blindness associated with this exposure. Although the case-control design is potentially useful for studying the efficacy of preventive strategies in diabetes care, the selection

Table 2 Principles of using case-control design to study the efficacy of screening in preventing an adverse outcome

Cases: all cases of the adverse outcome arising in a defined population
Controls: representative of the population from which the cases arose
Exposure under study: a diagnostic procedure applied while the subject was apparently healthy, as part of a screening programme
Possible confounders: any factor, such as social class, that is associated with participation in the screening programme and independently related to the chance of developing complications
Calculation of relative risk: odds ratio in a 2×2 table of cases and controls classified by exposure
Calculation of efficacy: $1 -$ relative risk

of suitable cases and controls requires careful consideration. The principles involved are summarized in Table 2 and discussed in more detail by Schlesselman [5].

Conclusion

Clinical trials in diabetes research have been successful in defining the effectiveness of laser treatment for retinopathy, and the risks and benefits of intensive insulin therapy in IDDM. Trials have been less successful in defining whether intervention is effective in reducing the incidence of nephropathy or cardiovascular disease.

The importance of randomization and blinding in trials are well appreciated, but other principles of trial design have sometimes been neglected in diabetes research. Many of the pitfalls of patient selection in diabetes research can be avoided by posing a research question in a way that is explicit and measurable. Defining a trial as primarily explanatory or pragmatic will guide patient selection criteria. Choice of trial end-points and realistic estimation of the magnitude of treatment effect will indicate the likely size and duration of study. Timely, large, simple trials with easily-determined clinical end-points offer the best scientific guide to improving diabetes care. Where randomized trials are not possible, we need to use alternative study designs, developed in other fields of research, to evaluate the effectiveness of diabetes care.

References

[1] University Group Diabetes Program. A study of the effects of hypoglycaemic agents on vascular complications in patients with adult-onset diabetes. Diabetes 1970; 19 (Suppl. 2): 747–830.

[2] Pocock SJ. Clinical Trials. A Practical Approach. John Wiley and Sons, 1983.

[3] Meinert CL. Clincial trials. Design, conduct and analysis. Oxford: Oxford University Press, 1986.

[4] Rothman KJ. Modern Epidemiology. Boston: Little, Brown and Co., 1986.

[5] Schlesselman JJ. Case-Control Studies. Design, Conduct, Analysis. Oxford: Oxford University Press, 1982.

[6] Cochrane AL. Effectiveness and efficiency. Random reflections on health services. London: The Nuffield Provincial Hospitals Trust, 1972.

[7] Mogensen CE. Long-term antihypertensive treatment inhibiting progression of diabetic nephropathy. Br Med J 1982; 285: 685–688.

[8] Parving H-H, Andersen AR, Smidt UM et al. Effect of antihypertensive treatment on kidney function in diabetic nephropathy. Br Med J 1987; 294: 1443–1447.

[9] DCCT Research Group. Are continuing studies of metabolic control and microvascular complications in insulin-dependent diabetes mellitus justified? N Engl J Med 1988; 318: 246–250.

[10] The DCCT Research Group. The diabetes control and complications trial (DCCT): Design and methodologic considerations for the feasibility phase. Diabetes 1986; 35: 530–545.

[11] Pirart J. Diabetes mellitus and its degenerative complications: a prospective study of 4400 patients observed between 1947 and 1973. Diabetes Care 1978; 1: 168–188.
[12] Chase PH, Jackson WE, Hoops SL et al. Glucose control and the renal and retinal complications of insulin-dependent diabetes. JAMA 1989; 261: 1155–1160.
[13] Klein R, Klein BEK, Moss SE et al. Glycoslated haemoglobin predicts the incidence and progression of diabetic retinopathy. Ophthalmology 1988; 260: 2864–2871.
[14] Andersen AR, Christiansen JS, Andersen JK et al. Diabetic nephropathy in type 1 (insulin-dependent) diabetes: an epidemiological study. Diabetologia 1983; 25: 496–501.
[15] Krolewski AS, Warram JH, Christlieb AR et al. The changing natural history of nephropathy in type 1 diabetes. Am J Med 1985; 78: 785–794.
[16] Kroc Collaborative Study Group. Blood glucose control and the evolution of diabetic retinopathy and albuminuria. A preliminary multicenter trial. N Engl J Med 1984; 311: 365–372.
[17] Feldt-Rasmussen B, Mathiesen ER, Deckert T. Effect of two years of strict metabolic control on progression of incipient nephropathy in insulin-dependent diabetes. Lancet 1986; II: 1300–1304.
[18] Viberti GC, Bilous RW, Mackintosh D et al. Long term correction of hyperglycaemia and progression of renal failure in insulin dependent diabetes. Br Med J 1983; 286: 598–602.
[19] Lauritzen T, Larsen H-W, Frost-Larsen K et al. The Steno Study Group: Effect of 1 year of near-normal blood glucose levels on retinopathy in insulin-dependent diabetics. Lancet 1983; 1: 200–204.
[20] Dahl-Jorgensen K, Brinchmann-Hanssen O, Hanssen KF et al. Aker Diabetes Group: Rapid tightening of blood glucose control leads to transient deterioration of retionpathy in insulin dependent diabetes mellitus: the Oslo Study. Br Med J 1985; 290: 811–815.
[21] Dahl-Jorgensen K, Brinchmann-Hanssen O, Hanssen KF. Effect of near normoglycaemia for two years on progression of early diabetic retinopathy, nephropathy, and neuropathy: the Oslo Study. Br Med J 1986; 293: 1195–1199.
[22] Hanssen KF, Dahl-Jorgensen K, Lauritzen T et al. Diabetic control and microvascular complications: the nnear-normoglycaemic experience. Diabetologia 1986; 29: 677–684.
[23] DCCT Research Group. Epidemiology of severe hypoglycaemia in the Diabetes Control and Complications Trial. Am J Med 1991; 90: 450–459.
[24] Diabetes Control and Complications Trial Research Group. The effect of intensive treatment of diabetes on the development and control of long-term complications in insulin-dependent diabetes mellitus. N Engl J Med 1993, 329: 977–81.
[25] Parving H-H, Hommel E. Prognosis in diabetic nephropathy. Br Med J 1989; 299: 230–233.
[26] Mathiesen ER, Borch-Johnsen K, Jensen DV et al. Improved survival in patients with diabetic nephropathy. Diabetologia 1989; 32: 884–886.
[27] DCCT Research Group. Diabetes Control and Complications Trial (DCCT): Results of Feasibility Study. Diabetes Care 1987; 10: 1–19.
[28] Yusuf S, Collins R, Peto R. Why do we need some large, simple randomized trials? Stat Med 1984; 3: 409–420.
[29] Marre M, Chatellier G, Leblanc H et al. Prevention of diabetic nephropathy with enalapril in normotensive diabetics with microalbuminuria. Br Med J 1988; 297: 1092–1095.
[30] Parving HH, Hommel E, Damkjaer Nielsen et al. Effect of captopril on blood pressure and kidney function in normotensive insulin dependent diabetics with nephropathy. BMJ 1989; 299: 533–536.
[31] Mathiesen ER, Hommel E, Giese J et al. Efficacy of captopril in postponing nephropathy in normotensive insulin dependent diabetic patients with microalbuminuria. Br Med J 1991; 303: 81–87.
[32] Brichard SM, Santoni JP, Thomas JR et al. Long term reduction of microalbuminuria after 1 year of angiotensin converting enzyme inhibition by perindopril in hypertensive insulin-treated diabetic patients. Diabete Metab 1990; 16: 30–36.

[33] Marre M, Leblanc H, Leobardo S et al. Converting enzyme inhibition and kidney function in normotensive diabetic patients with persistent microalbuminuria. Br Med J 1987; 294: 1448–1452.
[34] Bjorck S, Nyberg G, Mulec H et al. Beneficial effects of angiotensin converting enzyme inhibition on renal function in patients with diabetic nephropathy. Br Med J 1986; 293: 471–474.
[35] Abu Romeh SH, Nawaz MK, Ali JH et al. Short-term effect of angiotensin-converting enzyme inhibitor enalapril in incipient diabetic nephropathy. Clin Nephrol 1989; 31: 18–21.
[36] Cook J, Daneman D, Spino M et al. Angiotensin converting enzyme inhibitor therapy to decrease microalbuminuria in normotensive children with insulin-dependent diabetes mellitus. J Pediatr 1990; 117: 1,39–41,45.
[37] Hommel E, Parving H-H, Mathiesen E et al. Effect of captopril on kidney function in insulin-dependent diabetic patients with nephropathy. Br Med J 1986; 293: 467–470.
[38] Winocour PH, Waldek S, Anderson DC. Converting enzyme inhibition and kidney function in normotensive diabetic patients with persistent microalbuminuria. Br Med J 1987; 295: 391.
[39] Hay U, Ludvik B, Gisinger C et al. Lack of effect of ACE inhibition on severe proteinuria in diabetic nephropathy – a 6-month-long study. Schweiz Med Wochenschr 1988; 118: 165–169.
[40] Taguma Y, Kilamoto Y, Futaki G. Effect of captopril on heavy proteinuria in aoztemic diabetics. N Engl J Med 1985; 313: 1617–1620.
[41] Drummond K, Levy Marchal C, Laborde K et al. Enalapril does not alter renal function in normotensive, normoalbuminuric, hyperfiltering type 1 (insulin-dependent) diabetic children. Diabetologia 1989; 32: 255–260.
[42] Pedersen MM, Schmitz A, Pedersen EB et al. Acute and long-term renal effects of angiotensin converting enzyme inhibition in normotensive, normoalbuminuric insulin-dependent diabetic patients. Diabetic Med 1988; 5: 562–569.
[43] Jenkins DA, Cowan P, Collier A et al. Blood glucose control determines the renal haemodynamic response to angiotensin converting enyzme inhibition in type 1 diabetes. Diabetic Med 1990; 7: 252–257.
[44] Vora JP, Hendre TJ, Atiea J et al. Renal haemodynamics during short-term angiotensin converting enzyme inhibition in normotensive normoalbuminuric insulin dependent diabetics. Diabetes Res 1989; 11: 9–12.
[45] Passa P, Leblanc H, Marre M. Effects of enalapril in insulin dependent diabetic subjects with mild to moderate uncomplicated hypertension. Diabetes Care 1987; 10: 200–204.
[46] Mimran A, Insua A, Ribstein J et al. Comparative effect of captopril and nifedipine in normotensive patients with incipient diabetic nephropathy. Diabetes Care 1988; 11: 850–853.
[47] Melbourne Diabetic Nephropathy Study Group. Comparison between perindopril and nifedipine in hypertensive and normotensive diabetic patients with microalbuminuria. Br Med J 1991; 302: 210–215.
[48] Stephenson J. Should we be screening for early diabetic renal disease? J Epidemiol Comm Health 1991; 45: 177–179.
[49] Borch-Johnsen K, Wenzel H, Viberti GC et al. Is screening and intervention for microalbuminuria worthwhile in patients with insulin dependent diabetes? Br Med J 1993; 306: 1722–1725.
[50] Collins R, Gray R, Godwin J et al. Avoidance of large biases and large random errors in the assessment of moderate treatment effects: the need for systematic overviews. Stat Med 1987; 6: 245–250.
[51] Pocock SJ. The size of a clinical trial. In: Clinical trials. A practical approach. Wiley. 1983; 123–141.
[52] UK Prospective Diabetes Study Group. UK Prospective Diabetes Study (UKPDS) VIII. Study design, progress and performance. Diabetologia 1991; 34: 877–890.
[53] Hercules BL, Gayed II, Lucas SB et al. Peripheral retinal ablation in the treatment of proliferative diabetic retinopathy: a three year interim report of a randomized controlled study using the argon laser. Br J Ophthalmol 1977; 61: 555–563.

[54] British Multicentre Study Group. Photocoagulation for proliferative diabetic retinopathy: a randomized controlled clinical trial using the xenon arc. Diabetologia 1984; 26: 109–115.

[55] Diabetic Retinopathy Study Group. Photocoagulation treatment of diabetic retinopathy. Ophthalmology 1981; 88: 583–600.

[56] British Multicentre Study Group. Photocoagulation for diabetic maculopathy. A randomized controlled clinical trial using the xenon arc. Diabetes 1983; 32: 1010–1016.

[57] Rohan TE, Frost CD, Wald NJ. Prevention of blindness by screening for diabetic retinopathy a quantitative assessment. Br Med J 1989; 299: 1198–1201.

[58] The Coronary Drug Project Research Group. Influence of adherence to treatment and response of cholesterol on mortality in the Coronary Drug Project. N Engl J Med 1980; 303: 1038–1041.

[59] Ravid M, Savin H, Jutrin I et al. Long-term stabilizing effect of angiotensin-converting enzyme inhibition on plasma creatinine and on proteinuria in normotensive type II diabetic patients. Ann Intern Med 1993; 118: 577–581.

[60] Smith PG, Day NE. The design of case-control studies: the influence of confounding and interaction effects. Int J Epidemiol 1984; 13: 356–365.

[61] Klein R, Klein BEK, Moss SE. The Wisconsin epidemiological study of diabetic retinopathy: a review. Diabetes/Metabolism Reviews 1989; 5: 559–570.

[62] Orchard TJ, Dorman JS, Maser RE et al. Factors associated with avoidance of severe complications after 25 yr of IDDM. Pittsburgh Epidemiology of Diabetes Complications Study I. Diabetes Care 1990; 13: 741–747.

[63] Garcia MJ, McNamara PM, Gordon T et al. Morbidity and mortality in diabetics in the Framingham population. Sixteen-year follow-up study. Diabetes 1974; 23: 105–111.

[64] Barrett-Connor EL, Cohn BA, Wingard DL et al. Why is diabetes mellitus a stronger risk factor for fatal ischemic heart disease in women than in men? The Rancho Bernardo Study. JAMA 1991; 265: 627–631.

[65] Smith PG. Evaluating Interventions against Tropical Diseases. Int J Epidemiol 1987; 16: 159–166.

How to assess efficacy of oral antidiabetic agents

L. Groop

Introduction

Non-insulin-dependent diabetes mellitus (NIDDM) accounts for 85% of all the estimated cases of diabetes in the world. A majority of these patients are treated with sulfonylureas, which have represented the cornerstone of oral therapy of NIDDM for more than 30 years. However, only about 20–30% of these patients are considered to be in good glycemic control as defined by the European NIDDM Policy Group [1]. Treatment of newly-onset NIDDM is often successful while treatment of patients wich longstanding NIDDM has had a history of failures. Whereas primary sulfonylurea failure is usually due to incorrect use of sulfonylureas in patients with apparent IDDM, the causes of secondary sulfonylurea failure are less clear. Whether sulfonylurea failure is an inevitable phenomenon occurring in all patients with NIDDM is also unknown. It is, however, clear that fasting blood glucose rises about 0.25 mmol/l per year in NIDDM patients, despite current treatment with sulfonylureas and/or biguanides (Fig. 1) [2]. These facts demonstrate the obvious need for new treatment approaches to NIDDM.

Pathophysiology of hyperglycemia

Patients with manifest NIDDM are characterized by both insulin resistance and impaired beta-cell function, the former appearing in both the liver and muscle. Hepatic insulin resistance results in an overproduction of glucose in the basal state with fasting hyperglycemia as the clinical endpoint [3]. The therapeutic lowering of fasting blood glucose requires a means to suppress the elevated rate of hepatic glucose production. This is easily achieved with insulin therapy, since the liver is extremely sensitive to small increments in portal insulin concentration [4]. After being transported inside the cell and phosphorylated, glucose can be oxidized to carbon dioxide and water or stored as glycogen. In patients with manifest NIDDM, both pathways are resistant to the action of insulin, whereby defects in the latter predominate in the early stages [5]. Stimulation of glucose uptake in muscle requires insulin concentrations 4–5 times higher than those required for suppression of liver glucose production (the corresponding ED_{50} insulin values are 80–100 μU/ml vs 15–20 μU/ml). Apart from exercise, few treatment regimes have thus far been able to promote muscle glucose uptake.

Insulin resistance is frequently associated with other abnormalities, such as hyperinsulinemia, abdominal obesity, hypertension, hypertriglyceridemia, low HDL-cholesterol concentrations, the metabolic syndrome or the insulin resistance syndrome [6]. Although hyperglycemia infers nearly equal risk for

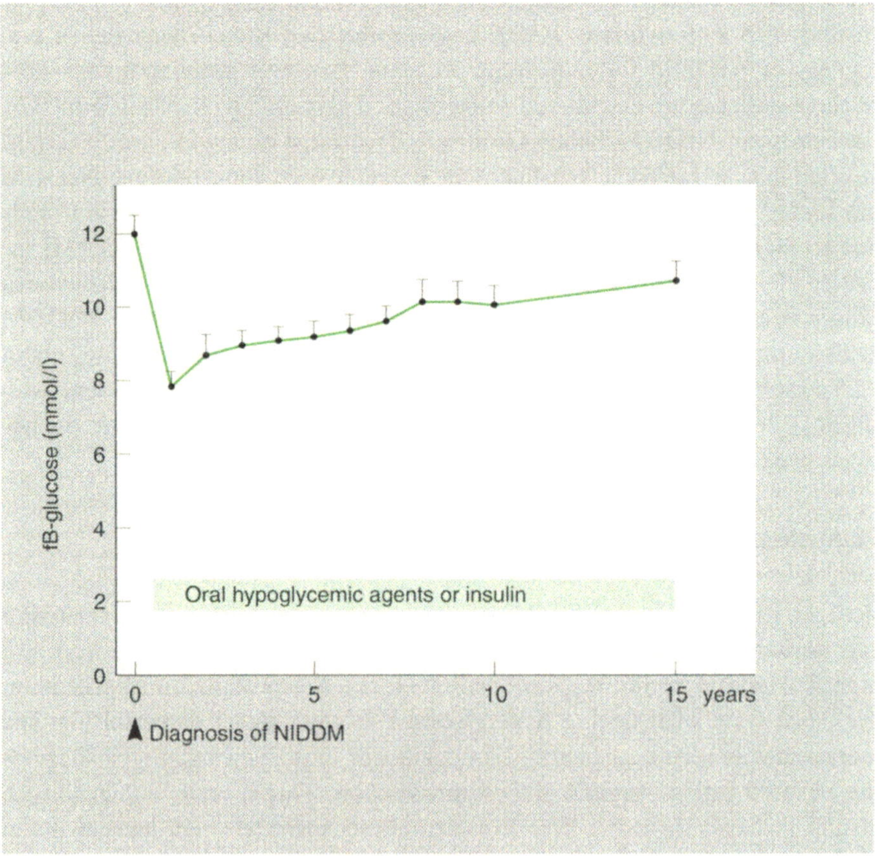

Fig. 1 Fasting blood glucose concentrations (annual means ± SE) in 156 patients with diagnosis of diabetes after the age of 35. Patients were treated with diet and/or oral antidiabetic agents. The annual increase in fasting blood glucose was 0.25 mmol/l [2]

the development of microangiopathic complications in NIDDM as in IDDM, the predominant cause of death in NIDDM is cardiovascular disease [7]. Insulin resistance is considered one of the major risk factors for the development of cardiovascular disease. The risk of cardiovascular disease increases even before glucose concentrations rise to values justifying a diagnosis of diabetes, e. g. the risk for patients with IGT is of almost the same magnitude as for patients with manifest diabetes [7]. Therefore, attempts to treat NIDDM should include a mean of reducing cardiovascular morbidity and mortality.

Finally, hyperglycemia per se can impair both insulin action and insulin secretion [8], and long-lasting hyperglycemia induces a state of metabolic insulin resistance (also referred to as glucose toxicity) on top of the most likely genetic insulin-resistance characteristic for NIDDM. Lowering glycemia by any treatment improves insulin sensitivity and insulin secretion. It is therefore extremely important in evaluating the effects of new agents to discern between drug-related and glycemia-related effects on metabolic parameters. In summary, new oral anti-diabetic agents should influence not only insulin secretion, but also peripheral insulin resistance and its concomitant disturbances in blood pressure and lipids.

Selection of patients

Age at onset of NIDDM

The selection of patients is one of the most crucial issues in evaluating the effect of new anti-diabetic agents. Although NIDDM patients may look phenotypically similar, there is considerable heterogeneity within the disease [9]. MODY (maturity-onset-diabetes of the young) is rare, but the disease can be diagnosed by its characteristic features, onset of the disease usually before the age of 20 years, autosomal dominant inheritance, impaired beta-cell function and characteristic mutations in the glucokinase gene [10]. It may be more pertinent to refer to a subgroup of MODY as glucokinase-deficient diabetes; such patients should not be included in studies evaluating the effect of new oral agents in NIDDM. It may therefore be useful to include age at onset of diabetes in the inclusion criteria. Since the onset of diabetes in most patients with NIDDM occurs after the age of 40, age at onset of diabetes could be set to 40–75 years. In populations with an earlier onset of NIDDM than in Scandinavia, the age range could be lowered to 35 years. After the age of 75 age-related effects begin to predominate over possible genetic effects.

Duration of diabetes

The duration of diabetes represents one of the major determinants of treatment responses. In newly-diagnosed patients, the duration of symptoms should be noted. The inclusion of patients with newly-diagnosed diabetes only is a safe way to obtain good treatment results, however, in my view, it produces a rather meaningless study, since these patients already respond nicely to current treatments. The new agents are supposed to improve treatment results in patients with a longer history of diabetes. Matching is necessary with respect to duration of diabetes (Table 1).

Table 1 Inclusion criteria for patients with NIDDM

– Even distribution of both sexes, including even distribution of pre- and postmenopausal women
– Age at onset of NIDDM 40(35)–75 years*
– Age 40(35)–75 years
– Duration of diabetes*
– BMI 22–32 kg/m^2*
– Glycemic control* Fasting blood glucose 7–15 mmol/l while off-treatment during run-in period regardless of previous treatment

* matching criterion

Body mass index

Body mass index (BMI) should be used instead of ideal body weight. The former can be calculated, the latter estimated from tables. The average BMI of Scandinavian patients with NIDDM is 27.5 ± 4.4 kg/m^2 ($N = 460$), but can be considerably higher, e. g. in USA. Because the patient population studied should be representative of the average NIDDM population, the BMI should also be representative of the average NIDDM population. For Scandinavian and most European patients this would include a BMI of 22 to 32 kg/m^2.

Glycemic control

The level of glycemic control is one of the most debatable issues. Firstly, if the treatment goal is to reduce the excess rate of hepatic glucose production and thereby ameliorate hyperglycemia, it may be pertinent to include patients with clearly-elevated fasting blood glucose concentration. However, if the fasting blood glucose concentration rises above 15 mmol/l, glucose toxicity will seriously influence the treatment responses. These patients may also display severe impairment of their beta-cell function. If the treatment goal is to alleviate insulin resistance and concomitant abnormalities including cardiovascular morbidity, treatment should be initiated at a much earlier stage, probably before the patients develop manifest diabetes.

The range of glycemic control allowed is therefore dependent upon the treatment goals, but it seems justified to match for glycemic control and to avoid patients with fasting blood glucose above 15 mmol/l.

Previous treatment

If the aim is to include patients with elevated fasting blood glucose, these patients are usually already treated with oral anti-diabetic agents. An attempt to include patients without previous treatment will bias the study against mild cases, which probably should not be studied. The same argument applies to previous insulin treatment. Given the present indication for starting insulin therapy in patients with NIDDM, there is no real need to treat these patients differently from those receiving sulfonylureas and metformin. It may be better to define a certain glycemic range that the patients should remain within during an off-drug run-in period (see later).

Exclusion criteria

The exclusion of patients with IDDM is an obvious requirement but not always easy. About 10−15% of patients with an apparent NIDDM phenotype may represent latent autoimmune diabetes [11, 12] characterized by the presence of islet-cell (ICA) or glutamic-acid-decarboxylase (GAD) antibodies. Especially the latter seem to correctly identify about 75−80% of those

Table 2 Exclusion criteria

- Patients with latent autoimmune diabetes or IDDM (or GAD antibody positive patients)
- Fasting blood glucose off-treatment above 15 mmol/l
- Treatment with steroids, other hormones, phenytoin or cytotoxic agents
- Acute or untreated disease
- Hepatic dysfunction (S-ALAT above 2× the upper limit of normal)
- Renal dysfunction (S-creatinine > 30% above normal and/or proteinuria of > 0.5 g/day)
- Pregnancy or breast feeding
- History of drug or alcohol abuse
- Mental condition rendering the patient unable to understand the nature, scope and possible consequences of the study

patients who subsequently will require insulin therapy [12, 13]. As these assays become more widely available, the question is raised as to whether GAD antibody screening should be introduced to exclude patients with a disease other than NIDDM (Table 2).

Such patients may also be characterized by gross hyperglycemia and ketoacidosis. Ketosis should not be used as an exclusion criterion for NIDDM. Obese NIDDM patients often present with ketosis when overnight fasting is extended.

Other drug treatment

It has been customary in many studies to avoid agents that may influence glucose control. Unfortunately, this has also included anti-hypertensive agents as thiazides, beta-blocking agents and angiotensin-converting enzyme inhibitors. Although these agents may influence glucose control in non-diabetic individuals, the impact on glucose control in diabetic patients is small if not negligible [14], and 50–60% of NIDDM patients have hypertension, which may require treatment. Under these circumstances, it seems more reasonable to keep treatment with anti-hypertensive agents unchanged throughout the study. Attempts to switch from one agent to another prior to the study should be abandoned.

Treatment with steroids, other hormones, phenytoin and cytotoxic agents should of course be avoided. With respect to hormone substitution, thyroxin replacement in a person with thyroid dysfunction may represent an exception. Hypothyreosis is common among NIDDM patients and appropriate replacement therapy should not constitute an exclusion criterion. On the other hand, any other unstable diseases should be considered as exclusion criteria. These include any acute or untreated disease, impaired hepatic (SGOT or S-ALAT 2 × the upper limit of normal) and/or renal disease (S-creatinine > 30% above normal and/or proteinuria > 0.5 g/day). Microalbuminuria is not an exclusion criterion, since microalbuminuria is observed among 20–25% of patients with NIDDM and reflects coexisting macroangiopathy rather than incipient nephropathy [15, 16].

Run-in period

In order to create as identical conditions as possible in the patients, a run-in period is necessary during which the patients are off their previous drug treatments. The length of this period can, however, be debated. If the run-in period is prolonged, the ensuing hyperglycemia will create metabolic insulin resistance (glucose toxicity), which may influence the results more than a carry-over effect from the previous drug treatment. One week off of the drug treatment is an acceptable compromise, but if the patient has been on chlorpropamide, the run-in period should be extended. Likewise, a second wash-out period should be added at the end of the study. This is especially important in uncontrolled studies. If the treatment period is 12 months or more, blood glucose concentrations during the second wash-out period will most likely be higher than during the first period. Prevention of this rise in blood glucose may be the only demonstrable effect of the agent.

No diet and other interventions should be allowed during the run-in period. Instead, after the patient has been recruited to the research unit, he or she should be seen during an observation period of 3–6 months in the research unit before randomized to the study. During this period, means should be taken to correct the diet and teach the patient about the disease and its monitoring. The patient should not be included in the study until blood glucose remains stable. It would be useful to provide data on blood glucose 3–6 months prior to the study and at the beginning of the run-in period.

Study design

It is obvious that studies should always be double-blind. Whether one should use a parallel or cross-over design can be discussed. The parallel design has many advantages, although it requires almost twice as many patients. Matching for inclusion criteria is mandatory. The cross-over design allows a reduction in the number of patients studied, but problems with carry-over effects are not easy to solve. Applying statistics testing for such carry-over effects (ANOVA with repeated measurements) may only partially solve the problem. Therefore, data from the different treatment periods should be given both separately and pooled.

Studies comparing two different agents should in general be carried out with a double-dummy design, rather than making "similar-looking" tablets of the other agent. The pharmacokinetics of this agent may be quite different from the pharmacokinetics of the original drug.

Drug dose and biological effect

The relationship between sulfonylurea dose and its biological effect is linear only within a rather narrow range of low plasma drug concentrations [17]. This issue was examined by performing euglycemic and hyperglycemic clamp studies in healthy control subjects with concomitant infusion of increasing concentrations of glibenclamide and relatively low drug concentrations [17]. Glibenclamide enhanced insulin secretion and glucose disposal only to drug levels of 100–200 nmol/l, corresponding to an oral dose of about 10 mg

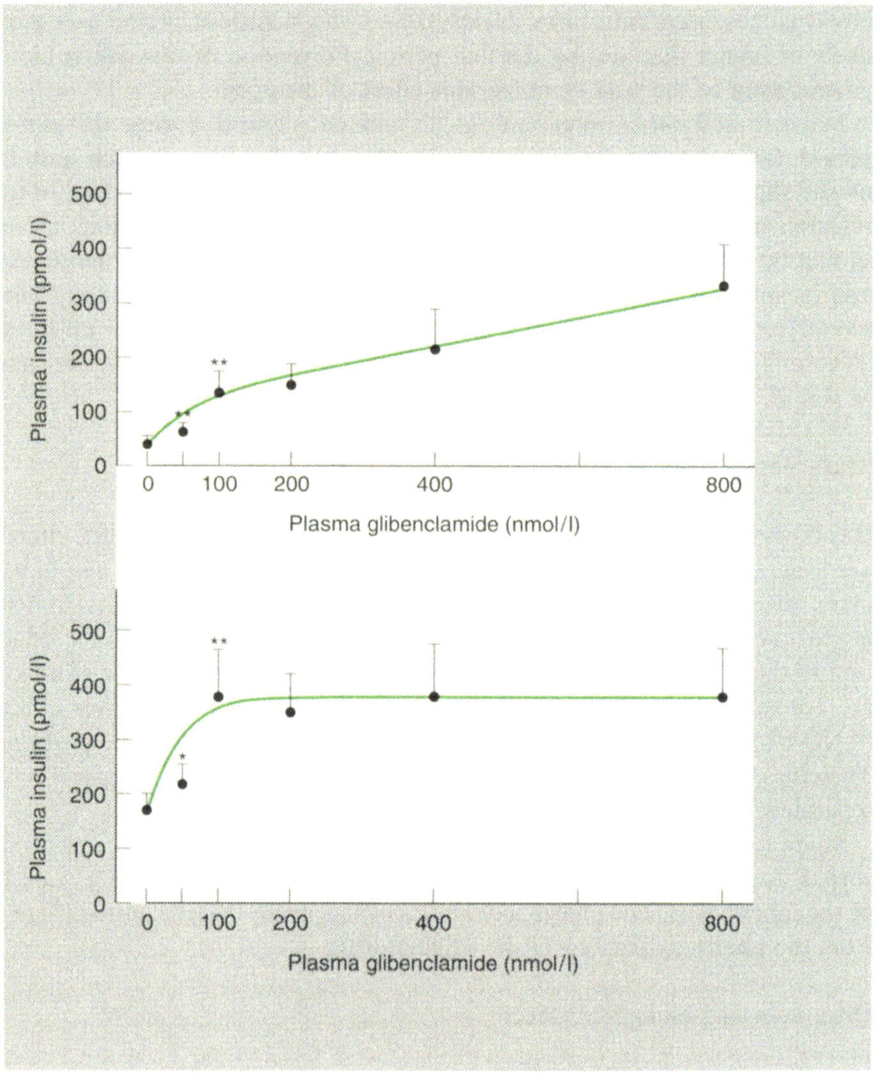

*Fig. 2 Dose response curves relating plasma insulin response during euglycemic (top) and hyperglycemic (bottom) periods to plasma glibenclamide concentration in 9 healthy subjects. Values are means ± SE. * $p < 0.05$, ** $p < 0.01$ compared with previous level [19]*

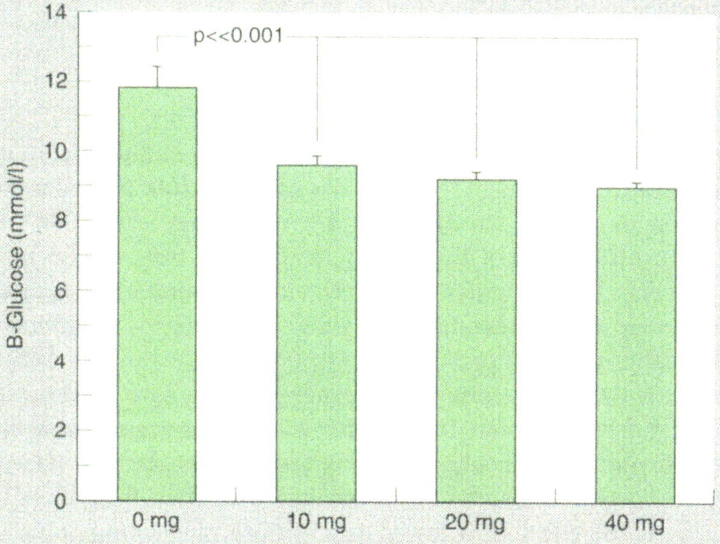

*Fig. 3 The effect of 3-month treatment with 10, 20 and 40 mg glipizide on mean blood glucose monitored at home in a double-blind fashion in 22 NIDDM patients. Time 0 denotes mean blood glucose during a 2-week placebo wash-out period in the beginning of the study. Values are means ± SE. * $p < 0.001$ compared with placebo*

(Fig. 2). Similarly, a placebo-controlled double-blind study, evaluating the effect of 10, 20 and 40 mg of glipizide on glycemic control in NIDDM patients, showed that maximal insulin response and blood glucose-lowering effect were achieved with a drug-dose of about 10 mg/day (Fig. 3) [18]. In most dose-titration studies, the drug dose is increased if the treatment goal is not achieved. Since few studies have evaluated the real benefit of such increases in drug dose, this usually results in higher than necessary recommended maximum dosages. In a dose titration study the drug dose should not only be increased, but also decreased when the "maximum" dose is achieved.

Most studies include a titration period, when the drug dose is allowed to increase by a certain amount per visit. Unfortunately, in many studies the patients are not seen frequently enough during this period to allow for this increase in drug dose. Therefore, the titration period should contain as many visits as necessary to allow an increase in the drug dose to the maximum dose recommended in the study.

Endpoints and efficacy variables

A study should be designed to test the effect on primary endpoints, in most cases glycemic control. Although the study design can include secondary (e. g. insulin secretion or insulin sensitivity) and even tertiary endpoints (body weight, blood pressure, lipids, cardiovascular events), they should not be allowed to influence the evaluation of the primary endpoint. To illustrate the problem, let us take a look at studies evaluating the efficacy of a combination of insulin and sulfonylurea or insulin and placebo [19]. The primary endpoint has in general been glycemic control, while many studies have used the insulin dose as secondary endpoint. Insulin plus sulfonylurea resulted in better glycemic control and lower insulin dose than insulin plus placebo. However, glycemic control is also a function of the insulin dose. Thus, the studies have in fact compared the effect of a lower insulin dose plus sulfonylurea with that of a higher insulin dose plus placebo on glycemic control.

Primary endpoints: glycemic control

How should the degree of glycemic control be estimated? Certainly measures of fructosamin and fasting blood glucose HbA_{1c} are necessary during visits to the research unit. HbA_{1c} assesses overall glycemic control, but does not, however, tell us anything about the day profile of action. For this, home monitoring of blood glucose using a blood glucose meter may add considerable information. Patients are asked to measure blood glucose four times a day (fasting in the morning, before lunch, before dinner) on two pre-determined weekdays. There is a strong positive correlation between the home-monitored blood glucose values and HbA_{1c} (Fig. 4). Given the time-dependent delay in the effects of change in glycemic control on HbA_{1c}, the home-monitored blood glucose concentrations are more sensitive to temporal changes in glycemic control.

It is also useful to define a "sufficient" treatment effect. The FDA considers a reduction in HbA_{1c} of at least 1% a sufficient effect.

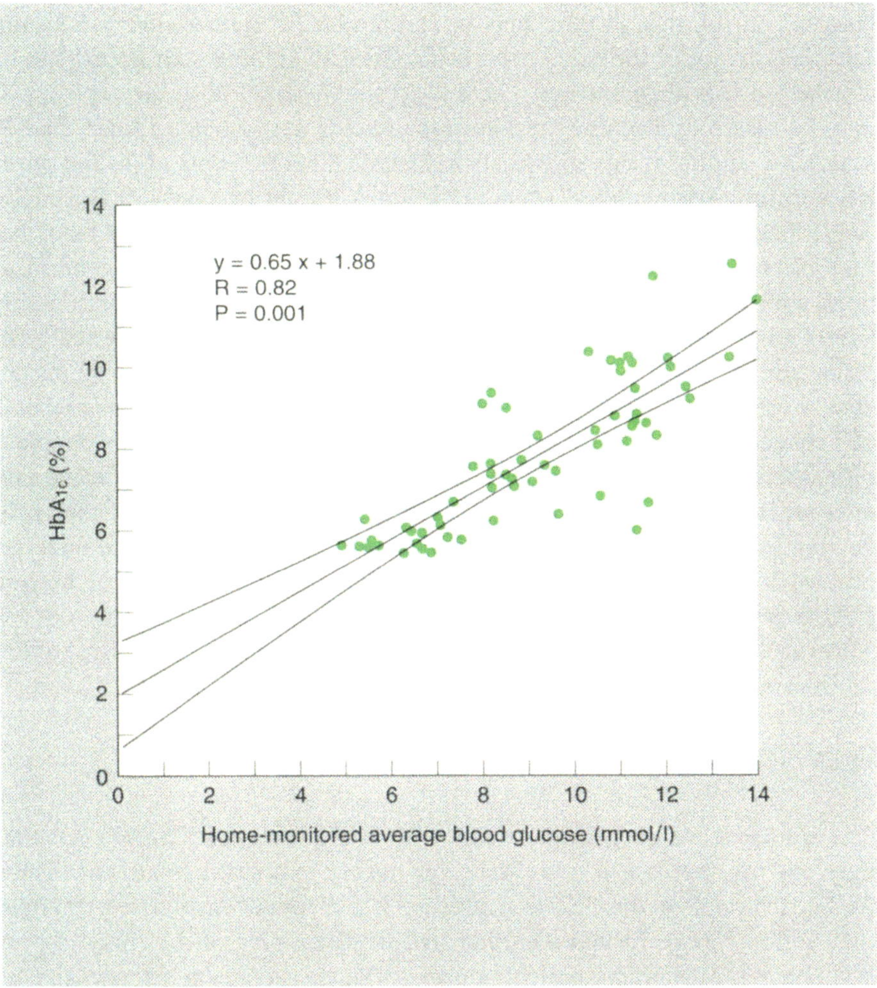

Fig. 4 Relationship between HbA_{1c} and blood glucose concentrations monitored at home twice a week (measurements before breakfast, lunch, dinner and bedtime) in NIDDM patients

Secondary endpoints

Insulin sensitivity

It is tempting to include measures of insulin secretion or insulin sensitivity as secondary endpoints in order to obtain some insight into the action mechanisms of drugs. This is not without problems. If the drug results in improved glucose control, this, in turn, may be responsible for improvement in insulin sensitivity. A lot of the extra-pancreatic effects of sulfonylurea agents can be ascribed to this phenomenon. There is no simple solution to the problem. It may be better to examine mechanisms in acute experiments rather than in long-term studies. If one still wants to include measurements of insulin sensitivity in long-term studies, some precautions should be taken. If the euglycemic insulin clamp is used to measure insulin sensitivity, measurements before and after treatment should be performed at identical glucose concentrations with the same duration of the clamp. Since it may take considerably longer to lower blood glucose to the euglycemic level in the pretreatment study, the clamp step should last at least 3–4 hours. If a low-dose insulin dose is used (e. g. plasma insulin concentrations < 50 μU/ml), measurements of hepatic glucose production are mandatory. Let us take as an example a case where the rate of total body glucose metabolism is similar before and after treatment. If the drug enhances suppression of hepatic glucose production by insulin, the effect of the drug on glucose disposal may be underestimated by an amount equivalent to the enhanced suppression of hepatic glucose production.

Regardless of these measures, it may not be possible from long term studies to discriminate between drug-related and glucose-related effects.

Insulin secretion

One argument for the extrapancreatic effects of sulfonylurea agents was that they did not increase insulin secretion during long-term treatment. These studies overlooked the fact that glucose is a stronger insulin secretagogue than sulfonylureas. Insulin secretion represents the sum of the effect of drug and glucose; re-studying patients during drug treatment on a lower glucose level is likely to underestimate the true effect on insulin secretion. Therefore, the glucose level should be raised to pretreatment levels when evaluating effects on insulin secretion regardless of whether the insulin response is measured during a hyperglycemic clamp, oral glucose tolerance test or a meal.

Several studies have demonstrated effects of sulfonylureas on insulin but not on C-peptide concentrations [20–24], suggesting effects on hepatic insulin clearance. Until this issue has been resolved, it may be useful to measure both insulin and C-peptide concentrations.

It should be kept in mind that we usually measure effects on peripheral hormone concentrations. To obtain an estimate of the effect on the insulin secretion rate, individual C-peptide kinetics are necessary [22].

Tertiary endpoints

Body weight

Body weight should be monitored throughout the study. Since weight changes can be due to changes in both fat and fat-free mass, it would be desirable to include estimates of the latter. Simple devices for accurate estimates of fat-free mass are available.

Blood pressure

Agents that improve insulin sensitivity could potentially lower blood pressure. Standardized readings of blood pressure are therefore necessary.

Lipids

Measurements of total and HDL-cholesterol and triglycerides should be performed in the fasting state. It is difficult to judge direct drug effects from indirect effects due to changes in glucose control or insulin sensitivity.

Monitoring of compliance

Patients are usually instructed to bring their study medication to every visit. Compliance is then assessed by tablet counting. This is a rather crude method, which if possible should be replaced by measurement of drug concentration in urine or blood.

References

[1] Alberti K, Gries A, eds. Management of noninsulin-dependent diabetes mellitus in Europe: a consensus view. Diabetic Med 1988; 5: 275–281.

[2] Groop LC. Sulfonylureas in NIDDM. Diabetes Care 1992; 15: 737–754.

[3] DeFronzo RA. The triumvirate: β-cell, muscle, liver: a collusion responsible for NIDDM. Diabetes 1988; 37: 667–687.

[4] Groop LC, Bonadonna RC, DelPrato S et al. Glucose and free fatty acid metabolism in non-insulin dependent diabetes mellitus. Evidence for multiple sites of insulin resistance. J Clin Invest 1989; 84: 205–213.

[5] Eriksson J, Franssila-Kallunki A, Ekstrand A et al. Early metabolic defects in persons at increased risk for non-insulin dependent diabetes mellitus. New Engl J Med 1989; 321: 337–343.

[6] Reaven GM. Role of insulin resistance in human disease. Diabetes 1988; 37: 1595–1607.

[7] Pyörälä K, Laakso M, Uusitupa M. Diabetes and atherosclerosis: an epidemiologic view. Diabet/Metab Rev 1987; 3: 463–524.

[8] Yki-Järvinen H. Acute and chronic effects of hyperglycemia on glucose metabolism. Diabetologia 1990; 33: 579–585.
[9] Groop L. Heterogeneity of Type 2 diabetes. A study of clinical, genetic, immunological and metabolic aspects. Helsinki: Thesis, 1982.
[10] Froguel P, Zouali H, Vionnet N et al. Familial hyperglycemia due to mutations in glucokinase. Definition of a subtype of diabetes. New Engl J Med 1993; 328: 697–702.
[11] Groop LC, Bottazzo GF, Doniach D. Islet cell antibodies identify latent type 1 diabetes in patients aged 35–75 years at diagnosis. Diabetes 1986; 35: 273–241.
[12] Tuomi T, Groop LC, Zimmet PZ et al. Antibodies to glutamic acid decarboxylase reveal latent autoimmune diabetes mellitus in adults with a non-insulin dependennt onset of disease. Diabetes 1993; 42: 359–362.
[13] Hagopian WA, Karlsen AE, Gottsäter A et al. Quantitative assay using recombinant human islet glutamic acid decarboxylase (GAD65) shows that 64K autoantibody positivity at onset predicts diabetes type. J Clin Invest 1993; 91: 368–374.
[14] Morales PA, Mitchell BD, Valdez RA et al. Incidence of NIDDM and impaired glucose tolerance in hypertensive subjects. The San Antonio Heart Study. Diabetes 1993; 42: 154–161.
[15] Tötterman K-J, Groop L, Groop P-H et al. Effect of beta-blocking drugs on beta-cell function and insulin sensitivity in hypertensive non-diabetic patients. Eur J Clin Pharmacol 1984; 26: 13–17.
[16] Pollare T, Lithell H, Berne C. A comparison of the effects of hydrochlorthiazide and captopril on glucose and lipid metabolism in patients with hypertension. New Engl J Med 1989; 321: 868–873.
[17] Groop L, Ekstrand A, Forsblom C et al. Insulin resistance, hypertension and microalbuminuria in patients with Type 2 (non-insulin-dependent) diabetes mellitus. Diabetologia 1993; 36: 642–647.
[18] Mogensen CE. Microalbuminuria predicts clinical proteinuria and early mortality in maturity-onset diabetes. N Engl J Med 1984; 311: 89–93.
[19] Groop L, Barzilai N, Ratheiser K et al. Dose-dependent effects of glyburide on insulin secretion and glucose uptake in humans. Diabetes Care 1991; 14: 724–727.
[20] Stenman S, Melander A, Groop P-H et al. What is the benefit of increasing the sulfonylurea dose? Ann Intern Med 1993; 118: 169–172.
[21] Groop LC, Groop P-H, Stenman S. Combined insulin-sulfonylurea therapy in treatment of NIDDM. Diabetes Care 1990; 13 (Suppl. 3): 47–52.
[22] Groop L, Groop P-H, Stenman S et al. Comparison of pharmacokinetics, metabolic effects and mechanisms of action of glyburide and glipizide during long-term treatment. Diabetes Care 1987; 10: 671–678.
[23] Scheen A, Castillo MJ, Lefébvre PJ. Decreased or increased insulin metabolism after glipizide in type II diabetes? Diabetes Care 1988; 11: 687–689.
[24] Shapiro ET, Van Cauter E, Tillil H et al. Glyburide enhances the responsiveness of the b-cell to glucose but does not correct the abnormal patterns of insulin secretion in noninsulin-dependent diabetes mellitus. J Clin Endocrinol Metab 1989; 69: 571–576.

Research methodologies of eicosanoid biosynthesis and function in diabetes

P. Patrignani, A Ganci, G. Davi, C. Patrono

Introduction

Eicosanoids are ubiquitous autacoids derived from arachidonate metabolism through various enzyme- or free-radical-catalyzed oxidative reactions [1–3].

At least 4 major series of biologically-active derivatives have been identified: 1. prostanoids, i. e. products of the so-called cyclooxygenase pathway of arachidonate metabolism; 2. hydroxy acids and leukotrienes, which are formed through various lipoxygenase reactions (e. g. 5-, 12-, 15-lipoxygenase); 3. epoxy fatty acids and dihydroxy fatty acids originating via the epoxygenase pathway; 4. isoprostanes, which include a series of prostaglandin (PG) F_2-like compounds produced by a non-cyclooxygenase, free-radical-catalyzed mechanism.

Although the *in vivo* production of all major series of eicosanoids has been demonstrated in humans, the bulk of the information on their biosynthesis and action has been obtained on prostanoids. These include PGD_2, PGE_2, PGF_{2a}, PGI_2 and thromboxane $(TX)A_2$.

Prostanoids are formed via the pathway depicted in Fig. 1. The coordinated sequence of enzymatic reactions involve: a) agonist-activated mobilization of esterified arachidonate from membrane phospholipids through the action of one or more lipases; b) conversion of free arachidonic acid to PGH_2, mediated by PGH-synthases; and c) cell-specific metabolism of PGH_2 by isomerases or reductases to form the various biologically active prostanoids. These substances are produced at a very low rate under physiological circumstances, and act in an autocrine or paracrine fashion through specific G protein-linked receptors present on the same prostanoid-producing cell or on neighboring cells [1].

Once synthesized and released *in vivo*, most eicosanoids undergo extensive enzymatic degradation to largely inactive metabolites. In the case of prostanoids, the methyl end side chain is modified first, leading to formation of the major circulating metabolites, 15-keto-13, 14-dihydro-PG_s. Further ω- and

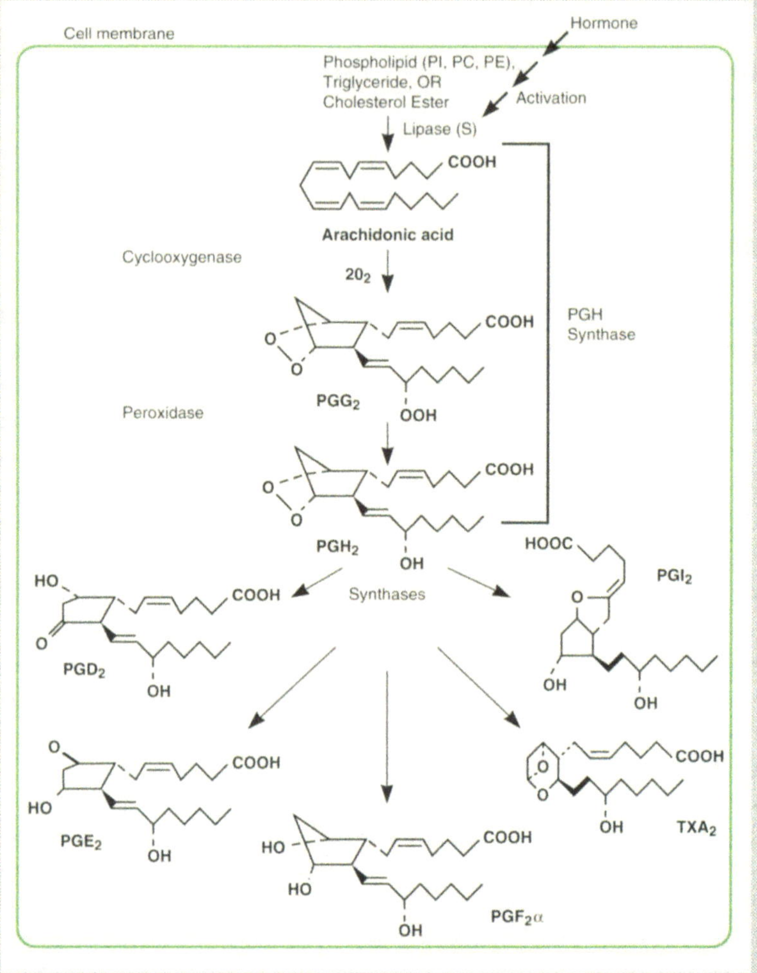

Fig. 1 Hormone-activated prostanoid biosynthesis in a model cell. Although all products of the "cyclooxygenase pathway" are depicted, usually only one prostanoid is formed as a major product by a given cell type.
PG, prostaglandin; TX, thromboxane; PI, PC, and PE, phosphatidyl-inositol, -choline, and -ethanolamine, respectively.
Reproduced from [1] with permission from the American Physiological Society

β-oxidation leads to chain-shortened products that are excreted in the urine. The majority of prostaglandin and thromboxane metabolites are thus C_{18} or C_{16} compounds, resulting from one or two cycles of β-oxidation.

Identification of major urinary eicosanoid metabolites has led to the development of analytical techniques based on gas chromatography/mass spectrometry (GC/MS) and radioimmunoassay (RIA). The availability of these methodologies for clinical investigation has allowed for considerable progress over the last 10 years in our understanding of the pathophysiologic significance of eicosanoid biosynthesis and action.

What follows is an overview of research methodologies related to prostanoid biosynthesis and action in 3 major areas of relevance to diabetes mellitus – platelet, vascular and renal arachidonate metabolism.

Studies of platelet arachidonate metabolism

Biosynthesis of TXA_2

TXA_2 is the major product of arachidonic acid metabolism in human platelets. Arachidonic acid, a ubiquitous constituent of membrane phospholipids, is mainly released by the activation of phospholipase A_2 as a consequence of the interaction with the platelet membrane of a wide variety of agonists, including thrombin, adenosine diphosphate (ADP), and platelet activating factor, (reviewed in [4]). The conversion of free arachidonic acid to the prostaglandin endoperoxide PGH_2 is mediated by the activity of PGH synthase-1 and PGH synthase-2 which exhibit both cyclooxygenase and peroxidase activities (reviewed in [1]). PGH synthase-1 and PGH synthase-2 have recently been cloned and their tissue distribution evaluated. PGH synthase-1 mRNA is present in platelets and in extracts of virtually all mammalian tissues. PGH synthase-2 mRNA, however, is detectable in prostate, brain, testis and lung but is undetectable in platelets and most other major organs. Due to the wide expression of PGH synthase-1, the cellular specificity of TXA_2 formation derives from the more restricted cellular distribution of TXA synthase. TXA synthase is a member of the cytochrome P450 family, and catalyzes the conversion of PGH_2 to TXA_2 (reviewed in [3]). Pharmacological studies have raised the possibility of tissue-specific TXA synthase isozymes [5]. Platelet TXA synthases have been cloned and sequenced, and two cDNAs of different length have been isolated; the larger cDNA species is designated TXA synthase I while the shorter cDNA is designated TXA synthase II (reviewed in [1]). During its catalytic activity TXA synthase can undergo suicide inactivation. Thus, as substrate is consumed to generate product, the enzyme is progressively inhibited. This phenomenon may represent an important mechanism limiting TXA_2 biosynthesis in platelets (reviewed in [4]).

Mechanism of action of TXA_2

Due to the evanescence of TXA_2 and its precursor PGH_2 (*in vitro* half-lives of 30 sec and 5 min, respectively), the biological actions induced by these substances on platelets have been characterized using chemically stable analogs. These studies have demonstrated that both eicosanoids have a similar affinity for a common receptor site on platelets which has been designated the TXA_2/PGH_2 receptor (reviewed in [6]). The interaction of these ligands with the receptor on isolated platelets produces shape change followed by an increase in intracellular calcium, phosphorylation of proteins, secretion of granular components, exposure of fibrinogen receptors and finally aggregation. TXA_2 acts as an amplifying signal for platelet agonists such as thrombin, ADP and epinephrine (reviewed in [4]). Pharmacological and biochemical studies suggest the existence of at least two distinct subtypes of the platelet TXA_2/PGH_2 receptor. One binding site evokes platelet shape change and an increase in intracellular calcium, the other site appears to be linked to the post-receptorial events that lead to platelet secretion and aggregation. It is unknown whether these sites represent distinct receptor isoforms or varied degrees of post-translational modification of a single receptor. Furthermore, it is unknown whether PGH_2 and TXA_2 differ in their affinity for the different binding sites.

The cDNA for a TXA_2 receptor has been recently cloned from a placental library [7]. Its deduced amino acid sequence suggests that it has 7 transmembrane-spanning domains, typical of a G protein-linked receptor. Pharmacological studies suggest that the platelet TXA_2/PGH_2 receptor(s) is linked to phospholipase C activation via pertussis-toxin-insensitive G proteins.

Desensitization of platelet TXA_2/PGH_2 receptor(s) due to receptor-G protein uncoupling and sensitization of platelet adenylate cyclase may represent mechanisms by which the response to receptor stimulation is regulated (reviewed in [4]).

Measurement of platelet TXA_2 biosynthesis

Various studies have shown that platelets from diabetic patients are "hyperfunctioning". In most of these studies platelet function was evaluated by studying platelet aggregation in stimulated platelet rich plasma (PRP) or in stimulated washed platelets (reviewed in [8]). Due to the role played by TXA_2 in modulating platelet function, the possible involvement of altered TXA_2 biosynthesis in the occurrence of platelet activation in diabetes has been extensively studied.

Enhanced biosynthesis of platelet TXA_2 has been demonstrated in diabetic patients both *in vitro* and *in vivo* (see [8] for a recent review).

Methods of studying platelet TXA_2 biosynthesis in vitro: a. Measurement of TXA_2 production in stimulated PRP: The production of TXA_2 during platelet aggregation induced in PRP stimulated by various agonists (such as ADP, sodium arachidonate, and thrombin) can be assessed by measuring the amount of TXB_2 (the stable hydration product of TXA_2) released from platelets into the plasma. The amounts of TXB_2 formed under these circumstances depend on the type and concentration of the aggregating agent used and on the time of incubation of platelets with the stimuli. Due to the possibility of isolating a subpopulation of platelets during the PRP preparation procedure, the biosynthesis of TXB_2 in this setting may not reflect the capacity of all circulating platelets to produce this eicosanoid. TXB_2 can be easily measured by RIA. Several kits are commercially available to provide adequate sensitivity and specificity for measurement of the relatively high concentrations of TXB_2 released under these conditions.
b. Measurement of platelet TXA_2 production in whole blood: We have described a relatively simple method which allows assessment of the production of TXB_2 during whole blood clotting at 37 °C by a specific RIA technique [9]. This is a time-dependent process achieving a steady-state TXB_2 level in serum within 60 min in healthy subjects. Serum TXB_2 concentrations measured under these circumstances averaged 300 ± 108 ng/ml (mean $\pm$ SD, $n = 177$) in healthy subjects, with no statistically significant differences between men and women [10]. Endogenous thrombin is the primary stimulus for platelet activation during whole blood clotting and the time-course of its formation closely parallels that of TXB_2. Since a statistically significant correlation exists between serum TXB_2 levels and the platelet count, the values of TXB_2 measured in the whole blood of patients characterized by an abnormal platelet count should be corrected for the platelet number [10].

Measurements of *ex vivo* TXB_2 production in whole blood or in stimulated PRP represent indexes of biosynthetic capacity that are unlikely to be relevant to changes occurring *in vivo*, except to reflect drug-induced changes in platelet cyclooxygenase or TXA synthase activity. In fact, there is a wide discrepancy between the capacity of human platelets to synthesize and release TXA_2 when maximally stimulated *ex vivo* and the actual rate of TXA_2 secretion into the human circulation [11]. Thus, the platelets present in 1 ml of human whole blood have the capacity to generate approximately the same amount of TXB_2 during 1 hour clotting *in vitro* as the total body synthesis *in vivo* over the same period of time [11]. The very low biosynthetic rate (approximately 0.1 ng/kg · min^{-1}) measured in healthy subjects suggests tight regulation of TXA_2 biosynthesis and low frequency and/or intensity of stimuli to its production.

Several studies have reported increased TXB_2 production in stimulated PRP of patients with type I and type II diabetes mellitus that can be reversed by strict glycemic control [12–17]. However, it is important to emphasize that because the maximal biosynthetic capacity of platelets is approximately 5,000-fold higher than the basal rate of production of TXA_2, the finding of enhanced capacity of platelets to produce TXB_2 in stimulated PRP does not necessarily imply changes in TXA_2 biosynthesis *in vivo.*

Methods of studying TXA_2 biosynthesis in vivo: Increased platelet TXA_2 production *in vivo* can result from local stimuli to platelet activation, as can occur at sites of endothelial injury, without the need for invoking enhanced metabolic properties or "hyper-reactive" platelets. Under such circumstances, where the stimuli are not in blood but in the vasculature, it is unlikely that one can detect alterations in TXA_2 biosynthesis by studying platelets *ex vivo.* Thus, analytical methods have been developed over the last 10 years for evaluating the biosynthesis of TXA_2 *in vivo* [18].

Due to its chemical instability, TXA_2 released into the circulation is rapidly transformed to TXB_2 via non-enzymatic hydrolysis. TXB_2 is then rapidly cleared from the bloodstream (plasma half-life: 5 min) due to extensive enzymatic degradation, involving β-oxidation and dehydrogenation of the hemiacetal alcohol group at C11. These processes in turn result in the appearance in the plasma of two major metabolites, 11-dehydro-TXB_2 and 2,3-dinor-TXB_2, characterized by longer plasma half-lives (45 min and 15 min, respectively). The enzymatic metabolites of TXB_2 are then cleared from the bloodstream by urinary excretion. The measurement of 11-dehydro-TXB_2 and 2,3-dinor-TXB_2 in plasma and urine represents a reliable approach for evaluating the biosynthesis of TXA_2 *in vivo* in man [18].

Analytical techniques for the measurement of these metabolites in plasma and urine have been developed [19, 20]. Two methods have been used: RIA and GC/MS. Although the latter represents the ultimate reference method for all eicosanoid measurements, comparable results can be obtained with the less cumbersome RIA, provided that adequate sensitivity and specificity of the antibodies is combined with appropriate sample extraction and separation of the immunoreactive species of interest from other cross-reacting eicosanoids. Detailed procedures for the extraction, purification and RIA measurement of 2,3-dinor-TXB_2 and 11-dehydro-TXB_2 are described in [11] and [19].

Several independent criteria have to be used in order to validate measurements of eicosanoids performed by RIA: a) adequate recovery of exogenously-added authentic standards to plasma and urine samples; b) identical immunologic behavior of the endogenous immunoreactive metabolite and the reference standard upon 10- to 50-fold dilution (i. e. apparent concentration of the unknown independent of the dilution factor); c) identical chromatographic behavior of the extracted plasma or urinary immunoreactivity and authentic metabolite on RP-HPLC (i. e. immunoreactivity detected only in the eluates corresponding to the retention time of the standard); d) statistically significant linear correlation between paired measurements performed by RIA and by GC/MS on a limited number of samples encompassing the range of clinically relevant concentrations [11, 19].

a. Plasma measurements: Plasma measurements of TXB_2 and its metabolites have been employed as indexes of the biosynthesis of TXA_2 in clinical investigation. The determinations of TXB_2 in plasma are invalidated by the inevitable artifactual formation of TXA_2 during and after blood sampling. In fact, due to the very high capacity of platelets to produce this eicosanoid when maximally stimulated *ex vivo* (i. e. approximately 200–400 ng/ml are formed during whole blood clotting at 37 °C), activation by as little as 0.1% of their maximal capacity during and after sampling would totally account for the putative circulating concentrations of TXB_2 reported by many investigators in physiological conditions (10–300 pg/ml). Maximal estimates of the endogenous plasma concentrations of TXB_2 based on urinary metabolite excretion are in the order of 1–3 pg/ml [11].

An alternative approach to the measurement of circulating levels of TXA_2 is to evaluate the plasma levels of the long-lived enzymatic metabolites of TXB_2, such as 11-dehydro-TXB_2 [21]. Since plasma or blood cells do not possess the enzymes necessary to metabolize TXB_2, the measurement of its enzymatic metabolites in plasma is not affected by *ex vivo* platelet activation during and after blood sampling [21]. Measurement of long-lived enzymatic metabolites of TXB_2 in the plasma of diabetic patients has been performed in very few studies. Alessandrini et al [22] found no change in 11-dehydro-TXB_2 plasma levels in type I diabetic patients without clinical evidence of macrovascular complications.

b. Urinary measurements: Studies of the infusion of exogenous TXB_2 into the systemic circulation of healthy volunteers have demonstrated that increased plasma levels of TXB_2 are followed by a significant increase in the urinary excretion of its major enzymatic metabolites, 2,3-dinor-TXB_2 and 11-dehydro-TXB_2 [11, 23]. A statistically significant linear correlation existed between the dose of TXB_2 infused and the excretion rates of both metabolites in urine. Moreover, the fractional conversion of infused TXB_2 (in a dose range up to 50-fold the endogenous rate of secretion) into its urinary metabolites was independent of the dose, demonstrating that over such range of entry rates of TXB_2 into the vasculature the enzymes involved in the metabolism of TXB_2 are not saturable [11, 23].

Thus, measurement of the major urinary enzymatic metabolites of TXB_2 represents a reliable, non-invasive index of the biosynthesis of TXA_2 *in vivo* in man. Potential limitations inherent to the interpretation of measurements of these metabolites in urine are related to: a) the cellular source(s) of TXB_2 metabolites; b) their vascular site(s) of origin and c) the timing of metabolite excretion in relation to altered biosynthesis.

Pharmacological studies have suggested that approximately 70% of the urinary excretion of 11-dehydro-TXB_2 and 2,3-dinor-TXB_2 may reflect a platelet source of TXA_2 biosynthesis. In fact, the administration of low-dose aspirin (20 mg/day), a relatively selective and irreversible inhibitor of platelet PGH synthase, to healthy volunteers caused a cumulative inhibition of the urinary excretion of the enzymatic metabolites of TXB_2 [24]. After 10 days of treatment, the urinary excretion of 2,3-dinor-TXB_2 and 11-dehydro-TXB_2 was reduced to less than 30% of control values [24]. Another piece of evidence supporting the predominant platelet origin of these metabolites is provided by their linear recovery over 10 days after discontinuing aspirin administration. This pattern is consistent with the time-dependent return of platelets with unacetylated PGH synthase to the systemic circulation [24].

Measurements of the excretion of enzymatic metabolites of TXB_2 have been reported in diabetic patients [17, 22, 25]. Thus, Davì et al [17] have described enhanced urinary excretion of 11-dehydro-TXB_2 in type II diabetic patients with clinical evidence of macrovascular disease. This alteration appeared to reflect persistently increased platelet synthesis of TXA_2, irrespective of the type of macrovascular complication [17]. On the contrary, the urinary excretion of 2,3-dinor-TXB_2 was unchanged in type I diabetic patients with or without retinopathy [22].

Whenever altered TXB_2 metabolite excretion is detected in a novel clinical setting, the following questions should be properly addressed: 1. is the identity of the metabolite unequivocally established?; 2. does metabolite excretion reflect changes in the rate of biosynthesis of TXA_2 or altered metabolic disposition?; 3. what is the cellular source(s) and mechanism(s) supporting these biochemical changes? Comparison of RIA measurements with GC/MS determinations can adequately address the first question. Measurement of both 2,3-dinor-TXB_2 and 11-dehydro-TXB_2 and exogenous TXB_2 infusion studies can provide answers to the second point. Pharmacological interventions (e. g. with low-dose aspirin) can indirectly address the third question. These approaches have been used for interpreting changes in TXB_2 metabolite excretion in diabetes mellitus and detailed protocols for these studies can be found in [17] and [22].

Methods of studying the action of TXA_2 on platelets: a. Characterization of platelet TXA_2/PGH_2 receptor(s) by radioligand binding studies: Determination of the equilibrium dissociation constant (K_D) and apparent maximum number of binding sites (B_{max}) of platelet TXA_2/PGH_2 receptor(s) can be obtained by the use of radioligand binding techniques.

Since both TXA_2 and PGH_2 are extremely labile, binding studies must be performed in intact platelets or platelet membranes using chemically stable radio-labeled agonists or antagonists. The use of tritium-labeled analogs of prostaglandin endoperoxides (e. g., U46619, 11,9-epoxymethano-PGH_2) has been limited by their low specific activity, high non-specific binding and modest K_D values. The synthesis of tritiated or iodinated antagonists ([^{3}H]-S-145, [^{3}H]-SQ-29,548 and [^{125}I]-PTA-OH) that possess high specific binding and high affinity and specificity for platelet TXA_2/PGH_2 receptors has permitted characterizing a single class of binding sites with a K_D in the nanomolar range (reviewed in [26]). Recently, the use of a novel and high potent [^{125}I]-labeled TXA_2 mimetic, I-BOP, has demonstrated the presence of two TXA_2/PGH_2 receptor subtypes in platelets with different affinities (K_D: 270 ± 60 pM and 3.9 ± 1.2 nM, respectively [27]).

In vitro studies have shown that the responses induced by occupancy of platelet TXA_2/PGH_2 receptors can be regulated by an initial rapid homologous desensitization due to uncoupling of the receptor from a G-protein that couples them to phospholipase C (reviewed in [4]). Prolonged exposure to agonists results in progressive loss of binding sites from the platelet surface. Thus, whenever platelets have been exposed to enhanced production of TXA_2 *in vivo*, TXA_2/PGH_2 receptor(s) are likely to be desensitized.

Desensitization of the platelet TXA_2/PGH_2 receptor can result in decreased number of binding sites despite normal binding affinity. Conflicting results have been obtained in diabetes (reviewed in [8]). In some studies the number of binding sites of TXA_2/PGH_2 receptors in platelets from type I diabetic patients was found decreased or unchanged, and receptor affinity was not affected. It should be mentioned that no single study has characterized receptor desensitization in platelets from patients with type II diabetes where enhanced platelet TXA_2 biosynthesis was demonstrated *in vivo*.

Another mechanism by which the response to TXA_2/PGH_2 receptor stimulation is regulated is by sensitization of platelet adenylate cyclase stimulation. Prostacyclin (PGI_2), the principal product of arachidonate metabolism in vascular cells, activates platelet adenylate cyclase to produce cyclic AMP thereby inhibiting platelet aggregation [28]. Thus, enhanced platelet TXA_2 biosynthesis should result in sensitization of PGI_2-dependent adenylate cyclase stimulation. On the contrary, several studies have reported diminished sensitivity of platelets to the anti-aggregatory effects of PGI_2 in both type I and type II diabetic patients whereas other studies showed no difference (see [8] for a recent review).

b. Intracellular Ca^{2+} mobilization: The activation of platelets by TXA_2 as well as by other agonists (vasopressin, thrombin and platelet activating factor) is associated with an increase in cytosolic Ca^{2+} that originates from the extracellular fluid through a putative receptor-operated Ca^{2+} channel and from one or more intracellular Ca^{2+} pools as a consequence of phospholipase C activation. Enhanced cytosolic free Ca^{2+} levels may regulate several platelet functional responses and the release and metabolism of arachidonic acid with the formation of TXA_2.

Cytosolic free Ca^{2+} concentrations can be measured using Ca^{2+} indicators such as fura 2 and aequorin in isolated washed platelets, both in the absence and in the presence of TXA_2 mimetics or other platelet agonists [29, 30].

The exposure of platelets to enhanced TXA_2 biosynthesis *in vivo* might be associated with desensitization of TXA_2/PGH_2 receptors and consequent reduction in Ca^{2+} release when platelets are stimulated with TXA_2 mimetics *in vitro*. However, no study has addressed the question of whether the handling of calcium that follows TXA_2/PGH_2 receptor stimulation is altered in diabetic platelets.

Enhanced intra-platelet calcium mobilization was found in platelets of type II diabetics both under basal conditions and after stimulation with thrombin and collagen (see [8] for a recent review). Alterations in phosphoinositide turnover and increased influx and diminished efflux rates of calcium across the platelet plasma membrane might be involved. Impaired exchange of calcium across the plasma membrane has been reported in type I diabetes [31]. However, the link between these biochemical changes in platelets and enhanced TXA_2 production *in vitro* or *in vivo* remains entirely hypothetical.

Studies of vascular PGI_2 biosynthesis

Mechanism of PGI_2 biosynthesis and action

PGI_2 is the most abundant product of arachidonic acid metabolism in a variety of vascular cells (mainly endothelial cells) [28]. In these cells, it is synthesized via the activity of three major enzymes: phospholipase A_2, which liberates arachidonic acid from phospholipids; PGH synthase, which converts arachidonic acid into PGG_2 and then PGH_2; and prostacyclin synthase, which generates PGI_2 from PGH_2 (Fig. 1). Both PGH synthase-1 and PGH synthase-2 mRNAs are expressed in vascular cells [32]. Prostacyclin synthase is a member of the cytochrome P450 family. PGI_2 synthesis is regulated by phospholipase activity and arachidonate availability and also by the steady-state level of PGH synthases which is determined by synthesis of the enzyme and its rate of loss, including suicidal inactivation of the enzyme during catalysis. Transcriptional, post-transcriptional and post-translational modifications may be important in regulating the enzyme level, but these events are not well characterized.

PGI_2 can also be generated through the metabolic cooperation of two different cell types. Human blood platelets are capable of synthesizing and releasing large amounts of PGH_2 but cannot convert PGH_2 into PGI_2. When platelets come in contact with other cells that possess prostacyclin synthase such as endothelial cells and lymphocytes, platelet-derived PGH_2 can be exported to these cells to produce PGI_2 [33].

PGI_2 inhibits platelet function by Gs-coupled stimulation of adenylate cyclase. Moreover PGI_2 inhibits tone and growth of vascular smooth muscle (reviewed in [34]).

The finding that the biosynthesis of PGI_2 is increased coincident with that of TXA_2 in clinical settings in which platelet-vascular interactions are likely to be increased suggests that PGI_2 might serve as a local homeostatic regulator of the platelet response to TXA_2 [35]. In fact, the sensitization of PGI_2-dependent stimulation of platelet adenylate cyclase, which follows TXA_2/PGH_2 receptor stimulation represents a phenomenon by which TXA_2-dependent platelet activation is regulated (reviewed in [4]).

Measurement of vascular PGI_2 biosynthesis

Soon after the discovery of PGI_2 as a major product of arachidonate metabolism in vascular tissue [28], pathophysiologic hypotheses were put forward linking reduced PGI_2 formation to endothelial dysfunction in diabetes (reviewed in [36]). In fact, decreased *ex vivo*-formation of PGI_2 by vascular fragments obtained from juvenile-onset diabetics was reported by Silberbauer et al [37]. Such reduced biosynthetic capacity of vascular tissue was not confirmed by later measurements of total body PGI_2 biosynthesis *in vivo*, as reflected by the urinary excretion of its major enzymatic metabolite 2,3-dinor-6-keto-$PGF_{1\alpha}$ [22, 35]. Such an apparent discrepancy can be reconciled by the very substantial difference between the high biosynthetic potential of vascular tissue, when challenged *ex vivo*, and the very low rate of endogenous PGI_2 biosynthesis measured in healthy subjects *in vivo* [38]. Thus, it has been calculated that the amount of PGI_2 synthesized by a fragment of human arterial tissue following 15-min incubation *in vitro* [39] approximates the total body production of PGI_2 *in vivo* [38]. Similar to the assessment of platelet TXA_2 production as discussed earlier, the evaluation of PGI_2 production by vascular fragments in response to various agonists added *in vitro* by no means reflects the actual rate of PGI_2 biosynthesis by untraumatized vascular tissue in response to stimuli operating *in vivo*. Furthermore, measurements of circulating levels of PGI_2 do not provide reliable information on its biosynthesis because: a) both unstable PGI_2 and its chemically stable derivative 6-keto-$PGF_{1\alpha}$ disappear rapidly from the systemic circulation [40]; b) spuriously elevated levels can be generated during blood sampling because of needle- or catheter-induced vascular trauma [18]. Thus, measurement of urinary metabolite excretion represents the only non-invasive approach for assessing *in vivo* PGI_2 biosynthesis in health and disease.

Both GC/MS [38] and RIA [40, 41] methods have been developed to quantitate plasma levels and urinary excretion of 6-keto-$PGF_{1\alpha}$, the non-enzymatic hydration product of PGI_2, and 2,3-dinor-6-keto-$PGF_{1\alpha}$, a major enzymatic metabolite.

All reagents necessary for these assays are commercially available and detailed analytical procedures have been published [38, 40, 41], including validation criteria for RIA measurements [40].

Much of the difficulty in ascertaining the pathophysiologic role, if any, of vascular PGI_2 in diabetes stems from the lack of selective inhibitors of PGI_2 biosynthesis or action. Thus, virtually all cyclooxygenase inhibitors will interfere, to a variable extent, with vascular PGI_2 biosynthesis. Possible exceptions are provided by very low doses (20–30 mg/day) of conventionally formulated aspirin as well as by recently-developed aspirin formulations with limited systemic bio-availability (reviewed in [42]). Inferring the clinical significance of vascular PGI_2 biosynthesis from the effects of biochemically selective (i. e. sparing PGI_2 formation) vs non-selective regimens of aspirin administration would require randomizing several thousand diabetic patients to long-term treatment with either regimen, with major vascular events (i. e. the combined incidence of non-fatal myocardial infarction, non-fatal stroke and vascular death) as primary end-points of the study. The rationale and feasibility of this approach have been discussed elsewhere [43].

Studies of renal arachidonate metabolism

Prostanoid synthesis and action within the kidney

Various prostanoids can be produced by isolated human glomeruli and renal epithelial and mesangial cells in culture [44]. The major renal cells express mainly PGH-synthase 1. Since PGH-synthase 2 can be up-regulated under conditions associated with increased cell replication or differentiation, expression of this isoenzyme might be expected to be induced in response to local inflammatory stimuli and/or in association with tissue repair [1]. Due to non-uniform distribution of TXA-synthase, PGI_2-synthase and other isomerases in different renal cells, the synthesis of various eicosanoids within the kidney is compartmentalized to specific areas and is not uniformly expressed throughout the nephron [44].

PGH_2 and TXA_2 exert multiple actions within the kidney which may contribute to the progression of renal disease. These include constriction of glomerular afferent and efferent arterioles, intraglomerular platelet aggregation, contraction of glomerular mesangial cells and proliferation of mesangial cell matrix (reviewed in [45]). These effects have been characterized using stable PGH_2/THA_2 analogs and, although radioligand binding studies suggest a single class of specific binding sites in glomeruli, it is unclear whether these are subtypes distinct from those in platelets and vascular smooth muscle cells and whether their affinity for PHG_2 and TXA_2 is similar. As demonstrated for the platelet receptor, PGH_2/TXA_2 receptors present on isolated renal glomeruli undergo homologous desensitization.

In addition, both PGI_2 and PGE_2 have multiple tubular and vascular actions in the kidney. In cortical collecting tubule cells and cortical and medullary thick limb cells, PGE_2 has been shown to act through pharmacologically distinct stimulatory (EP2) and inhibitory (EP3) receptors to stimulate and inhibit cAMP formation, respectively (reviewed in [1]). Tubular actions of PGE_2 mediated via an EP1 receptor coupled to Ca^{2+} mobilization and protein-kinase C activation have also been described.

Given the compartmentalized nature of prostanoid synthesis and action within the kidney, largely unsatisfactory tools are available for clinical investigation. These include measurement of urinary unmetabolized prostanoids (i. e. PGE_2, $PGF_{2\alpha}$, 6-keto-$PGF_{1\alpha}$ and TXB_2) and use of synthesis inhibitor and/or receptor antagonists.

Measurement of renal prostanoid biosynthesis

Largely indirect evidence supports the notion that the urinary excretion of primary unmetabolized eicosanoids, including TXB_2, may represent a fraction of intra-renal eicosanoid production in man (reviewed in [46]). The evidence concerning urinary TXB_2 derives from infusion studies of exogenous TXB_2 in healthy subjects [11], from the investigation of patients with lupus nephritis [47] and from pharmacologic studies of selective and nonselective cyclooxygenase inhibitors in health and disease [46, 48]. These human studies have measured the urinary excretion of TXB_2 and 2,3-dinor-TXB_2 and have demonstrated a dissociation of their excretory pattern possibly suggestive of a renal vs extra-renal origin, respectively.

Problems in the assessment of renal prostanoid production through measurements of urinary prostanoid excretion are related to: a) reliable identification and quantization of picomolar concentrations of the unmetabolized compound of interest amongst nanomolar concentrations of numerous potentially cross-reacting prostanoid metabolites (up to 20 in the case of TXB_2); b) uncertainty as to the renal vs extra-renal origin of unmetabolized prostanoids under pathophysiological circumstances associated with enhanced extra-renal prostanoid biosynthesis (e. g. increased platelet TXA_2 production); c) contamination of urine with trace amounts of seminal fluid or blood possibly contributing substantial amounts of the prostanoid of interest and/or structurally related cross-reacting eicosanoids [46]. The first problem can only be adequately addressed through a comparison of RIA measurements with GC/MS determinations on a limited number of urine samples. Addressing the second issue requires a more complex approach, involving measurements of both the unmetabolized prostanoid of interest and its major enzymatic metabolites (e. g. TXB_2 and 11-dehydro-TXB_2 or 2,3-dinor-TXB_2) as well as the use of selective inhibitors of extrarenal prostanoid production (e. g. low-dose aspirin). As for the third problem, this may invalidate measurements of PGE_2 and, to a lesser extent, TXB_2 performed in male urine as well as urinary prostanoid assessment in the presence of menstruation, trauma or lower urinary tract infection. A careful clinical history should lead to appropriate exclusions.

Detailed procedures for RIA measurements of urinary PGE_2 [49], $PGF_{2\alpha}$ [49], 6-keto-$PGF_{1\alpha}$ [40], and TXB_2 [47] have been published. Their validation criteria have been reviewed previously [46]. A valid alternative to RIA is provided by enzyme immunoassay (EIA) of the same compounds [50]. Most reagents are now commercially available for both RIA and EIA [50].

Arachidonic acid is also metabolized by means of P450 isoenzymes to form epoxyeicosatrienoic acids (EETs) and their corresponding dihydroxy derivatives (DHETs). Catella et al [51] have reported the presence in human urine of 8,9-, 11,12-, and 14,15-EETs and their corresponding DHETs, and provided preliminary evidence to suggest that urinary DHETs largely derive from the kidney. Quantitative assays based on negative ion, chemical ionization GC/MS have been described for these compounds [51].

Measurement of other eicosanoids

Besides being a substrate for PGH-synthase- and epoxygenase-catalyzed reactions, arachidonic acid can be a source of other biologically active eicosa-

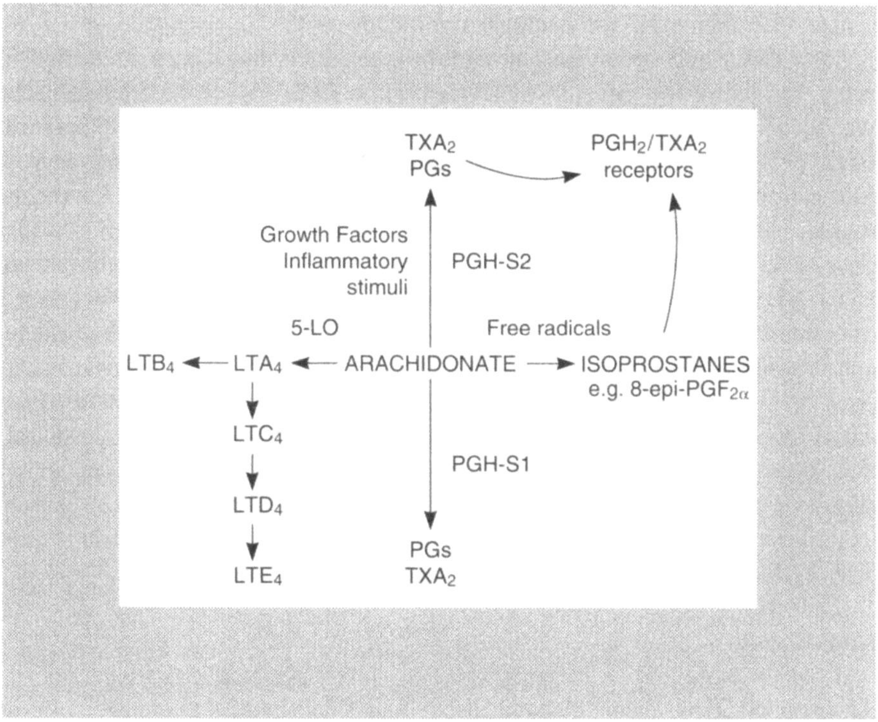

Fig. 2 Schematic representation of arachidonate metabolism through the constitutive and inducible PGH-synthases (PGH-S1 and PGH-S2, respectively), 5-lipoxygenase (5-LO) pathway and through free radical-catalyzed lipid peroxidation. The scheme also depicts isoprostanes acting on PGH_2/TXA_2 receptors

noids, including leukotrienes (LTs) originating via the 5-lipoxygenase pathway and isoprostanes produced by a non-cyclooxygenase mechanism involving free-radical-catalyzed peroxidation of arachidonic acid (Fig. 2). What follows is a brief outline of current knowledge on their formation in humans and the availability of analytical methods for their measurement.

Sulfidopeptide leukotrienes

The sulfidopeptide LTC_4, LTD_4 and LTE_4 are potent mediators of smooth muscle cell contraction and may be responsible for a wide variety of disorders, including bronchoconstriction in asthma, vasoconstriction in cardiovascular disease, or vasopermeation such as that observed in inflammatory or allergic syndromes (reviewed in [52]). The role of leukotrienes in diseases has been suspected mainly because of their pharmacologic properties. Assessment of their production *in vivo*, in relationship to disease states, should provide insight into their pathophysiologic significance.

Both LTE_4 and its ω- and β-oxidation products have been identified in urine, following the infusion of LTC_4 [53] or LTE_4 [54] in healthy subjects. We recently measured the excretion of LTE_4 during the infusion of exogenous LTC_4 over a 25-fold dose range to enable estimation of the rate of entry of endogenous LTC_4 into the bloodstream of normal humans [55]. Our results suggest that a) LTC_4 is produced at a low rate ($0.06\ pmol/kg \cdot min^{-1}$) under physiologic circumstances and is rapidly converted in the vasculature to LTE_4; b) changes in the urinary excretion of LTE_4 may reliably reflect short-term changes in the rate of secretion of LTC_4; and c) measurement of the ω- and β-oxidation products may reflect long-term changes in cysteinyl leukotriene biosynthesis [55]. Both RIA and EIA methods have been described for measurement of urinary LTE_4 and all reagents are commercially available [55]. It is still unclear to what extent urinary LTE_4 excretion may reflect leukocyte activation and/or the process of transcellular metabolism of neutrophil-derived LTA_4 by other cells endowed with glutathione-S-transferase (e. g. platelets, endothelial cells) [56].

Isoprostanes

Recently, Morrow et al [2] have discovered that there is a unique class of PGF_2-like compounds that are formed *in vitro* from arachidonyl-containing lipids in plasma by a free-radical catalyzed mechanism. These prostanoids are also produced *in vivo* in humans by a similar non-cyclooxygenase mechanism. Levels of these PGF_2 compounds detected by a GC/MS assay in normal human plasma and urine range from approximately 5–50 pg/ml and 500–3000 pg/mg creatinine, respectively. Circulating levels of these compounds were shown to increase by as much as 200-fold in animal models of free radical-induced lipid peroxidation [2]. These findings suggest that quantification of these prostanoids may provide a new approach to assessing oxidative stress *in vivo* in humans [57].

One of these PGF_2-like compounds, 8-epi-$PGF_{2\alpha}$, has been further characterized and shown to be a potent pre-glomerular vasoconstrictor, acting principally through TXA_2 receptor activation [58]. Thus, the beneficial effects of PGH_2/TXA_2 receptor antagonists may be related not only to blockade of vasoconstrictor products of PGH-synthases but also to partial interference with this novel pathway (Fig. 2). Besides the original GC/MS method developed by Morrow et al [2], an EIA kit for 8-epi-$PGF_{2\alpha}$ has recently become commercially available from Cayman Chemical Company.

RIA methods are currently being developed by several laboratories. Given the large series of compounds potentially originating via lipid peroxidation of arachidonic acid, the specificity of EIA and RIA methods for 8-epi-$PGF_{2\alpha}$ should be accurately verified through a comparison with GC/MS determinations in the appropriate biological fluids. Furthermore, the potential *ex vivo* formation of these compounds in biological fluids containing lipids should be prevented by appropriate handling of the samples [57].

Acknowledgments

The expert editorial assistance of Alessandra Migliavacca is gratefully acknowledged.

References

[1] Smith WL. Prostanoid biosynthesis and mechanisms of action. Am J Physiol 1992; 263: F181–F191.

[2] Morrow JD, Hill KE, Burk RF et al. A series of prostaglandin F_2-like compounds are produced *in vivo* in humans by a non-cyclooxygenase, free radical-catalyzed mechanism. Proc Natl Acad Sci USA 1990; 87: 9383–9387.

[3] Smith WL, Marnett LJ, DeWitt DL. Prostaglandin and thromboxane biosynthesis. Pharmacol Ther 1991; 49: 153–179.

[4] FitzGerald GA. Mechanism of platelet activation: Thromboxane A_2 as an amplifying signal for other agonists. Am J Cardiol 1991; 68: 11B–15B.

[5] Patrignani P, Filabozzi P, Catella F et al. Differential effects of dazoxiben, a selective thromboxane synthase inhibitor on platelet and renal prostaglandin-endoperoxide metabolism. J Pharm Exp Ther 1984; 228: 472–477.

[6] Morinelli TA, Halushka PV. Thromboxane A_2/prostaglandin H_2 receptors, characterization and antagonism. Trends Cardiovasc Med 1991; 1: 157–161.

[7] Hirata M, Hayashi Y, Ushikubi F et al. Cloning and expression of cDNA for a human thromboxane A_2 receptor. Nature 1991; 389: 617–620.
[8] Ishii H, Umeda F, Nawata H. Platelet function in diabetes mellitus. Diabetes/Metabolism Reviews 1992; 8: 53–66.
[9] Patrono C, Ciabattoni G, Pinca E et al. Low-dose aspirin and inhibition of thromboxane B_2 production in healthy subjects. Thromb Res 1980; 17: 317–327.
[10] Alessandrini P, Avogaro P, Bittolo Bon G et al. Physiologic variables affecting thromboxane production in human whole blood. Thromb Res 1985; 37: 1–8.
[11] Patrono C, Ciabattoni G, Pugliese F et al. Estimated rate of thromboxane secretion into the circulation of normal humans. J Clin Invest 1986; 77: 590–594.
[12] Halushka PV, Rogers RC, Loadholt CB et al. Increased platelet thromboxane synthesis in diabetes mellitus. J Lab Clin Med 1981; 97: 87–96.
[13] Lagarde M, Burtin M, Berciaud P et al. Increase of platelet thromboxane A_2 formation and its plasmatic half-life in diabetes mellitus. Thromb Res 1980; 19: 823–830.
[14] Davì G, Rini GB, Averna M et al. Thromboxane B_2 formation and platelet sensitivity to prostacyclin in insulin-dependent and insulin-independent diabetics. Thromb Res 1982; 26: 359–370.
[15] Mayfield RK, Halushka PV, Wohltmann HJ et al. Platelet function during continuous insulin infusion treatment in insulin-dependent diabetic patients. Diabetes 1985; 34: 1127–1133.
[16] Abbate R, Pinto S, Panetta A et al. Platelet synthesis of cyclooxygenase and lipoxygenase products in type I and type II diabetes. Prostaglandins Leukot Essent Fatty Acids 1988; 31: 9–15.
[17] Davì G, Catalano I, Averna M et al. Thromboxane biosynthesis and platelet function in type II diabetes mellitus. N Engl J Med 1990; 322: 1769–1774.
[18] FitzGeral GA, Pedersen AK, Patrono C. Analysis of prostacyclin and thromboxane biosynthesis in cardiovascular disease. Circulation 1983; 67: 1174–1177.
[19] Ciabattoni G, Patrignani P, Patrono C. Radioimmunoassay of 11-dehydrothromboxane B_2. Methods Enzymol 1990; 187: 34–42.
[20] Catella F, FitzGerald GA. Measurement of thromboxane metabolites by gas chromatography-mass spectrometry. Methods Enzymol 1990; 187: 42–50.
[21] Catella F, Healy D, Lawson JA et al. 11-dehydrothromboxane B_2: A quantitative index of thromboxane A_2 formation in the human circulation. Proc Natl Acad Sci USA 1986; 83: 5861–5865.
[22] Alessandrini P, Mcrae J, Geman S et al. Thromboxane biosynthesis and platelet function in type I diabetes mellitus. N Engl J Med 1988; 319: 208–212.
[23] Ciabattoni G, Pugliese F, Davì G et al. Fractional conversion of thromboxane B_2 to urinary 11-dehydro-thromboxane B_2 in man. Biochim Biophys Acta 1989; 992: 66–70.
[24] Catella F, FitzGerald GA. Paired analysis of urinary thromboxane B_2 metabolites in humans. Thromb Res 1987; 47: 647–656.
[25] Katayama S, Inaba M, Maruno Y et al. Increased renal TXA_2 synthesis in diabetes mellitus: simultaneous determination of urinary TXB_2 and 2,3-dinor-TXB_2. Prostaglandins Leukot Essent Fatty Acids 1990; 39: 47–51.
[26] Arita H, Nakano T, Hanasaki K. Thromboxane A_2: Its generation and role in platelet activation. Progr Lipid Res 1989; 28: 273–301.
[27] Dorn GW, Dejesus A. Human platelet aggregation and shape change are coupled to separate thromboxane A_2-prostaglandin H_2 receptors. Am J Physiol 1991; 260: H327–H334.
[28] Bunting SR, Gryglewski R, Moncada S et al. Arterial walls generate from prostaglandin endoperoxides a substance (prostaglandin X) which relaxes strips of mesenteric and coeliac arteries and inhibits platelet aggregation. Prostaglandins 1976; 12: 897–913.
[29] Murray R, FitzGerald GA. Regulation of thromboxane receptor activation in human platelets. Proc Natl Acad Sci USA 1989; 86: 124–128.
[30] Yamaguchi A, Suzuki H, Tanoue K et al. Simple method of aequorin loading into platelets using dimethyl sulfoxide. Thromb Res 1986; 44: 165–174.

[31] Bergh CH, Hjalmarson H, Holm G et al. Studies on calcium exchange and uptake in human diabetes. Eur J Clin Invest 1988; 18: 92–97.
[32] Hla T, Neilson K. Human cyclooxygenase-2 cDNA. Proc Natl Acad Sci USA 1992; 89: 7384–7388.
[33] Marcus AJ, Weksler BB, Jaffe EA et al. Synthesis of prostacyclin from platelet-derived endoperoxides by cultured human endothelial cells. J Clin Invest 1980; 66: 979–986.
[34] Thiemermann C. Biosynthesis and interaction of endothelium-derived vasoactive mediators. Eicosanoids 1991; 4: 187–202.
[35] FitzGerald GA, Smith B, Pedersen AK et al. Increased prostacyclin biosynthesis in patients with severe atherosclerosis and platelet activation. N Engl J Med 1984; 310: 1065–1068.
[36] Vallance P, Calver A, Collier J. The vascular endothelium in diabetes and hypertension. J Hypertension 1992; 10 (Suppl. 1): S25–S29.
[37] Silberbauer K, Schernthaner G, Sinzinger H et al. Decreased vascular prostacyclin in juvenile-onset diabetes. N Engl J Med 1979; 300: 366–367.
[38] FitzGerald GA, Brash AR, Falardeau P et al. Estimated rate of prostacyclin secretion into the circulation of normal man. J Clin Invest 1981; 68: 1272–1276.
[39] Weksler BB, Pett SB, Alonso D et al. Differential inhibition by aspirin of vascular and platelet prostaglandin synthesis in atherosclerotic patients. N Engl J Med 1983; 308: 800–805.
[40] Patrono C, Pugliese F, Ciabattoni G et al. Evidence for a direct stimulatory effect of prostacyclin on renin release in man. J Clin Invest 1982; 69: 231–239.
[41] Ciabattoni G, Boss AH, Daffonchio L et al. Radioimmunoassay measurement of 2,3-dinor-metabolites of prostacyclin and thromboxane in human urine. Adv Prost Thromb Leuk Res 1987; 17: 598–602.
[42] Patrono C. Aspirin as an antiplatelet drug. N Engl J Med, 1994; 330: 1287–1294.
[43] Patrono C, Davì G. Antiplatelet agents in the prevention of diabetic vascular complications. Diabetes/Metabolism Reviews, 1993; 9: 177–188.
[44] Schlondorff D. Renal prostaglandin synthesis: sites of production and specific actions of prostaglandins. Am J Med 1986; 81: 1–11.
[45] Remuzzi G, FitzGerald GA, Patrono C. Thromboxane synthesis and action within the kidney. Kidney Int 1992; 41: 1483–1493.
[46] Patrono C, Dunn MJ. The clinical significance of inhibition of renal prostaglandin synthesis. Kidney Int 1987; 32: 1–12.
[47] Patrono C, Ciabattoni G, Remuzzi G et al. Functional significance of renal prostacyclin and thromboxane A_2 production in patients with systemic lupus erythematosus. J Clin Invest 1985; 76: 1011–1018.
[48] Ciabattoni G, Boss AH, Patrignani P et al. Effects of sulindac on renal and extrarenal eicosanoid synthesis. Clin Pharmac Ther 1987; 41: 380–383.
[49] Ciabattoni G, Pugliese F, Spaldi M et al. Radioimmunoassay measurement of prostaglandins E_2 and $F_{2\alpha}$ in human urine. J Endocrinol Invest 1979; 2: 173–179.
[50] Pradelles P, Grassi J, Maclouf J. Enzyme immunoassays of eicosanoids using acetylcholinesterase. Methods Enzymol 1990; 187: 24–34.
[51] Catella F, Lawson JA, Fitzgerald DJ et al. Endogenous biosynthesis of arachidonic acid epoxides in humans: increased formation in pregnancy-induced hypertension. Proc Natl Acad Sci USA 1990; 87: 5893–5897.
[52] Lewis RA, Austen KF, Soberman RJ. Leukotrienes and other products of the 5-lipoxygenase pathway: biochemistry and relation to pathobiology in human diseases. N Engl J Med 1990; 323: 645–655.
[53] Orning L, Kaijsier L, Hammarstrom S. *In vivo* metabolism of leukotriene C_4 in man: urinary excretion of leukotriene E_4. Biochem Biophys Res Commun 1985; 130: 214–220.
[54] Sala A, Voelkel N, Maclouf J et al. LTE_4 elimination and metabolism in normal human subjects. J Biol Chem 1990; 265: 21771–21778.
[55] Maclouf J, Antoine C, De Caterina R et al. Entry rate and metabolism of leukotriene C_4 into vascular compartment in healthy subjects. Am J Physiol 1992; 263: H244–H249.

[56] Maclouf JA, Murphy RC. Transcellular metabolism of neutrophil-derived leukotriene A_4 by human platelets. A potential cellular source of leukotriene C_4. J Biol Chem 1988; 263: 174–181.
[57] Morrow JD, Roberts LJ. Quantification of non-cyclooxygenase derived prostanoids as a marker of oxidative stress. Free Radic Biol Med 1991; 10: 195–200.
[58] Takahashi K, Nammour TM, Fukunaga M et al. Glomerular actions of a free radical-generated novel prostaglandin, 8-epi-prostaglandin $F_{2\alpha}$, in the rat. Evidence for interaction with thromboxane A_2 receptors. J Clin Invest 1992; 90: 136–141.

Measurement of components of the renin angiotensin system in humans: relationship with diabetic complications and antihypertensive treatment

F. H. M. Derkx, J. A. M. J. L. Janssen, M. A. D. H. Schalekamp

Biochemistry of the renin angiotensin system

Renin is synthesized via preprorenin and prorenin, and is stored in cytoplasmatic granules of the juxtaglomerular cells in the kidney, where it can be secreted on demand [1, 2]. The secretion of prorenin does not seem to occur in a regulated fashion but rather constitutively by the extrusion of juvenile granules [3].

Plasma from bilaterally nephrectomized subjects contains little or no renin, whereas the concentration of prorenin can be as high as in normal individuals [4]. Thus, plasma renin originates from the kidney, whereas a large proportion of plasma prorenin originates from extrarenal sites. Synthesis of prorenin is known to occur in the reproductive organs and in the adrenal gland [5].

The spatial conformation of renin shows a bilobar structure. The two lobes are separated by a deep cleft containing the enzyme's active site [6]. In prorenin, the active site is covered by the carboxyl terminus of the prosegment. Prorenin is generally considered to be a relatively inactive zymogen although it may have some degree of intrinsic activity against angiotensinogen as judged from its ability to specifically bind active site-directed renin inhibitors [7].

Prorenin can be activated in vitro by a number of proteases, such as trypsin, plasmin, tissue-type plasminogen activator and plasma kallikrein, which causes the prosegment to be cleaved from the renin part of the molecule [8]. There is no direct evidence to support the claim that prorenin-to-renin conversion takes place in the circulation.

Prorenin can also be activated by exposure to low pH or low temperature [9, 10]. Both acid- and cryo-activation are reversible at pH 7.4 and 37 °C, because, in this case, cleavage of the prosegment does not occur. Non-proteolytic activation of prorenin is caused by a conformational change, by which the cleft is uncovered so that the scissile bond of angiotensinogen can obtain access to the active site. Incubation of prorenin with active site-directed renin inhibitors also induces a conformational change of prorenin, which can be detected by a monoclonal antibody that recognizes active renin but not inactive prorenin [7]. This observation may provide a model for substrate-mediated activation of prorenin and suggests that some "open forms" may have proteolytic activity.

Renin is a highly selective protease that only hydrolyses a specific substrate, angiotensinogen, to release angiotensin Ang I (Fig. 1). Angiotensinogen is an α-2 globulin synthesized mainly by the liver, but it is also synthesized in extrahepatic tissues such as brain and kidney [1]. The decapeptide Ang I (Ang 1-10) is converted to Ang II (Ang 1-8) by angiotensin I converting

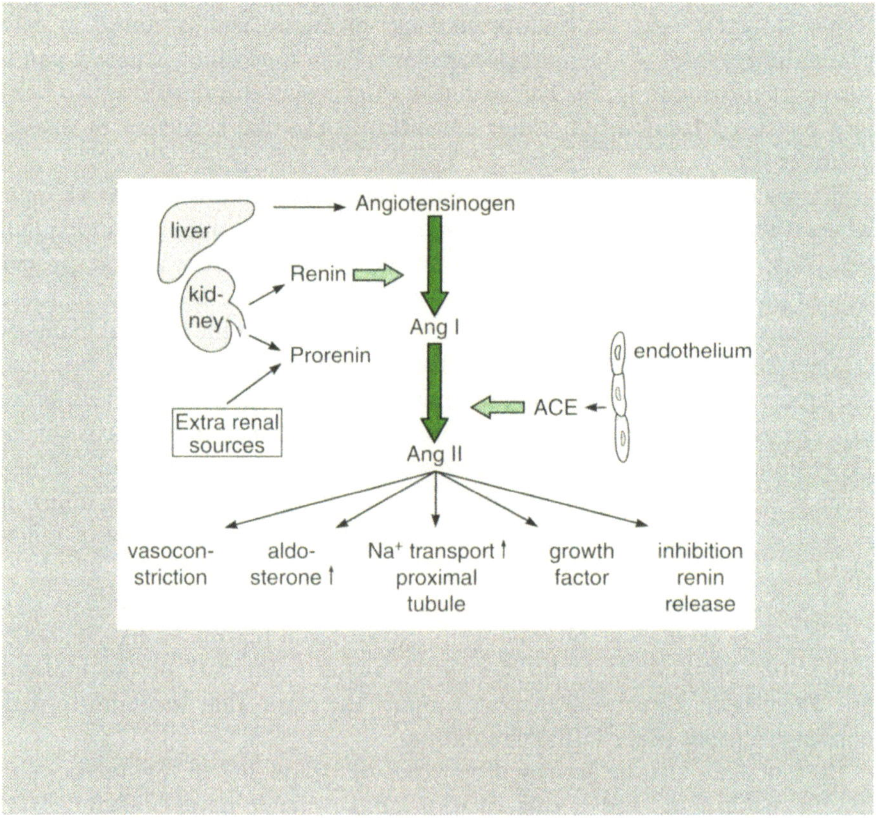

Fig. 1 The components of the renin angiotensin system. Ang I = angiotensin I, Ang II = angiotensin II. ACE = angiotensin converting enzyme

enzyme (ACE), a dipeptidyl carboxypeptidase, located on the plasma membrane of endothelial cells. This zinc-dependent enzyme is identical to kininase II, a bradykinin-degrading protease.

The Ang II thus formed is transported to peripheral tissues where its binds to specific receptors on target cells. Ang II is converted to smaller inactive peptide fragments by a series of aminopeptidases, also summarized under the general term of angiotensinases. The plasma half life of Ang II is 15−30 seconds. Some of the Ang I and II peptide fragments Ang 2-8 (Ang III) and Ang 1-7 may serve physiological functions [11].

Because the cleavage of the Leu10-Val11 bond of angiotensinogen by renin is the first rate limiting step in the formation of Ang II, a highly potent vasoconstrictor and aldosterone-releasing hormone, renin is a key hormone in blood pressure regulation and sodium and water homeostasis. Ang II also has other functions, which are summarized in Table 1.

Table 1 Actions of angiotensin II

Tissue or organ	Effect
Smooth muscle cell	Constriction, hypertrophy, mitogenic activity
Blood vessels	Neovascularization
Adrenal cortex	Aldosterone synthesis
Adrenal medulla	Catecholamines secretion
Kidney	Constriction efferent more than afferent
	Increase filtration fraction
	Mesangial contraction
	Increase tubular sodium transport
	Inhibition renin release
Heart	Hypertrophy. positive inotropy
Brain	Thirst, NaCl apatite
Anterior pituitary	Inhibition release AVP and ACTH
Autonomic nervous system	Presynaptic facilitation release catecholamines
Reproductive organs	Steroidgenesis

The primary mechanisms regulating the renal release of renin are: 1. a baroreceptor sensor in the afferent arteriole, and 2. NaCl delivery to the region of the macula densa of the renal tubule [1, 2]. Renal renin is secreted into the circulation in response to a fall in blood pressure and following a decreased delivery of sodium to the macula densa. The renin-secreting juxtaglomerular cells have adrenoceptors on their surface and activation of these receptors stimulates renin secretion by stimulation of β1-adrenoceptors on the juxtaglomerular cells. Local factors that may stimulate renin release are kinins and prostaglandins. Renin secretion is inhibited by elevation of blood pressure, by high sodium delivery to the macula densa, by β1-adrenoceptor blockade and by Ang II, atrial natriuretic peptide and vasopressin.

All the components of the renin angiotensin system have been identified in various tissues by a variety of techniques, including immunohistochemistry and modern molecular biological methodology [1, 2, 12]. The renin angiotensin system acts both as a classical circulating endocrine system and as an autocrine or paracrine system [12, 13]. The formation of Ang I at tissues sites in extrarenal tissues appears to depend both on kidney-derived renin and, in some organs, on in situ synthesized renin [14, 15].

A substantial fraction of Ang I in circulating plasma is derived from Ang I that is generated at tissues sites, whereas virtually all Ang II in plasma is derived from circulating Ang I [16–18].

Enzyme-kinetic and immunological assays of renin and prorenin

It seems logical to use the plasma level of Ang II as a measure of the activity of the renin angiotensin system in vivo. However, the plasma level of Ang II is low. The antibodies that are used are insufficiently sensitive to measure subnormal levels of Ang II accurately, and most Ang II antibodies crossreact with Ang I and some degradation peptides of Ang I or II. Plasma Ang II measurements are therefore not widely used.

Most laboratories use the enzyme-kinetic assays of renin to assess the activity of the renin angiotensin system. The assays are highly sensitive and it is possible to measure renin accurately, despite its low level in plasma. The plasma concentration of renin is in the order of picomoles/l [1, 2, 4]. The concentration of prorenin in normal plasma is about ten times the concentration of renin [4]. Until the development of monoclonal renin antibodies, it was not possible to measure the low renin levels in plasma directly by an immunological assay.

Enzyme-kinetic assay of renin

In the so-called plasma renin activity (PRA) assay plasma samples are incubated at 37 °C for periods up to 3 h and in some cases for longer periods. The amount of Ang I generated during incubation from endogenous angiotensinogen is measured by radioimmunoassay [19, 20].

A number of factors may influence the PRA assay results:

Physiological factors: The plasma level of renin is strongly influenced by factors that interfere with the control of the release of renin from the kidney.

Such factors are, for example, sodium intake, posture, menstrual cycle, pregnancy and drugs (Table 2). These factors should be strictly controlled to ensure interpretable results.

Table 2 Physiological and pharmacological factors affecting the plasma level of renin and prorenin

Factor	Effect on plasma renin or prorenin
Sodium intake	Decrease renin and prorenin as sodium intake increases and vice versa
Posture	Upright 2-fold increase and sitting 1.5-fold increase of renin as compared to 45 min supine. No or small effect on prorenin
Blood pressure	Acute fall in blood pressure increases renin no effect prorenin and vice versa. (see antihypertensive drugs)
Age	Decrease renin and prorenin
Race	Low renin and prorenin in blacks
Menstrual cycle	Increase in prorenin in early luteal phase
Pregnancy	Increase prorenin, renin, angiotensinogen
Oral contraceptives	Decrease prorenin, renin, increase angiotensinogen
Antihypertensive drugs	
Diuretics, ACE inhibitors vasodilators, α blockers spironolactone	Increase renin and prorenin
clonidine, α-methyl DOPA	Decrease renin and prorenin
β blockers	Decrease renin, prorenin may increase
Ca-antagonists	No effect or small increase

Renin substrate concentration: The K_m of the reaction of human renin with human angiotensinogen is 1.25 μM and the normal angiotensinogen concentration is approximately 1 μM [20–22]. Ang I generation in the PRA assay therefore depends on both renin and angiotensinogen concentrations. Angiotensinogen concentration is increased during pregnancy and is also increased in women taking oral contraceptives [22]. This leads to an "overestimation" of renin when PRA is used as a measure of its concentration [19, 20, 22]. Besides oestrogens, glucocorticoids and thyroid hormone increase angiotensinogen [23]. Angiotensinogen is also elevated after bilateral nephrectomy. Low angiotensinogen concentrations are found in patients with liver disease, adrenal insufficiency or during ACE inhibitor treatment.

To avoid these problems it is possible to run parallel samples with known quantities of a human kidney renin standard. The renin concentration (pg/ml) can also be calculated by entering PRA (pmol Ang I/ml/h), angiotensinogen (pmol/ml) and K_m (pmol/ml) in the Michaelis Menten equation to determine V_{max} (pmolAng I/h per pg of renin) [22].

An alternative approach for measuring renin concentration is to add saturating amounts of purified exogenous angiotensinogen from human or animal sources [21, 24]. This is the so-called plasma renin concentration (PRC) method. We use substrate prepared from plasma of nephrectomized ewes. The K_m of the reaction of human renin with sheep angiotensinogen is four to five times lower than the K_m of the reaction of human renin with human angiotensinogen [21, 22]. The V_{max} of the reaction of human renin with sheep substrate at neutral pH is three times higher than the V_{max} of the reaction of human renin with human substrate. Thus the sensitivity of the renin assay is increased by using sheep angiotensinogen.

Standardization of the renin assay: Despite the fact that pure recombinant human renin is now available, the renin standard 68/356 prepared from human cadaver kidney introduced in 1974 is still used [25]. Each ampule of this standard contains 188.7 mg of the International Reference Preparation 68/356 and is equivalent to 0.1 U. One μU of this standard is approximately 1 pg pure renin [22, 25].

Activation of prorenin during processing of the plasma samples: Prorenin can be activated when it is exposed to low temperature. In a purified system cryoactivation of prorenin is a unimolecular non-proteolytic process. Prorenin activated in this way again becomes inactive after incubation at 37 °C [10]. In crude plasma however, non-proteolytically activated prorenin is irreversibly activated to renin by the endogenous factor XII-kallikrein pathway [26].

Inadvertent cryoactivation results in an overestimation of the in vivo level of plasma renin and in an underestimation of the in vivo level of prorenin [22]. This is especially a problem in plasma samples with high levels of prorenin and low or normal levels of renin. The combination of low plasma renin and high prorenin is seen in pregnant women, in ovarian-stimulated women, and in diabetic patients. In plasma from patients with very low renin, for instance in Conn's syndrome and after bilateral nephrectomy, inadvertent cryoactivation can also cause falsely higher renin levels.

To avoid these problems, blood and plasma should be handled at room temperature. Plasma can be stored at −20 °C or lower. Frozen plasma samples should be thawed rapidly and not placed on ice or in a refrigerator prior to assay.

pH of the assay: The pH optimum for the reaction of human renin with human angiotensinogen is about pH 5.7 [19, 21]. One prefers to perform the assay at this pH rather than at neutral pH, in order to increase Ang I generation. The pH is often adjusted to 5.7 by adding maleic acid to plasma [19].

If one prefers to perform the assay at neutral pH, one has to be aware of the fact that pH may increase from 7.4 to 7.9 or higher during incubation for 3 hours. The rate of Ang I generation decreases at these higher pH values, and renin is destroyed at pH 8 or higher [19–20]. Stabilization of pH to 7.4 is possible by adding imidazole buffer prior to incubation [14]. Aliquots to measure Ang I should be taken after different time periods of incubation to ensure linear Ang I generation. Blanks at zero time incubation should be included in order to correct for non-specific substances.

Pseudorenins: Cathepsin D and other enzymes are capable to generate Ang I at pH 5.7 but much less so at pH 7.4 [20]. To differentiate between these pseudorenins and true renin one can use highly specific renin inhibitors that inhibit renin in the nanomolar range and have no effect on pseudo renins [27].

Breakdown of angiotensin I: During incubation of plasma at 37 °C, Ang I is rapidly converted to Ang II by ACE and some of it is broken down to smaller peptide fragments by angiotensinases. Several enzyme inhibitors are used to inhibit ACE and angiotensinase activity without interfering with the reaction of renin with its substrate [19–23]. We use a combination of 8-hydroxyquinoline sulphate 3.4 mM, phenylmethylsulfonyl fluoride 1.4 mM, aprotinin 100 Kallikrein inhibiting units/ml and EDTA 5 mM (final concentrations). Neomycine sulphate 1 mg/ml is added to prevent destruction of Ang I by bacteria.

Another possibility for inhibiting Ang I breakdown is to add high concentrations of Ang I antibodies. This is the so-called antibody trapping technique [28].

In patients treated with a renin inhibitor, one encounters a special problem with the use of angiotensinase inhibitors in the PRA assay because the inhibitors may displace the renin inhibitor from protein binding sites. This causes an increase in the free fraction of the renin inhibitor and an overestimation of the in vivo inhibition of renin [29].

Enzyme-kinetic assay of prorenin

Prorenin can only be measured with the enzyme-kinetic assay after its conversion to renin. The implicit assumption that in vitro activated prorenin has the same K_m and V_{max} as naturally occurring renin appears to be correct [21,

22]. Prorenin can be activated in vitro 1. by exposure to low temperature, 2. by exposure to low pH, and 3. by proteolytic enzymes [19–24]. Incubation of prorenin at neutral pH and 4 °C (cryoactivation) leads to slow and incomplete activation. Incubation of prorenin at pH 3.3 and 4 °C for 24 h (acid-activation) leads to more complete activation. A problem with these methods for activation is not only that the activation is not complete, but also that it is possibly reversible during the incubation with angiotensinogen. These procedures result therefore in gross underestimations of the true amount of prorenin.

For the proteolytic activation of prorenin, most laboratories are now using trypsin. The concentration of trypsin added to the plasma samples ranges from 0.25 to 5 mg/ml for optimal prorenin activation. These high trypsin concentration are required because of the presence of protease inhibitors in plasma. However, at these high trypsin concentrations, some prorenin and renin may be destroyed, which leads to erroneously low results. Trypsin may also attack renin substrate and may interfere with the radioimmunoassay of Ang I. Trypsin activity must therefore be blocked by adding a serine protease inhibitor prior to the incubation with renin substrate. We developed an assay of prorenin, in which prorenin is converted to renin by Sepharose-bound trypsin, which can be quantitatively removed by centrifugation prior to the incubation step [21].

Immunological assay of renin

Monoclonal antibodies with different affinity constants for renin and of prorenin are available and allowed Simon et al [30] to design an immunoradiometric assay for renin in plasma. There are now two commercially-available kits for the immunoradiometric assay of renin. The first kit (Diagnostics Pasteur, Marnes de La Coquette, France) uses, as a primary antibody an antibody that recognizes both renin and prorenin and is coupled to polyacrylamide-agarose beads containing ferrous oxide (Magnogel). With this antibody, renin and prorenin in the plasma samples are bound to the Magnogel beads. Bound renin is then measured with a secondary radiolabeled antibody that recognizes renin but does not cross-react with inactive prorenin. Bound and free radioactivity are separated by means of a magnetic ruler placed in close contact with the tubes.

A similar sandwich-type immunoradiometric renin assay (Nichols Institute, Wychen, Netherlands) has recently been introduced [31]. In this assay, the primary antibody is conjugated covalently to biotin and the secondary antibody, which is radiolabeled, is again specific for renin. Free and bound radioactive antibody can be easily separated by using avidin-coated polystyrene beads.

Most of the problems mentioned in the section on the enzyme kinetic assay of renin are circumvented by using immunoradiometric assays. Inadvertent cryoactivation however, remains a problem. Results of the two types of assays show a good correlation but, in the immunoradiometric assay the intra- and interassay variability is rather high in plasma samples with low renin content [32].

Plasma may contain truncated forms of prorenin in addition to fully inactive prorenin [33]. Antibody reacting with renin, and not with inactive prorenin, may show cross-reactivity with these truncated forms of prorenin and this may lead to some discrepancy between the results of the immunoradiometric assay and the enzyme-kinetic assay [32].

Immunological assay of prorenin

Several groups have reported on a sensitive immunoradiometric assay for total renin (renin plus prorenin). In these assays both the primary and secondary monoclonal antibodies recognize renin as well as prorenin [22, 34]. Prorenin can also be measured with an immunoradiometric assay in which the secondary antibody is renin-specific. In the latter type of assay, prorenin has to be converted to renin prior to the assay.

We observed that active site-directed low molecular weight renin inhibitors induce a conformational change in the prorenin molecule, which also occurs during the proteolytic activation of prorenin. The inhibitor-"activated" prorenin is detected by a monoclonal antibody that reacts with renin and not with inactive prorenin [7]. This observation was the basis of developing a novel immunoradiometric assay of prorenin [32]. In this assay plasma is incubated with renin inhibitor Ro 42-5892 (Remikiren, Hoffmann La Roche, Basel, Switzerland), in a final concentration of 100 μmol/l, for 24 h at 4 °C. This leads to the complete conversion of prorenin into the form that is recognized by the secondary antibody, which recognizes renin and not inactive prorenin.

Monoclonal antibodies directed against synthetic peptides corresponding with the C-terminal portion of the prorenin prosegment have been developed [35] and it may possible to use such antibodies to measure activated forms of prorenin in plasma.

Measurements of angiotensinogen, ACE and angiotensins

The enzyme-kinetic assay of plasma angiotensinogen is based on the maximal amount of Ang I that is generated during incubation with added renin, and the generated Ang I is measured by RIA [23]. A direct immunological assay of angiotensinogen has also been described [36]. The latter method gives higher results because the antibody reacts with both des-Ang-I-angiotensinogen and complete angiotensinogen.

ACE is measured with an enzyme kinetic assays using synthetic substrates [36]. Since the active site of ACE contains zinc, it is important that no chelating agents are used when the blood samples are collected. ACE can also be measured with radioinhibitor binding assays [37]. These assays make use of radiolabeled inhibitors directed to the active site of ACE. The binding is saturable, reversible, and displaceable by non-radioactive ACE inhibitor in a concentration-dependent manner.

Plasma levels of Ang I and II are measured with RIA. It is mandatory to extract the angiotensins from plasma prior to RIA in order to prevent non-specific binding. In the past, many laboratories relied on measurements of crude plasma extracts. However, it is now realized that such crude methods can greatly overestimate the true angiotensin levels [38]. Separation of the angiotensin peptides from the plasma extracts, for example by high-performance liquid chromatography, yields more accurate results.

The pitfalls encountered when measuring plasma Ang I and II are discussed elsewhere [39]. Ang II antibodies may cross-react with Ang I and with degradation products of Ang I and, depending on the method used, the concentration of "true Ang II" is only approximately 50% of "immunoreactive" Ang II [38]. This is important in situations where Ang II is low and Ang I is high, such as is the case after treatment with ACE inhibitor. A major problem is the continued ex vivo formation and breakdown of Ang I and II during blood sampling and during handling of the samples prior to RIA. Blood for Ang I or II measurements must be rapidly drawn with syringes already containing inhibitors of renin, ACE and angiotensinases.

The renin angiotensin system in patients with diabetes mellitus

Renin

Low, normal or high PRA has been reported in patients with type I or type II diabetes mellitus [40, 41]. Numerous confounding factors may explain part of the discrepancies (see Table 2). In carefully performed studies, PRA is often on the low side in diabetics, and this is usually interpreted as evidence of reduced renin secretion by the kidney. Factors that may contribute to abnormal renin secretion are: elevation of blood pressure, retention of sodium and water, the existance of autonomic diabetic neuropathy with decreased β-adrenoceptor-mediated renin release. Plasma levels of atrial natriuretic peptide may be increased in diabetics and this may contribute to a low renin state. Finally, the capacity of the kidneys to produce renin may be reduced because juxtaglomerular cells are damaged or destroyed by hyalinosis.

As depicted in Fig. 2, we also found somewhat lower levels of renin in type I diabetes patients no matter microvascular complications were present

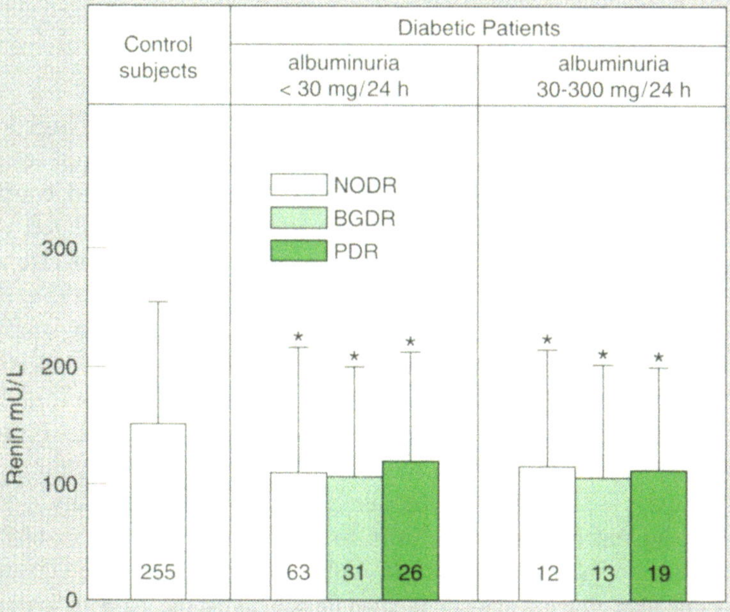

*Fig. 2 Plasma renin in diabetic patients with and without microalbuminuria (albuminuria 30–300 mg/24 h). The patients are subdivided into those without diabetic retinopathy (NODR), with background retinopathy (BGDR) and with proliferative retinopathy (PDR). Results are expressed as geometric mean times tolerance factor. * $p < 0.05$ for difference from control subjects. The numbers in the bar diagram refer to the numbers of patients. (Adapted from [42] and [43])*

or not [42]. Several groups reported somewhat higher levels of PRA in patients with increased albumin excretion [41]. As will be discussed below, prorenin is often elevated in diabetic patients with microvascular complications. It is possible that inadvertent activation during collection and the processing of plasma samples causes artifactually high PRA.

In normal subjects, an oral glucose load results in a small increase in plasma renin [41]. In patients with type I or II diabetes mellitus we found no correlation between plasma renin and blood glucose. We also did not observe a correlation with the degree of metabolic control of the diabetes as judged from the level of glycated hemoglobin A1c [43].

Hyperglycaemia with concomitant alterations in acid-base homeostasis may influence renin secretion and may contribute to the increased levels of renin, Ang II and aldosterone that are found in diabetic ketoacidosis [41].

Prorenin

Luetcher et al [44] were the first to report an association between a high level of plasma prorenin and the presence of microvascular diabetic complications in patients with longstanding diabetes mellitus. Our group could confirm these findings, and found that a high plasma prorenin was associated with the level of serum creatinine, with 24 h urinary albumin excretion rate and with the presence of diabetic retinopathy, retinopathy of the proliferative type in particular (Fig. 3) [42, 43]. Multiple logistic regression analysis showed that the association of the presence of retinopathy, increased albumin excretion, and increased serum creatinine were independent of confounding factors such as age, sex, duration of diabetes, blood glucose, HbA1c, insulin-dependency, and blood pressure. Moreover, the association with retinopathy was at least in part independent of the association with nephropathy.

The underlying mechanism that leads to a selective increase in plasma prorenin without an increase in renin in diabetics remains unclear. Usually, when the renin angiotensin system is stimulated, as is the case in patients with renal artery stenosis, after sodium deprivation or after ACE inhibitor treatment, both renin and prorenin are increased [4]. Under these circumstances, the increase in renin is more pronounced than the increase in prorenin, so that the percentage of total renin (renin + prorenin) that is in the active form rises from approximately 10% under normal conditions to levels as high as 50–60% under conditions of stimulated renin release (Fig. 4).

High plasma prorenin may be explained by increased renal or extrarenal synthesis, by reduced clearance or by a combination of the two. It has been proposed that coexisting autonomic neuropathy may lead to decreased secre-

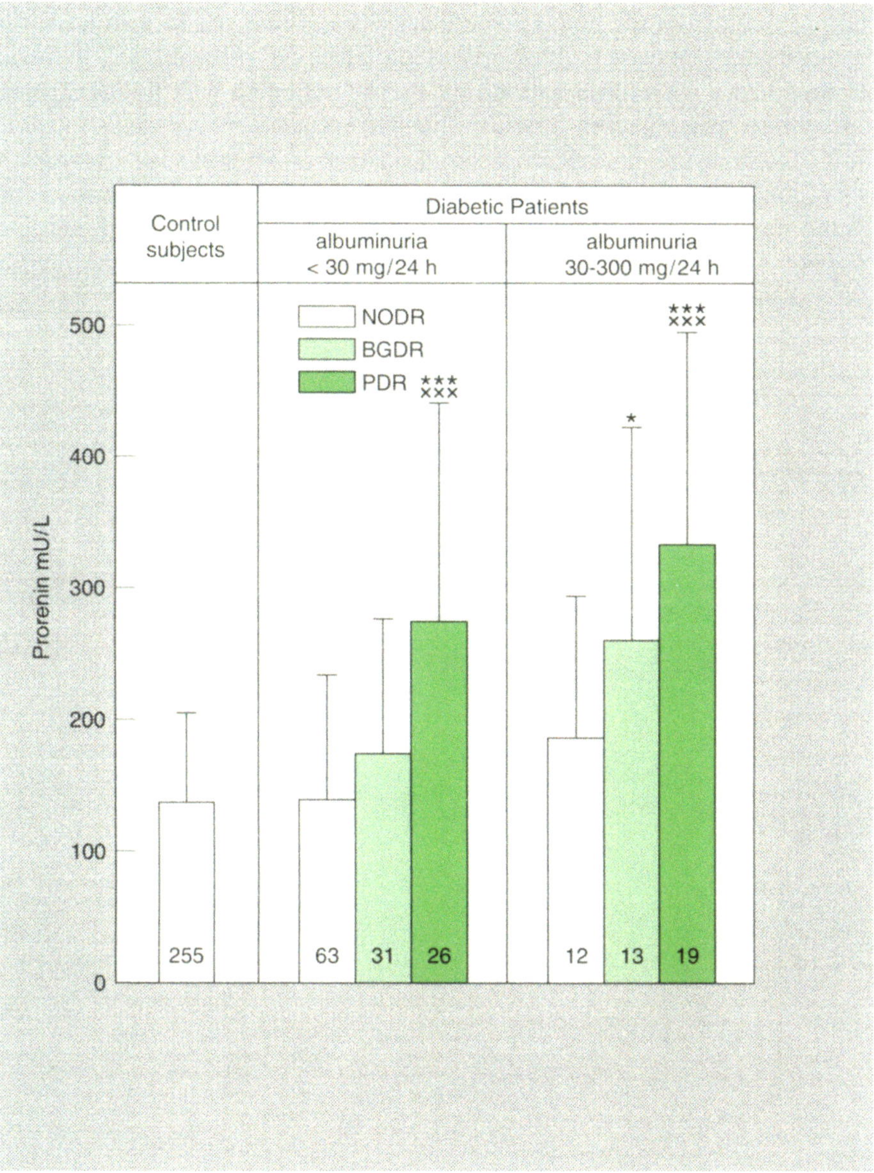

*Fig. 3 Plasma prorenin in diabetic patients with and without microalbuminuria (albuminuria 30–300 mg/24 h). The patients are subdivided into those without diabetic retinopathy (NODR), with background retinopathy (BGDR) and with proliferative retinopathy (PDR). Results are expressed as geometric mean times tolerance factor. x $p < 0.05$ for difference from diabetics without retinopathy, xxx $p < 0.001$ for difference from diabetics without retinopathy. *** $p < 0.001$ for difference from diabetics with background retinopathy. The numbers in the bar diagram refer to the numbers of patients. (Adapted from [42] and [43])*

tion of renin from the juxta-glomerular cells and that this in turn leads to a compensatory increase in the synthesis and release of prorenin [45]. In favour of this theory is the observation that during treatment with β-adrenoceptor antagonists, plasma renin concentration decreases whereas prorenin increases [46]. However, the increase in prorenin observed with β-blocker treatment is small and never reaches the values measured in diabetics. Furthermore, we found no association between elevated plasma prorenin and the presence of diabetic autonomic neuropathy and, more importantly, plasma prorenin is not elevated in non-diabetics with autonomic neuropathy [43].

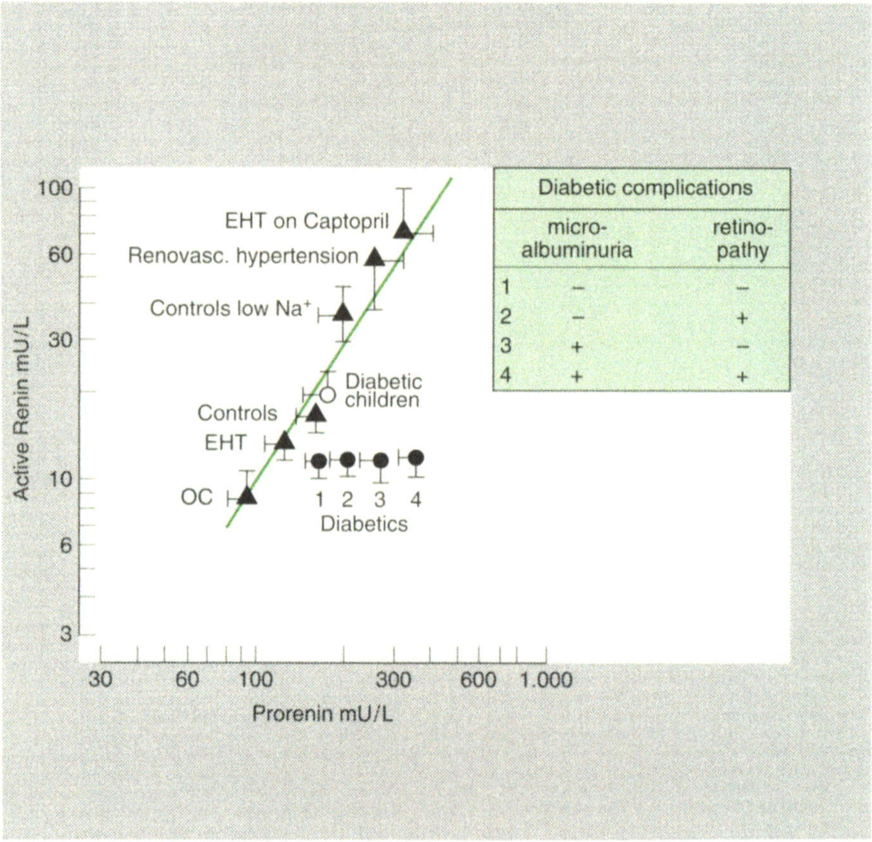

Fig. 4 Relationship between plasma levels of renin and prorenin in type I diabetics and in different other groups of patients. Data are expressed as geometric mean and SEM. EHT = essential hypertension. OC = women on oral contraceptives. Number of patients: diabetic, group 1, n = 63; group 2, n = 57; group 3, n = 12; group 4, n = 45; controls n = 250; controls on low sodium intake, n = 16; OC, n = 47; EHT, n = 66; EHT on captopril, n = 68, renovascular hypertension; n = 92. (Adapted from [4])

In order to collect more direct evidence in diabetics for increased release of prorenin from the kidney, we measured the plasma prorenin levels across the kidneys in diabetic patients with advanced nephropathy and proliferative retinopathy who were prepared for renal transplantation. The renal vein renin sampling was performed at the time of renal arteriography, prior to the injection of the contrast [43]. The renal vein-to-artery ratio of prorenin was not elevated in these patients, despite the fact that their peripheral plasma prorenin was grossly elevated and renal plasma flow was very low. The results therefore, do not support the idea that plasma prorenin was high in these patients exclusively because of increased release of prorenin from the kidney.

As mentioned, we observed an association between the plasma level of prorenin and the presence of diabetic retinopathy. Implantation of Ang II in the cornea of the rabbit leads to neovascularization originating from the limbus of the cornea [47]. Neovascularization is a hallmark of proliferative diabetic retinopathy and it is possible that local generation of Ang II in the eye may contribute to its pathogenesis.

We measured the prorenin levels in ocular vitreous fluid. Vitreous prorenin was up to 100 times higher than expected on the basis of its serum protein content (Fig. 5). In vitreous fluid obtained from patients with retinal detachment due to proliferative diabetic retinopathy, the prorenin-to-albumin ratio was significantly higher than in vitreous fluid from non-diabetic patients with spontaneous retinal detachment (Table 3) [48].

In the bovine eye, prorenin shows a gradient; posterior vitreous fluid > anterior vitreous fluid > aqueous humor, suggesting that the main source of extracellular prorenin is the posterior eye [27]. More direct evidence for intraocular production of prorenin (and possibly renin) is provided by the demon-

Table 3 Proteins in vitreous fluid of diabetics with proliferative retinopathy and in non-diabetics with spontaneous or traumatic retinal detachment

Protein		Vitrous fluid Nondiabetics (n = 16)	Diabetics (n = 15)
Prorenin	mU/L	34.5 (17.4–61.9)	61.0* (19.0–172)
Renin	mU/L	2.4 (0.9–6.4)	2.0 (nd–2.5)
Angiotensinogen	nmol/L	54.5 (3.0–630)	61.0 (7.0–1,000)
Albumin	g/L	1.55 (0.11–20.2)	1.51 (0.32–17.1)
IgG	g/L	0.19 (0.03–0.70)	0.19 (0.04–0.96)
Transferrin	g/L	0.18 (0.02–1.74)	0.14 (0.06–0.37)

Results are expressed as geometric mean and range. * $p < 0.001$ for difference from non-diabetics. (Adapted from [48])

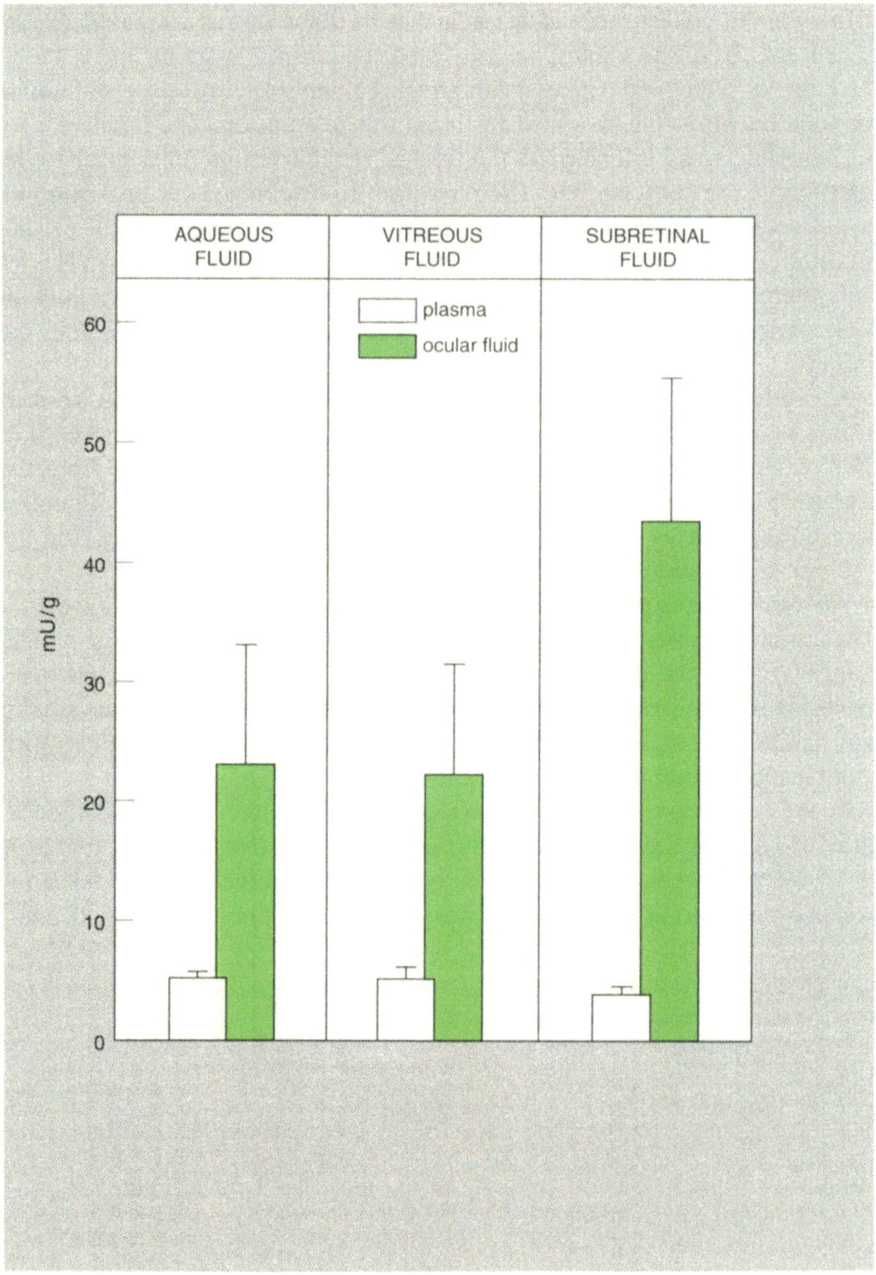

Fig. 5 Prorenin-to-albumin concentration ratio in ocular fluids and in plasma of non-diabetics. Results are expressed as mean ± SEM. Number of patients: aqueous fluid, n = 21; vitrous fluid, n = 16; subretinal fluid, n = 18. (Adapted from [48])

stration of renin mRNA expression in the human eye, which was highest in the choroideal layer [48]. Angiotensinogen mRNA and ACE mRNA have also been detected in human eyes [49]. Thus, local production of prorenin and renin, with subsequent generation of Ang I and II in the eye may play a role in the pathogenesis of retinopathy.

Theoretically, one might speculate that eyes affected by diabetic retinopathy may release prorenin into the circulation and thus may contribute to an elevation of plasma prorenin. The blood flow, however, is only 0.4–0.5 ml/min per eye [50]. If indeed prorenin from the eye makes a substantial contribution to contribute to the level in circulating plasma, the veno-arterial gradient of prorenin across the eye must be very high. One would therefore expect to find high levels in some part of the eye, levels much higher than in the circulation. In normal bovine eyes at least, such high levels have not been found [27].

Studies on the clearance of prorenin in diabetics are not available. The normal half-life of renin in non-diabetic patients after bilateral nephrectomy is 10–30 min and for prorenin it is 60–120 min [4]. Because of this short half-life it is unlikely that non-enzymatic glycation of prorenin may explain the high prorenin levels in diabetics.

Enzymatic glycosylation, rather than non-enzymatic glycation, may influence the clearance of prorenin. Different enzymatically glycosylated forms of prorenin and renin have been demonstrated in the rat and such differences indeed influence the clearance rate of renin and prorenin from the circulation [51].

Angiotensinogen, ACE and Ang II

The plasma level of angiotensinogen appears to be normal in diabetics [41]. Studies on Ang II are scarce. Feldt-Rasmussen [52] found low immunoreactive Ang II levels in diabetic patients, and this was the case in patients both with or without nephropathy. In patients with diabetes mellitus, ACE activity in serum has been reported to be about up to two times the normal values particularly in diabetics with microvascular complications [53].

Summary

Human plasma contains both renin and its biosynthetic precursor prorenin. In healthy subjects, the molar concentration of prorenin is approximately 10 times that of renin. In patients with diabetes mellitus, plasma prorenin is more than 20 times higher than renin, due to a selective increase in prorenin, and this is the case both in type I and type II diabetes. High plasma levels of prorenin are associated with the presence of microvascular complications, and the highest levels are found in patients with combined proliferative retinopathy and advanced nephropathy. The association of prorenin with microvascular retinal and renal disease is independent of age, metabolic control of diabetes, insulin-dependency, and blood pressure.

Until recently, prorenin was usually measured with the enzyme-kinetic assay, which is based on the in vitro generation of angiotensin I from angiotensinogen, after the enzymatically inactive prorenin has been converted to active renin by the addition of trypsin. Angiotensinogen is added to plasma in large excess, so that the enzyme substrate reaction is zero-order with respect to substrate.

Inadvertent activation of prorenin during the preparation and handling of blood samples prior to the addition of trypsin or other activating enzymes may result in falsely high renin and falsely low prorenin levels. To a large extent appropriate precautions can prevent inadvertent activation of prorenin.

In recent years, highly specific and sensitive immunoradiometric assays of renin and prorenin have been developed. It is expected that this newly introduced technology will contribute to our understanding of the role of the renin angiotensin system in diabetes mellitus and other disease states.

References

[1] Hackenthal E, Paul M, Ganten D et al. Morphology, physiology and molecular biology of renin secretion. Physiological Reviews 1990; 70: 1067–1116.

[2] Skøtt O, Jensen BL. Cellular and intrarenal control of renin secretion. Clin Sci 1993; 84: 1–10.

[3] Galen FX, Deveaux C, Houot AM et al. Renin biosynthesis by human tumoral juxtaglomerular cells. Evidence for a renin precursor. J Clin Invest 1984; 73: 1144–1155.

[4] Derkx FHM, Schalekamp MADH. Human Prorenin: pathophysiology and clinical implications. Clin Exp Hypertension 1988; A10: 1213–1225.

[5] DeSchepper CF, Mellon SH, Cumin F et al. Analysis by immunohistochemistry and in situ hybridization of renin and its mRNA in kidney, testis, adrenal gland and pituitary of the rat. Proc Natl Acad Sci USA 1986; 83: 7552–7556.

[6] Blundell T, Sibanda BL, Pearl L. Three-dimensional structure, specificity, and catalytic mechanism of renin. Nature 1983; 304: 273–275.

[7] Derkx FHM, Deinum J, Lipovski M et al. Nonproteolytic "activation" of prorenin by active site-directed inhibitors as demonstrated by renin-specific monoclonal antibody. J Biol Chem 1992; 267: 22837–22842.

[8] Schalekamp MADH, Derkx FHM. Biochemistry of prorenin. In: Robertson JIS, Nicholls MG, eds. The renin-angiotensin system. London: Gower Medical Publishing, 1993; 6.1–6.13.

[9] Derkx FHM, Schalekamp MPA, Schalekamp MADH. Two-step prorenin–renin conversion. Isolation of an intermediary form of activated prorenin. J Biol Chem 1987; 262: 2472–2477.

[10] Pitarresi T, Rubattu S, Heinrikson R et al. Reversible cryoactivation of recombinant human prorenin. J Biol Chem 1992; 267: 11753–11759.

[11] Campagnole-Santos MJ, Diz OI, Santos RA et al. Cardiovascular effects of angiotensin 1-7 injected into the dorsal medulla of rats. Amer J Physiol 1989; 257: H324–H329.
[12] Johnston CI. Renin-angiotension system: a dual tissue and hormonal system for cardiovascular control. J Hypertension 1992; 10 (Suppl. 7): S13–S27.
[13] Campbell DJ. The site of angiotensin production. J Hypertension 1985; 3: 199–207.
[14] Admiraal PJJ, Derkx FHM, Danser AHJ et al. Metabolism and production of angiotensin I in different vascular beds in subjects with hypertension. Hypertension 1990; 15: 44–55.
[15] Admiraal PJJ, Derkx FHM, Danser AHJ et al. Intrarenal de novo production of angiotensin I in subjects with renal artery stenosis. Hypertension 1990; 16: 555–563.
[16] Danser AHJ, Koning MMG, Admiraal PJJ et al. Metabolism of angiotensin I by different tissues in the intact animal. Am J Physiol 1992; 263: H418–H428.
[17] Danser AHJ, Koning MMG, Admiraal PJJ et al. Production of angiotensins I and II at tissues sites in the intact pigs. Am J Physiol 1992; 263: H429–H437.
[18] Admiraal PJ, Danser AHJ, Jong MS et al. Regional angiotensin II production in essential hypertension and renal artery stenosis. Hypertension 1993; 21: 173–184.
[19] Sealey JE. Plasma renin activity and plasma prorenin assays. Clin Chem 1991; 37: 1811–1819.
[20] Poulsen K, Nielson AH. The measurement of renin. In: Robertson JIS, Nicholls MG, eds. The renin-angiotensin system. London: Gower Medical Publishing, 1993; 13.1–13.12.
[21] Derkx FHM, Tan-Tjiong HL, Wenting GJ et al. Asynchronous changes in prorenin and renin secretion after captopril in patients with renal artery stenosis. Hypertension 1983; 5: 244–256.
[22] Derkx FHM, Stuenkel C, Schalekamp MPA et al. Immunoreactive renin, prorenin, and enzymatically active renin in plasma during pregnancy and in women taking oral contraceptives. J Clin Endocrinol Metab 1986; 63: 1008–1015.
[23] Robertson JIS. Angiotensinogen measurement. In: Robertson JIS, Nicholls MG, eds. The renin-angiotensin system. London: Gower Medical Publishing, 1993; 14.1–14.8.
[24] Skinner SL. Improved assay methods for renin 'concentration' and 'activity' in human plasma. Methods using selective denaturation of renin substrate. Circ Res 1976; 20: 392–402.
[25] Poole S. Renin and angiotensin standards. In: Robertson JIS, Nicholls MG, eds. The renin-angiotensin system. London: Gower Medical Publishing, 1993; 17.1–17.5.
[26] Derkx FHM, Bouma BN, Schalekamp MADH. Prorenin–renin conversion by the contact-activation system in plasma: role of plasma protease inhibitors. J Lab Clin Med 1984; 103: 560–573.
[27] Deinum J, Derkx FHM, Danser AHJ et al. Identification and quantification of renin and prorenin in the bovine eye. Endocrinol 1990; 126: 1673–1682.
[28] Poulson K, Jorgensen J. An easy radioimmunological microassay of renin activity, concentration and substrate in human plasma and tissues based on angiotensin I trapping by antibody. J Clin Endocrinol Metab 1974; 39: 816–825.
[29] Derkx FHM, van den Meiracker AH, Fischli W et al. Nonparallel effects of renin inhibitor treatment on plasma renin activity and angiotensins I and II in hypertensive subjects. An assay-related artifact. Amer J Hypertension 1991; 4: 602–609.
[30] Simon D, Hartmann DJ, Badouaille G et al. Two-site direct immunoassay specific for active renin. Clin Chem 1992; 38: 1959–1962.
[31] Rosmalen FMA, van Hoek MJC, Jilesen LEJM et al. An immunoradiometric assay for the quantification of active renin in plasma. Amer J Hypertension 1993; 6: 126A.
[32] Derkx FHM, de Bruin RJA, van Gool JMG et al. A novel assay of plasma prorenin using a renin inhibitor. J Hypertension 1993; (Suppl 5): S. 240–241.
[33] Shinagawa T, Do YS, Baxter J, Hsueh WA. Purification and characterization of human truncated prorenin. Biochemistry 1992; 31: 2758–2764.
[34] Nielsen MD, Rasmussen PH, Giese J. A highly sensitive and reproducible immunoradiometric assay for total human renin using monoclonal antibodies, iodogen labelling and polystyrene star tubes. Clin Exp Hypertension 1987; A9: 1391–1414.

[35] Schumacher M, Nanninga A, Delfs T et al. A direct immunoradiometric assay for human plasma prorenin: concentrations in cycling women and in women taking oral contraceptives. J Clin Endocrinol Metab 1992; 75: 617–623.
[36] Mizrahi J, Coezy E, Auzan C et al. Monoclonal antibodies to human angiotensinogen: development of an ElISA for measurement of hepatocyte cultured cell content. Clin Exp Hypertension 1987; 9A: 1479–1492.
[37] Perich RB, Jackson B, Johnston CI. Measurement of angiotensin converting enzyme. In: Robertson JIS, Nicholls MG, eds. The renin-angiotensin system. London: Gower Medical Publishing, 1993; 16.1–16.7.
[38] Nussberger J, Brunner DB, Waeber B et al. Specific measurement of angiotensin metabolites and in vitro generated angiotensin II in plasma. Hypertension 1986; 8: 476–482.
[39] Schalekamp MADH, Derkx FHM, van den Meiracker AH. Renin inhibitors, angiotensin converting enzyme inhibitors and angiotensin II receptor antagonists: relationship between blood pressure responses and effects on the renin angiotensin system. J Hypertension 1992; 10 (Suppl. 7): S157–S164.
[40] Björck S. The renin angiotensin system in diabetes mellitus. Scan J Urology Nephrol 1990; 126 (suppl.): 1–51.
[41] Weidmann P, Ferrari P, Shaw SG. Renin in diabetes mellitus. In: Robertson JIS, Nicholls MG, eds. The renin-angiotensin system. London: Gower Medical Publishing, 1993; 75.1–75.26.
[42] Franken AAM, Derkx FHM, Blankenstijn PJ et al. Plasma prorenin as an early marker of microvascular disease in patients with diabetes mellitus. Diabete Metab 1992; 18: 137–143.
[43] Franken AAM, Derkx FHM, Man in't Veld AJ et al. High plasma prorenin in diabetes mellitus and its correlation with some complications. J Clin Endocrinol Metab 1990; 71: 1008–1015.
[44] Luetscher JA, Kraemer FB, Wilson DM et al. Increased plasma inactive renin in diabetes mellitus. A marker of microvascular complications. N Eng J Med 1985; 312: 1412–1417.
[45] Misbin RI, Grant MB, Pecker MS et al. Elevated levels of plasma prorenin (inactive renin) in diabetic and non-diabetic patients with autonomic dysfunction. J Clin Endocrinol Metab 1987; 64: 964–968.
[46] Derkx FHM, Gool van JMG, Wenting GJ et al. Inactive renin in human plasma. Lancet 1976; 2: 496–499.
[47] Fernandez LA, Twickler J, Mead A. Neovascularization produced by angiotensin II. J Lab Clin Med 1985; 105: 141–145.
[48] Danser AHJ, van den Dorpel MA, Deinum J et al. Renin, prorenin, and immunological renin in vitreous fluid from eyes with and without diabetic retinopathy. J Clin Endocrinol Metab 1989; 68: 160–167.
[49] Wagner J, Danser AHJ, Derkx FHM et al. Demonstration of renin-, angiotensinogen-, and converting enzyme mRNA expression in the human eye. 1993; submitted.
[50] Robinson R, White M, McCann P et al. Effect of aneasthesia on intraocular blood flow. Brit J Ophthalmology 1991; 75: 92–93.
[51] Kim S, Hiruma M, Ikemoto F et al. Importance of glycosylation for hepatic clearance of renal renin. Am J Physiol 1988; 255: E642–E651.
[52] Feldt-Rasmussen B, Mathiesen ER, Deckkert T et al. Central role for sodium in the pathogenesis of blood pressure changes independent of angiotensin, aldosteron and catecholamines in type I (insulin-dependent) diabetes mellitus. Diabetologia 1987; 30: 610–617.
[53] Toop MJ, Dallinger KJ, Jennings PE et al. Angiotensin-converting enzyme (ACE): relationship to insulin-dependent diabetes and microangiopathy. Diabetic Medicine 1986; 3: 455–457.

Research methods of cerebrovascular disease in diabetes

M. Daffertshofer, W. Rautenberg, M. Hennerici

Diabetes and stroke

A variety of studies have indicated that diabetics are at increased risk of ischemic stroke, with diabetes as an independent risk factor for ischemic stroke at an adjusted relative risk of 1.5–2.0 [2, 4, 13].

Cerebral ischemia is closely related to atherosclerosis and its associated major risk factors like diabetes. Ischemic events are precipitated by cardiac, aortic, large and small vessel diseases.

Large-vessel diseases may cause both hemodynamic insufficiency and artery-to-artery embolism. Identification of these lesions and follow-up studies of their natural progression provide adequate data for estimating the prognosis of a particular lesion and for the scientific study of the best treatment.

Small-vessel diseases involve penetrating arteries originating from the choroid, middle cerebral, anterior and posterior cerebral, posterior communicating, basilar and vertebral arteries. Occlusion of these branches gives rise to small deep infarcts of the lacunar type in the putamen, thalamus, caudate nucleus, internal capsule, corona radiata, cerebellum and the brainstem. It is a common type of stroke, and one particular subtype is closely correlated with both diabetes and arterial hypertension [3, 16, 37]. Blockage of small penetrating arteries (< 200 µm in diameter) due to lipohyalinosis produces quite small infarcts (< 500 µm diameter) that remain asymptomatic unless strategically placed in a clinically sensitive tract (pure motor or pure sensory strokes). In contrast, blockage of larger penetrating arteries (~ 900 µm in diameter) produces infarcts of 0.5–1.5 cm in diameter that are more often symptomatic. They are most frequently due to atherosclerotic plaques and thromboembolism at the origin of one or more branching penetrating arteries, and hence "miniature lesions" similar in etiology and pathomechanism to those seen in large-vessel diseases.

White matter lesions are demonstrable with increasing age and in patients with demented illnesses – association with diabetes has been suggested but so far not proved [7, 22].

Diagnostic instruments

Scientific investigations of pathophysiology and the treatment of cerebrovascular diseases have been promoted considerably by non invasive diagnostics. A variety of such non invasive techniques (ultrasound and MRA) have been developed to display the cerebrovascular system for the detection of both extra- and intracranial large artery diseases. They are currently used for the diagnosis of symptomatic patients with a history, signs or symptoms of cerebrovascular, cardiovascular or peripheral vascular diseases. According to recent clinical trials, patients with severe extracranial carotid disease may benefit from surgery, whereas those who, as a coincidental result of a check-up examination or because of manifestation of atherosclerosis in the non-cerebrovascular tree, provide evidence of asymptomatic carotid disease do not seem to benefit from prophylactic carotid endarterectomy but rather from risk factor reduction.

Non invasive technologies have also been applied to image the brain tissue by means of ultrasound (in infancy), computerized tomography (CT) and magnetic resonance imaging (MRI).

Non-invasive ultrasound techniques

Continuous-wave and pulsed-wave Doppler sonography assess the hemodynamics according to the Doppler shift [19]. Both are used for the evaluation of blood flow velocity in extracranial vessels. Continuous-wave systems use two transducers, one of which emits while the other receives ultrasound continuously. This system is useful for the detection of a broad range of flow velocity alterations including very high blood flow velocities such as those occurring in severe stenosis. However, it does not provide any information about the topographic origin of the ultrasound reflecting source in the tissue. To detect the source of the signals, pulsed-wave Doppler systems are used which both emit and receive ultrasound from a piezocrystal in a single transducer. Pulsed-wave Doppler is the only method useful for the evaluation of intracranial blood flow velocities within the major basal cerebral arteries because knowledge of the tissue depth from which the signal is derived is crucial for estimating the artery being insonated. Pulsed-wave Doppler techniques have been extended for two-dimensional display and eventually three-dimensional reconstruction of the circle of Willis and the major vessels within the posterior fossa. It has also been introduced for the assessment of intrathoracic, supraaortic and submandibular segments of the cranially bound arteries. Both systems may be combined with real-time brightness-modulated

(B-mode) sonography, imaging tissue and vessel structure in a two-dimensional gray scale display (duplex sonography): Color-coded Doppler flow imaging (CDFI) represents the most recently developed combination of Doppler-mode and B-mode technologies.

Extracranial circulation

Indirect tests were used for the detection of severe obstructive lesions within the carotid system. They are still useful as the equipment can be easily transported, can almost be carried in the pocket and are quickly available for use. They provide some information regarding the movement of blood through vessels, even in the hand of a poorly trained examiner. However, these tests fail to detect hemodynamically significant ipsilateral carotid artery obstructions in > 20%; therefore, direct tests of the extracranial carotid artery system are necessary. The interpretation of these direct tests provides valuable information on the extent, site and degree of atherosclerotic lesions of > 40% lumen-narrowing with a sensitivity of 92 to 100% and a specificity of 93 to 100% of that of arteriography as compared in a large series studied. Various degrees of carotid artery stenosis and occlusion may be separated on the basis of hemodynamic criteria such as turbulences, increased flow velocities, spectral broadening etc. Vertebral artery stenosis and occlusion can be directly assessed if they are located at the origin or at the atlas loop. The criteria used for the classification of the degree of vertebral stenosis are similar to those used for the carotid system. Doppler methods are excellent noninvasive tools for the detection of associated flow alterations in the vertebral arteries in patients with proximal subclavian and innominate artery obstructions such as the subclavian steal phenomenon.

Carotid artery plaques producing less-encroaching lesions (< 40%) are better displayed by B-mode echotomography rather than by hemodynamic methods. The echogenicity of the plaque, surface structure, and extent may all be repeatedly visualized during follow-up to assess the development of a lesion. Using this system, the very early stages of atherosclerotic disease, e. g. alterations in the intima, may be detected even far below the physical resolution power of the ultrasound systems applied. This demonstrates the efficacy of modern imaging procedures for investigating the treatment or prevention of progressive and regressive atherosclerosis.

Duplex scanning of the carotid and vertebral arteries has been greatly improved by recent advances in color Doppler flow imaging (CDFI). It provides two-dimensional, real-time information about intravascular blood flow superimposed on the gray scale image of the vessel anatomy. Compared to conventional duplex scanning, CDFI has several advantages such as simultaneous real-time imaging of blood flow and vessel anatomy, simplification of vessel identification, faster data acquisition, shorter examination time, improved estimation of plaque surface structure and residual vessel lumen, facilitated localization of the point of maximal intrastenotic frequency shift, display of the morphologic hemodynamic interaction, and higher intra- and interobserver reproducibility. Limitations are due to the variability of the interpretation of signals associated with reversed flow, undisturbed flow towards the transducer, turbulences and aliasing phenomena, the detection of very slow flow velocities, and the poor temporal resolution of color-coded flow patterns.

Intracranial circulation

The application of Doppler methods for the insonation of intracranial vessels has long been believed impossible. A high energy bi-directional pulsed-wave Doppler system operating at low frequencies (1−2 MHz) was, however, used 10 years ago for the first time and allowed the non invasive recording of flow velocities from arteries at the base of the skull. Identification of intracranial vessels critically depends on flow direction, depth control of the range-gated Doppler signal, position and tilting of the probe, and compression tests in selected cases. Three different approaches allowed the recording of intracranial flow velocity: 1. the transtemporal, using the temporal "window", 2. the transorbital, and 3. the nuchal. Recently, real-time transcranial color-coded Duplex sonography has been introduced. This method allows imaging of the basal intracranial vessels through the scull. Knowledge of the extracranial non invasive studies is essential for the interpretation of the transcranial findings. In addition, velocities of intracranial vessels vary with age, hematocrit, end tidal CO_2 partial pressure, anemia, glucose levels, and other variables. These variables should be considered. Intracranial collateralization of significant extracranial lesions as well as the detection of intracranial arterial disease represents the most frequent application of this technique. The possibility of assessing the intracranial reserve capacity by using a CO_2 or azetazolamide test has long been known and has also been introduced for the diagnosis of cerebrovascular diseases. These tests have been suggested for the detection of patients at risk for hemodynamic stroke. Hypercapnia leads to vasodilatation of the peripheral vessels and consequently to an increased flow velocity in the more proximal arteries at the circle of Willis, whereas hypocapnia causes vasoconstriction and a reduced blood flow velocity in the more proximal artery segments. Results of cerebral investigations of the intracranial reserve capacity in patients with significant extracranial disease have shown that normal or reduced cerebral vasomotor reactivity is independent of the degree of carotid artery obstruction. Thus, the severity of the extracranial lesion does not predict the hemodynamic relevance for the intracranial circulation.

Monitoring of cerebral hemodynamics during orthostasis

Diabetic neuropathy commonly affects autonomic nerve fibres that may become clinically relevant if orthostatic dysregulation results in syncope due to a deficit of brain perfusion. Brain perfusion, physiologically, is regulated independently of systemic circulation. Cerebral blood flow is kept constant throughout a wide range of systemic blood pressure (50–150 mmHg) by cerebrovascular regulation (CR) mechanisms which are not totally understood but are definitely different from the mechanisms in systemic autoregulation [5, 11, 27]. Since some patients with autonomic failure also have orthostatic problems despite systemic blood-pressure regulation within physiological ranges, CR may be disturbed even in the presence of normal blood pressure regulation. Thorough descriptions exist on peripheral cardiovascular regulation disorders, including autonomic incompetence of peripheral vascular innervation [25, 27, 34]. However, only limited knowledge exists regarding orthostatic dysfunction of CR – causing an additional and topographically distinct mismatch of brain perfusion [9, 16, 17, 34].

Methods for testing autonomic innervation of cardiac or peripheral vascular function are well established. With the Schellong test [36] the systemic regulation of blood pressure and heart rate can be tested. The analysis of the heart rate variability during hyperventilation, Valsalva manoeuver, handgrip or other techniques, test parasympathetic innervation of the heart. Skin-evoked responses are taken as indicators of peripheral sympathetic activity and laser Doppler methods are used to measure the peripheral vascular autonomic function of both the sympathetic and parasympathetic autonomic branches.

Previous methods for measuring cerebral perfusion had several limitations, such as invasiveness, poor time resolution and analysis restricted to the arteriolar regulation [18]. Although transcranial Doppler sonography can only register instantaneous flow velocities of the main intracranial arteries with an approximation of volume flow as an indicator of brain perfusion [1, 25], the possibility to monitor these values over a longer period compensates for this disadvantage [6, 8]. Polygraphic monitoring of heart rate, blood pressure and cerebral blood flow velocity during an orthostatic paradigm has been shown to provide valid information about cerebral blood flow regulation [10]. Patients are placed on a tilt table in a horizontal position. After 5 minutes at rest, the table is tilted into a vertical position so that the patient stands up for an additional 15 minutes. The table is again tilted in a horizontal position for 5 minutes to complete the investigation. Orthostatic dysregulation with fainting occurs clinically during a wide time interval after standing up. A decrease in blood pressure as well as in cerebral blood flow can occur directly after getting up or after a period of several minutes in an upright position, which may reflect disturbance of different mechanisms involved in orthostatic regulation. Thus, changes in the position of the table should be completed rapidly (within 2–3 seconds), while the standing paradigm should last at least 15 minutes. All variables can be transformed into relative values, using the mean value during the last three minutes in the first supine phase

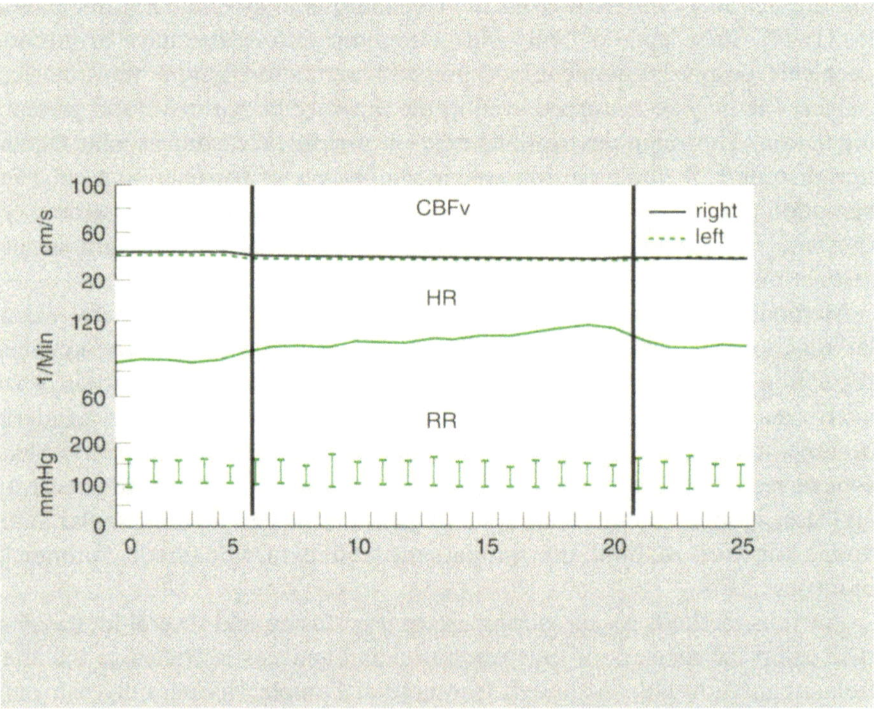

Fig. 1A Normal orthostatic regulation with an increase of heart rate during upright position while blood pressure and CBFV remain constant. Blood pressure (RR), heart rate (HR), CBFV in the left middle cerebral artery and CBFV in the right middle cerebral artery (MCA) in an orthostatic paradigm: In the first five minutes, the patient lies in a horizontal position; in the next 15 minutes, the patient is standing up; in the last five minutes, the patient is in a horizontal position again. The point of position change is marked with a vertical line

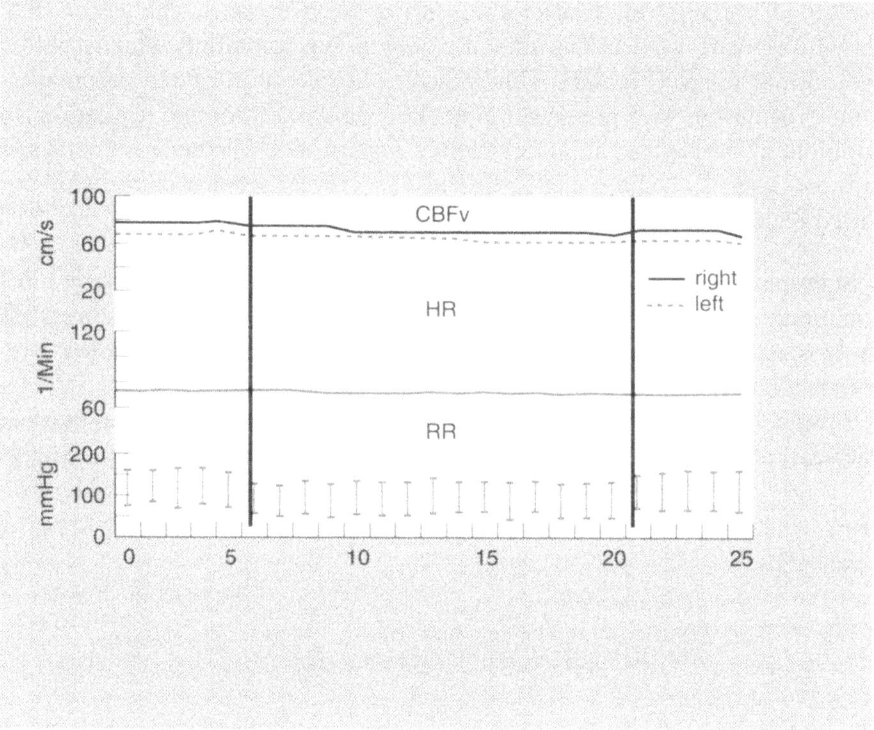

Fig. 1B RR, HR and CBFV in the left and right MCA during orthostatis in a diabetic patient without a history of syncope but tests indicating autonomic neuropathy. RR and CBFV are kept constant during the upright position although HR is fixed

as a reference (= 100%). The amount of data can then be reduced by calculating for each variable 22 successive mean values (one per minute).

In normal subjects (Fig. 1A), an increase in heart rate occurs after changing from a horizontal to a vertical position. Blood pressure is slightly reduced after standing but generaly remains constant throughout the entire procedure. In contrast, the intracranial blood flow velocity shows a mild decrease during the standing position with normalization after lying down again. Pulsatility index (PI) values increase slightly after tilting the table to a vertical position [24]. Standard deviations range from 30% in the pulsatility measurements to 3% in single heart rate values. Due to two standard deviations, the normal deviation range for blood pressure and cerebral blood flow velocity (CBFV) while standing is 20% from the mean of the blood pressure and CBFV during the initial supine period. Patients with diabetic neuropathy and a history of orthostatic syncopes commonly have a fixed heart rate while the blood pressure mildly decreases during the orthostatic changes. CBFV shows a tendency to decrease after standing up but commonly remains within the normal range (Fig. 1B). This indicates an affection of the cardioautonomic regulation with preservation of the vascular autonomic regulation. In addition, normal intracranial flow values suggest that CR remains unaffected in most cases. In some patients, this test can reveal specific patterns of distorted orthostatic cerebrovascular dysregulation.

Subtype I: CBFV decreases parallel to a decrease in blood pressure, most commonly while the heart rate is fixed (Fig. 1C). These patients sometimes show signs of syncope during the investigation as a result of exceeding cerebrovascular regulation capacities.

Subtype II: In less severe cases, patients show a pathological and marked decrease of blood pressure while the cerebral blood flow velocity remains

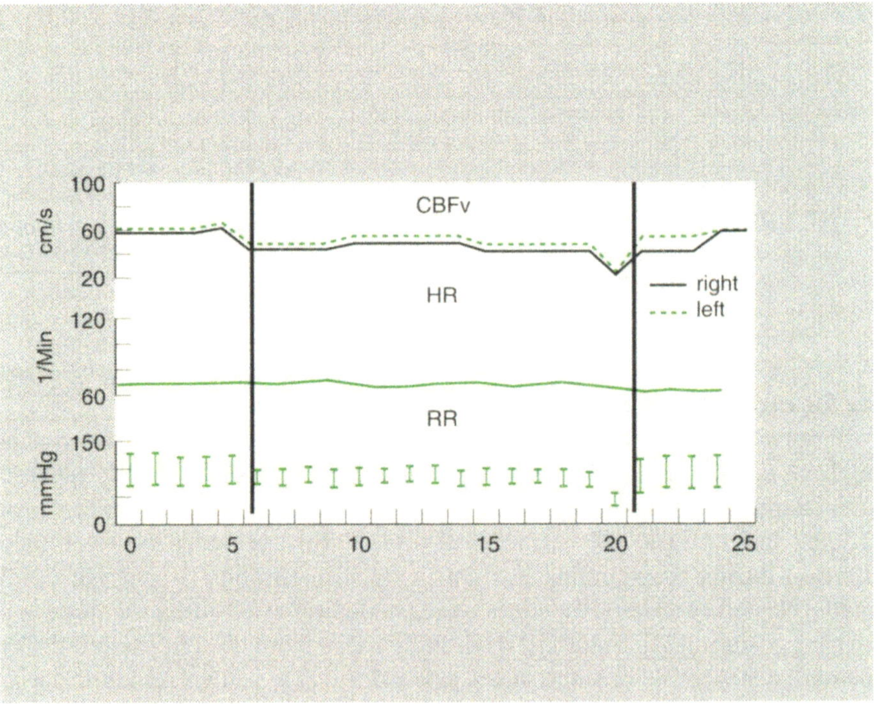

Fig. 1C RR, HR and CBFV in the left and right MCA during orthostasis in a diabetic patient with a history of syncope and autonomic neuropathy evidenced by a pathological heart rate variability and infrared pupillometry. HR is fixed, and RR shows a decrease during an upright position with consecutive CBFV reduction

within normal ranges (Fig. 1D), due to compromised systemic but sufficiently compensated cerebrovascular regulation.

Subtype III: In contrast, some patients show a pathological decrease in CBFV while the blood pressure and the heart rate remain within a normal range (Fig. 1E). In the course of the CBFV decrease, these patients often report warning signs for syncope. A selective disturbance of cerebrovascular regulation can be hypothesized for this pattern.

Particularly subtypes II and III can only be diagnosed if combined CBFV and systemic blood pressure/heart rate polygraphic recordings are made. Registration of CBFV using this experimental design is sensitive in discriminating patients with orthostatic dysregulation [20]. In particular, subjects with orthostatic dysregulation can be differentiated according to whether or not they show repeated decreased blood flow velocity in the MCA. Moreover, measurement of MCA flow, in addition to cardiovascular parameters,

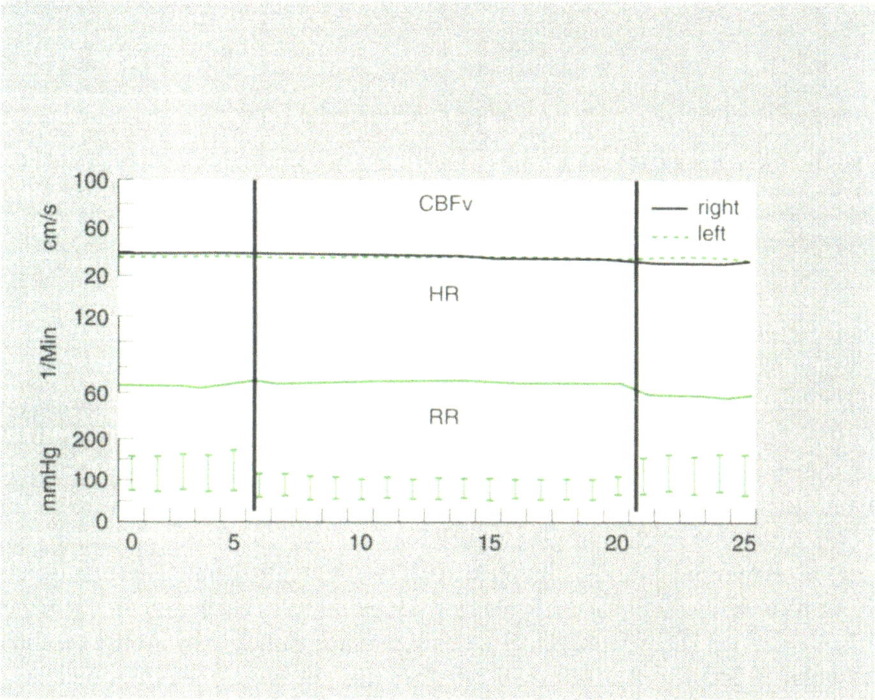

Fig. 1D RR, HR and CBFV in the left and right MCA during orthostatic paradigm in a patient with diabetes without history of syncope but a pathological Schellong test. RR decreases when the patient is standing up – but CBFV is kept constant as an indicator of cerebrovascular autoregulatory compensation (subtype I)

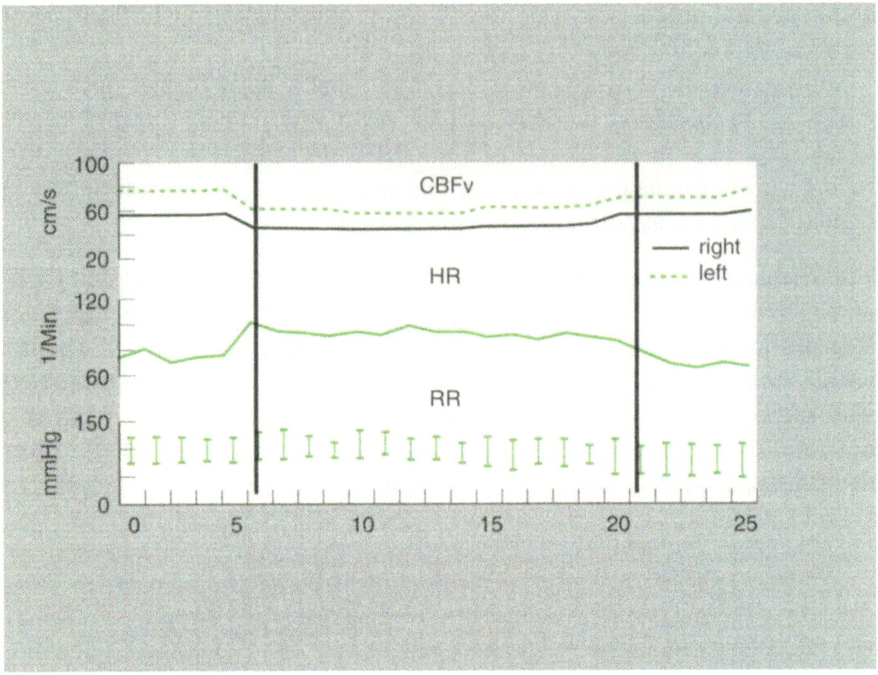

Fig. 1E RR, HR and CBFV in the left and right MCA during an upright position in a patient with diabetes and a history of syncope but a normal Schellong test. HR increases, and RR is kept normal during the upright position, but CBFV decreases significantly as an evidence for circumscribed cerebrovascular dysregulation (subtype II)

can detect an orthostatic flow dysregulation in the MCA without systemic cardiovascular dysregulation or a severely disturbed cardiovascular control with nearly normal regulation of MCA flow. In diabetics, the measured CBFV parameters predict whether or not the patient has a decreased CBFV in the upright position, which may lead to syncope. It is also possible to demonstrate a sufficient cerebrovascular regulation compensating for an already disturbed cardiovascular regulation.

Our studies indicate that the disturbance of the autonomic nervous system is an important factor in orthostatic dysregulation in diabetics. Its influence mainly acts on the peripheral vascular resistance rather than on the cerebrovascular resistance. It is not clear whether this autonomic regulation is parallel to or different from that of the peripheral vascular resistance. Future studies should, therefore, measure parameters for the peripheral resistance. Furthermore, for better prediction of cerebrovascular regulation, these studies should provide data about intracranial blood pressure. Müller et al

[28] have attempted this by measuring blood pressure with the index positioned at the level of the MCA. Obviously, blood flow does not depend only on blood flow velocity but also on the structural parameters of the vessel in which the measurement is made.

Since Doppler signals recorded from the MCA may be influenced by both changing diameters and flow velocities a controversy has arisen as to whether flow velocity interpretation alone is misleading [1, 25]. Aaslid et al. showed that there were only negligible changes in diameter during systemic blood pressure variations in the insonated vessel segment of the MCA. Based on previous angiographic studies by Huber and Handa [21], it is unlikely that alterations of vessel caliper in large arteries such as the MCA significantly modify flow velocity data, as is the case in smaller vessels (0.5–1 mm diameter) outside the area directly accessible by TCD techniques. This issue, however, needs to be more thoroughly addressed in experimental investigations.

Functional investigations assessing changes in blood flow during neuronal activation by mental activity, light exposure and visual stimulation have been reported. These findings are useful for the investigation of the metabolic and hemodynamic reserve capacities.

Hypoglycemia and cerebral blood

In humans, cerebral blood flow (CBF) during hypoglycemia has been studied by a variety of techniques. Cross-cannulation studies, using the nitrous oxide method for measuring CBF during insulin-induced hypoglycemia, reported conflicting results showing no change in CBF [14, 23] and a significant increase in schizophrenic patients [30]. Neil et al [29] reported a significant increase in cerebral blood flow in diabetic patients using an intravenous xenon clearance technique. These results suggest that in young diabetic patients cerebral vessels dilate normally in response to hypoglycemia. Other authors reported abnormal cerebrovascular reactivity using CO_2 stimulation [12] or azetazolamide [32]. Shapiro et al [33] showed in a PET study that the brain extracts an increased fraction of 2-DFG from the blood in the presence of mild hypoglycemia. This compensatory increase in fractional glucose uptake results in a constant cerebral metabolic rate. This can be interpreted as a mechanism to protect the brain from mild reductions in plasma glucose levels. Using iv xenon SPECT, Tallroth et al [35] found an increase of CBF, showing the highest increases in frontal and parietal cortex during hypoglycemia.

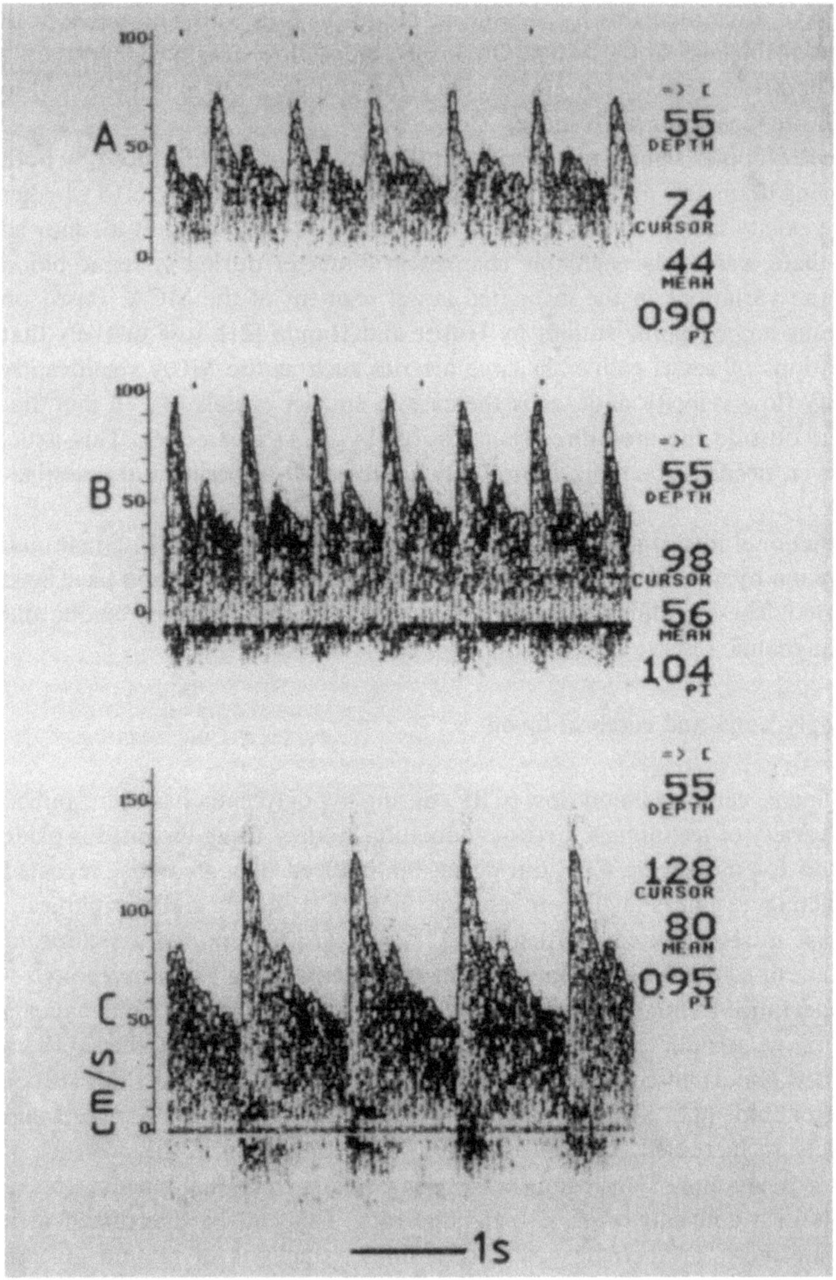

Fig. 2 Doppler spectra from the middle cerebral artery in a patient with diabetes during step-wise lowering of blood glucose at 5.0 (A), 3.6 (B) and 2.5 mmol/l (C) showing a marked increase of peak and mean flow velocities during hypoglycemia

Transcranial Doppler was used to study the effect of severe hypoglycemia on cerebral hemodynamics in 8 healthy volunteers and in 16 type I diabetic patients (8 patients with good and 8 with moderate metabolic control) [31]. Blood glucose concentration was lowered stepwise by insulin infusion and clamped for 45 minutes at 5.0, 3.6 and 2.5 mmol/l. Blood pressure, heart rate, endexpiratory CO_2, blood glucose and P300 latencies were monitored. Blood pressure, and endexpiratory CO_2 remained constant during hypoglycemia in all groups. The heart rate only mildly increased.

Peak velocities in the middle cerebral artery increased by 12 cm/s in the control group ($p < 0.004$), by 22.8 cm/s in patients with good ($p < 0.004$) and by 25.8 cm/s in patients with moderate metabolic control during blood glucose reduction from 5.0 to 2.5 mmol/l (Fig. 2). The increase of mean flow velocity in the middle cerebral artery was more than threefold that of normal controls. Hypoventilation or cardiac failures were not responsible for the increase of blood velocity. The stimulus for cerebral vasodilation during hypoglycemia remains unclear. The significant difference in the increase of velocity between diabetics and controls may be interpreted as a protective factor in patients at frequent risk of hypoglycemia.

Magnetic resonance

Studies on MR techniques form a large part of the recent publications in the field of cerebrovascular disease. Since standard MRI has been well established during recent years, methodological studies now explore special issues such as the hyperacute phase of stroke for an improved estimate of the development and prognosis of tissue recovery within the very first hours after onset of symptoms. In addition, the measurement of perfusion and diffusion has been assessed by imaging cytotoxic edema within hypoxic brain tissue. Another goal of MRI is to image lesions due to microangiopathy.

Magnetic resonance angiography (MRA) is the most recent development of MR technology, and it is increasingly used as a standard investigation versus the already-established ultrasound technique and conventional arteriography. The quality of the images is generally good, and problems related to the detection of very slow blood flow and turbulent flow components have been recently reduced by application of time-of-flight techniques or two-dimensional spinecho sequences with flow presaturations and by the usage of thin sections post-processed with a minimum intensity protection algorithm. In a recent study, the sensitivity of MRA vs. conventional arteriography was reported to be 86% with a specificity of 92%, which is only slightly above the accuracy of ultrasound techniques. The combination of MRA,

CDFI and Doppler ultrasound tests is particularly useful for providing supplementary information on both morphology and function of the cerebral circulation.

References

[1] Aaslid R, Lindegaard KF, Sorteberg W et al. Cerebral autoregulation dynamics in humans. Stroke 1989; 20: 45–52.
[2] Abbott RD, Donahue RP, MacMahon SW et al. Diabetes and risk of stroke. The honolulu heart program. Jama 1987; 257: 949–952.
[3] Arboix A, Marti-Vilata JL, Garcia JH. Clinical study of 227 patients with lacunar infarcts. Stroke 1990; 21: 842.
[4] Barrett-Connor E, Khaw KT. Diabetes mellitus: An independent risk factor for stroke? Am J Epidemiol 1988; 128: 116–123.
[5] Berne RM, Winn HR, Ruplo R. The local regulation of cerebral blood flow. Progress in Cardiovascular Diseases 1981; 24: 243–260.
[6] Briebach T, Fischer PA. Kreislaufphysiologische Untersuchungen und transcranielle Dopplersonographie bei orthostatischen Regulationsstörungen. Ultraschall 1988; 9: 223–226.
[7] Brott T, Mouradin M, Uthman B. Dementia, ventricular enlargement, and hypertension associated with periventricular hypodensity by CT. Ann Neurol 1986; 20: 129.
[8] Brunhölzl C, Müller HR. Transcranielle Doppler-Sonographie in Orthostase. Ultraschall 1986; 7: 248–252.
[9] Caronna JJ, Plum F. Cerebrovascular regulation in preganglionic and postglanglionic autonomic insufficiency. Stroke 1973; 4: 12–19.
[10] Daffertshofer M, Diehl RR, Ziehms GU et al. Orthostatic changes of cerebral blood flow velocity in patients with autonomic dysfunction. J Neurol Sci 1991; 104: 32–38.
[11] Daffertshofer M, Hennerici M. Synkopen bei neurologischen Erkrankungen. Herz 1993; 18: 187–201.
[12] Dandona P, James IM, Newbry PA et al. Cerebral blood flow in diabetes mellitus: evidence of abnormal cerebrovascular reactivity. British Medical Journal 1978; 2: 325–326.
[13] Davis PH, Dambrosia JM, Schoenberg BS et al. Risk factors for ischemic stroke: A prospective study in Rochester, Minnesota. Ann Neurol 1987; 22: 319–327.
[14] Eisenburg S, Seltzer HS. The cerebral metabolic effects of acutely induced hypoglycemia in human subjects. Metabolism 1962; 11: 1162–1168.
[15] Fisher CM. Thalamic pure sensory stroke: a pathologic study. Neurology 1978; 28: 1141.
[16] Fitch W, MacKenzie ET, Murray Harper A. Effects of decreasing arterial blood pressure on cerebral blood flow in the baboon. Circulation Research 1975; 37: 550–556.
[17] Gotoh F, Ebihara SI, Toyoda M et al. Role of autonomic nervous system in autoregulation of human cerebral circulation. Cerebral blood flow and intracranial pressure. Proc 5th int Symp, Roma–Siena Part I Europ Neurol 1971; 6: 203–207.
[18] Halsey JH. Measurement of cerebral blood flow. In: Toole JF, ed. Handbook of Clinical Neurology. Vol. 10 (54): Vascular Diseases Part II. Amsterdam: Elsevier Science Publishers BV, 1989; 139–155.
[19] Hennerici M, Mohr JP, Rautenberg W et al. Ultrasound imaging and Doppler sonography in the diagnosis of cerebrovascular diseases. In: Barnett HJM, Mohr JP, Stein BM et al, eds. Stroke. New York: Churchill Livingstone, 1992; 241–268.
[20] Hennerici M, Daffertshofer M. Imaging in cerebrovascular disease. Current Opinion in Neurology and Neurosurgery 1992; 5: 49–57.
[21] Huber P, Handa J. Effect of contrast material, Hypercapnia, Hyperventilation hypertonic glucose and papaverine on the diameter of the cerebral arteries. Investigative Radiology 1967; 2: 17–32.

[22] Kertesz A, Black SE, Tokar G et al. Periventricular and subcortical hyperintensities on MRI: rims, caps, and unidentified bright objects. Arch Neurol 1988; 45: 404.
[23] Kety SS, Schmidt CF. Cerebral blood flow and metabolism in schizophrenia. The effects of barbiturate semi-narcosis, insulin and electroshock. Am J Psychiat 1948; 104: 765–770.
[24] Kirkham FJ, Padayachee TS, Parson S et al. Transcranial measurement of blood velocities in the basal cerebral arteries using pulsed Doppler ultrasound. Ultrasound in Med & Biol 1986; 12: 15–21.
[25] Kontos HA. Validity of cerebral arterial blood flow calculations from velocity measurements. Stroke 1989; 20: 1–3.
[26] Kontos HA, Richardson DW, Norvell JE. Mechanisms of circulatory dysfunction in orthostatic hypotension. Trans Am Clin Climatol Assoc 1976; 87: 26–33.
[27] Low PA. Autonomic neuropathy. Seminars in Neurology 1987; 7: 49–57.
[28] Müller HR, Casty M, Moll R et al. Response of MCA volume flow to orthostasis. Cerebrovascular Diseases 1991; 1: 82–89.
[29] Neil HA, Gale EAM, Hamilton SJC et al. Cerebral blood flow increases during insulin-induced hypoglycaemia in Type I (insulin dependent) diabetic patients and control subjects. Diabetologia 1987; 30: 305–309.
[30] Porta PD, Maiolo AT, Negri VU et al. Cerebral blood flow in metabolism in therapeutic insulin coma. Metabolism 1964; 13: 131–140.
[31] Rautenberg W, Heinemann L, Starke AAR et al. Cerebral blood velocity during hypoglycemia. Washington: Second world congress of Stroke, 1992; S31 (Abstract).
[32] Rodriguez G, Hassan K, Nobili F et al. Regional cerebral blood flow and cerebrovascular reactivity in IDDM. Diabetes Care 1993; 16: 462–468.
[33] Shapiro T, Cooper M, Chen C et al. Change in hexose distribution volume and fractional utilization of (18F)-2-deoxy-2-Fluoro-D-Glucose in brain during acute hypoglycemia in humans. Diabetes 1990; 39: 175–180.
[34] Skinhoe E. The sympathetic nervous system and the regulation of cerebral blood flow in man. Stroke 1982; 3: 711–716.
[35] Tallroth G, Ryding E, Agard CD. Regional cerebral blood flow in normal man during insulin-induced hypoglycemia and in the recovery period following glucose infusion. Metabolism 1992; 41: 717–721.
[36] Thulesius O. Pathophysiological classification and diagnosis of orthostatic hypotension. Cardiology 1976; 61: 180–189.
[37] Tuszynski MH, Petito CK, Levy DE. Risk factors and clinical manifestation of pathologically verified lacunar infarctions. Stroke 1989; 20: 990.

World Medical Association Declaration of Helsinki

Recommendations guiding physicians in biomedical research involving human subjects.

Adopted by the 18th World Medical Assembly, Helsinki, Finland, June 1964, and amended by the 29th World Medical Assembly, Tokyo, Japan, October 1975, and the 35th World Medical Assembly, Venice, Italy, October 1983, and the 41st World Medical Assembly, Hong Kong, September 1989.

Introduction

It is the mission of the physician to safeguard the health of the people. His or her knowledge and conscience are dedicated to the fulfillment of this mission.

The Declaration of Geneva of the World Medical Association binds the physician with the words, "The health of my patient will be my first consideration", and the International Code of Medical Ethics declares that, "A physician shall act only in the patient's interest when providing medical care which might have the effect of weakening the physical and mental condition of the patient."

The purpose of biomedical research involving human subjects must be to improve diagnostic, therapeutic and prophylactic procedures and the understanding of the aetiology and pathogenesis of disease.

In current medical practice most diagnostic, therapeutic or prophylactic procedures involve hazards. This applies especially to biomedical research.

Medical progress is based on research which ultimately must rest in part on experimentation involving human subjects.

In the field of biomedical research a fundamental distinction must be recognized between medical research in which the aim is essentially diagnostic or therapeutic for a patient, and medical research, the essential object of which is purely scientific and without implying direct diagnostic or therapeutic value to the person subjected to the research.

Special caution must be exercised in the conduct of research which may affect the environment, and the welfare of animals used for research must be respected.

Because it is essential that the results of laboratory experiments be applied to human beings to further scientific knowledge and to help suffering humanity, the World Medical Association has prepared the following recommendations as a guide to every physician in biomedical research involving human subjects. They should be kept under review in the future. It must be stressed that the standards as drafted are only a guide to physicians all over the world. Physicians are not relieved from criminal, civil and ethical responsibilities under the laws of their own countries.

Basic principles

1. Biomedical research involving human subjects must conform to generally accepted scientific principles and should be based on adequately performed laboratory and animal experimentation and on a thorough knowledge of the scientific literature.
2. The design and performance of each experimental procedure involving human subjects should be clearly formulated in an experimental protocol which should be transmitted for consideration, comment and guidance to a specially appointed committee independent of the investigator and the sponsor, provided that this independent committee is in conformity with the laws and regulations of the country in which the research experiment is performed.
3. Biomedical research involving human subjects should be conducted only by scientifically qualified persons and under the supervision of a clinically competent medical person. The responsibility for the human subjects must always rest with a medically qualified person and never rest on the subject of the research, even though the subject has given his or her consent.
4. Biomedical research involving human subjects cannot legitimately be carried out unless the importance of the objective is in proportion to the inherent risk to the subject.
5. Every biomedical research project involving human subjects should be preceded by careful assessment of predictable risks in comparison with foreseeable benefits to the subject or to others. Concern for the interests of the subject must always prevail over the interests of science and society.
6. The right of the research subject to safeguard his or her integrity must always be respected. Every precaution should be taken to respect the privacy of the subject and to minimize the impact of the study on the subject's physical and mental integrity and on the personality of the subject.

7. Physicians should abstain from engaging in research projects involving human subjects unless they are satisfied that the hazards involved are believed to be predictable. Physicians should cease any investigation if the hazards are found to outweigh the potential benefits.
8. In publication of the results of his or her research, the physician is obliged to preserve the accuracy of the results. Reports of experimentation not in accordance with the principles laid down in this Declaration should not be accepted for publication.
9. In any research on human beings, each potential subject must be adequately informed of the aims, methods, anticipated benefits, and potential hazards of the study and the discomfort it may entail. He or she should be informed that he or she is at liberty to abstain from participation in the study and that he or she is free to withdraw his or her consent to participation at any time. The physician should then obtain the subject's freely-given informed consent, preferably in writing.
10. When obtaining informed consent for the research project the physician should be particularly cautious if the subject is in a dependent relationship to him or her or may consent under duress. In that case the informed consent should be obtained by a physician who is not engaged in the investigation and who is completely independent of this official relationship.
11. In case of legal incompetence, informed consent should be obtained from the legal guardian in accordance with national legislation. Where physical or mental incapacity makes it impossible to obtain informed consent, or when the subject is a minor, permission from the responsible relative replaces that of the subject in accordance with national legislation.
    Whenever the minor child is in fact able to give a consent, the minor's consent must be obtained in addition to the consent of the minor's legal guardian.
12. The research protocol should always contain a statement of the ethical considerations involved and should indicate that the principles enunciated in the present declaration are complied with.

Medical research combined with professional care (clinical research)

1. In the treatment of the sick person, the physician must be free to use a new diagnostic and therapeutic measure, if in his or her judgement it offers hope of saving life, reestablishing health or alleviating suffering.

2. The potential benefits, hazards and discomfort of a new method should be weighed against the advantages of the best current diagnostic and therapeutic methods.
3. In any medical study, every patient – including those of a control group, if any – should be assured of the best proven diagnostic and therapeutic method.
4. The refusal of the patient to participate in a study must never interfere with the physician-patient relationship.
5. If the physician considers it essential not to obtain informed consent, the specific reasons for this proposal should be stated in the experimental protocol for transmission to the independent committe (1, 2).
6. The physician can combine medical research with professional care, the objective being the acquisition of new medical knowledge, only to the extent that medical research is justified by its potential diagnostic and therapeutic value for the patient.

Non-therapeutic biomedical research involving human subjects (non-clinical biomedical research)

1. In the purely scientific application of medical research carried out on a human being, it is the duty of the physician to remain the protector of the life and health of that person on whom biomedical research is being carried out.
2. The subjects should be volunteers – either healthy persons or patients for whom the experimental design is not related to the patient's illness.
3. The investigator or the investigating team should discontinue the research if in his/her or their judgement it may, if continued, be harmful to the individual.
4. In research on man, the interest of science and society should never take precedence over considerations related to the well-being of the subject.

Subject Index

Bei Fragen zur Produktsicherheit wenden Sie sich bitte an:
If you have any questions regarding product safety,
please contact:

Walter de Gruyter GmbH
Genthiner Straße 13
10785 Berlin
productsafety@degruyterbrill.com